INTEGRATIVE CARDIOLOGY

INTEGRATIVE CARDIOLOGY
Complementary and Alternative Medicine for the Heart

Edited by

John H. K. Vogel, MD, MACC, FSCAI, FESC

Former Chairman
Cardiology Department
Santa Barbara Cottage Hospital and Former President American Heart Association
Santa Barbara, California

Mitchell W. Krucoff, MD, FACC, FCCP

Professor, Medicine/Cardiology
Duke University Medical Center
Director, Cardiovascular Devices Unit
Duke Clinical Research Institute
Durham, North Carolina

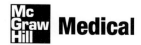 **Medical**

New York Chicago San Francisco Lisbon London Madrid Mexico City
Milan New Delhi San Juan Seoul Singapore Sydney Toronto

The *McGraw-Hill* Companies

INTEGRATIVE CARDIOLOGY: Complementary and Alternative Medicine for the Heart

1 2 3 4 5 6 7 8 9 0   DOC/DOC   0 9 8 7

ISBN-13: 978-0-07-144337-1
ISBN-10: 0-07-144337-1

This book was set in Janson by International Typesetting and Composition.
The editors were Ruth Weinberg and Christie Naglieri.
The production supervisor was Phil Galea.
Production management was provided by International Typesetting
    and Composition.
The cover designer was Mary McKeon.
RR Donnelley, Crawfordsville was printer and binder.

This book is printed on acid-free paper.

Cover photo credits: Left inset and background: Don Farrall/GettyImages; center inset: George Doyle/GettyImages; right inset: istock.

Library of Congress Cataloging-in-Publication Data

Vogel, John H.K., 1932-
Krucoff, Mitchell.
    Integrative cardiology / edited by John H.K. Vogel, Mitchell W.
Krucoff.—1st ed.
        p. ; cm.
    Includes bibliographical references and index.
    ISBN 13: 978-0-07-144337-1
    ISBN 10: 0-07-144337-1
    [DNLM: 1. Cardiology.   2. Integrative medicine.   3 Heart—Diseases—
Alternative treatment.   4. Cardiovascular Diseases—therapy.
5. Complementary Therapies—methods.   WG 166 I608   2007]
RC669.I63   2007
616.1/206 22   2006046970

DEDICATION

This book is dedicated to my wife Cynthia, my children, Kristen, Nancy, Carrie, and John Jr. It is also dedicated to all of those health-care providers who have enhanced my sensitivity and compassion in providing health care. This results in a greater trust of the true physician in providing total care of the mind, body, and spirit. It is also dedicated to all the authors of this text book who have given so much time and effort in providing a meaningful text to enhance the ability of physicians to provide total care for their patients.

John H. K. Vogel, MD, MACC, FSCAI

This book is dedicated to my father, Morris, whose life as a father and physician has inspired me through his love of his profession, patients and family; to my mother Sylvia, who in her life provided the most extraordinary example of how the mind, the body and the spirit vitalize one another; and to my wife Carol and our children Max and Rae, whose hearts and love continually point me to the need for health-care paradigms of present and future to be driven by compassion, wholeness and wellness. Finally, this book is the dedicated product of our authors, all committed to this book's creation not as a departure from modern high-tech cardiovascular medicine, but as an embrace and a celebration of its return to the transformation of human suffering as a scientifically and humanistically driven healing art.

Mitchell W. Krucoff, MD, FACC, FCCP

Childhood Disappearances

It's hard to know
If his footsteps were echoes,
or if they were constantly changing,
time after time.
She'd see a shadow depart down the stairs,
To help others find a tomorrow or just a dawn.
Those unlucky ones would just see
the sunrise,
but if he disappeared into the night,
faster than the beat of a heart,
he could capture them from the glittering clouds
and bring them back so they could
push the sun behind the curtains
of the horizon,
to go play amongst the stars in their dreams.
He would come home,
tired,
satisfied,
and she saw his footsteps,
and wondered whom he helped,
as she heard his shadow pass.

Kristen Marie Richmond (Vogel) Blabey

Dedicated to my Dad and all physicians devoted to their patients.

CONTENTS

PART 1
INTRODUCTION / 1

PART 2
BASICS / 11

PART 3

CAM TREATMENT MODALITIES: NCCAM CATEGORIES / 87

PART 4

MECHANISTIC AND PHYSIOLOGICAL LINKS BETWEEN CAM AND THE CARDIOVASCULAR SYSTEM / 357

PART 5

SPECIAL CONSIDERATION AREAS / 423

PART 6

APPENDIX / 573

CONTRIBUTORS

Earl E. Bakken, MD *(Chapter 1)*
Founder and Director Emiritus
  Medtronic, Inc.
President, Board of Directors
Five Mountain Medical Community
Kamuela, Hawaii

George A. Beller, MD, MACC *(Prologue)*
Ruth C. Heede Professor of Cardiology
Cardiovascular Division
University of Virginia Health System
Attending Physician
University of Virginia Medical Center
Charlottesville, Virginia

Josh Berman, MD, PhD *(Chapter 5)*
Assistant Professor of Clinical Psychiatry
Department of Psychiatry
Columbia University Medical Center
New York, New York

Steven F. Bolling, MD *(Chapter 24)*
Professor of Surgery
University of Michigan
Ann Arbor, Michigan

Robert Allan Bonakdar, MD *(Chapter 8)*
Scripps Center for Integrative Medicine
La Jolla, California

Robert O. Bonow, MD, FACC *(Prologue)*
Goldberg Distinguished Professor of
  Cardiology
Northwestern University Feinberg School
  of Medicine
Chief Division of Cardiology
Northwestern Memorial Hospital
Chief Division of Cardiology
Northwestern University Medical School
Chicago, Illinois

Jeffrey Brantley, MD *(Chapter 29)*
Director, Mindfulness-Based Stress
  Reduction
Duke Center for Integrative Medicine
Duke University
Durham, North Carolina

Michael H. Cohen, JD, MBA *(Chapter 3)*
Attorney-at-law
Assistant Clinical Professor of Medicine
Department of Medicine
Harvard Medical School
Assistant Professor
Department of Health Policy & Management
Harvard School of Public Health

Rebecca B. Costello, MD, PhD
  (Chapters 8, 23, Appendix)
Deputy Director
Office of Dietary Supplements
National Institutes of Health
Bethesda, Maryland

Suzanne W. Crater RN, ANP-C
  (Chapters 12, 28)
Duke University Medical Center
VA Medical Center
Durham, North Carolina

Michael S. Cuffe MD, FACC
  (Chapters 12, 25)
Duke Medical Center
Durham, North Carolina

Cheryl Dileo, PhD, MT-BC
  (Chapter 15)
Professor of Music Therapy
Director, Arts and Quality of Life Reasearch
  Center
Director of Music Therapy
Temple University Hospital
Clinical Music Therapist
Compassionate Care Hospice
Philadelphia, Pennsylvania

Pamela S. Douglas, MD, MACC (Prologue)
Past President of ACC
Ursula Geller Professor of Research in
  Cardiovascular Diseases
Chief, Cardiology Division
Duke University Medical Center
DUMC 3943
Durham, New Carolina

Johanna T. Dwyer, DSc, RD *(Chapter 23)*
Professor, Friedman School of Nutrition
  Science and Policy
Tufts University
Boston, Massachusetts

Jennifer L. Francis, Ph.D *(Chapter 18)*
Department of Medical and Clinical
  Psychology
Uniformed Services University of the Health
  Sciences
Bethesda, Maryland

M. Kay Garcia, DrPH, MSN, RN, Lac
  (Chapter 13)
Clinical Faculty, Community Health
The University of Texas Health Science
  Center at Houston
School of Nursing, Advanced Practice Nurse
Integrative Medicine
MD Anderson Cancer Center
Houston, Texas

Erminia Guarneri, MD, FACC
  (Chapters 8, 11)
Scripps Center for Integrative Medicine
Scripps Clinic
La Jolla, California

Maryann Ivons, RN, ND *(Chapter 17)*
Clinical Faculty
Bastyr Center for Natural Health
Seattle, Washington

Rauni Prittinen King *(Chapter 11)*
RN, CHTI
Program Director, Scripps Center for
  Integrative Medicine
La Jolla, California

Willem J. Kop, PhD *(Chapter 18)*
Division of Cadiology
University of Maryland Medical Center
Baltimore

Mitchell W. Krucoff, MD, FACC, FCCP
  (Chapters 12, 29, Preface)
Professor, Medicine/Cardiology
Duke University Medical Center
Director, Cardiovascular Devices Unit
Duke Clinical Research Institute
Durham, North Carolina

David C. Leopold, MD *(Chapter 14)*
Director of Integrative Medical Education
Scripps Center for Integrative Medicine
La Jolla, California

John C. Longhurst, MD, PhD
  (Chapter 4, 7, 19)
Professor and Chair, Department of Medicine
University of California at Irvine
Irvine, California

Shahla J. Modir, MD *(Chapter 14)*
Medical Director, Summit Centers Malibu
Torrance Memorial Medical Center
Torrance, California

Richard L. Nahin, PhD *(Chapter 5)*
Division of Extramural Research
National Center
Complementary and Alternative Medicine
Bethesda, Maryland

Brian Olshansky, MD *(Chapters 6 and 26)*
Professor of Medicine and Director of
   Cardiac Electrophysiology
Department of Internal Medicine
University of Iowa Healthcare
Iowa City, Iowa

Barbara Reuer, PhD, MT-BC, NMT
   (Chapter 15)
Director, Musicworx of California
San Diego, California

Martin L. Rossman, MD, Diploma Ac,
   NCCAOM *(Chapter 10)*
Clinical Faculty, University of California
San Francisco Medical School
Adjunct Faculty, California School of
   Professional Psychology
Consultant, Stanford Corporate Health
   Program
Co-Founder of the Academy for Guided
   Imagery
Director, Collaborative Medicine Center
   Mill Valley, California

Victor S. Sierpina, MD *(Chapter 13)*
WD and Laura Nell Nicholson Family
   Professor of Integrative Medicine
Associate Professor of Family Medicine
University of Texas Medical Branch,
   Galveston, Texas

Martinus T. Spoor, MD *(Chapter 24)*
University of Michigan Integrative
   Medicine Program
Ann Arbor, Michigan

Catherine M. Stoney, PhD *(Chapter 5)*
National Center for Complementary and
   Alternative Medicine
National Institutes of Health
Bethesda, Maryland

Christopher Suhar, MD *(Chapter 11)*
Cardiology Fellow
Integrative Cardiology, Scripps Clinic
La Jolla, California

Martin J. Sullivan, MD *(Chapter 29)*
Executive Director, Institute for Healing in
   Society and Medicine
Chapel Hill, North Carolina

H. Robert Superko, MD, FACC, FAHA,
   FACSM *(Chapter 21)*
Chair of Molecular, Genetic and Preventive
   Cardiology
Medical Director, Fugua Heart Center
   for Prevention
Piedmont Hospital

Stephanie C. Tjen-A-Looi, PhD
   (Chapter 19)
Project Scientist, School of Medicine
University of California
Irvine, California

Michael Traub, ND, DHANP, CCH
   (Chapter 16)
Director, Lokahi Health Center
North Hawaii Community Hospital
Naturopathic Medicine
Kailua Kona, Hawaii

John H.K. Vogel, MD, MACC, FSCAI
   (Chapters 27, 28, Preface)
Former Chairman, Cardiology Department
Santa Barbara Cottage Hospital
Former President American Heart
   Association, Santa Barbara
Santa Barbara, California

Robert A. Vogel, MD *(Chapter 9, 20)*
University of Maryland Hospital
Division of Cardiology
Baltimore, Maryland

Sara L. Warber, MD *(Chapters 22, 24)*
Assistant Professor, Department of Family
    Medicine
University of Michigan Integrative
    Medicine
Ann Arbor, Michigan

Julie H. Webster MN, APRN-C
    (Chapter 28)
Nurse Practitioner
Fuqua Heart Failure Resource Center
Piedmont Hospital
Atlanta, Georgia

Andrew T. Weil, MD *(Foreword)*
Director, Program in Interactive Medicine
University of Arizona College of Medicine
Clincal Professor of Medicine
University of Arizona
Vail, Arizona

Shan S. Wong, PhD *(Chapter 5)*
Program Officer
National Center for Complementary and
    Alternative Medicine
National Institutes of Health
Bethesda, Maryland

Gloria Y. Yeh, MD, MPH *(Chapter 13)*
Integrative Medical Therapies
Harvard Medical School, Osher Institute
Boston, Massachusetts

Cathy Young, RN, MBA *(Chapter 2)*
Queens Medical Center
Honolulu, Hawaii

Katrina Zapotulko, MHA *(Chapter 2)*
Administrative Director, Cardiac Research
    and Education
Newark Beth Israel Medical Center
Newark, New Jersey

Douglas Zipes, MD, MACC *(Prologue)*
Past President of ACC
Distinguished Professor
Director Emiritus
Krannert Institute of Cardiology
Indianapolis, Indiana

FOREWORD

Cardiology and integrative medicine belong together. Cardiology treats diseases that are multifactorial in origin, in which lifestyle choices have great influence, in which mind/body interactions are prominent, and where alternative treatments, from dietary supplements to spiritual interventions, have something to offer.

Integrative medicine is healing-oriented medicine that takes account of the whole person—body, mind, and spirit—as well as all aspects of lifestyle. It emphasizes the therapeutic relationship and makes use of all appropriate therapies, both conventional and alternative. Integrative medicine is emphatically not synonymous with complementary and alternative medicine (CAM). It differs from CAM in its broader philosophical orientations, its commitment to use conventional medicine appropriately, and its insistence on a good evidence base for any CAM interventions it uses.

I believe that integrative medicine is the way of the future. Not only is it the kind of medicine that our patients want, it can restore the core values of the profession, which have so eroded in the present era of for-profit practice. As the health-care crisis deepens—with total collapse of the system a real possibility—integrative medicine is poised to become mainstream for one simple reason: it has the potential to lower costs while preserving outcomes. It can do this by bringing lower cost treatments into conventional medical settings.

For the past 10 years the Program in Integrative Medicine that I founded and continue to direct at the University of Arizona has provided intensive training to physicians, residents, medical students, nurse practitioners, and others. It has done this by means of residential fellowships, distance-learning fellowships, and rotations. We have trained physicians from many specialties, including cardiologists. Many of our graduates now direct integrative medicine clinics and training programs at other academic institutions; others are providing clinical services; some have authored textbooks in this new field.

As integrative medicine develops, there are pressures to set standards for training, practice, and research for example, to organize an American College of Integrative Medicine, as if this were a new subspecialty. I oppose that course of action, because I feel training in integrative medicine should be foundational in all specialties, as important to surgeons as to physicians, to dermatologists as much as to internists.

One of the more recent accomplishments of the Arizona Program has been the design of a joint family medicine residency/integrative medicine fellowship that weaves training in the latter through years 2 to 4 of a 4-year program. We have partnered with five family medicine residency programs throughout the United States to offer this experience, and we look forward to adding new sites. I think this is a much better way to proceed than offering training in integrative medicine as a subspecialty. My hope is that collaborations with other residency and fellowship training programs will soon come about, and I have a special hope that we will soon see joint training in cardiology and integrative medicine.

Integrative cardiology practice offers benefits to both doctors and patients. It gives physicians the chance to partner with patients in teaching them lifestyle skills, such as how to form better habits of eating, physical activity, and stress management, how to use dietary supplements wisely, and how to improve their mental and emotional health. It allows patients to experiment with nonpharmacological methods of mitigating cardiac risk factors, from botanical remedies to breath control to Chinese medicine. Integrative approaches in cardiology may result in less need for invasive procedures, lower utilization of medication, fewer adverse reactions to treatment, and lower costs of treatment.

In fact, this approach has so much to offer that one may wonder why there is any resistance to it. How can anyone object to focusing on the body's innate potential for healing, emphasizing preventive lifestyle choices, taking account of the emotional and spiritual dimensions of patients, and restoring the sanctity of the physician–patient relationship? Most resistance centers on the incorporation of ideas and therapies that are now outside the mainstream and are not taught in medical schools and residency programs, especially on a perceived lack of research and evidence to support them.

Leaving aside that many conventional treatments, some of them potentially harmful, lack a solid evidence base, I must state my own bias about the nature of evidence for medical interventions. My experience as a long-time practitioner and teacher of integrative medicine is that physicians and patients more often than not have to deal with uncertainty, and we are not trained to do that. We are always gambling, trying to evaluate often inconsistent data, and making the best choices we can based on our past experience and expertise of colleagues. I have suggested that a course in gaming theory be part of the core curriculum in medicine, and am working to develop one. If we must live with uncertainty, we can certainly benefit from learning what mathematicians know about how to place bets wisely so that we can help patients do the same.

We hear much today about the lack of randomized controlled trials (RCTs) of CAM therapies. Of course, we could use more—more well-designed ones that is. But I have to tell you that we will never have good studies of all the interventions out there that our patients are using. We do not have the time or money to do them, especially in an era of dwindling resources. Besides, the RCT may not be the best instrument to evaluate the efficacy and cost-efficacy of integrative treatment for the management of cardiovascular and other diseases. What we most need are outcomes studies, in which conventional and integrative treatments are compared head-to-head in large populations, in order to compare both medical outcomes and bottom-line costs.

The problem here is that integrative treatment is complex by nature. An integrative treatment plan for managing congestive heart failure, for example, would include, in addition to appropriate medications: dietary recommendations, use of selected dietary supplements and botanicals, exercise, stress-management techniques, and possibly treatments from energy medicine, Chinese medicine, or Ayurvedic medicine. We want to know how such a complex package of treatment, which will differ from patient to patient, stacks up against conventional treatment, not how any single intervention compares to placebo in an RCT.

Conventional researchers seem unable or unmotivated to take on this kind of research, particularly because of the issue of complexity. But it is the data from such outcomes studies that we really need right now, when we are trying to contain health-care costs that are escalating beyond control. My hope is that the private sector—large corporations for example—perhaps in partnership with government agencies, will take this task on. Corporations are being hobbled by health-care costs and are highly motivated to find solutions.

In the meantime, I offer this operating principle as a way of coping with uncertainty about treatments: the greater the potential of a treatment to cause harm, the stricter the standards of evidence it should be held to for efficacy. My colleagues and I in integrative medicine always make our prescriptions and recommendations with this in mind, and it works well for us. If I recommend a breathing exercise to a patient to lower blood pressure, based on my clinical experience with it, I do not feel I have to wait for definitive evidence from an RCT to make that recommendation, as long as I am not using it in place of a needed pharmaceutical intervention.

Publication of this text on Integrative Cardiology is a milestone in the inevitable merging of the two fields. It follows on the Expert Consensus Document, "Integrating Complementary Medicine into Cardiovascular Medicine," that appeared in the *Journal of the American College of Cardiology* earlier this year. I am well aware of the amount of work it took to prepare that document, but I hope and believe that such efforts will get easier in the near future, as cardiologists become more aware of what integrative medicine can offer them, and as integrative medicine makes more headway in academia. I have always said that the success of this movement will be that one day we will be able to drop the word "integrative." This will just be good medicine—medicine that serves the needs of our patients and maximizes outcomes, while containing harm and costs.

Andrew T. Weil, MD

PROLOGUE

Today, we physicians need to remember that a sizable number of our patients, more than a third of all Americans, turn to preventive and therapeutic resources beyond the mainstream of Western medicine. Many are searching for alternative medicine—practices used instead of conventional medical care; they are also exploring complementary medicine—practices used alongside conventional care; and they are using integrative medicine—what proponents see as the best of both worlds. While some medical facilities have developed specialized complementary and alternative medicine (CAM) centers to investigate its potential benefits for integration into care and lifestyle management, little CAM is used in most major hospitals, there is lack of teaching CAM at most major medical schools, and little good research.

Many of these therapies have real potential. For example, some cardiologists are already urging their patients to use meditation to lower their blood pressure. Others are suggesting that patients try yoga as a way of managing congestive heart failure symptoms or acupuncture to relieve pain. Still others are prescribing soy or garlic for patients' high cholesterol or St. John's Wort for neurocardiogenic syncope. Some cardiovascular surgeons are becoming interested in having patients practice self-hypnosis to reduce depression, fatigue, and tension following heart surgery.

But there is a potential downside. CAM can be dangerous because most dietary supplements have not been tested in any sort of a scientific fashion, and if they are called a "dietary supplement," the Food and Drug Administration (FDA) does not monitor them closely. This means that a bottle of herbal medicine may contain the substances in the amount stated on the label, but it may not. While it may be that many or most untested herbal remedies are harmless, examples of adverse responses abound. Patients who use a natural form of ephedrine called "ma huang" to lose weight and boost their energy levels are at increased risk for stroke, myocardial infarction, and sudden death, leading to its commercial removal by the FDA. Patients can unknowingly consume preparations contaminated with arsenic, lead, or other toxins, or supplements that interact adversely with prescription medications or interfere with test results. Or they can delay their visit to a physician and lose precious time in the diagnosis and treatment of an illness.

A lot of physicians do not routinely ask their patients whether they are "complementing" their prescriptions. Inquiring about garlic, ginkgo, ginger, and ginseng can be important because these compounds can inhibit clotting and thus should not be used with blood thinners such as aspirin, heparin, or warfarin. Likewise, there can be potential interactions between such popular supplements as St. John's Wort and gingko and anesthetic drugs used during surgery because such supplements can deepen the effect of anesthesia or cause blood pressure or bleeding problems.

Physicians suspicious or ignorant of complementary medicine can inadvertently put their patients at risk. When patients are silent about using complementary therapies, perhaps fearing derision, the physician–patient relationship is damaged. And even worse, such physicians might offend or scare off complementary medicine adherents who may be in dire need of the conventional treatment only physicians can provide.

Part of the appeal of CAM is that its practitioners give their patients *time*, averaging 30 minutes in a session. In addition to giving patients a chance to talk about what is on their minds, being open and able to discuss complementary therapies with patients helps transform them from passive recipients of care to true partners in care.

That relates to another of CAM's attributes, which is a holistic approach. CAM practitioners acknowledge the crucial roles of the body *and the mind* in health. CAM tends to focus on staying well, not treating illness, and stresses the role of self-care. Many patients want to be involved in their own care. They want to be empowered to make decisions that affect their health, and they want to believe in the outcomes. While we physician researchers acknowledge the role of the "placebo effect" in clinical trials and other studies, CAM practitioners often take it one step further. Instead of merely acknowledging that the placebo can influence results, they believe in the power of this effect to help patients feel better and even get well. The power of the mind as a tool for healing is an extraordinary but elusive attribute, often unsupported by conventional scientific data. And no less miraculous may be the inner peace that comes with yoga or meditation or the benefits that seem to accompany sipping tea or undergoing acupuncture. We do not understand why these approaches may work, and some defy biological mechanisms that we have been taught must underlie acceptable medical practices; but we must resist the temptation to discard all of them out of hand just because we do not understand them. Experience one of them personally and you become a believer.

Of course, there's still a great need for research and new knowledge in this area. The National Center for Complementary and Alternative Medicine (NCCAM) at the National Institutes of Health is already working to fill that void, as is this book. Here, editor/authors Vogel and Krucoff capture the latest information about CAM, including its basics, treatment modalities, mechanistic and physiological links to the cardiovascular system, and management of common problems. This is the most complete and up-to-date source about integrative medicine.

It is clear that the time has come not only for us to acknowledge the potential of some forms of CAM but also for physicians and CAM practitioners to learn from each other. Both groups share a common mission—to help people get well, to help them feel healthy, and to prevent disease in the first place. CAM practitioners are gradually accepting that they need controlled studies to demonstrate the effectiveness of their treatments, and physicians are opening their minds to the potential benefit of these unproven therapies. If these groups put their minds together, the result could be the best of both worlds for our patients.

Douglas Zipes, MD, MACC
George A. Beller, MD, MACC
Robert O. Bonow, MD, FACC
Pamela S. Douglas MD, MACC

PREFACE

In 2000, nearly 50% of all Americans sought the help of an alternative health care practitioner. This represents over 600 million visits. Nearly $30 billion was spent in the year 2001 on CAM. Many CAM interventions, including numerous herbal supplements have been employed in an attempt to treat cardiovascular disease. Of prime importance is putting CAM into perspective with potential benefits and knowledge of important interactions with traditional cardiovascular medicines. Communication between patients and health-care providers is extremely important with regard to CAM because of the potential interaction of certain CAM therapies with other traditional cardiovascular therapies. It is important for cardiologists and other health-care providers who care for cardiovascular patients to be familiar with CAM therapies so as to promote this dialog. Because many patients hesitate to discuss CAM usage with their physicians, a certain level of knowledge will allow for a more open and honest discussion about these therapies.

The most complete and comprehensive findings to date of Americans' use of CAM were released on May 27, 2004, by the National Center for Complementary and Alternative Medicine (NCCAM) and the National Center for Health Statistics (NCHS, part of the center for disease control and prevention). The new data came from a detailed survey on CAM and included for the first time in 2002 in the National Health Interview Survey. The NHIS done annually by the NCHS interviews people in tens of thousands of American households about their health and illness-related experiences. The findings are yielding and will continue to yield through future analysis, a wealth of information on who uses CAM, what they use, and why. In addition, researchers can examine CAM uses that relate to many other factors such as age, race/ethnicity, place of residence, income, educational level, marital status, health problems, and the practice of certain behaviors that impact health such as smoking cigarettes or drinking alcohol.

The survey showed that a large percentage of American adults are using some form of CAM (36%). When prayer, specifically for health reasons, is included in the definition of CAM, that figure rises to 62%. Dr Stephen E. Strauss, NCCAM director, said, "The survey will provide new and more detailed information about CAM use and the characteristics of people who use CAM." One benefit will be to help us target NCCAM's research, training, and outreach efforts, especially as we plan NCCAM's 5 years, 2005 through 2009.

There is little doubt that CAM represents a revolution within our health-care delivery system. Nevertheless, our traditional views of the medical establishment do not fully support CAM. There is a lack of significant instruction of CAM in medical schools although at this time, there are now approximately

25 medical centers involved in CAM and several private hospitals are now becoming involved. Unfortunately, compensation by insurance companies for CAM is limited at this time.

Integrating CAM into medicine must be guided by compassion but enhanced by science and made meaningful through solid doctor–patient relationships. Most importantly, CAM involves a commitment to the core mission of caring for patients on a physical, mental, and spiritual level. This book attempts to enable us to fulfill these objectives.

John H. K. Vogel, MD, MACC, FSCAI
Mitchell W. Krucoff, MD, FACC, FCCP

P A R T

1

INTRODUCTION

1

HIGH TECH/HIGH TOUCH: HEALING ENVIRONMENT IN BLENDED MEDICINE AT NORTH HAWAII COMMUNITY HOSPITAL

Earl E. Bakken

INTRODUCTION

I gave this talk with a PowerPoint presentation to American College of Cardiology (ACC) Integrated Cardiology meeting that was held in October 2004 on the Island of Hawaii, which is my home. There were many great scholars on complementary and alternative medicine as lecturers, and I thought "what in the world can I teach these experts?" For many years we have heard of the importance of integrated medicine or alternative medicine, as it is often called. I don't like that term. It implies that you have to use either one or the other. I used complementary medicine for a number of years to explain the importance using high tech and high touch, but I found that there was often another aspect that was overlooked. That is, the importance of a healing environment.

So, I have added the healing environment to high tech and high touch, and coined the phrase "blended medicine." This chapter discusses all three aspects of blended medicine: the importance of high tech, the importance of high touch or the human side of caring, and the importance of a healing environment. In addition, I will use the model of blended medicine that I have been a part of creating at the North Hawaii Community Hospital (NHCH) in Waimea on Hawaii Island. NHCH opened, after 9 years of community planning and development, in 1996. There had never been a hospital in Waimea prior to that time.

At NHCH, we use the best of high tech and the best of high touch, those that have been proven effective. The design and layout of the physical plant were thoughtfully planned, not only in accordance with important principles of physics, but also in alignment with our cultural wisdom. Consultants were used from both of these spheres, and we ended up with blended medicine.

Science (high tech) has much to teach us about healing environments. Cultural wisdom (high touch) and the aloha spirit are also important elements. During our planning and design phase at NHCH, we also used Feng Shui. From our Hawaiian experts, we have learned about the concept of lokahi, which is the balance of body, mind, spirit, nature, and community. All these must be addressed for a total healing environment. We have blended these principles of physics and cultural wisdom with our architecture and design to create a total healing environment at NHCH.

WHAT YOU CAN SEE

Obviously, there are elements of a healing environment that can be seen as well as those that are unseen. First, I will address what can be seen.

- The hallways are wide, so we don't trigger the "fight or flight" phenomenon—most hospitals do not use wide hallways.
- There are windows and skylights all over to keep people, including patients, in sync with the sun, according to principles of chronobiology. Chronobiology is the study of the innumerable rhythms and cycles in nature, large and small, that effect is on many levels.
- We have fluorescent lights that use the 30,000-cycle electronic ballasts, which are way above "flicker fusion" rates for people (vs. the 60-cycle lights that flicker 120 times per second and can make people sick).
- The color of the lights (warm or cool colors) is also important and we use different shades in different areas.

WHAT YOU CANNOT SEE

There are also many things that you cannot see that are vitally important to a healing environment. For example:

- During construction, we saw that the power cables are buried deeper than the building code required, reducing harmful effects of electrical-magnetic fields (EMFs).
- There is clean mountain air moving throughout the hospital as we are able to open the doors and windows during the day. We also have very high-quality high efficiency particulate air (HEPA) filters that circulate this air, which is important, especially at night when all doors and windows are closed and secured.
- There is a special water filtration system so that we know our water is free of all possible contaminants.

CULTURAL WISDOM—LOKAHI

According to the Hawaiian culture, lokahi is the balance and harmony of body, mind, spirit, nature, and community. Where our hospital was built in Waimea, we are surrounded by five majestic volcanic mountains, which are spiritual icons for us all. Each of these mountains speaks to one of the five aspects I have just mentioned. They are Hualalai, Mauna Kea, Haleakala, Mauna Loa, and Kohala.

BODY

"I am Hualalai. I am the physical embodiment of grace and beauty. It is important to cherish the things around you."

- The "body" of the hospital (physical plant) is designed as a healing instrument versus most hospitals, which are likened to "warehouses" or "prisons" for sick bodies rather than places for people to be cared for or to heal.

- Its geographic location, building footprint, floor plans, and spatial relationships were all taken into consideration for the optimum care and movement of patients, as well as operational efficiency. Of course, future expansion was also considered.

- Waimea, where the hospital is located, is centrally located and accessible within the golden hour for all the people in our North Hawaii service area—an area that is larger than all of the other islands combined, and home to approximately 30,000 people.

- Upon visiting, you will see serene landscapes with rainbows hovering over lush green misty foothills, streams and waterfalls, animals grazing in pastures, and sometimes snow-capped mountains.

- Many people who come from other places comment that Waimea feels "like home" or is "spiritual."

- Makahikilua (the land the hospital is on) was a gathering place for Ancient Hawaiians, as early as AD 700. Peace was celebrated there during the Makahiki season, which is the time each year between October and January that the Hawaiian people traditionally celebrated peace.

- The footprint of the hospital aligns the front of the building with Kohala Mountain, and the back with Mauna Kea. According to Feng Shui experts and cultural practitioners, this is a positive alignment for energy flow.

- Before the hospital was built and opened, our tagline was "Not Just Another Hospital."

- All decisions relating to design and planning were made based on the philosophy of patient-centered care. We asked "what is best for the patient?" This philosophy still holds strong through the ninth year of operation.

- Patient respect and privacy are extremely important. Our patient rooms are designed so that a person walking by cannot see the patients' faces through the door as they lie in bed, but the patients can see the door. This is an important principle of Feng Shui.

- Each patient room has windows to see outdoors—the view is so important to the sick patient. For Hawaiian people especially, it is important for them to keep their connection to the land or "aina" and to their community, even while they are hospitalized.

- Sleep chairs or extra beds are available for guests to stay overnight and there are no limits on the number of visitors or visiting hours.

- A primary nursing model was used to plan nurses' desks. Instead of one big, noisy nursing station, there are five smaller ones spread throughout the unit. They were designed with a lowered visual barrier, and each desk is surrounded by seven or eight patient rooms.

- Our hospital is committed to ecological responsibility. Attention is paid to recycling, environmentally friendly construction materials and nontoxic cleaning substances, the dangers of polyvinyl chlorides, and the risks of medical waste management.

MIND

"I am Mauna Kea. I look into the eyes of the gods and whisper the knowledge of life. Understand why. Imitate how. Know when."

We know the importance of the mind's influence on our health status, and we understand how environmental elements affect our emotional well-being, comfort levels, feelings of safety, privacy, and respect.

- Our lobby gives the people who enter their first impression. It is open, with windows and sunlight, and the design and décor makes it feel like someone's home.

- There are smiling volunteers who greet and welcome with "aloha," introducing our culture of caring and sharing of spirit. In Hawaii, people who meet will often put their faces together and share a breath. This is called "honi" and Hawaiian people believe that the breath is the essence or spirit of life.

- Once again, Feng Shui principles were used as they relate to color, textures, materials, and spatial relationships.

- There are warm colors and carpeting on the floors for warmth since Waimea has a cool, moist climate at 3000-ft elevation.

- There are familiar patterns/textures used in the wallpaper, carpeting, and furniture coverings. Since many of our indigenous people are familiar with weaving patterns, or plant patterns, there are many of these used throughout.

- There is an open feeling in the patient rooms. Doors that open to the outdoors can be unlocked and kept open during the day.
- There is an array of healing art, which is culturally and historically meaningful.
- Each patient room has a place to display artwork that can be changed, according to the patient's preference.
- There is the CARE Channel 2 on all TVs in patient rooms and wait areas, which shows soothing nature video with background music specially designed without lyrics, tunes, or distinct rhythms that may bring back bad memories.
- There is a commitment to noise reduction, and therefore there is very little overhead paging. Carpeted hallways reduce the sounds of traffic and equipment.
- There is an array of complementary healing modalities available to the patients that include acupuncture, chiropractic, naturopathy, massage therapy, guided imagery, and healing touch. The hospital has an on-demand video system whereby patients can choose from a number of educational programs, including one on these complementary therapies that is narrated by the hospital's CEO.
- We have a healing services department with staff that visits each patient to introduce these concepts. Over 50% of all patients at NHCH receive healing touch at any given time.
- We believe in the healing power of humor, and agree that laughter can be some of the best medicine.

SPIRIT

"I am Haleakala that awaits each new day. I am Haleakala that greets the sun and warms the heart of man. The spirit of aloha that spreads as the rays of the sun embrace the coolness of the sleeping sky."

We know the importance of the intangible, of faith, and of honoring our past and the Hawaiian host culture. We know we must also honor each individual's basic human dignity and personal spiritual practices. At NHCH, we have created the space for the spirit of aloha to thrive and warm our hearts.

- There are numerous spiritual icon representative of our diverse cultural mix. We honor the spiritual wisdom of our many cultures through our artwork, décor, and practices.
- Ti plants have been planted at all entrances and corners of the building to "filter out the bad spiritual energy." This was in accordance with the advice of a native Hawaiian healer. The Ti leaf is used in sacred ceremonial practices in Hawaii.

- There is a bamboo garden filled with bamboo plants or "ohe." These plants are the overall spiritual protective plant for our hospital, as advised by the late Papa Henry Auwae. Papa Henry was our states' foremost practitioner of native Hawaiian herbal healing, or "laau lapaau." For the Hawaiians, bamboo is representative of bones and bodily strength.

- Our chapel is named Hale Manaolana, which translates to House of Hope. It is a quiet place; open to nature, physically separated from the building by a corridor, not "buried" within the building as many hospital chapels are. It is multipurpose, and has even been used for weddings. The staff has many spontaneous prayer or meditation sessions there.

- We have a code that is called "Patient Lavender" for prayer or sending healing intention. It is used instead of the word "code" as in Code Red or Code Blue, since the word "code" can provoke a sense of urgency or emergency with the hospital staff. "Patient Lavender Room 350" is softly announced through the paging system (one exception to our no-paging practice) and that way people can pray or think positively for that patient.

- We try to honor the diverse spiritual practices of our patients, families, and staff. There are religious scriptures and books available in the chapel for the main 14 religions in our area.

- There is an oshibori service that takes place each morning. Warm, moist towels using aromatherapy are passed to staff going off the night shift from the emergency room (ER), birthing unit, or medical-surgical, and occasionally to patients and families.

- The concept of healing intention is used in the dietary department and food services. The dietary staff is told that they can put aloha into the food during preparation, and they are encouraged not to prepare food if they are upset.

- Many of our staff are local, so they live the aloha spirit. All staff, including housekeepers, food service, engineering, and accounting, consider themselves part of the healing team.

- The hospital's vision statement is "to be the most healing hospital in the world."

NATURE

"I am Mauna Loa. I am nature and life. I create and bring forth the elements from the center of creation. Behold the patterns of life that embrace and support each other's existence."

In Hawaii and at NHCH, we are always reminded of the healing forces of creation, the beauty of nature that surrounds us, and the patterns of life that embrace and support our existence. For our local people, nature is a powerful healer, and their daily lives and spiritual and religious practices are closely interwoven with nature's rhythms and patterns.

- There are views of nature and the outdoors from everywhere inside the hospital. There are no visual barriers between the patients and the outdoors, no typical views of parking lots or brick walls.

- Our mountains are the source of spiritual strength for most of us, and patients can see them from their room. They can also see the pastures with cattle, horses, and sheep, and nature's many patterns of life, which remind them of home, and of "life going on" out there.

- Because of the windows and doors that open to the outdoors, there is *no hospital smell*. In addition, our housekeepers are meticulous in their work.

- Essential oils and aromatherapy are used in the house-keeping practices and in some patient care areas such as the family birthing unit, where nurses help patients relax and relieve pain and nausea through the use of lavender and peppermint in aromatherapy.

- Hawaiian medicinal plants were used as an overall guiding design theme, as advised by the late Papa Henry Auwae, kahuna pookela la`au lapa`au (Hawaiian herbal medicine specialist of the highest order).

- Papa Henry, who passed away a few years ago at age 95, was a dear friend and cultural guide. He taught us that in healing, 80% of the success is a result of spirituality, and 20% is a result of the medicine.

- The NHCH logo is a Hawaiian quilt pattern based on the noni (Indian Mulberry) plant, which was a Hawaiian "cure-all."

- Some herbal supplements and homeopathics are included on the formulary in the pharmacy. Patients bring their own herbal remedies to use with permission from their doctors.

- There are healing garden landscapes surrounding the hospital with flowers, trees, and water features.

- The Maluhia Labyrinth Garden, dedicated to peace and meditation, is paved with ceramic tiles designed with Hawaiian nature elements, each one expressing a message of remembrance, love, or peace.

COMMUNITY

"I am Kohala.........God, nature, man, relationships. Ke kahi a me ke kahi. One to another, man to God, man to nature, and man to man—community. We are not alone. We are a family."

The concept of community teaches us about the importance of accountability, self-determination, and our relationships with ourselves, our families, our cultures, and our neighbors—that which ties us all together. Prior to the hospital being built in Waimea, patients in North Hawaii had to travel long distances on our big island or to Honolulu for their care.

- Our patient rooms are oversized to allow the family to be there. The birthing rooms are particularly large for our larger families.

- Our waiting rooms are called "ohana rooms." Ohana means family in the Hawaiian language.
- There is one larger ohana room with a kitchenette, TV, piano, and couches for families to rest, prepare special meals, or even play some of their own music.
- Suzanne's Corner is the name of a small room for quiet contemplation, or for doctors/nurses to talk with families, instead of in the corridors. It was named in memory of a family counselor from our community that was loved by many.
- A Celebration of Life meal is served to each "new family" when a baby is born in our family birthing unit, complete with a special menu, battery-operated candle-light, and nonalcoholic champagne.
- NHCH allows its conference space for community meetings at no charge.
- We pride ourselves in offering "not just more hospital food." The hospital café is so popular that people come from all over town to have their meals there and the nutritional services department caters parties, meetings, and events.
- There are many community programs that include an Artist in Residence program, celebrity presentations, labyrinth walks, community health education and health fairs for children and seniors, and interesting blended continuing medical education (CME) offerings.

PROCESS

How did we get to this? We asked our community and listened to their ideas, and we researched the best science had to offer. We did things right for the local people—we did the right things for our patients. We continue to honor our cultural traditions such as the practice of "honi," which is to exchange breath and share your spirit.

There are many measures of success. We have high patient satisfaction results on surveys and people from other locations on our island choose to come to our hospital when they could choose others, and then they choose to come back. We've had people from around our state and even from Japan who chose our hospital for their care. Joint Commission on Accreditation of Healthcare Organizations (JCAHO), the national health-care quality expert, has acknowledged our innovation and leadership.

CONCLUSION

Even though "lokahi" may be a specific Hawaiian concept that has deep meaning for our people here, it is the idea of reconnecting with one's cultural wisdom that is a vital key to the healing process. Reconnecting to cultural wisdom can happen in urban inner cities, heartland farming communities, or any neighborhood anywhere.

P A R T

2

BASICS

2

INTEGRATING COMPLEMENTARY/ALTERNATIVE MEDICINE INTO YOUR CARDIAC PROGRAM

Cathy Young and Katrina Zapotulko

INTRODUCTION

In January 2002, two medical facilities in northern New Jersey, began offering complementary and alternative medicine (CAM) therapies as a part of their routine care. At Newark Beth Israel Medical Center and Saint Barnabas Medical Center, affiliates of the Saint Barnabas Health Care System (SBHCS), all patients scheduled to undergo cardiothoracic surgery were offered to participate in a cardiac integrative medicine (IM) program. Since the program inception in 2002, 2987 patients received holistic consultations and therapies* free of charge.

Located 9 miles away from each other, Newark Beth Israel and Saint Barnabas Medical Center offered 250 dedicated cardiac beds, 5 cardiothoracic operating rooms, 9 digital catheterization and electrophysiology laboratories, and a host of state-of-the-art cardiac diagnostic and therapeutic modalities well complemented by highly trained and dedicated medical and clinical staff. The cardiac service-line at the two acute-care facilities, formerly known as the Heart Hospital of New Jersey, was governed by the Cardiac Services Executive Committee which, in 2001, included vice president for Cardiac Services, chairman of Cardiothoracic Surgery, chief of Cardiology, and medical director of Invasive Cardiovascular Laboratories for the SBHCS. The mission of Cardiac Services called for a single standard of care for the two medical centers.

---

*Program utilization and other data reported herein pertain to period of January 7, 2002–December 31, 2004

In 2001, prior to initiation of the IM program, the risk-adjusted mortality rate for coronary artery bypass graft (CABG) procedures performed at Newark Beth Israel and Saint Barnabas Medical Center was reported by a national cardiac surgical database at 1.81%, with 70.9% of CABG procedures performed off-pump. The cardiac transplantation program at Newark Beth Israel has also experienced excellent clinical outcomes, with a 1-year survival rate of 83.7% for male and 80.8% for female transplant recipients, 2000–2002.*

PATH TO CARDIAC INTEGRATIVE MEDICINE

Once upon a time, in 1998, the authors were introduced to the inpatient application of CAM modalities by the new chairman of the Department of Cardiothoracic Surgery, Craig R. Saunders, MD, who thought to implement guided imagery for the cardiac surgery patients. In the long run, the guided imagery project was not successful due to lack of dedicated staff, as the philanthropic funding only covered the cost of supplies (tapes and players). However, it provided us with the first taste of an integrative approach to cardiac care and a valuable insight into the operations of a small adjunct program.

Around the same time, the Medtronic Foundation, under the leadership of Bill George, then CEO, and M. Bridget Duffy, MD, who at the time was medical director of the Medtronic Foundation, organized several forums to raise awareness and share knowledge of the IM approaches to patient care. In 1999 and 2000, Cathy Young, then vice president of Cardiac Services for the SBHCS, and Gary J. Rogal, MD, FACC, chief of Cardiology, SBHCS, had an opportunity to attend two of the Medtronic meetings which proved to be highly educational. Inspired by the experiences of the forums, the Cardiac Executive Committee decided to establish a cardiac IM program at the Saint Barnabas facilities (see Fig. 2-1). A cardiac IM steering committee was created, which included members of cardiac executive team, a physician specializing in IM, and a project manager for Cardiac Services.

Vision and planning

The leadership team envisioned a comprehensive program—inpatient and outpatient—combining the best of traditional medical care with the appropriate, evidence-based CAM modalities that would be offered to all cardiac patients admitted to the Heart Hospital of New Jersey facilities, free of charge. Initiated in an acute-care setting, the program was intended to enable patients to take an active role in their postoperative recovery, as well as make changes toward life-long

---

*One-year transplant survival rate as reported by The United Network for Organ Sharing (UNOS)/ Organ Procurement and Transplantation Network (OPTN), Kaplan-Meier Survival Rates for Transplants Performed in 1997–2002.

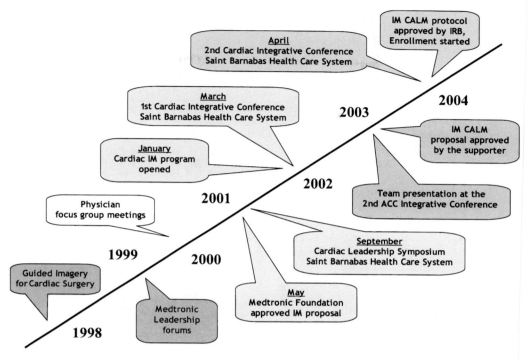

FIGURE 2-1   *Path to cardiac integrative medicine.*

wellness and disease prevention. By continually educating patients and health-care professionals on the principles of healthy lifestyle, the program was meant to empower patients to enhance their quality of life, at present and in the future. In addition, the authors hoped to collect scientific evidence of efficacy of the integrative cardiac care.

The key concepts of the program, in addition to the best medical care, included nutrition, exercise, stress management/relaxation, and spirituality. Initially, the IM committee focused on the development of an operational model of the program (see Fig. 2-2), which was later presented to groups of cardiologists and cardiothoracic surgeons practicing at the two hospitals. These focus group meetings proved invaluable in ensuring physician support of the program.

In keeping with the program vision, the committee developed a proposal, titled *Making the Conversation Happen*, which was approved by the Medtronic Foundation in May 2001. At that point, the generous, yet finite, amount of funding dictated the need to limit the program scope. The committee selected cardiothoracic surgery patients as the program target population. The choice was driven by a combination of factors, including high acuity of care and likelihood of need for a lifestyle modification within the chosen patient population, as well as sufficient length of hospital stay to allow for repeated staff-patient

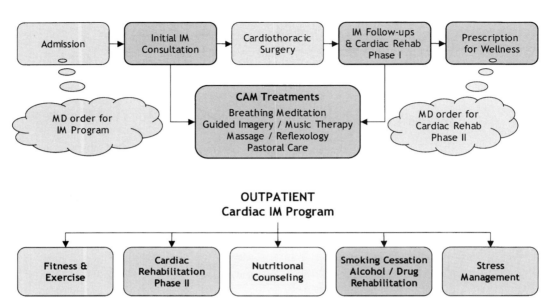

FIGURE 2-2   *Cardiac integrative medicine program—operational model.*

interaction. No less important was the strong support of the chairman of Cardiothoracic Surgery, Dr. Craig Saunders, whose contribution to the program continued to make it possible to this day.

Staff credentials and recruitment

Once the funding was secured, we began the laborious process of recruiting staff for the one-of-a-kind—at least, in New Jersey—program. It would be fair to say that no other recruitment experience, before or since, have been quite as educational. What started with open snickering at our new job titles—mind-body-spirit specialist, subsequently changed to holistic clinical nurse specialist—and a complete bafflement of the medical staff office when asked about privileging massage therapists, quickly changed into a procession of CAM professionals and enthusiasts who introduced us to modalities we could not have imagined. We were pleasantly surprised by the abundant response and awed by the dedication that was clearly required in order to pursue "alternative" qualifications within the traditional health-care and educational systems of the United States.

Based on our experience, the CAM "educational system" was highly fragmented, which created considerable challenges when evaluating and comparing professional credentials. Some states recognized and credentialed certain types of professionals. When state-approved credentials were not available, we found professional organizations that maintained lists of recognized practitioners. We were fortunate to find a graduate of the New York University (NYU) Program in Holistic Nursing (NP) as our program manager. New York University was one of the few institutions offering master and post-master education in holistic disciplines at that time. Subsequently, Newark Beth Israel and Saint Barnabas Medical Center hosted NYU holistic students on their clinical rotations.

Sharing the good news

In September 2001, before the program opened, the IM steering committee held a retreat for the cardiac physician and clinical leadership to introduce the program and solicit input on the proposed operational design. The symposium, which also included several presentations by expert guest speakers, was well received by the attendees. It brought together and energized the cardiac team as well as helped various disciplines understand their role in the new initiative.

In keeping with the educational mission of the IM program, two regional cardiac IM conferences were held in March 2002 and April 2004. Both included demonstrations of CAM modalities, from guided visualization to qi gong, as well as national IM updates and a host of other topics ranging from safety of herbal use to experiences of other CAM programs throughout the country. In April 2004, the audience was mesmerized by heart transplant recipients who spoke about their life-saving treatment and experience with the IM program. The conferences, attended by over 250 health-care professionals, indicated strong interest and need for more evidence-based education in Complementary/Alternative and Integrative Medicine.

THE PROGRAM

Organizational structure

The cardiac IM was envisioned as a hospital-based program with extensive referral network of outpatient services. Interestingly enough, the operational model developed in the planning stages of the project proved viable and remained largely unchanged throughout program operations (refer to Fig. 2-2). The key component of the program, which is largely responsible for the considerable number of patients served, was the inclusion of IM consultation into preoperative orders for cardiothoracic surgical patients.

The IM consultation (see Figure 2-3) provided by the program staff was a comprehensive holistic health assessment of patient's health habits designed to identify focal issues and to give patients ample opportunity to voice concerns that may not have been sufficiently addressed by their physicians or other caregivers. It quickly became apparent that majority of patients welcomed an

```
┌─────────────────────────────────────────────────────────────────────────┐
│          Integrative Cardiac Medicine Worksheet              1 of 2       │
│                                                                           │
│   Date:_____          Medical record #_____  │
│   Patient name:_____   Phone #_____  │
│   Age:_____      Residence:_____   Religion:_____  │
│   Surgical proc:_____   Date:_____   Surgeon:_____  │
│   Cardiologist:_____   Community hospital:_____  │
│   History                                                                 │
│   MI_____   CAD_____CHF_____HTN_____  IDDM_____ NIDDM____↑Chol_____ EF____%│
│   Valve disease_____   PCI_____ Stents____COPD____Obesity___Renal disease_____│
│   Other:_____ │
│   Initial IM consult Date:_____ Out Pt visit (PAT)_____ In Pt referral_____│
│   Follow-ups                                                              │
│   Date:_____  _____ │
│   Date:_____  _____ │
│   Date:_____  _____ │
│   Date:_____  _____ │
│   Predischarge visit    Date:_____ _____ │
│   Inpatient therapies [dates]                                             │
│   Reflexology:_____ _____ _____ _____ _____ Massage:_____ _____ _____│
│   Massage/Reflexology:_____ _____ _____ _____ _____ _____ _____ __  │
│   Inpatient therapies and patient evaluation                              │
│   Breathing meditation    Therapy      Yes_____ No_____ Unsure_____        │
│   Guided imagery          promoted     Yes_____ No_____ Unsure_____        │
│   Music therapy           relaxation?  Yes_____ No_____ Unsure_____        │
│   Massage                               Yes_____ No_____ Unsure_____        │
│   Reflexology                           Yes_____ No_____ Unsure_____        │
└─────────────────────────────────────────────────────────────────────────┘
```

FIGURE 2-3   *Template of IM consultation documentation.*

unrushed conversation with a health-care professional, frequently bringing the entire family into the process, or sharing private thoughts they did not want to unburden onto their loved ones. One of the patients, a psychiatrist, described his experience during his IM consultations as "cathartic."

Depending on the patients' condition, their first encounter with the program could take place prior to hospital admission—for elective cases, during hospitalization but before their surgical intervention—for "in-house" patients and transfers from other facilities, or after the procedure. Having the IM consultation in "standing" preoperative orders allowed the IM staff open access to

Integrative Cardiac Medicine Worksheet   2 of 2

Health & Wellness/Lifestyle Modification

Alcohol: Y_____ N_____ Frequency (f)_____

Smoking: Y_____ N_____ Type_____ Amount_____ Quit_____

Drugs: Y_____ N_____ Type_____

Diet/Nutrition Type_____

Eat out (f)_____ Order in (f)_____ Fast food (f)_____

Supplements:_____ Current needs:_____

Exercise Y_____ N_____ Type_____ Frequency (f)_____
Recreation/Hobbies:_____

Stress High_____ Moderate_____ Low_____ Source_____
Symptoms:_____

Coping / Relief of stress:_____

Stress management: Very well_____ Well_____ Fairly well_____ Poorly_____
Support systems:_____

Spirituality Pastoral care: Visit requested_____ Referral made_____

Higher power: Y_____ N_____ Meaning & purpose:_____

Quality of Life Excellent_____ Good_____ Fair_____ Poor_____ Satisfied? Y_____ N_____
Changes would like to make:_____

Effects of illness:_____

Employment/Retirement Retired_____ Returning to work_____ Retiring_____
          Unemployed_____ Disability_____

Previous CAM exposure_____

Discharge Date:_____ Home_____ Rehab_____ New residence_____

Frequency (f): Monthly or less, 2–4 per month, 2–3 per week, 4 or more per week

FIGURE 2-3   (*Continued*)

all cardiac surgical patients, including ventricular assist device (VAD) recipients and transplant candidates.

The cardiac IM program was staffed by a full-time program manager, a holistic NP, several part-time holistic clinical nurse specialists, all registered nurses (RNs) with a variety of CAM qualifications, and a group of per diem massage therapists, who were certified by the State of New Jersey and had prior inpatient experience. The services offered by the IM program included:

- Initial IM consultation, inpatient follow-up visits and predischarge wellness consultation provided by the core program staff.
- Breathing meditation teaching, guided imagery and music therapy (for patients who were not receptive to guided imagery) introduced by the holistic RNs during initial IM consultation.
- Massage, reflexology or combination treatments designed to familiarize patients with both therapies—delivered by either massage therapists or the core staff. We found it practical to recruit CAM professionals who were cross-trained in different treatment modalities.
- Pastoral care—offered by holistic RNs during consultations and delivered by full-time or volunteer clergy. Not surprisingly, the program required reliable pastoral support.

Early in the program, the steering committee explored the possibility of delivering CAM treatments perioperatively—healing words and guided imagery—but the efforts were abandoned due to complexity of implementation in the operating room environment.

Another important factor contributing to the success of the program was consistent support of the Cardiac Rehabilitation programs, phase I. The outpatient, phase II, programs were also available at both facilities and strongly recommended by the holistic RNs.

The final patient interaction with the IM professionals prior to discharge included preparation of a "prescription for wellness" (see Figure 2-4), a summary of outpatient activities recommended by the holistic nurses given to patients along with a list of organizations offering recommended services near their homes.

Administration and financial management

The IM program manager reported directly to the vice president for Cardiac Services, who was intricately involved in all aspects of program operations. In order to accurately track program finances, a separate grant account was established, and detailed records of all program-related funding and expenditures were kept. The program finances were managed by Katrina Zapotulko, then project manager for Cardiac Services. The project manager also prepared progress reports to sponsors, as the program was supported by several organizations.

Securing funding sources for a program is always a challenge. The IM committee applied to the Medtronic Foundation in hope that the grant would cover the first few years of program operations. Within 9 months later we were excited to learn of the grant, but it covered only a portion of our anticipated costs. The annual cost of supporting 1,100 patients at two hospitals was approximately $250,000 per year. The Cardiac Executive Committee worked with the vendors of our catheterization laboratories and cardiac operating rooms (ORs) to

Prescription for Health & Wellness

_____ Cardiac rehabilitation (in approximately 6 weeks)

Facility: _____

Phone # _____

_____ Emotional support

Facility: _____

Phone # _____

_____ Nutritional counseling

Facility: _____

Phone # _____

_____ Stress management

Facility: _____

Phone # _____

_____ Breathing meditation

_____ Guided imagery

_____ Massage therapy/reflexology

_____ Other _____

_____

_____

FIGURE 2-4   *Template of prescription for wellness.*

improve our rebate programs. The physicians were supportive and SBHCS gave approval to use the rebate dollars for funding of the IM program.

Environment of care

Prior to starting the program, we had the benefit of a capital project approval to renovate the cardiothoracic ICU at one of the Heart Hospital facilities. After some research, we decided to employ an architectural designer who had the knowledge of an ancient Chinese art and science of living in harmony with the environment and could use it to create and direct the flow of "chi," or energy.

We thought it critical to develop a process that allowed patients to stay in the same area or, at least, not to be transferred more than once during their hospitalization. The renovated unit had private rooms only, with decorative colors, fabrics, and artwork in pleasing earth tones selected to resemble the aspects of nature. Decentralized nursing pods and curved geometric shapes replaced traditional square furniture and nursing stations. A walking track was built to encourage patients and staff to keep the commitment to active postoperative recovery ("We do your surgery, you do the walking"). The use of aromatherapy—lavender— became the standard in the Heart Hospital of New Jersey units.

Data management

Since 1999, the Department of Cardiothoracic Surgery utilized a cardiovascular patient-oriented clinical information system, Clinical Automated Office Solutions (CAOS), developed by Intelligent Business Solutions, Inc. (IBS), Winston-Salem, North Carolina.[1] Mark Shill, the president of IBS, partnered with the program to develop an IM module of the CAOS system, which was completed in May 2002 (see Fig. 2-5).

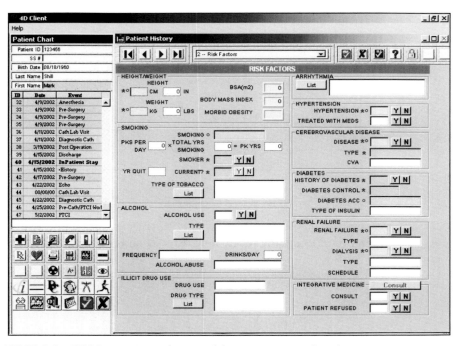

FIGURE 2-5 *CAOS integrative medicine module, version 2.90—selected screen captures.* (Printed by permission of Intelligent Business Solutions, Inc.)

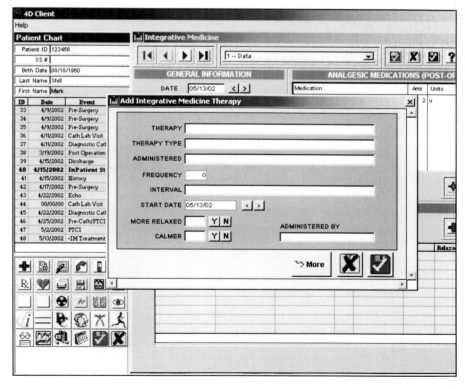

FIGURE 2-5 (Continued)

The IM-specific data was collected by the holistic nurses and entered into CAOS, where it became fully integrated with a wealth of clinical data collected for all cardiothoracic surgery patients. The CAOS system is certified by the American College of Cardiology, the Society of Thoracic Surgery and offers extensive data-mining capabilities.

Outcomes

Since January 2002,[1] 2,987 individuals were offered CAM services, which constituted 93.9% of all patients who underwent cardiothoracic surgery at the Heart Hospital facilities during that period (see Table 2-1). The remaining 6.1%

TABLE 2-1

CARDIAC IM PROGRAM ACCEPTANCE RATE, MEAN AGE, AND GENDER DEMOGRAPHICS AT NEWARK BETH ISRAEL MEDICAL CENTER AND SAINT BARNABAS MEDICAL CENTER, 2002–2004

Cardiothoracic (CT) Surgery	2002–2004 Total	IM Offered[*]	IM Not Offered	2001 Total (No IM)
Activity (cases) (% of total)	3,312 (100%)	3,111 (93.93%)	201 (6.07%)	1,100
Mean age (years)	66.3	66.4	64.2	64.7
Female (cases) (% of subgroup total)	1,110 (33.83%)	1,042 (33.49%)	68 (33.83%)	322 (29.27%)
Breakdown of IM Offered	IM Offered	IM Accepted[†]	IM Refused	
Activity (cases) (% of offered)	3,111 (100%)	2,987 (96.01%)	124 (3.99%)	
Mean age (years)	66.4	66.4	68.1	
Female (cases) (% of subgroup total)	1,042 (33.49%)	1,007 (33.71%)	35 (28.23%)	

[*]IM offered group included IM accepted and IM refused.
[†]IM accepted includes all patients who participated in the program and received holistic consultations and/or therapies.

included critically ill, emergency cases, or patients who were not able to communicate with holistic RNs. About 96.0% of patients who were offered the program accepted all or some of the services. Based on our experience, when financial restraints were alleviated, 96% of cardiac patients agreed to try CAM treatments! In addition, with an increase in the average age of patients from 2002 to 2004, the demand for the program has not diminished.

The utilization of CAM services was as follows (see Table 2-2 and Fig. 2-6):

- Initial and follow-up IM consultations comprised the majority of program activity (54.6%); predischarge visits were counted as follow-up consultations.
- Massage, reflexology, and massage/reflexology combination treatment accounted for 28.9%, of which reflexology was, by far, the most common therapy (25.4%) as it was the less invasive of the two and could be utilized shortly after open-heart surgery.

TABLE 2-2

UTILIZATION OF CAM SERVICES AT NEWARK BETH ISRAEL MEDICAL CENTER AND SAINT BARNABAS MEDICAL CENTER, 2002–2004

IM Modality	Activity	% of Total Activity	Mean Interactions/Case[*]
Holistic consultations (visits)			
Initial IM consult	2,987	16.02%	
Follow-up visits	7,192	38.58%	
Subtotal	10,179	54.60%	3.4
Massage and reflexology (1/2 and 1/4 hour treatments)			
Reflexology	4,736	25.40%	
Massage and reflexology	565	3.03%	
Massage	94	0.50%	
Subtotal	5,395	28.94%	1.8
Guided imagery and music therapy (tape sets)			
Guided imagery[†]	2,976	15.96%	
Music therapy	92	0.49%	
Subtotal	3,068	16.46%	n/a
Total activity	18,642	100.00%	n/a

[*]Mean interaction/case is calculated with respect to 2,987 total number of patients who participated in the program ("IM accepted" group depicted in Table 2-1).

[†]Guided imagery and music therapy activity was counted by the number of tapes distributed. In some cases, different programs (tapes) were used pre- and postoperatively, which accounts for the subtotal number of guided imagery and music therapies being higher than the total number of patients in the program.

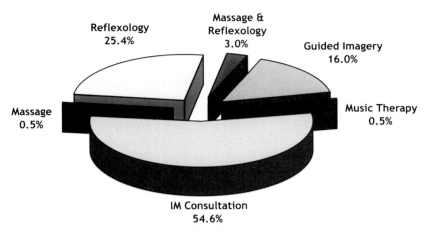

FIGURE 2-6   *CAM services utilization at Newark Beth Israel Medical Center and Saint Barnabas Medical Center, 2002–2004.*

- Guided imagery and music therapy—16.5%—all patients were encouraged to use guided imagery tapes which they took home after discharge. Music therapy proved a useful alternative for patients who did not understand English, or were slightly confused.

- All patients were taught, and given written directions for, breathing meditation during their initial consultation—the IM team decided not to keep a separate count of these activities.

Patients who participated in the program received, on average, 5.2 CAM treatments/interactions during their inpatient stay. Considering the relatively short period of time in which the interactions took place, the IM team hoped to have provided sufficient learning opportunity and reinforcement to assist participants in making long-term changes toward a healthier lifestyle.

On the other hand, acutely ill heart-failure patients sometimes spent weeks, and even months, at Newark Beth Israel Medical Center waiting for their transplantation procedures. While not originally intended as the target population for the IM program, transplant candidates were often in desperate need of CAM services to help them battle anxiety and depression that was, unfortunately, common in such circumstances. The IM team quickly adapted to the needs of this unique group, many of whom became the most devoted advocates of the program.

It was one of the transplant recipients who had first mentioned that reflexology helped him sleep better and, eventually, enabled him to stop taking anti-anxiety medications (Xanax). Intrigued by his experience, the Newark Beth Israel Pharmacy department compared the use of Xanax, before and after opening of the IM program (2001 vs. 2002), on the cardiothoracic ICU and stepdown units where patients recovered postoperatively. Since Xanax was not on the units standard orders, the overall use was relatively low for both years (less than 0.25 doses per patient-day), but there was a notable 29.95% drop in Xanax use (0.25- and 0.5-mg doses combined) in 2002 with respect to 2001 use, while physician practice on the units remained largely unchanged.

Patient satisfaction scores for areas where majority of patients received CAM therapies have consistently stayed well above the hospital average, and regularly rose above other cardiac units; at both hospitals the quarterly mean unit nursing scores gathered by a leading national company for IM units ranged 87.7–95.1% of the highest score, while the hospitals' averages for all units ranged 84.0–88.3%. Program-specific patient satisfaction scores collected by the IM staff have also been very positive: 8.8 out of 10, in a sample of 200 patients. Within a year of program operations, the IM committee had to develop a policy for the massage therapists asked by patients to continue therapy at home; some of the treatments have been continuing for years.

The cardiac nursing staff eagerly embraced the IM program from its inception. The physicians, overall, took a more neutrally supportive approach, and we were pleasantly surprised by lack of apparent resistance. However, as more patients received services, both nursing and medical staff repeatedly noted to us that the IM patients seemed more relaxed, as well as less anxious and fearful. The CAM therapies seemed to help patients sleep better and made them more comfortable and positive throughout their hospital stay. As the word of the program spread, we received several requests for CAM services, mostly massage and reflexology, from other clinical disciplines. Sadly, due to financial restraints, we were not able to expand the program beyond open-heart surgical population.

In 2003, the vice president of Cardiac Services led local electrophysiology specialists in the development of a CAM utilization protocol for the implantable cardiac defibrillator (ICD) patients. The proposal, titled "*Integrative Medicine* Approach to Medi*cal* Care of ICD Patients: A Prospective Study of the Effects of CA*M* Treatments on Anxiety, Depression, Device Acceptance and Quality of Life in ICD Recipients (IM CALM)," was promptly supported by Medtronic, Inc. The investigator-initiated protocol was approved by the local IRB in September 2004 and begun patient enrollment later that year.

CONCLUSION

Components of successful execution

Looking back on our experience, we realized that having to narrow the scope of the program to the open-heart surgical population provided us with a sharper focus and a better chance of effective implementation. A well-chosen patient population for a pilot program would need to have sufficient interaction time with the program staff (inpatient length of stay or regular outpatient visits) and a consistent, preferably pathway-driven, plan of care delivered by physicians who practice exclusively at the program facilities. Having full support of the medical staff who treat the selected patient population is essential. The degree of physician support is best assessed early in the planning stages and further developed through varied educational activities. Operationally, having program staff who are solely dedicated to the project is critical for the success of the program.

In planning stages and through the first years of the program, the IM team met weekly with the vice president for Cardiac Services, following a structured agenda and evaluating the progress with respect to the implementation timeline developed early and followed closely throughout the program start-up. A commitment of high-level administrators and physicians, as well as allocation of staffing resources, was essential for effective execution of the project that did not readily fit into the existing infrastructure. Creating a closely knit team, by meeting frequently and productively, and performing activities as a group (e.g., staff interviews), instilled a sense of individual responsibility for the success of the program.

From the initial stages of the project, the steering committee emphasized financial self-sufficiency and accountability of the program, which could only have been achieved by creating a separate program account and designating a program CFO, who maintained detailed financial records. In the current healthcare environment, few institutions would be able to dedicate sufficient internal resources to CAM initiatives; locating and securing external sources of funding is likely to continue being a priority and a challenge.

As program initiators, we strongly believe that the cardiac IM program enhanced the quality of care and improved patients' hospitalization experience. There was clear evidence that CAM services strengthened patient, physician, and staff satisfaction, and we hope that the program helped some patients and staff to make a change toward a healthier lifestyle. On the other hand, we have also heard from patients for whom, in their own words, the availability of CAM therapies had made a difference between life and death.

ACKNOWLEDGMENTS

The authors would like to express their deepest gratitude to the Medtronic Foundation and Medtronic, Inc. for providing funding and inspiration without which the cardiac IM program would not be possible. We would also like to recognize and thank the Healthcare Foundation of New Jersey and St. Jude Medical, Inc. for their support of the cardiac IM conferences.

REFERENCES

1. Intelligent Business Solutions (IBS), Inc. Website:*www.ecaos.com*

3

LEGAL AND ETHICAL ISSUES IN INTEGRATIVE CARDIOLOGY

Michael H. Cohen

INTRODUCTION

As detailed elsewhere,[1–6,7–10] the clinical integration of complementary and alternative medical (CAM) therapies generally—such as acupuncture and traditional oriental medicine, chiropractic, herbal medicine, massage therapy, and "mind-body" therapies such as guided imagery—into conventional health care raises important legal and risk management issues for clinicians and institutions. Integration of CAM therapies in care of patients with cardiac disease is no exception. Some may see legal issues as presenting overwhelming obstacles to clinical integration of potentially viable therapies, while others are finding ways to surmount institutional roadblocks and manage legal risks effectively.[1]

Frequently, the process of selectively and judiciously integrative CAM therapies that may be safe and effective involves delicate negotiations between clinicians and patient, bringing out differences in legal, ethical, and clinical perspectives.[2] Patients may underreport existing use of CAM therapies. Alternatively, patients may be interested in trying a broad variety of approaches, while clinicians may view the existing evidence for safety and efficacy of specific therapies championed by the patient as insufficient to justify recommending these therapies. Yet again, the medical literature may suggest that potential adverse interactions with conventional treatment may result.

To date, few hospitals have created guidelines for their clinicians seeking to advise patients in response to requests for information about use or avoidance of CAM therapies.[3] Professional medical groups often offer little guidance other than cautioning against potential safety and liability risks. This chapter addresses the salient liability issues and offers risk management suggestions (with relevant case examples) for clinicians treating patients with cardiac disease.

HEALTH-CARE LAW RELEVANT TO CAM

The law related to CAM therapies is evolving, but the basic principles of health law would seem to apply whether a therapy is labeled "conventional" or "CAM".[4] Health-care law generally governs the provision of CAM therapies, as its principles apply across therapies, whether considered "conventional" or not. Seven critical areas relating to CAM are: (1) licensure, (2) scope of practice, (3) malpractice liability, (4) professional discipline, (5) access to treatments, (6) third-party reimbursement, and (7) fraud. These areas are broadly described with case examples elsewhere.[4] In brief, licensure refers to the requirement in most states that health-care providers maintain a current state license to practice their professional healing art. While a few states recently have enacted statutes authorizing nonlicensed CAM providers to practice,[5] in most states, licensure serves as the first hurdle to professional practice. Licensure of CAM providers varies by state; chiropractors, for example, are licensed in every state, whereas massage therapists and acupuncturists are licensed in well over half the states, and naturopaths in about a dozen states.[6]

Scope of practice refers to the legally authorized boundaries of care within the given profession. State licensing statutes usually define a CAM provider's scope of practice, regulations promulgated by the relevant state licensing board (such as the state board of chiropractic) often supplement or interpret the relevant licensing statute, courts interpret both statutes and administrative regulations.[4] For example, chiropractors can give nutritional advice in some states but not others; and typically, massage therapists are prohibited from mental health counseling.

Malpractice refers to negligence, which is defined as failure to use due care (or follow the standard of care) in treating a patient, and thereby injuring the patient. Generally, each CAM profession is judged by its own standard of care—for example, acupuncture; chiropractic; physical therapy; massage therapy.[4] In cases where the provider's clinical care overlaps with medical care—for example, the chiropractor who takes and reads a patient's X-ray—then the medical standard may be applied.[4]

An in-depth discussion of the intricacies of malpractice insurance is beyond the scope of this chapter. It should be noted, however, that states vary in their requirements for malpractice coverage,[11] and individual insurers vary in their coverage of CAM therapies. The individual practitioner should determine the coverage available and the amount, if any, required by his or her state.

Professional discipline refers to the power of the relevant professional board—in the psychiatrist's case, the state medical board—to sanction a clinician, most gravely by revoking the clinician's license. The concern over inappropriate discipline, based on medical board's antipathy to inclusion of CAM therapies, has led consumer groups in many states to lobby for "health freedom" statutes—laws providing that physicians may not be disciplined solely on the basis of incorporating CAM modalities.[4] More recently, the Federation of State Medical

Boards has issued Model Guidelines for Physician Use of Complementary and Alternative Therapies, reaffirming this same principle.[12]

Third-party reimbursement involves a number of insurance policy provisions, and corresponding legal rules, designed to ensure that reimbursement is limited to "medically necessary" treatment; does not, in general, cover "experimental" treatments; and is not subject to fraud and abuse.[4] In general, insurers have been slow to offer CAM therapies as core benefits—largely because of insufficient evidence of safety, efficacy, and cost-effectiveness—though a number of insurers have offered policyholders discounted access to a network of CAM providers.

Health-care fraud refers to the legal concern for preventing intentional deception of patients. Overbroad claims sometimes can lead to charges of fraud, and its related legal theory, misrepresentation.[4] If the clinician or institution submits a reimbursement claim for care that the clinician knew or should have known was medically unnecessary, this also might be grounds for a finding of fraud and abuse under federal law.[4]

MALPRACTICE CONSIDERATIONS

The area that primarily concerns many clinicians is malpractice liability for clinical inclusion of CAM therapies, particularly as the research for such therapies is less extensive than for many conventional modalities. Indeed, because the research base is smaller, conclusions seem to swing rapidly as new discoveries respectively enhance or diminish validation for such therapies as St. John's Wort to treat moderate depression. Few judicial opinions address malpractice and CAM therapies; the legal landscape is relatively new and subject to rapid change as CAM therapies increasingly penetrate mainstream health care.[13] Yet, as suggested, we can extrapolate general principles from malpractice in conventional care, since theoretically the same legal concepts and standards should apply, whether the therapy is considered "conventional" or "CAM".[7]

Medical malpractice (or negligence) generally consists of two elements: (1) providing clinical care below generally accepted professional standards and (2) thereby causing the patient injury. The plaintiff (who is suing) usually hires a medical expert to testify that the defendant physician practiced below generally accepted standards of care.

There are multiple possible claims of health-care malpractice, including misdiagnosis, failure to treat, failure of informed consent, fraud and misrepresentation, abandonment, vicarious liability, and breach of privacy and confidentiality.[8] This chapter will focus on several of these theories of liability, with examples of potentially problematic practices relating to treatment of cardiac disease.

Misdiagnosis refers to failure to diagnose a condition accurately, or at all; it is malpractice when the failure occurred by virtue of providing care below generally accepted professional standards, and the patient was thereby injured. A provider who fails to employ conventional diagnostic methods, or who substitutes CAM diagnostic methods for conventional ones, risks a malpractice verdict.

Thus, adding complementary diagnostic systems (such as those of chiropractic and acupuncture) is not itself problematic, so long as the conventional bases are covered.[7] For example, it would be perilous to treat headaches as "subluxations" or "displaced *chi*" if the patient turns out to have a brain tumor, just as it would probably be malpractice to misdiagnose chest pain as a muscular ache when it might be a warning sign of cardiac arrest. Continuing to monitor conventionally, while maintaining a healthy system of conventional referrals, may be useful in dispelling this type of liability risk.[7]

Failure to treat by following conventional standards of care also can lead to malpractice liability if the patient is thereby injured. Again, it is not the use of CAM therapies that is problematic in itself, but rather overreliance on such therapies, to the exclusion of necessary medical care. Following the earlier first example, if a chiropractor continued to treat headaches without referring the patient to a medical doctor to rule out the possibility of a neurological or cancerous condition, this could constitute failure to treat (or more specifically for the chiropractor, failure to refer to a medical doctor) and thereby malpractice; similarly, the massage therapist who ignores signs and angina and fails to refer to a cardiologist (or the internist who refers the patient for massage and misses the diagnosis or need to refer to a cardiac specialist) could potentially be liable for malpractice.

SOME CLINICAL SCENARIOS AND A LIABILITY FRAMEWORK

Understanding which CAM therapies patients use is legally prudent, if not mandatory as a means of understanding how conventional treatment advice may interact with patients' own efforts toward self-care. Some CAM therapies, such as mind-body techniques, have been shown safe and/or effective for conditions such as chronic pain and insomnia.[14] Specifically, in cardiac care, some have suggested that integrating CAM therapies may be beneficial so as to create "an optimal healing environment" in which the "intrapersonal/interpersonal characteristics of the health care provider and patient, mind/body/spirit wholeness and healing versus curing are discussed, as is the impact psychosocial factors may have on atherosclerosis and cardiovascular health".[15] And likewise, therapies such as audiovisual relaxation training treatment involving deep breathing, exercise, muscle relaxation, guided imagery, and meditation were shown to compare favorably with routine nursing care for reducing anxiety, improving sleep, and promoting relaxation in adults with cardiac disease;[16] studies have also suggested that relaxation and music therapy are effective modalities to reduce stress in patients, such as those in a coronary care unit admitted with the presumptive diagnosis of acute myocardial infarction.[17]

On the other hand, inclusion of some CAM therapies can raise the specter of direct harm from the therapy or from adverse interactions with conventional care, or of indirect harm from diverting the patient from necessary conventional care. For example, herbal products may contain "undisclosed drugs or heavy metals, interaction with the pharmacokinetic profile of concomitantly administered drugs, or association with a misidentified herbal species".[18]

In general, the following framework may help the clinician (or institution) classify any given therapy into one of four regions:[7]

A. The medical evidence supports both safety and efficacy.

B. The medical evidence supports safety, but evidence regarding efficacy is inconclusive.

C. The medical evidence supports efficacy, but evidence regarding safety is inconclusive.

D. The medical evidence indicates either serious risk or inefficacy.

In region A, clinicians clearly should feel comfortable recommending the CAM therapy, as a therapy deemed both safe and effective could be recommended regardless of whether it is classified as conventional or CAM.

Similarly, in D, clinicians should avoid and discourage patient use of the CAM therapy. Again, the proposition is self-evident: a therapy that is either seriously risky or ineffective should be avoided and discouraged, whether labeled conventional or CAM.

This notion of applying the framework across the board is consistent with the key recommendation of the recent report by the Institute of Medicine (IOM) at the National Academy of Sciences on complementary and alternative medicine:[19]

> *The committee recommends that the same principles and standards of evidence of treatment effectiveness apply to all treatments, whether currently labeled as conventional medicine or CAM.*

It should be clear that in region A, liability is unlikely, since inclusion of the therapy is unlikely to fall below prevailing standards of care (since it is effective), and unlikely to injure the patient (since it is safe). In D, on the other hand, liability is likely, since the converse is true: the therapy is likely to fall below prevailing standards of care (since it is ineffective), and likely to injure the patient (since it is seriously risky).

Many CAM therapies will fall within either B or C. Liability is conceivable but probably unlikely, particularly in B, where the product presumably is safe.[7] If, however, the patient's condition deteriorates in either case B or C, then the physician should consider implementing a conventional intervention, or risk potential liability if the patient becomes injured through reliance on the CAM therapy.[7] The best strategy in B and C is to caution the patient and, while accepting the patient's choice to try the CAM therapy, continue to monitor efficacy and safety respectively.[7]

Consider, for example, use of chiropractic to treat low back pain, a therapy widely used within the United States for a condition that afflicts millions of patients and for which conventional care offers few reliable "cures." There is sufficient evidence of safety and efficacy (at this date) that treatment with chiropractic would probably be warranted.[7,9] On the other hand, there is poor evidence regarding use of St. John's Wort to treat severe depression; a clinician who relies on herbal formulas in such a case may risk malpractice if the patient continues to slide deeper into the depression, and particularly if that results in a physical injury to (or by) the patient.

More relevant to cardiac care are the "serious or potentially serious cardiovascular adverse effects of herbal medicines".[20] In other search of five electronic literature databases, case reports and case series indicated that:[20]

> *Life-threatening adverse effects of herbal medicines occur. Potentially serious adverse effects are arrhythmias, arteritis, cardiac glycosides overdose, chest pain, congestive heart failure, hypertension, hypotension, myocardial infarction, overanticoagulation, pericarditis and death. The problems relate to toxic herbal ingredients, adulteration and contamination of herbal medicinal products, and herb-drug interactions. Herbal medicines that have been implicated repeatedly include aconite, ephedra and licorice.*

According to this study:[20]

> *Because of the anecdotal nature of the evidence, it is impossible to estimate the incidence of adverse effects. In conclusion, herbal medicinal products are regularly associated with serious cardiovascular adverse events but the size of this problem cannot be estimated at present. Vigilance and research seem to be the best way forward.*

Such findings readily lend themselves to categorization of the selected therapies such as the herbal medicines in question, either alone or in combination with the conventional treatment in place to fall within regions (D) (avoid and discourage) or perhaps C (caution and monitor for safety). On the other hand, a therapy such as intercessory prayer could be considered safe with uncertain efficacy,[21] falling into category B (monitor for efficacy, and do not substitute for necessary conventional care).

UNDERSTANDING CAM AS PART OF COMPREHENSIVE CARE

As suggested, if a condition readily can be cured by conventional care, there is a strong imperative to provide such care. Delay in itself is not negligent—but delay that aggravates the patient's condition or leads to irreversible progression of the disease might be considered negligent. This goes back to the earlier definition of malpractice as providing substandard care, and in so doing, creating patient injury.

On the other hand, engaging the patient in a conversation about options, and suggesting or agreeing to a trial run with a CAM therapy that may have some evidence of safety and/or efficacy in the medical literature, while continuing to monitor conventionally, is a strategy that makes sense. Indeed, the IOM report suggested:

> The goal should be the provision of comprehensive medical care that is based on the best scientific evidence available regarding benefits and harm, that encourages patients to share in decision making about therapeutic options, and that promotes choices in care that can include CAM therapies, when appropriate.[19]

In short, comprehensive is evidence informed, patient centered, and mindful of the possibility that CAM therapies may in some cases be recommended as useful, in others discouraged as unsafe or ineffective, and in many others, be accepted for a time with a readiness to intervene conventionally if the CAM therapy turns out to be either unsafe or ineffective.

What happens if the patient does not abandon conventional therapy, but rather, has a complication from the interaction of conventional therapy with the CAM therapy, and there is little, if any, medical literature to inform the clinician? The above liability framework presents a good guide for the clinician. Unless there is clear evidence of a potential adverse interaction, the clinician can allow the CAM therapy while continuing to monitor conventionally. If the CAM therapy turns out to be either unsafe or ineffective in combination with the conventional therapy, then the clinician accordingly should advise the patient to discontinue use of the CAM therapy. Since research regarding CAM therapies is ongoing and the medical evidence can change rapidly, the clinician should communicate regularly with the patient regarding any new developments and reconsider therapeutic decisions accordingly.

DIETARY SUPPLEMENTS: ESPECIALLY PROBLEMATIC

As suggested earlier, the current evidence suggests that some recommendations involving herbal products remain especially problematic. Under the Dietary Supplement Health Education Act of 1994, "dietary supplements"—containing vitamins, minerals, amino acids, and herbs—generally are regulated as foods, not drugs, and therefore can be sold in interstate commerce without prior proof of safety or efficacy. Further, the federal Food and Drug Administration (FDA) rarely interferes with individual clinicians' practices, since the FDA is a federal agency and health-care practice is regulated under state law.

The medical literature is full of reports about safety concerns associated with various herbal products. In addition to issues of contamination and adulteration, and lack of batch-to-batch consistency, clinicians have to consider the possibility of adverse herb-herb as well as herb-drug interactions. The literature on efficacy is sparse compared to comparable pharmaceutical medications, and concerns have been raised about adverse reactions from patient use of dietary supplements.[22]

For example, one study examined patient use of dietary supplements prior to surgery, particularly in terms of potential interactions with anesthetics. The survey revealed that of 500 patients, 51% preoperatively took herbs, vitamins, dietary supplements, or homeopathic medicines (range, 1–22 per patient); 24% of surveyed patients consumed 50 different herbs, 41% took 9 types of vitamins, 44% took 31 types of dietary supplements, and 1% of patients took the homeopathic arnica.[23] Thus:

> *Classification by potential adverse effects revealed that 27% of surgical patients consumed alternative medicines that may inhibit coagulation, affect blood pressure (12%), cause sedation (9%), have cardiac effects (5%), or alter electrolytes (4%).*[23]

In light of all these potential dangers, clinician in-office sales of dietary supplements as ancillary to treatment also are especially troublesome. So, too are any arrangements whereby clinicians receive any percentage or profit from sales of supplements recommended to patients. Such sales can trigger legal antikickback considerations. Sales of dietary supplements also can suggest that the clinician has been not only negligent, but potentially reckless, a higher state of culpability, triggering the possibility of punitive as well as compensatory damages.[10]

But in addition to legal culpability are ethical questions pertaining to conflict of interest. The American Medical Association has opined that physician sale of dietary supplements for profit may present an impermissible conflict of interest between good patient care and profit, and thus be ethically objectionable. Several states have enacted laws limiting or prohibiting physician sales of dietary supplements.[24]

Yet another concern is potential discipline by the relevant state regulatory boards—such as the state medical board for physicians. Many of the relevant statues contain generic provisions that allow physician discipline, for example, for such acts as "failure to maintain minimal standards applicable to the selection or administration of drugs, or failure to employ acceptable scientific methods in the selection of drugs or other modalities for treatment of disease".[25] Some state medical boards have applied these generic (or catch-all) statutory provisions to physicians offering nutritional treatments.

It should be noted that there is also evidence to suggest that some dietary supplements may be effective in treatment of cardiac disease, and thus could be allowed or even recommended (depending on the current state of the evidence), according to the liability risk framework presented earlier. Thus, for example, one recent study has found a number of possible antiarrhythmic actions from long-chain polyunsaturated omega-3 fatty acids in "animal and laboratory studies, mainly on ventricular arrhythmias," observing:

These include reducing pro-arrhythmic eicosanoids and inhibiting sodium and calcium currents. If found to be beneficial to these patients, dietary advice to eat more oil-rich fish, or take LCn3 supplements, could be part of a package of care for people with this arrhythmia.[26]

It may be appropriate to state overall that, as "herbs and dietary supplements can have significant physiological effects...there is a need for definitive research on the potential risks and benefits of these compounds, including appropriate dosages and formulations, and delineation of adverse events and interactions".[22] Thus:

Garlic (Allium sativum) has shown beneficial lipid effects in a majority of trials; dried garlic preparations are superior to oil preparations. There is preliminary evidence that indicates that hawthorn (Crataegus species) may provide benefits in congestive heart failure. Coenzyme Q also may be of benefit in congestive heart failure. Although observational studies indicate a protective effect of dietary or supplemental vitamin E, controlled trails have not shown a beneficial effect on angina and have been mixed on whether supplementation decreases major cardiac events. Although several observational studies have noted that fish intake protects against cardiovascular disease, prospective studies are less impressive. Fish oil supplementation may have a mild beneficial effect on hypertension, but there is no effect on total cholesterol levels. Trials are inconsistent on whether fish oil reduces restenosis rates following coronary angioplasty. Carnitine appears to have beneficial effects on congestive heart failure and angina; there is also preliminary evidence that arginine may benefit patients with congestive heart failure or angina. Herbs and supplements have been associated with adverse effects and interactions; for example, garlic inhibits platelet aggregation and can cause significant anticoagulation, and the Chinese herb danshen (Salvia miltiorrhiza) appears to potentiate warfarin. Several herbs and supplements hold promise as adjuncts in the prevention and treatment of cardiovascular disease.

This mixed picture suggests that the evidence could place dietary supplements in any of regions B, C, or possibly D within the liability risk framework, depending on the supplement and/or its interaction with a given conventional therapy; at the least, caution and close monitoring are always advised.

INFORMED CONSENT

The legal obligation of informed consent is to provide the patient with all the information material to a treatment decision—in other words, that would make a difference in the patient's choice to undergo or forgo a given therapeutic protocol. This obligation applies across the board, whether CAM or conventional therapies are involved.[9] Materiality refers to information about risks and benefits that is reasonably significant to a patient's decision to undergo or forgo a particular therapy; about half the states judge materiality by the "reasonable patient's" notion of what is significant, while the other half judge materiality by the "reasonable physician".[9] Presumably, materiality in the latter half means evidence-informed judgments concerning what therapies may be potentially useful.[9]

The principle of shared decision-making takes informed consent a step further, by ensuring that there are not only disclosures by physicians to patients, but also full and fair conversations in which patients feel empowered and participatory. The IOM report, as noted above, encouraged shared-decision as a means of patient empowerment. Updating the patient about changes in medical evidence also is an important part of the informed consent obligation. If the discussion involves a herbal product, the physician should try to deconstruct the notion that "natural" necessarily means "safe".[27,28] Some patients are more deferential or compliant to clinical authority whereas others are resistant. In any event, informing the patient about the changing medical evidence may shift (in one direction or another) the patient's willingness to accept the known risks and benefits of the CAM therapy, or even to use this therapy.

An interesting question is how the law might treat clinicians who fail to make recommendations for patients regarding nutrition, mind–body, and other readily accepted CAM therapies as adjuncts to conventional care. If/as medical evidence begins to show safety and efficacy for such therapies, and these therapies become more generally accepted within the medical community, there may be liability for clinicians who fail to make helpful, adjunctive recommendations involving CAM therapies.[4,29] The case would likely depend on the court's view of whether the medical profession generally accepted the CAM therapy as safe and effective for the patient's condition, and possibly, as a safer and more effective therapeutic option than the conventional drug or treatment route otherwise prescribed.[4]

For example, clinical research has demonstrated that "guided imagery, a simple form of relaxation, can reduce preoperative anxiety and postoperative pain among patients undergoing surgical procedures;" thus, "guided imagery is now considered a [valid] complementary means to reduce anxiety, pain, and length of stay among our cardiac surgery patients".[30] One might say the same about inclusion of acupuncture and self-education, found in one study to be beneficial in patients with advanced angina pectoris.[21]

Of course, risks as well as benefits of potential avenues of treatment should be described; so, too, should risks of adverse reactions between conventional and CAM therapies. For example, in cardiac care, bleeding is one of the primary concerns for patients using both kinds of modalities;[31] patients should therefore be advised of this risk.

FRAUD AND MISREPRESENTATION

Fraud and misrepresentation involve the knowing inducement of reliance on inaccurate or false information for the benefit of the person committing the fraud and to the detriment of the victim. The practitioner must know the information or representation is false, or must recklessly fail to discover its falsity; and the victim must reasonably rely on the representation.

Because it involves intentionality or recklessness, as opposed to lack of due care, fraud presents a higher level of culpability than the negligence in most malpractice cases. As such, a fraud claim typically opens the defending physician to the possibility of punitive damages. At the same time, fraud is harder to prove, since it requires proving a mental state (intention or recklessness) and not simply a negligent act. Nonetheless, fraud can serve as a potent tool to curb overreaching and abusive conduct in provision of CAM therapies.[5]

PATIENT ABANDONMENT

Abandoning patients is ethically proscribed and legally yet another ground for suit. Abandonment refers to the unilateral and unjustified termination of the treatment relationship by the physician that results in patient injury. As the term "unjustified" indicates, there are situations in which it is reasonable and appropriate for treating clinicians to unilaterally terminate the treatment relationship. These include threatening or violent patients, patients who repeatedly fail to keep appointments, and patients who are noncompliant to the point where the clinician can no longer justify seeing them.[32] Even where termination of the relationship may seem justified to the clinician, however, it is advisable (1) to consult with one or more colleagues to see how they assess the situation, (2) make arrangements for emergency coverage until the patient can find another physician, and (3) wherever possible, help facilitate the identification of a new physician and transfer of patient care. Ideally, the patient should be transferred to a provider who feels comfortable with the patient's preference yet can offer evidence-based guidance, monitoring, and treatment.[33]

REFERRALS AND VICARIOUS LIABILITY

A major concern involves the potential liability exposure for referral to a CAM provider. While there are few judicial opinions setting precedent regarding referrals to CAM therapists, the general rule in conventional care is that there is no liability merely for referring to a specialist. There is no particular reason why this rule should not be applied to any referral, whether for conventional or CAM care.[10]

One of the exceptions to this general rule, however, involves "joint treatment," in which various clinicians collaborate to develop a treatment plan and to monitor and treat the patient. Such coordinated care is a premise of integrative care. It suggests that liabilities may be shared within the integrative care team—for example, between the psychiatrist and the acupuncturist.[7] Ensuring that referred-to providers have competence and a good track record in their area of expertise will help reduce potential liability risk.

Liability risk management

As suggested, a principal strategy to help reduce liability risk involves paying attention to the therapeutic relationship, as bad outcomes compounded by bad feelings can lead to litigation. Good communication with patients, which includes tailoring the communication content and style to the needs of the individual patient, has been shown to enhance the perception of the physician's competence and decrease the risk of malpractice.[34]

Next, good clinical care includes monitoring for potential adverse reactions between conventional and CAM therapies—such as, monitoring for adverse herb-drug interactions, particularly where the patient is ingesting dietary supplements concurrent with medication or surgery. Certainly, the cases have emphasized the importance of conventional diagnosis and monitoring when CAM therapies are recommended or allowed. This is probably the most important means of ensuring that patients do not receive substandard care.[7] Continuing to monitor conventionally, and intervene conventionally when medically necessary, means that the standard of care will have been met, and the possibility of patient injury minimized. For example, the physician and patient may wish to try a CAM therapy for a predefined period of time instead of conventional care (e.g., a combination of herbal products and lifestyle changes) and return to conventional care (e.g., medication) when it becomes necessary.

From a liability perspective, the more acute and severe the condition, the more important it would be to monitor and treat conventionally. Again, the definition of medical malpractice emphasizes failure to follow the standard of care, and patient injury. The greater the disease's severity, the more likely patient injury will result from over relying on a CAM therapy, and thus the greater possibility for a lawsuit with concomitant malpractice liability; as well, the more likely the psychiatrist will be held liable for failure to insist on standard, conventional care. Further, the more curable the condition conventionally, the more likely a court would see failure to provide (or even, perhaps, insist) on such care as negligent.

Another risk reduction measure is the practice of obtaining consultation. Ongoing supervision, as well as occasional "curbside" consultations regarding a specific case should be documented in the patient's record. These serve to establish the standard of care in the community, can provide valuable input into clinical decision-making, and show that the clinician is willing to take extra steps for the benefit of the patient.[35]

Third, poor medical records can suggest negligence to a jury. In general, it is advisable to keep complete and accurate medical records that include documentation of the patient's medical history concerning use of CAM therapies, and of conversations with patients concerning potential inclusion of such therapies. Such thorough documentation can help physicians prove that informed consent requirements were satisfied, and also may help protect against undue disciplinary action by state medical boards concerned with use of CAM therapies.[7] If the physician recommends or allows use of a CAM therapy based on the medical literature, it is a good idea to keep a back-up file of the medical literature supporting the specific medical recommendation. On the other hand, if the physician believes that, based on the medical literature the patient's continued use of one or more CAM therapies is medically inadvisable, and yet the patient insists on using such therapies against medical advice, this event should be documented in the medical record.

Physicians also should familiarize themselves with documentation standards suggested by the Federation of State Medical Board Guidelines, and whether these are applicable in their state or home institution. Finally, there is a legal doctrine known as "assumption of risk"; the doctrine can, under some circumstances, provide a defense to medical malpractice where the patient has chosen a therapeutic course despite the physician's efforts to dissuade and discourage.[10] In some states, if patients continue to use a CAM therapy against the physician's advice, and this is documented in the medical record, there may be a defense to a malpractice action.[10]

Assumption of risk has been allowed as a defense in at least one case involving patient election of a CAM therapy instead of conventional care (i.e., of a nutritional protocol in lieu of conventional oncology care).[10,36] In this case, the court allowed the patient's signing of an appropriate consent form to serve as an "express" assumption of risk and therefore a complete defense to the claim of medical malpractice. In another case, a New York court found that the patient had "impliedly" assumed the risk because she was aware of and voluntarily chose a CAM protocol for cancer care, even without signing the requisite form.[37]

Based on these cases, some attorneys might advise physicians to have the patient sign a waiver, expressly stating that the patient knowingly, voluntarily, and intelligently chose the CAM therapy or regimen—for example, energy healing and a nutritional protocol—instead of the recommended conventional treatment. Courts, however, tend to disfavor waivers of liability in medical malpractice cases, taking the perspective that medical negligence cannot be waived away, and that the physician remains responsible for the patient's treatment.[38] Physicians should, nonetheless, engage in clear conversations with patients concerning options involving CAM therapies, since such an approach and is likely to satisfy informed consent concerns, respect an ideal of shared decision-making, and encourage positive relationships that can help mitigate the prospect of litigation.

FEDERATION OF STATE MEDICAL BOARD GUIDELINES

As noted, the federation has passed model guidelines for: "(1) physicians who use CAM in their practices, and/or (2) those who comanage patients with licensed or otherwise state-regulated CAM providers".[39] These guidelines are not binding, but rather offer a framework for individual state medical boards to regulate physicians integrating CAM therapies. They should be read in conjunction with existing medical board guidelines in the state in which the physician practices, as the guidelines may provide ways for medical boards to think about integrative practices.

In general, the guidelines "allow a wide degree of latitude in physicians' exercise of their professional judgment and do not preclude the use of any methods that are reasonably likely to benefit patients without undue risk".[39] The guidelines also recognize that "patients have a right to seek any kind of care for their health problems," and that "a full and frank discussion of the risks and benefits of all medical practices is in the patient's best interest".[39] To this extent, the guidelines implicitly recognize both shared decision-making and patients' interest in integrative care.

At the same time, in trying to assess whether an integrative care practice is violative and should trigger physician discipline, the guidelines ask whether the therapy selected is

- Effective and safe? (Having adequate scientific evidence of efficacy and/or safety or greater safety than other established treatment models for the same condition)
- Effective, but with some real or potential danger? (Having evidence of efficacy, but also of adverse side effects)
- Inadequately studied, but safe? (Having insufficient evidence of clinical efficacy, but reasonable evidence to suggest relative safety)
- Ineffective and dangerous? (Proven to be ineffective or unsafe through controlled trials or documented evidence or as measured by a risk/benefit assessment)

Some of these standards may be difficult to meet. For example, the first category is stated in terms of the CAM therapy having greater evidence of safety and/or efficacy than the applicable conventional treatment; there may or may not be available evidence to suggest whether this condition is met. Moreover, the guidelines list these four categories but do not offer suggestions for how to utilize the categories in clinical decision-making.

In addition to the above standards, the guidelines provide an extensive checklist of items to which the physician must attend when providing CAM therapies. The psychiatrist practicing integrative care should review these items with legal counsel and determine which are advisable and practical. For example, these items include documentation regarding:[39]

- What medical options have been discussed, offered, or tried, and if so, to what effect, or a statement as to whether or not certain options have been refused by the patient or guardian
- That proper referral has been offered for appropriate treatment; that the risks and benefits of the use of the recommended treatment to the extent known have been appropriately discussed with the patient or guardian
- That the physician has determined the extent to which the treatment could interfere with any other recommended or ongoing treatment

The guidelines also provide that the CAM treatment should

- Have a favorable risk/benefit ratio compared to other treatments for the same condition
- Be based upon a reasonable expectation that it will result in a favorable patient outcome, including preventive practices
- Be based upon the expectation that a greater benefit will be achieved than that which can be expected with no treatment

Again, the guidelines are suggestive but not binding in any given state, unless adopted by that state's medical board.

ETHICAL ANALYSIS

Adams et al. offer seven factors to consider in assessing the ethics of whether or not to offer the patient CAM therapies:[33]

- Severity and acuteness of illness
- Curability with conventional treatment
- Invasiveness, toxicities, and side effects of conventional treatment
- Quality of evidence of safety and efficacy of the CAM treatment
- Degree of understanding of the risks and benefits of conventional and CAM treatments
- Knowing and voluntary acceptance of those risks by the patient
- Persistence of patient's intention to utilize CAM treatment

These factors dovetail with the liability approach described earlier. Thus, if the illness is not severe or acute, and not easily curable with conventional treatment, and/or the conventional treatment is invasive and carries toxicities or side effects that are unacceptable to the patient, then, assuming the CAM therapy is not proven unsafe or ineffective, it may be ethically compelling to try the CAM approach for a limited period of time, while monitoring conventionally.[33] The ethical posture is even further improved if the patient understands the risks and benefits, is willing to assume the risk of trying such an approach, and insists on this route. In this case, a monitored, "wait-and-see" approach respects the patient's autonomy interest, while satisfying the clinician's obligation to do no harm.[33]

Consider, for example, the use of hypnotism in an effort to reduce the need for pain-killers and anesthesia, and to reduce anxiety.[40] Such a therapeutic technique, in conjunction with conventional care, if likely safe and potentially effective, would be ethically compelling, assuming the clinician held a full and fair conversation with the patient about the potential benefits and risks of such an approach.

On the whole, integrative care suggests the need for such conversations.[9] Even though the legal obligation of informed consent *mandates* disclosure of risks and benefits, the premise of integrative care suggests the importance of engaging patients in shared decision-making.[19] Rather than choosing between the three possibilities suggested in the liability analysis above—recommend, tolerate, or reject—clinicians should review all the clinical options with each patients, and, in the scenario of "tolerating" (or accepting) the patient's persistent interest in using CAM therapies, be ready to step in with conventional medical care if, as, and when appropriate, in shared decision-making with the patient.

Notably, the IOM report[19] cited this framework with approval. In broader terms, the report highlighted five ethical values to be held in balance in public policy conversations about integration of CAM therapies: a social commitment to public welfare; a commitment to protect patients and the public from hazardous health practices; a respect for patient autonomy; recognition of medical pluralism; and public accountability.[19] While autonomy, a commitment to protect patients from harm (nonmaleficence), and a commitment to public welfare (beneficence) are more familiar ethical values, the report defined medical pluralism and public accountability, respectively, as follows:

> *Serious consideration of the safety, efficacy and potential integration of CAM therapies into conventional medicine means acknowledgement of multiple valid modes of healing, and a pluralistic foundation for health care....[P]ublic accountability, like medical pluralism, must include some consideration of the vast array of perspectives that constitute the national (and even international) heritage of healing traditions.[19]*

Without disclaiming the importance of considerations of safety and efficacy, the IOM report also placed a new emphasis on the importance of factoring in multiple perspectives about health and human healing.

CONCLUSION

Decision as to how to guide the cardiac care patient deserves serious discussion, and requires consideration of a combination of clinical and legal/ethical judgments. Historically, many characterized CAM therapies as a whole as "unproven" and the matter ended there. But the medical evidence regarding safety and efficacy changes rapidly, and both research and legislative developments reflect a shifting environment in which it becomes increasingly important to track information and communicate responsibly with patients. Most profoundly, the IOM's report on Complementary and Alternative Medicine has given impetus to efforts toward integrative cardiology that apply an evidence-based, patient-centered approach toward realizing the best of conventional and complementary care. One way to state the ideal is to respond to patient interest in CAM therapies in a way that is "clinically responsible, ethically appropriate, and legally defensible".[41] To do so, clinicians who are practicing within in a hospital may have the benefit of guidance from the hospital's legal counsel; and those in free-standing integrative care clinics, from their attorneys. Rather than a black-and-white, yes/no response to a therapy labeled as "CAM," the preferred approach is to investigate the literature and advise the patient accordingly. The clinician can then decide whether to recommend, approve, or avoid and discourage a given CAM therapy. It is also imperative to ask patients, as part of the medical history, what dietary supplements and other CAM therapies they are currently using; to evaluate the extent to which such concurrent regimens may either accelerate or interfere with conventional care; and to advise the patient accordingly.

In guiding the patient, the clinician may wish to bear in mind the ideal of "shared decision making between patient and clinician, in which patient preferences are actively considered and valued," as recently articulated by the IOM report.[21] Shared decision-making suggests that the conversation goes well beyond the legal and ethical requirement of informed consent toward a respectful exchange in which both parties bear the weight of determining the optimal clinical course. Patients who favor CAM therapies despite medical advice to the contrary should not be abandoned, but should be monitored and encouraged to utilize medically necessary, conventional therapies, and full documentation should be made of relevant conversations and decisions in the medical record. As a last resort, if a clinician feels the patient is choosing a therapeutic route that is not clinically supportable, the patient may be referred to another medical specialist who can offer evidence-based care and monitoring in a manner more consistent with the patient's requests. At the same time, it is important to point out specified risks of various CAM therapies as well as what is unknown, including potential adverse reactions with concurrent conventional therapies.

ACKNOWLEDGMENTS

This paper was supported by grants from the Greenwall Foundation, and gifts from the Rudolph Steiner Foundation and the Bernard Osher Foundation.

REFERENCES

1. Cohen MH, Ruggie M. Overcoming legal and social barriers to integrative medicine. Medical Law Intl. 2004;6:339–93.
2. Cohen MH. Negotiating integrative medicine: a framework for provider-patient conversations. Negotiation J. 2004;30(3):409–33.
3. Cohen MH, Ruggie M. Integrating complementary and alternative medical therapies in conventional medical settings: legal quandaries and potential policy models. Cinn L Rev. 2004;72(2):671–729.
4. Cohen MH. Complementary and alternative medicine: legal boundaries and regulatory perspectives. Baltimore (MD): Johns Hopkins University Press; 1998.
5. Cohen MH. Healing at the borderland of medicine and religion: regulating potential abuse of authority by spiritual healers. J Law Relig. 2004;18(2):373–426.
6. Eisenberg DM, Cohen MH, Hrbek A, Grayzel J, van Rompay MI, Cooper RA. Credentialing complementary and alternative medical providers. Ann Intern Med. 2002;137:965–73.
7. Cohen MH, Eisenberg DM. Potential physician malpractice liability associated with complementary/integrative medical therapies. Ann Intern Med. 2002;136:596–603.
8. Schouten R, Cohen MH. Legal issues in integration of complementary therapies into cardiology. In: Frishman WH, Weintraub MI, Micozzi MS, editors. Complementary and integrative therapies for cardiovascular disease. Elsevier. 2004; p. 20–55.
9. Ernst EE, Cohen MH. Informed consent in complementary and alternative medicine. Arch Intern Med. 2001;161(19):2288–92.
10. Cohen MH. Beyond complementary medicine: legal and ethical perspectives on health care and human evolution. Ann Arbor (MI): University of Michigan Press. 2000;47–58.
11. American Medical Association IL. Liability insurance requirements. Available at http://www.ama-assn.org/ama/pub/category/print/4544.html Last accessed 2004, Sept 3.
12. Federation of State Medical Boards. Model guidelines for physician use of complementary and alternative therapies in medical practice. Available at www.fsmb.org Accessed 2004, May 2.
13. Studdert DM, Eisenberg DM, Miller FH, Curto DA, Kaptchuck TJ, Brennan TA, et al. Medical malpractice implications of alternative medicine. JAMA. 1998;280(18): 1620–25.
14. NIH Technology Assessment Statement. Integration of behavioral and relaxation approaches into the treatment of chronic pain and insomnia. Bethesda, National Institutes of Health; 1995. NIH Publication No. PB96113964.
15. Marshall DA, Walizer E, Vernalis MN. Optimal healing environments for chronic cardiovascular disease. J Altern Complement Med. 2004;10 (Suppl 1):S147–55.
16. Tsai SL. Audio-visual relaxation training for anxiety, sleep, and relaxation among Chinese adults with cardiac disease. Res Nurs Health. 2004 Dec;27(6):458–68.
17. Guzzetta CE, Effects of relaxation and music therapy on patients in a coronary care unit with presumptive acute myocardial infarction. Heart Lung. 1989 Nov;18(6): 609–16.
18. Isnard Bagnis C, Deray G, Baumelou A, Le Quintrec M, Vanherweghem JL. Herbs and the kidney. Am J Kidney Dis. 2004 Jul;44(1):1–11.
19. Institute of Medicine (Board on Health Promotion and Disease Prevention). Complementary and alternative medicine in the United States. Washington (WA): National Academies Press, 2005.
20. Ernst E. Cardiovascular adverse effects of herbal medicines: a systematic review of the recent literature. Can J Cardiol. 2003 Jun;19(7):818–27.

21. Aviles JM, Whelan SE, Hernke DA, Williams BA, Kenny KE, O'Fallon WM, et al. Intercessory prayer and cardiovascular disease progression in a coronary care unit population: a randomized controlled trial, Mayo Clin Proc. 2001 Dec;76(12):1192–8.

22. Fugh-Berman A. Herbs and dietary supplements in the prevention and treatment of cardiovascular disease. Prev Cardiol. 2000 Winter;3(1):24–32.

23. Norred CL, Zamudio S, Palmer SK. Use of complementary and alternative medicines by surgical patients. AANA J. 2000 Feb;68(1):13–8.

24. Dumoff A. Medical board prohibitions against physician supplements sales. Altern Complement Ther. 2000;6(4):226–36.

25. Ohio Rev. Code Ann. § 4731.22 (18).

26. Harrison RA, Elton PJ. Is there a role for long-chain omega3 or oil-rich fish in the treatment of atrial fibrillation? Med Hypotheses. 2005;64(1):59–63.

27. Ernst E. Second thoughts about safety of St John's wort. Lancet. 1999;354:2014–16; Fugh-Berman A. Herb-drug interactions. Lancet. 2000;355:134–8.

28. Piscitelli SC, Burstein AH, Chaitt D, Alfaro RM, Falloon J. Indinavir concentrations and St John's wort. Lancet. 2000;355:547–8.

29. Moore v. Baker, 98 F.2d 1129 (11th Cir. 1993).

30. Halpin LS, Speir AM, CapoBianco P, Barnett SD. Guided imagery in cardiac surgery. Outcomes Manag. 2002 Jul-Sep;6(3):132–7.

31. CAM a special challenge for cardiac care. Healthcare Benchmarks Qual Improv. 2003 Nov;10(11):129–30.

32. Fentiman LC, Kaufman G, Merton V, Teitell EF, Zonana H. Current issues in the psychiatrist-patient relationship: outpatient civil commitment, psychiatric abandonment and the duty to continue treatment of potentially dangerous patients—balancing duties to patients and the public. Pace Law Rev. 2000;20(2):231–62.

33. Adams KE, Cohen MH, Jonsen AR, Eisenberg DM. Ethical considerations of complementary and alternative medical therapies in conventional medical settings. Ann Intern Med. 2002;137:660–4.

34. Adamson TE, Tschann JM, Guillon DS, Gullion DS, Oppenberg AA. Physician communication skills and malpractice claims: a complex relationship. West J Med. 1989; 150(3):356–60.

35. Gutheil TG, Simon RI. Abandonment of patients in split treatment. Harv Rev Psychiatry. 2003;11(4):175–9.

36. Schneider v. Revici, 817 Federal Reporter 2d 987 (2d Cir. 1987).

37. Charell v. Gonzales, 660 New York Supplement 2d 665, 668 (S.Ct., N.Y. County, 1997), affirmed and modified to vacate punitive damages award, 673 New York Supplement 2d 685 (App Div., 1st Dept., 1998), reargument denied, appeal denied, 1998 New York Appellate Division LEXIS 10711 (App. Div., 1st Dept., 1998), appeal denied, 706 Northeastern Reporter 2d 1211 (1998).

38. Tunkl v. Regents of the Univ. of Calif., 383 Pacific Reporter 2d 441 (Cal. 1963).

39. Federation of State Medical Boards. Model guidelines for physician use of complementary and alternative therapies in medical practice. Available at www.fsmb.org. Accessed on May 2, 2004).

40. Sanjida O'Connell. It won't hurt you one bit. The Times (London), 2002, Jun 24.

41. Cohen MH. Legal issues in integrative medicine: a guide for clinicians, hospitals, and patients. Gig Harbor, WA: National Acupuncture Foundation; 2005.

C H A P T E R

4

ACADEMIC INTEGRATIVE MEDICAL CENTERS OF EXCELLENCE

John C. Longhurst

Over the last 20 years, there has been a groundswell of interest in complementary and alternative medicine (CAM), which has been more aptly renamed integrative medicine (IM), with increasing recognition that the goal is not to use these therapies as alternatives but rather in a complementary fashion with traditional allopathic medicine to better treat the whole individual. In fact, many of the therapies are now thought to provide approaches to diseases that are not well treated by usual strategies available in western medicine. For example, chronic pain, stress reduction, and weight management are a few of the areas that we do not optimally treat using standard allopathic medical approaches. However, acceptance of these CAM or IM therapies has been much less well received by our academic medical community, including both scientists and physicians, than by the public in general. In response to the differences in public attitude versus clinical and academic acceptance, a number of centers throughout the United States have begun to develop programs in IM that variably focus on education, research, and clinical care. In fact, a consortium of academic medical centers, the Consortium of Academic Health Centers for Integrative Medicine (Table 4-1), has been established to provide a more cohesive approach to these new areas of medicine and health care. This chapter describes the experience at the Susan Samueli Center of Integrative Medicine at the University of California, Irvine (UCI), as one example of an academic IM center.

HISTORY

Most of today's faculty in academic medicine were not exposed during their medical school training to any of the areas that we currently define as CAM or IM. In fact, it is more likely that they were taught that these areas were studied incompletely and represent unproven methods of therapy. This was clearly my

TABLE 4-1

CONSORTIUM OF ACADEMIC HEALTH CENTERS FOR INTEGRATIVE MEDICINE

Center	Education				Research		Clinic/Conference		
	Clinical Training Program	Didactic Courses	Local Comm.	Professional Meetings	Clinical	Basic	CAM	Herbal	Women's Health
University of California, Irvine Susan Samueli Center for Integrative Medicine www.ucihs.uci.edu/com/samueli	–	+	+	+	+	+	+	+	+
Univ of Arizona Program for Integrative Medicine http://www.integrativemedicine.arizona.edu/	+	+	+	+	+	+	+	+	+
UCLA Collaborative Center for Integrative Medicine http://www.mbcrc.med.ucla.edu/	–	+	+	+	+	+	+	+	+
UCSF Osher Center http://www.osher.ucsf.edu/	–	+	+	+	+	+	+	+	+
Columbia University Rosenthal Center http://www.rosenthal.hs. columbia.edu/ Sister center in Shanghai, China	–	–	+	+	+	+	+	+	+
Univ of Connecticut http://www.uchc.edu/	–	–	+	–	–	–	+	–	+

Duke University Duke Center for Integrative Medicine http://dukehealth1.org/health-services/integrative–medicine.asp	–	+	+	+	+	+	+	–	+
Albert Einstein COM Continuum Center for Health and Healing http://www.healthandhealingny.org/	–	–	+	+	+	+	–	+	+
George Washington University Center for Integrative Medicine www.integrativemedicinedc.com	–	–	+	+	+	+	–	+	+
Georgetown University Kaplan Clinic www.georgetown.edu/schmed/cam	–	+	–	–	–	–	–	–	–
Harvard Medical School Osher Institute www.osher.hms.harvard.edu http://www.osher.hms.harvard.edu/pe_partners.asp (partnership)	–	+	+	+	–	+	+	Clinical research	–
Oregon Health and Science University Women's Primary Care and Integrative Medicine, Center for Women's Health www.ohsu.edu/orcamind	–	+	–	+	+	+	+	–	+
Thomas Jefferson University Center for Integrative Medicine www.jeffersonhospital.org/cim	–	+	+	+	+	+	+	–	–

(Continued)

TABLE 4-1

CONSORTIUM OF ACADEMIC HEALTH CENTERS FOR INTEGRATIVE MEDICINE (*CONTINUED*)

Center	Education				Research		Clinic/Conference		
	Clinical Training Program	Didactic Courses	Local Comm.	Professional Meetings	Clinical	Basic	CAM	Herbal	Women's Health
University of Hawaii at Manoa Program in Integrative Medicine www.uhm.hawaii.edu	–	–	–	–	+	+	–	–	–
University of Maryland Center for Integrative Medicine www.compmed.umm.edu	–	+	–	+	+	+	+	+	+
University of Massachusetts Center for Mindfulness http://www.sscim.uci.edu/index.asp	–	+	+	+	+	–	+	–	–
University of Michigan Michigan Integrative Medicine www.med.umich.edu/mim	–	–	+	+	+	+	+	–	+
University of Minnesota Center for Spirituality and Healing www.csh.umn.edu	–	+	+	+	+	+	+	–	–
University of Medicine and Dentistry of New Jersey Institute for Complementary & Alternative Medicine www.umdnj.edu/icam	–	–	+	+	+	+	+	–	–

Institution										
University of New Mexico — Health Science Center — hsc.umm.edu/medicine/Integrative_med	–	+	+	–	+	+	–	+	+	–
University of Pennsylvania — Office of Complementary Therapies — www.med.upenn.edu/penncam	–	+	–	+	+	+	+	–	+	+
University of Pittsburgh — Center for Complementary Medicine — integrativemedicine.upmc.com	–	–	–	+	?	+	+	–	+	–
University of Texas Medical Branch — UTMB Integrative Health Care — cam.utmb.edu	–	+	+	+	?	+	+	+	+	+
University of Washington — Department of Family Medicine — www.fammed.washington.edu/predoctoral/cam	–	+	–	+	?	+	+	–	+	–
Wake Forest University — Holistic and Integrative Medicine — www1.wfubmc.edu/phim/	–	+	+	+	+	+	+	+	–	–

Question marks indicate inconclusive information.

understanding when I first traveled to China in 1992. At that time and during subsequent trips I was asked to participate in acupuncture research, a proposition that I rejected until it became apparent that worthwhile research was being conducted and published in high-quality journals. Subsequent events led to joint collaboration with a respected Chinese scholar that resulted in publications in journals such as *Circulation*, *American Journal of Physiology*, *Autonomic Neuroscience: Basic and Clinical*, and *Journal of Applied Physiology and Brain Research*. Once it became clear that it was possible to define mechanisms of action for acupuncture that could be described in modern western scientific concepts, my orientation and belief began to change. In fact, when I had the opportunity to join the UCI, where a number of other faculty were beginning to study various areas in IM, I began to see possibilities for extension of my early CAM research and to develop an educational approach.

In 1999, the College of Medicine at UCI received a gift from Henry and Susan Samueli that allowed creation of the Samueli Center for Integrative Medicine. Susan Samueli had practiced homeopathy and was very interested in working with an academic center to increase knowledge and to provide education in the general area of IM. The original purpose was to create an informal center at the university that was devoted to research, education, and analysis. Three years later, a clinical component was added. This experience is typical of a number of IM academic centers in the United States and Canada (Table 4-1), which were started as a result of a benefactor interested in promoting health and unconventional areas of medicine. Other centers developed as a result of interested faculty who have been funded to conduct research and have reached out to establish collaborations with other like-minded individuals. Although university administration rarely has decided de novo to start an IM program, there is increasing recognition of the public's desire to see these programs develop and flourish.

VISIONS OF CENTERS OF EXCELLENCE

As western medicine in general and academic centers specifically have begun to engage the broad discipline of IM, several issues have emerged that clearly need to be addressed. The first is that the older generation of scientists and physicians have not been exposed to these areas in their formal curriculum and hence they have little understanding or appreciation for their significance. Furthermore, as these individuals begin to review the literature and see what is offered by the CAM community itself, there is a widespread view that research and practice of many, if not all, CAM modalities have been approached much less rigorously than the accepted standards for western medical therapies. For example, western medicine has embraced the concept of rigorous prospective, blinded, randomized, placebo-controlled clinical trials, while many areas of CAM in the community are practiced without a foundation of information supporting efficacy and awareness of potential toxicity. This lack of information has led to substantial skepticism among many allopathic physicians and scientists. The other side of this issue is the much wider acceptance of CAM by the public for a variety of reasons. IM provides a low-cost, low-tech alternative, although those of us in western medicine would like to think not of alternatives but of complementary therapies that provide added value. Also, the perception by the public is that many of these therapies have no downside, that is, IM is not associated with side effects or toxicity. While it is true that the incidence of complications in IM is low, all CAM therapies carry with them either documented or a real potential for side effects, even if it is a diversion from accepted standard medical practice that has been well documented to be efficacious.

Second, there is a problem with communication. The description of many aspects of unconventional medicine uses a vocabulary and sometimes a whole language that is quite foreign to that normally used in western medical practice. Furthermore, there are concepts in IM that have no analogy to modern biology, including anatomy, physiology, pharmacology, biochemistry, and molecular biology, which students, practitioners, and educators in medicine and science hold as the fundamental principles underlying our understanding and practice of modern medicine. The problem with communication goes even deeper. Because there is the feeling that most aspects of CAM therapy are not evidence-based, physicians provide either subliminal or liminal messages to their patients that limit conversation about CAM practice (Eisenberg, Kessler, et al. 1993 1551 /id). As a result, patients don't tell their physician what integrative medical therapies they are using and physicians don't ask.

Third, the practice of many CAM therapies rests on anecdotal evidence, which is not construed as either acceptable or sufficient by the western medical community. Yet, this is precisely how many of these unconventional therapies are used by CAM practitioners and this is how the public develops their collective opinion of benefit.

Fourth, until recently, academic centers in the United States have not had the infrastructure that would allow careful assessment and application of these many areas of CAM. In fact, until just a few years ago, there were very few faculty who were sufficiently interested or knowledgeable to move the field forward. Resources that are always scarce were simply not directed at this emerging field. It was and remains today a low priority for most deans and hospital directors. However, due to the public's and more recently legislative interest this trend has begun to reverse, significantly because of the creation by congress of the Office of Alternative Medicine that has evolved into the National Center for Complementary and Alternative Medicine (NCCAM). Although this branch of the National Institutes of Health has undergone growing pains and continues to be constrained by its budget, it does provide funding specifically directed to many unconventional areas of medicine that traditionally have not been well supported by the older established institutes. Funding of research and clinical trials by NCCAM has raised the level of consciousness and interest in this area, although there continues to be substantial scrutiny by western scientists and clinicians about the types of projects that are supported. Such governmental support adds to philanthropic support from interested individuals such as the Samueli family and together they have begun to provide for the infrastructure that provides education, fosters research, and rigorously assesses clinical care and practice in CAM.

EDUCATION

The Samueli Center at UCI provides education at many levels to its constituency. These include programs for students, faculty, staff, and clinical housestaff. Like many academic medicine centers, lectures on various topics in IM have been incorporated into the regular curriculum for first- and second-year medial students. These include, for example, a broad overview of CAM, acupuncture, herbals, and mind-body modalities. In addition, elective courses are provided in selected areas such as mediation and qi gong as well as clinical rotations in our integrative medical clinic. A number of grand rounds on special topics in CAM are given in clinical departments. A special interest group in CAM has been formed by the students and they host a yearly symposium usually on a selected topic of interest in IM. Combined with the monthly seminar series sponsored by the Samueli Center that is open to students, faculty, practitioners, and the public as well as research rotations, these educational offerings provide a framework of material that supplement the standard curriculum in allopathic medicine. This program is funded by a grant from the American Medical Student Association, which surveys faculty and student attitudes and understanding of CAM each year.

Although not currently part of the Samueli Center, a few members of the Consortium of Academic Health Centers for Integrative Medicine provide residency and fellowship training programs in IM. For example, the University of Arizona provides a 2-year program for allopathic and osteopathic physicians that includes clinical and research components in their associate fellowship program. The program incorporates courses on philosophical foundations, lifestyle practice, therapeutic systems as well as personal development (clinical integration and research). There is neither board requirement nor recognition by the American Board of Medical Specialties, which is the umbrella organization that incorporates all boards responsible for establishing educational standards, evaluating candidates' knowledge, and awarding certification in western medicine.

Equally important are programs offered to professionals, including physicians and other practicing professions, in both standard allied health specialties and in the CAM community. Because many physicians know little about IM and because programs in many training schools and programs that offer course work leading to licensure do not teach these modalities from a twenty-first century perspective of modern biology and medicine, there is a need for such education. Furthermore, there is a strong need to bring CAM practitioners into the proximity of western physicians to encourage communication around common areas of interest such as management of stress, chronic pain, and the many difficult-to-treat diseases that cross disciplines in medicine like fibromyalgia or chronic fatigue syndrome. The conversations between attendees that take place at these meetings provide an introduction between both groups of health-care workers, western clinicians, and IM practitioners, and encourage development of a better understanding of therapeutic strategies, referrals, and eventually more communication and understanding of their respective disciplines.

Education also occurs at our scientific conferences, including local, national, and international meetings. The Samueli Center has hosted an international conference every 12–18 months for the last several years on a variety of topics, but most commonly in the field of acupuncture and Traditional Chinese Medicine (TCM). These conferences provide a platform for information exchange that not only assists in raising the quality of the science, but also provides local faculty and students with an opportunity to hear about the latest advances in research and to put this new knowledge into a framework that can be compared with other "classical" areas of science and medicine. Not only are collaborations fostered, but such meetings can form the basis of agreement about underserved areas of IM research and areas of consensus. Because there is a tendency by western scientists and physicians to ignore or neglect much of the foreign literature from non-European countries because it is not in English, not available on PubMed, or perceived to be low quality, it is important to bring international scientists together to critically evaluate progress in CAM research. Optimally, these meetings provide introductions, identify high- and low-quality research, train students and faculty, and foster new research directions that should be pursued.

The lay community clearly is very interested in learning more about the latest advances in IM research. Much communication about IM practices occurs anecdotally by word of mouth, from one friend to another. Otherwise, the public knows only what it reads, hears on the radio, sees on television, or learns from their practitioners. Printed and visual media, particularly the advertisements, are filled with hyperbole and clinicians may be variably trained and therefore unknowledgeable about the many CAM practices available to and accessed by their patients. All too often, there are deceptive marketing practices that promise much more than can be delivered. The Samueli Center has addressed this problem in two ways. First, they host a regular monthly colloquium or seminar series on a variety of integrative medial topics that would be of interest to the lay public, students, and clinicians alike. Second, the center hosts yearly conferences typically aimed at one or more specific segments of our community, for example, a Women's Wellness Conference, as well as special seminars on IM topics of interest to the lay community. The Women's Wellness Conference, for example, has grown from 110 to over 300 participants who come to hear a 1-day series of lectures, tutorials, and workshops on topics ranging from acupuncture to herbals and nutrition, to mind-body. There is a need for the public to hear about the advances in research and to put the areas of IM into perspective so that they can make more informed choices in their selection of these CAM therapies for their health care.

Education from centers of excellence, such as the Samueli Center not only educates our students, faculty, and staff, but provides an ideal model for academic institutions in the United States to reach out to colleagues abroad to educate them on the principles of evidence-based medicine, including fundamental concepts such as hypothesis testing, adequate controls, power analysis, and blinding. Likewise, integrative medical centers in the U.S. academic community have a unique opportunity to better educate CAM practitioners in the United States, including those trained abroad, so that they can place their CAM practice into a framework that can be understood by all, incorporating not just ancient methods and theory but also an enlightened perspective brought about by new knowledge and techniques gain in western science and medicine. This enlightened understanding will assist, not only in the acceptance of these holistic practices by academic and clinical communities in the United States but also will encourage communication and appropriate referrals.

RESEARCH

Like many other academic medical centers (Table 4-1), the Samueli Center at UCI has developed a broad range of research programs, as well as a clear focus. TCM, including acupuncture, and to a lesser extent, herbal medicine, is the major focus with a thrust toward definition of mechanisms. In fact, understanding IM from a fundamental perspective is the major focus of research on this campus. For example, the neurobiology of acupuncture's mechanism of action with respect to regulation of cardiovascular performance is funded by several NIH grants. The approaches used in these studies incorporate experimental models that can be studied with respect to responses in the intact organism, processing of information by organ systems such as the brain, peripheral nervous and cardiovascular systems as well as human and clinical studies that are more translational in nature.

A number of laboratories located in departments spread throughout the medical school and the general campus at UCI address research in other areas of IM, including mediation and healing touch; counter irritation; garlic and other botanicals, including fundamental neurobiology of stress; herbal influence on cellular energetics, cancer, longevity, and immune function; exercise in aging and Alzheimer's disease; neural-cardiovascular mechanisms of qi gong; yoga; IM epidemiology and in health-care policy; and psychoneuroimmunology, among others. In addition, clinical protocols in the IM clinic (see below) prospectively assess herb efficacy, herb–drug interactions, and other herbal toxicities.

Each of the research programs occurs under the guidance of one or more faculty members who conduct IM research as part of a larger program of research sponsored by the NIH, NCCAM, foundations or private funding that typically is oriented mainly toward western medicine and biology. Rarely is CAM research the sole area of investigation. The research programs train pre- and postdoctoral students, including undergraduate students, medical students, and occasionally allopathic and CAM practitioners. Hence there is a good opportunity for information transfer as well as for critique of research protocols from multiple perspectives. Of particular issue, however, is the large discrepancy in approach to the patient as well as research standards between most CAM therapists and western physicians and scientists. Thus, it is important to calibrate protocols so that they are performed not only with the exacting standards applied to research in academic medicine in the United States, but also account for variations in approach to the patient, including systems of evaluation and diagnosis and the range of therapeutic options used in CAM. Standardization of individual protocols is particularly important. Without a collaborative approach, resulting outcomes may not be applicable to the IM discipline as it is practiced clinically. For example, an upper respiratory viral infection or the common cold typically is classified as a single disease in western medicine, although it is recognized that multiple viruses may cause this problem. In contrast, TCM may classify a cold be as wind heat or wind cold depending upon the pattern diagnosis, the two of which are treated quite differently. A careful categorization of patients allows a more accurate assessment of different therapeutic strategies applied in these CAM practices. Cooperative research programs between the CAM and allopathic communities needs to become a high priority.

CLINICAL CARE

The third arm of most academic IM centers of excellence is clinical care. In some centers, this can be the predominate component with little in the way of research or education. An important aspect of clinical care is the added value IM clinics provide for the overall center's program in both education and research. Not only do they serve a clinical need for the community, especially students, staff, and faculty of the academic institution and not only do such clinics attract individuals from the surrounding community who desire this form of therapy, but they also educate students and faculty about the incorporated CAM practices and provide an excellent opportunity for clinical research.

The Samueli Center began its clinic approximately 2 years ago in the Gottschalk Plaza next to the school of medicine on the UCI campus, which is located approximately 12 miles from the university hospital. This small clinic is part of a multispecialty group practice specifically located in the family practice section of the building. It was formed after discussions with our sister campuses at UCLA and UCSF, which had active IM clinics. It was established as a fee-for-service TCM clinic offering acupuncture, with the idea of incorporating herbals as soon as practical. Although it has successfully incorporated both education and research into its structure, it has experienced growing pains that are typical of these types of clinics in academic medical centers.

Space for the clinic has been inadequate both in terms of availability and the type of space. As part of a clinic that serves multiple needs (mostly in allopathic medicine), the environment is not conducive to comfort or a relaxed atmosphere. Those institutions that enjoy stand-alone IM clinics or wellness centers have the opportunity to develop an atmosphere that patients and practitioners expect.

Referrals are the lifeblood for any clinic's success, yet our clinic initially received few internal referrals. Most patients were attracted by word-of-mouth and through talks and discussions at health fairs and conferences. The volume of internal referrals has increased slowly as staff physicians gradually begin to appreciate the areas of health care that TCM benefits. A related problem is the absence of promotion of our clinic by the UCI heath system. The hospital is focused on high revenue-producing specialties such as surgery and technical procedures rather than nontraditional specialties like CAM that provide less revenue. As such, marketing for the clinic has depended fully on print and media advertisements developed by the center.

Most CAM modalities are not well covered by insurance. Eisenberg's early study (Eisenberg, Kessler, et al. 1993 1551 /id) indicated that most patients are willing to pay out-of-pocket for these unconventional therapies. Advice from our sister schools indicated that it would not be cost effective for us to bill insurance. Therefore, our clinic began as a fee-for-service program. This has allowed the clinic to remain financially solvent. We provide a superbill for patients that they can present to their insurance providers to regain their expenses. We presently are reconsidering the issue of insurance mainly to be able to offer our services to patients who cannot afford the out-of-pocket expense. Our decision, however, will be purely financial since we need to remain not only financially viable but actually fund other programs from clinical revenue.

An important issue in development of an IM clinic is how large it should be and how many services should be offered. On the advice of our sister campuses, we began small and have remained so today. We are presently considering expansion in a few other areas including manipulative medicine (massage) and naturopathy. We have selected these areas for expansion for two reasons. First, they have been shown in other IM clinics to be cost effective and revenue producing. Second, in academic medicine we constantly try to maintain a balance between allopathic and CAM philosophies. Since most western medical practices do not treat chronic conditions well, including for example, weight or stress management, there is a rationale for introducing those disciplines that supplement western medical practices in managing weight loss and reducing stress. Obesity is the cause of many forms of cardiovascular, pulmonary, and endocrine diseases. Stress is universally a component, sometimes a major component, of almost all diseases, but plays a particularly important role in chronic disease, heart disease and cancer. Stress in these disorders contributes to poor outcomes, including excess morbidity and mortality. Massage works very well in reducing stress, while naturopathy with its strong foundation in nutrition is well positioned to assist with weight control. Thus, initial acceptance of massage and naturopathy, like acupuncture, will be potentially higher than other areas of IM in an academic medical center such as ours.

We proposed to provide herbals when we first introduced acupuncture and TCM as our initial CAM modality. Herbals are important because they are within the scope of practice of acupuncture as defined by the state board in California and are a major component of acupuncturist's therapy, occurring in about two-thirds of all treatment regimens. Furthermore, they are a major source of income production for most acupuncturists and hence we would like to help finance the clinic through herbal sales. Finally, we wanted to study herbals, to learn more about these complex substances, as they are used in our IM clinic in treatment of patients. Since our current clinic is a hospital-based clinic (site of service 22), it comes under the jurisdiction of the hospital and must meet all of its standards, including those imposed by the Joint Commission of Hospital Accreditation (JACO). The joint commission has indicated that in the near future it will require oversight of herbals in a manner similar to that provided for western drugs. Therefore, we have applied for and received approval for providing herbals by the Pharmacy and Therapeutics Committee of the hospital. However, we agreed to provide herbals under a human subjects research protocol and to use companies that had been certified by independent third party review. Herbals are not regulated by the Food and Drug Administration but rather fall under the Office of Dietary Supplements. Currently, the FDA is considering upgrading the standards of manufacturing to require a good manufacturing process for all dietary supplements, including herbals. At present, we have not been able to find companies that meet all requirements of the Pharmacy and Therapeutics Committee and have not yet begun to provide herbals. However, if we locate our clinic outside the Gottschalk Plaza, it will fall outside the scope of hospital jurisdiction (site of service 11) and we will have the opportunity to sell and provide herbals like any independent practitioner. Providing herbs as part of an IM clinic that falls under the jurisdiction of an academic medical center hospital clearly is a complex matter that has yet to be resolved. If we do sell herbs we need to do in a conscientious manner keeping risks to a minimum, avoiding herbals like ma huang and St. John's Wort that have been shown to cause side effects or interact with drugs or to be contaminated. This is an ongoing issue, yet to be resolved, that we will continue to address in a very careful manner.

SUMMARY

Academic medical centers serve an important role in the evaluation and the eventual acceptance of those areas of IM that are found to have a beneficial effect in disease over and above placebo. The process of acceptance will be through several mechanisms. First, will be rigorous research programs to define mechanisms of action of the CAM modalities. Second, will be adequately powered prospective randomized and blinded clinical trials that are properly constructed to fairly evaluate the IM practices from the perspective of both the modality itself and modern clinical trial theory and practice. Translational research should be a collaborative effort between the IM community, including schools, students in training, CAM practitioners, and allopathic medical and science communities. Third, the academic centers of excellence will educate students, faculty, and CAM practitioners on the outcomes of the basic and clinical studies. In both communities, it will be necessary to take fresh perspectives and to not hold onto preconceived notions that cannot be proven using rigorous scientific methods to create a basis of evidence that can be prospectively applied and verified. This approach will be difficult for both organizations, but the public deserves to know what works, what doesn't, what is placebo, what is unproven dogma and hyperbole, and what is dangerous. Thus, academic programs of excellence like the Samueli Center for Integrative Medicine are well positioned to not only develop the evidence for causality and efficacy, but they can help move the largely undocumented area of unconventional medicine to a level of understanding and acceptance that currently does not exist. Twenty years from now, we should be able to reflect on the gradually diminishing area of IM that has become a commonly accepted and therefore a natural part of medical curricula and practice.

CHAPTER

5

APPROACHES TO CLINICAL TRIALS OF COMPLEMENTARY AND ALTERNATIVE MEDICINE

Richard L. Nahin, Josh Berman,
Catherine M. Stoney and Shan S. Wong

INTRODUCTION

Despite many advances in conventional cardiovascular therapies in the past 30 years, cardiovascular disease (CVD) and its sequelae, including heart disease and stroke, are still leading causes of mortality and morbidity in the United States. Because medical and surgical therapies for CVD are often invasive, are perceived by many patients to lead to substantial side effects, and may offer only limited efficacy for many individuals, patients often seek complementary and alternative medicine (CAM) treatments to either complement or replace conventional medical approaches. The types of CAM therapies sought and used for CVD encompass a wide range of strategies, including acupuncture and other components of traditional, indigenous systems of medicine, mind-body interventions (meditation, guided imagery), herbal treatments, high-dose vitamins and other types of dietary supplements, and various types of "energy" healing (e.g., Reiki, Qi Gong).

Demographic data on the use of CAM for treating CVD are limited but growing. A randomized household telephone survey conducted in 1997 revealed that 9% of individuals over age 65 years use CAM to treat their heart disease, but the survey did not indicate which particular therapies were used.[1] The survey also found that, among those sampled who had elevated blood pressure, about 12% used a CAM therapy. Dietary supplements (e.g., coenzyme Q10, the botanical product hawthorn, and vitamin E) and relaxation techniques were the most frequent types of therapies used to treat high blood pressure.[2] A recent Centers for Disease Control and Prevention (CDC) national survey, the National Health Interview Survey (NHIS), which annually draws information from more than

100,000 randomly selected individuals, included questions on CAM use.[3] The NHIS revealed that many adults use CAM to manage risk factors associated with CVD—for instance, 1.9 million adults used CAM to help them manage weight problems, 1 million used CAM to treat high cholesterol, and 890,000 adults used CAM to treat their hypertension. Furthermore, CAM is also used to treat existing heart disease, with 214,000 using CAM for their irregular heartbeat, 165,000 for coronary heart disease (CHD), 107,000 for angina, and 59,000 for congestive heart failure. Finally, CAM is also employed to manage peripheral vascular disease, with 400,000 individuals using CAM for intermittent claudication.

Because of this substantial public use, the National Institutes of Health (NIH) supports about 50 cardiovascular research projects involving some form of CAM. The National Center for Complementary and Alternative Medicine (NCCAM) supports 30 of these projects, which are listed in Table 5-1. More than 75% of these projects are clinical studies. Since 1997, there have been 15 systematic reviews and meta-analyses of 12 types of CAM interventions for CVD performed by either the Cochrane Collaboration* or the Agency for Healthcare Research and Quality (AHRQ) Evidence-Based Practice Centers (EPCs)[†] (Table 5-2). All but one of these reviews examined the use of biologically based CAM therapies such as omega-3 fatty acids, garlic, herbal medicine, or chelation therapy. Of these reviews, 3 concluded that a given CAM therapy worked to improve an intermediate marker or prevent a clinical event; 3 concluded that a given therapy did not work; but 12 judged that the existing evidence was insufficient to say whether a given therapy worked or not.[‡] In all cases, those reviews not able to reach a conclusion on efficacy and safety noted the low quality of the clinical trials reviewed. Among the methodological weaknesses noted in these clinical trials were small sample sizes, with resulting low statistical power; inadequate randomization; poor choice of control groups (e.g., placebos that did not account for the strong smell of fish oil or garlic); poor blinding; and inadequate description and/or justification of the product used or of the treatment parameters (e.g., dose, schedule). It is NCCAM's goal in its clinical trial program to address these and other methodological issues that have plagued earlier clinical trials of CAM interventions.

---

*The Cochrane Collaboration is an international nonprofit and independent organization that produces and disseminates systematic reviews of health-care interventions, chiefly through its publication *The Cochrane Database of Systematic Reviews.*

[†]About 13 EPCs are currently supported by AHRQ to develop evidence reports and technology assessments on topics relevant to clinical, social science/behavioral, economic, and other health-care organization and delivery issues. Topics are nominated by both federal partners, such as NIH or the Center for Medicare and Medicaid Services, and nonfederal partners such as professional societies, health plans, insurers, employers, and patient groups.

[‡]Since each review might make multiple conclusions based on different outcome measures, the total number of conclusions is greater than 15.

TABLE 5-1

CARDIOVASCULAR RELATED RESEARCH PROJECTS SUPPORTED BY NCCAM IN FISCAL YEAR 2005

Grant Mechanism	Project Title	Principal Investigator/Institute
U01	Trial to Assess Chelation Therapy	Gervasio A. Lamas, Mount Sinai Medical Center, Miami Beach, FL
U01	Ginkgo Biloba Prevention Trial in Older Individuals	Steven DeKosky, Rush-Presbyterian-St. Lukes Medical Center, Chicago, IL
U01	Phytoestrogens and Progression of Atherosclerosis	Howard Hodis, University of Southern California, Los Angeles, CA
P50	Center for CAM Research in Aging	Fredi Kronenberg, Columbia University College of Physicians and Surgeons, New York, NY
P50	Alexander Center for CAM, Minority Aging and CVD	Robert Schneider, Maharishi University of Management, Fairfield, IA
P50	Botanical Center for Age-Related Diseases	Connie Weaver, Purdue University, West Lafayette, IN
P01	CER on CAM Antioxidant Therapies (CERCAT)	Balz Frei, Oregon State University, Covallis, OR
R01	Tai Chi Mind-Body Therapy for Chronic Heart Failure	Russell Phillips, Beth Israel Deaconess Medicine Center, Boston, MA
R01	Comparing Effects of Three Sources of Garlic on Serum Lipids	Christopher Gardner, Stanford University School of Medicine, Palo Alto, CA
R01	The Safety and Efficacy of Low- and High-Carbohydrate Diet	Gary D. Foster, University of Pennsylvania, Philadelphia, PA
R01	High-Dose Alpha Tocopherol on Carotid Atherosclerosis	Ishwarlal Jialal, University of Texas Southwestern Medical Center, Dallas, TX
R01	Effects of Meditation on Mechanism of CHD	C. Noel Bairey Merz, Cedars-Sinai Medical Center, Los Angeles, CA

(Continued)

TABLE 5-1

CARDIOVASCULAR RELATED RESEARCH PROJECTS SUPPORTED BY NCCAM IN FISCAL YEAR 2005 (CONTINUED)

Grant Mechanism	Project Title	Principal Investigator/Institute
R21	Flax: Safety & Efficacy in Reducing Cardiovascular Risk	Phillippe Szapary, University of Pennsylvania, Philadelphia, PA
R21	Cardiovascular Effects of Iyengar Yoga	Phillippe Szapary, University of Pennsylvania, Philadelphia, PA
R21	Mechanisms of Hawthorn Action in Heart Failure	Barry Bleske, College of Pharmacy, University of Michigan, MI
R21	Effects of Energy Healers on Atherosclerosis	Joan E. Fox, Cleveland Clinic Foundation, Cleveland, OH
R21	Grape Seed Extract— Cardiac Impact and Drug Interaction	Steven Bolling, University of Michigan, Ann Arbor, MI
R21	Evaluation of Antioxidant Supply in Focal CNS Ischemia	Wayne Clark, Oregon Health Science University, Portland, OR
R21	Carioprotective Effects of American Ginseng	Chun-Su Yuan, University of Chicago, Chicago, IL
R21	Efficacy of Healing Touch in Stressed Neonates	Sharon McDonough-Means, University of Arizona, Tucson, AZ
R21	Exploring the Effect of Meditation on Hypertension	Sarah Reiff-Hekking, University of Massachusetts, Worcester, MA
R21	Flavonoids in the Amelioration of Hypertriglyceridemia	Andre Theriault, University of Hawaii at Manoa, Honolulu, HI
R21	Use of Herbs and Dietary Supplements in Four Ethnicities	Anette Fitzpatrick, University of Washington, Seattle, WA
R21	Do High- Dose B-Vitamins Delay Age-Related Decay	Bruce Ames, Children's Hospital Oakland Research Institute, Oakland, CA

TABLE 5-1

CARDIOVASCULAR RELATED RESEARCH PROJECTS SUPPORTED BY NCCAM IN FISCAL YEAR 2005 (CONTINUED)

Grant Mechanism	Project Title	Principal Investigator/Institute
R21	Relevance of Herbal Products in Transplantation	Dilip Kittur, Suny Upstate Medical University, NY
R03	Race and Herbal Medications Among Medicare Recipients	William Lafferty, University of Washington, Seattle, WA
R25	Integrative Curriculum for Medicine and Allied Health	Sara Warber, University of Michigan, Ann Arbor, MI
K23	Ayurvedic Herbals: Effects on Lipids & Atherosclerosis	Phillippe Szapary, University of Pennsylvania, Philadelphia, PA
K24	Clinical Studies in Nutrition and Metabolism	Ishwarlal Jialal, University of California, Davis, TX
K24	Midcareer Investigator Award—Patient-Oriented Research	Iris Bell, University of Arizona, Tucson, AZ

NCCAM uses the same approach to clinical evaluation of CAM interventions as used for approved conventional drugs and devices. In particular, fundamental data regarding safety and efficacy are obtained so that health-care providers and consumers will have confidence in the information and ultimately be able to make informed decisions regarding CAM use. The remainder of the chapter will discuss design issues facing clinical trials of CAM interventions, especially for CVD and review some of NCCAM's CVD-related clinical trials.

NCCAM CLINICAL TRIAL METHODOLOGY AND PROTOCOLS

Clinical considerations for all CAM interventions

Many of the disorders for which CAM modalities are prescribed have variable natural histories and are highly subjective, such as chronic pain syndromes, depression, and anxiety.[3] These features make study of these disorders relatively difficult. Consequently, particular attention should be paid to several essential

TABLE 5-2

AHRQ-EPC OR COCHRANE COLLABORATION SYSTEMATIC REVIEWS OF CAM FOR CARDIOVASCULAR DISEASE THROUGH JUNE 2005

Intervention	Disease or Condition	Outcome of Interest	Author's Conclusion	Reference
Acupuncture	Stable angina	Angina Myocardial infarction	Inconclusive	AHRQ #10[4]
Artichoke leaf extract	Hypercholesterolemia	Cholesterol levels	Inconclusive	Pittler et al., 2002[5]
Calcium supplements	Pregnancy	Blood pressure	Effective	Atallah et al., 2002[6]
Chelation therapy	Peripheral vascular disease	ABPI, walking distance, or pain-free walking distance	Inconclusive	Villarruz et al., 2002[7]
CoQ 10	Cardiovascular disease	Total mortality Cardiovascular mortality Myocardial infarction Blood lipid levels	Inconclusive	AHRQ # 83[4]
Garlic	Cardiovascular disease	Triglyceride levels Cholesterol levels Blood pressure Pain-free walking distance	Inconclusive	AHRQ #20[4]
Garlic	Arterial occlusive disease	Pain-free walking distance Blood pressure Heart rate Ankle and brachial pressures	Inconclusive	Jepson et al., 1997[8]

Intervention	Condition	Outcome	Result	Reference
Herbal medicine	Stable angina	Angina Myocardial infarction	Inconclusive	AHRQ #10[4]
Herbal medicine (multiple)	Viral myocarditis	Arrhythmia Cardiac function Creatine phosphokinase	Inconclusive	Liu et al., 2004[9]
Herbal medicine (Dan Shen)	Acute ischaemic stroke	Neurological deficit	Inconclusive	Wu et al., 2005[10]
Horse chestnut seed extract	Chronic venous insufficiency	Leg pain Edema Pruritus Leg volume	Inconclusive	Pittler and Ernst, 2004[11]
Omega-3 fatty acid supplements	Cardiovascular disease	Total mortality All-fatal and nonfatal cardiovascular events	Effective Effective	AHRQ # 94[4]
Omega-3 fatty acid supplements	Cardiovascular disease	Triglyceride levels Cholesterol levels Blood Pressure	Effective Ineffective Ineffective	AHRQ #93[4]
Omega-3 fatty acid supplements	All cardiovascular disease	Total mortality; numbers of cardiovascular events	Inconclusive	Hooper et al., 2004[12]
Omega-3 fatty acid supplements	Intermittent claudication	Triglyceride levels Cholesterol levels Pain–free walking distance Ankle brachial pressure index	Effective Ineffective Ineffective Ineffective	Sommerfield and Hiatt, 2003[13]

(Continued)

AHRQ–EPC OR COCHRANE COLLABORATION SYSTEMATIC REVIEWS OF CAM FOR CARDIOVASCULAR DISEASE THROUGH JUNE 2005 (CONTINUED)

Intervention	Disease or Condition	Outcome of Interest	Author's Conclusion	Reference
Vitamin C	Cardiovascular disease	Total mortality Cardiovascular mortality Myocardial infarction Blood lipid levels	Ineffective	AHRQ # 83[4]
Vitamin E	Cardiovascular disease	Total mortality Cardiovascular mortality Myocardial infarction Blood lipid levels	Ineffective	AHRQ # 83[4]
Vitamin E	Intermittent claudication	Various measures of pain-free walking and standing	Inconclusive	Kleijnen and Mackerras, 1997[14]

features of study design: dose, choice of control groups, entry criteria and outcome variables, randomization, and adherence.

DOSE AND DOSAGE

A first step in the evaluation of any CAM intervention is to determine how much to give (dose), and how often and how long to give it (dosage). This is a critical step since an underdosed intervention, or an intervention given too infrequently, or for too short a time may be inappropriately judged as ineffective, while an intervention given in too high a dose may be mistaken as too toxic (biological agents), too physically painful (manipulative and body-based interventions), or unnecessarily costly (all interventions). NCCAM's goal is to identify the optimum dose, defined as that dose with full clinical value (efficacy) but with an acceptable safety, adherence, and cost profile. Once the apparent optimum dose is determined in phase 1 and phase 2 trials, larger phase 3 trials can compare the optimum dose to an appropriate control group and/or a conventional intervention. It is important to emphasize that:

> *Use of a suboptimal dose that is safe but ineffective does not serve the larger goals of NCCAM or the CAM community. Although the trial indicates only that the tested dose of the intervention was ineffective, the community may conclude that all doses of the intervention are ineffective, and patients will be denied possible benefit from the intervention. The inappropriate rejection of an intervention, because Phase 1 and 2 studies did not precede a Phase 3 trial and a suboptimal dose was used in the Phase 3 trial, is common for CAM modalities... (http://nccam.nih.gov/ research/policies/guideonct.htm)*

An excellent example of this issue is our experience with the herbal product, saw palmetto, which is used by the public to alleviate symptoms associated with benign prostatic hyperplasia (BPH). Initial data with a standard dose (160 mg twice daily) of saw palmetto has been positive in some studies but negative in other studies.[15] Instead of testing the standard dose in a large phase 3 study, and possibly finding that the standard dose has insubstantial efficacy, NCCAM and the National Institute of Diabetes and Digestive and Kidney Diseases are sponsoring a dose-escalation trial of saw palmetto to identify the optimally effective dose for a future phase 3 trial.

CONTROL GROUPS

One control group that is particularly important, given the variability and subjectivity of endpoints for which CAM interventions are generally used, is a placebo group (for dietary supplements) or sham group (for procedure-based CAM). Placebo and sham controls are intended to account for the nonspecific effects of an intervention, as well as for the natural history of the disease/condition in question. To take an example from psychiatry, St. John's wort demonstrated partial responses (50% improvement in the standard Hamilton Depression Rating

Scale) or full responses in 38% of patients with major depression, but 43% of placebo recipients also demonstrated such responses.[16] Importantly, not only patients taking St. John's wort but also those taking sertraline had improvements in depression that were similar in magnitude to that of the patients in the placebo group. Both St. John's wort and sertraline would have appeared to be substantially effective for this disorder if a placebo group had not been included in the study.

ENTRY CRITERIA, PATIENT POPULATION, AND OUTCOME VARIABLES

In design of clinical trials, the investigators have to consider if there is a subset of patients and outcomes for which the intervention might be particularly effective. For example, cranberry might be a more effective prophylaxis for urinary tract infections in younger women rather than older women, or Echinacea might be more effective as a treatment for colds rather than as prophylaxis for colds. Since it may be difficult to completely blind the intervention for some CAM therapies, the choice of outcome measure may be critical. Improvements may be seen when using subjective outcome measures but not when using objective measures, or visa versa. For instance, in clinical trials of Echinacea or cranberry, the use of subjective measures such as patient or physician symptom severity scales may lead to different trial outcomes compared to objective measures such as changes in immune markers or bacteria counts.

RECRUITMENT AND RANDOMIZATION

Experience suggests it is difficult to recruit participants into some CAM trials.[17–19] Many CAM users have specific philosophical perspectives, world views, or life experiences that make them skeptical of science.[20] These negative beliefs about science, as well as positive views about specific CAM interventions, may reduce their willingess to be randomized to conventional treatment or placebo (sham) controls. For instance, the National Cancer Institute and NCCAM cosponsor a study of the Gonzalez regimen for pancreatic cancer (ClinicalTrials.gov). Many potential participants refused randomization because of strong treatment preference for either the Gonzalez regimen or conventional therapy, with the result that the study was converted from a randomized, controlled trial, to an observational study (CAPCAM Minutes, May 21, 2001—http://nccam.nih.gov/about/advisory/capcam/minutes/2001may.htm).

Even after agreeing to randomization, participants who strongly favor CAM may subsequently take steps that can invalidate study blinding and randomization. The easy access to dietary supplements and other CAM interventions in the open market greatly increases the likelihood of "cheating" by the control group. In addition, inadvertent crossover of control participants to active treatment can occur because participants become aware of treatment options by their participation in the trial. For example, although not a CAM study, the NIH-supported MRFIT trial,[21] which studied integrated lifestyle modifications to prevent CHD, is an example of control group participants incorporating some of the interventions randomized to the treatment group. Much of this crossover began when the media began touting the benefits of the various lifestyle modifications. Thus studies need to be carefully designed to minimize such patient-created crossover.

In addition to philosophic differences, the treatment burden required in some CAM trials may discourage participation. For example, the large number of study visits required of participants increased the difficulty of recruiting individuals into the Trial to Assess Chelation Therapy (TACT).

ADHERENCE

In any intervention trial, significant efforts are spent on ensuring that patients adhere to the treatment regimen once the trial begins. In the case of the classic randomized clinical trial, efforts to improve adherence generally involve ensuring that participants understand the treatment schedule, the treatment is readily available, side effects to the treatment are minimized, treatment effects are maximized, and patients are reminded to take their treatment. Careful thought regarding these issues during the design phase of a study can put into place effective strategies to minimize nonadherence. Such strategies include minimizing participant burden by making interventions as easy to understand and implement as possible, maximizing participant benefit by ensuring maximum treatment effects and building additional benefits into the trial, and planning on strategies to maintain regular contact with participants. It is also essential to assess adherence directly. This assessment can be as simple as pill counts for dietary supplements and patient diaries for mind-body therapies, or as complex as blood or urine analyses to measure some metabolite of a dietary supplement.

Additional challenges to studies of mind-body interventions and procedure-based therapies

In addition to the above considerations, which are common to all trials of CAM, trials investigating the efficacy of mind-body therapies (e.g., meditation, hypnosis, guided imagery) and procedure-based CAM interventions (e.g., acupuncture, chiropractic manipulation, massage therapy) have added challenges in the design and implementation of clinical trials.

STUDY DESIGN

Blinding Double blinding is usually not possible in mind-body and procedure-based intervention trials, as well as trials of special diets. Assignment to group may be visible to both the practitioner delivering the treatment and to the patient. As such, specific strategies such as the use of detailed manual of operations and specific treatment protocols that reduce patient-provider interactions must be put into place to minimize potential sources of bias. Most importantly, experimenters who are not involved with treatment delivery, including those making assessments regarding posttreatment diagnosis, should ideally remain blinded to assignment. Similarly, study coordinators who are responsible for randomization to treatment should also remain blinded.

Control group Decisions regarding how to construct a control or placebo group are particularly complex with regard to some CAM interventions because the treatment is often multifaceted. This is illustrated in the combined transcendental meditation and herbal antioxidant trial cited below. Decisions must be made with regard to which aspects of the intervention, whether deliberate or not, are necessary to control. For example, many mind-body interventions and all procedure-based CAM therapies involve frequent interaction with a practitioner and, sometimes, a group of other patients. Apart from any effects specific to the intervention, there can be a significant social support component to such interventions, and in these cases it is imperative to include an attention control group in the study design. Such a group would be matched for contact time between participants and practitioners, but no active treatment component would be included. Another option is to employ a psychoeducational control group, which is also matched for contact time, but includes an educational component as well. This group essentially serves as a "placebo" control, because participants are randomized to a group where there is active contact, although not active treatment. Whichever type of attention control that is chosen should always be piloted to ensure there is adequate adherence and minimal dropout.

A placebo control group for procedure-based CAM interventions is typically a sham control. As with all placebo control groups, including sham and psychoeducational controls, one must consider the possibility that these placebo controls may, themselves, produce a physiological response. This has been documented for "sham" acupuncture,[22] "sham" manipulation,[23] and a variety of other placebo control groups. The end result is to reduce the ability to detect a significant difference between real and placebo groups and potentially to judge an intervention as ineffective when, in fact, it is effective. Therefore, placebo controls should always be validated before their use in a clinical trial.

It might be suggested that "usual care" or "no treatment" controls might be more appropriate for procedure-based interventions because they would avoid the problem of a potentially physiologically active sham group. However, "usual care" and "no treatment" controls don't control for nonspecific effects of the intervention.

Preference trials Another design option that is particularly salient with regard to mind-body interventions and procedure-based therapies is the preference trial.[24] In this three-arm design, some portion of participants is randomly assigned to either the control or active treatment group. The remaining participants are allowed to enter either group according to their preference. This design allows researchers to examine both the effects of treatment, as well as the potential benefits of "matching" treatment to participant in the preference arm of the trial. Such trials, although larger and more expensive, can be particularly valuable for high-burden interventions such as some trials of mind-body or procedure-based therapies.

Attrition and adherence Mind-body and procedure-based CAM therapies are almost always more time-intensive or burdensome to patients than more conventional biomedical interventions with the exception of some diet studies. In particular, mind-body therapies usually involve a training phase, followed by regular practice on ones own, homework, and periodic "booster" sessions. Therefore, attrition and adherence rates are a concern. In addition, attrition and adherence problems can occur because of a high degree of unpleasant side effects, or because of low perceived efficacy. A high degree of participant burden is a common side effect in many mind-body interventions; less commonly but importantly, some participants may experience significant distress when interacting in a group setting, as is common in many mind-body therapies. Thus, designs incorporating mind-body and procedure-based CAM therapies must reduce excess burden whenever possible by, for example, making intervention groups readily accessible at convenient places and times, and by carefully considering optimal dosing of the intervention. Regarding efficacy, it is important to recognize that perceived efficacy is as important as actual efficacy.

Take, for example, a mind-body intervention to reduce blood pressure in hypertensive individuals. Blood pressure reduction is not detectable without a measurement device, so perceived efficacy will be determined by a combination of (relatively infrequent) blood pressure readings along with other, perceived positive benefits, which may or may not be related to blood pressure control. Relaxation for the treatment of hypertension may have actual benefit for blood pressure management, but may have other, additional perceived benefits related to stress management and consequent improved quality of life. To the extent that perceived benefits can be maximized, attrition will likely be minimized.

IMPLEMENTATION ISSUES

Therapeutic allegiance   Therapeutic allegiance or clinician bias can be present in any type of intervention trial, and simply refers to the potential for bias for a favored treatment strategy among the practitioner administering the intervention. However, the previously mentioned difficulty in double-blinding trials of mind-body and procedure-based CAM therapies exacerbates the potential for therapeutic allegiance. Therefore, the degree of therapeutic allegiance should be measured and controlled as much as possible in all such investigations. Strategies to do so include optimizing practitioner training and considering the value of having several practitioners deliver treatment. While this latter strategy may increase the danger of differential treatment, it has the significant advantage of allowing for testing of therapeutic allegiance. Finally, the use of manuals to clearly articulate the precise components of the treatment intervention[25] to be delivered can be particularly useful for minimizing therapeutic allegiance. Such manualized therapies, although generally less powerful than tailored interventions, allow the highest degree of treatment standardization.

Administration of the intervention   Some dietary supplements, such as herbal products, may be difficult to manufacture reproducibly, but they are simple to administer to patients. In contrast, other CAM modalities such as manipulative and body-based interventions, mind-body interventions, and energy therapies, have no manufacturing issues but (like conventional interventions such as surgery and psychotherapy) are more difficult to administer reproducibly. For CAM interventions other than dietary supplements, studies need to have a set of standard operating procedures, such as the use of manuals (see section titled "Therapeutic allegiance"), so that the interventions are performed in a reproducible manner. Meditation may be highly useful for many diseases including stress-related cardiovascular problems. However, for the scientific community to believe study results and for others to duplicate these results, meditation would have to be administered according to standardized methods. This generally requires a detailed step-by-step description of the procedures, exercises, and training to be performed, and review of sessions (by videotape or audiotape) to verify that the procedures have been followed.

Additional challenges for studies of botanical products

For biologically active agents such as dietary supplements, results of their production must be reproducible. Unlike synthetic drugs, botanical products used as CAM are complex mixtures. The active ingredient can be hypothesized but is not definitively known. For example, soy isoflavones are hypothesized to prevent atherosclerosis based on the diminished incidence of this problem in Asian populations who consume large quantities of soy.[26, 27] Assuming that soy products do have this benefit, which soy constituents, alone or in combination, are responsible? Is it soy protein, or the isoflavones, or both, and if the isoflavones, which one—genisten, diazin, or as yet unidentified isoflavones? For this formulation and other natural products, consistent synthesis of the many identified and not yet identified components is needed. Thus, all the processes leading to the final clinical product—species, geographic location, harvest, extraction, and manufacturing of the final product—must be controlled. In 2003, the Food and Drug Administration (FDA) proposed new chemistry-manufacturing-control (CMC) standards for marketed botanical dietary supplements. Published in 2004, these standards, known as the *Botanical Drug Guidance* will make manufacturing controls more like those seen for conventional drugs [http://www.fda.gov/cder/guidance/index.htm]. A key feature of the new standards is the introduction of manufacturing process controls to supplement analysis of the final product.

With respect to the final properties of botanicals resulting from the above manufacturing processes and used as CAM in NCCAM clinical trials, NCCAM has published its requirements on its website (http://nccam.nih.gov/research/policies/naturalproducts.htm#2). NCCAM's requirements paraphrase FDA's *Botanical Drug Guidance*. Since these products may have been in clinical use for many years, even centuries, and because phase 1 and phase 2 trials involve only small numbers of patients under carefully monitored conditions, there is an assumption that the products will be relatively safe during evaluation, and that any rare adverse events that might occur will be quickly recognized and addressed. In brief, the following are essential components required by the FDA and NCCAM prior to initiation of phase 1 and phase 2 clinical trials: (1) description of the plant and the extraction procedure; (2) analysis of the clinical formulation for putative active ingredient(s), including chemical fingerprinting of both identified and unidentified ingredients; and (3) analysis for the presence of pesticides, heavy metals, and synthetic drugs. Phase 3 trials involve a much larger number of patients and are penultimate to registration and marketing for conventional drug products. Although the FDA Botanical Drug Guidance is not clear as to specific CMC requirements for phase 3 trials, it is likely that full conventional drug Good Manufacturing Practices (GMP) will need to be followed. NCCAM requires GMP practices be followed in all of the "stages" leading to the final clinical trial product: cultivation/harvesting of the plant, and extraction, analysis, and manufacturing of the clinical product.

ONGOING NCCAM CLINICAL TRIALS

NCCAM is currently managing several single or multisite randomized, controlled trials (RCTs) considering cardiovascular outcomes. Although data are not yet available from these on-going trials, the design and implementation of these trials address many of the issues already discussed. Selected examples are detailed in the following sections.

Chelation therapy

BACKGROUND

In August 2002, NCCAM, in close collaboration with the National Heart, Lung, and Blood Institute (NHLBI), initiated a multisite, randomized, placebo-controlled trial to investigate the efficacy and safety of ethylenediaminetetraacetic acid (EDTA) chelation therapy in individuals suffering from coronary artery disease (CAD). The FDA has approved EDTA chelation therapy as a prescription drug to treat heavy metal poisoning. An FDA investigational new drug application (IND) is on file for the present investigational use of EDTA chelation therapy. The principal investigator (PI) of this study, known as the TACT, is Gervasio Lamas, MD of the Mount Sinai Medical Center in Miami.

DESIGN

TACT is designed as a 7-year, 1950-patient, randomized, placebo-controlled, factorial trial testing whether EDTA chelation therapy and/or high-dose vitamin therapy is effective for the treatment of CAD. It is estimated that up to 200 clinical sites will be necessary to fully enroll the trial. Patients are eligible if they are at least 50 years of age and have had an acute myocardial infarction (MI) more than 3 weeks prior to enrollment. The primary endpoint of this trial is a composite endpoint that combines all cause mortality, MI, stroke, coronary revascularization, and hospitalization for angina.

The EDTA chelation therapy or placebo solution will be delivered through 40 intravenous infusions that are administered over a 28-month course of treatment.

The first 30 infusions will be delivered on a weekly basis and the last 10 will be delivered bimonthly. The protocol for the trial was developed using a model protocol for EDTA chelation therapy endorsed by the American College for the Advancement of Medicine (ACAM). Chelation practitioners use the ACAM protocol worldwide. It is the intent of this study to ensure that the most widely practiced method of delivering EDTA chelation is rigorously tested.

EDTA chelation therapy, as practiced in the community, often includes administration of high doses of antioxidant vitamin and mineral supplements. Thus, it is possible that effects of the therapy could be connected to these supplements. In order to test whether some of the therapy's effect may be attributable to vitamin/mineral supplements, or to the EDTA solution itself, the investigators will first randomly assign participants to receive either EDTA chelation solution or placebo. Then the patients in these two groups (about 975 in each) will again be randomly selected to receive either low-dose or high-dose vitamin/mineral supplements. The trial will have greater than 85% power to detect a 25% reduction in the primary endpoint for each treatment factor in the 2×2 factorial design.

In addition, because one purported claim for chelation therapy is enhanced quality of life, TACT has a fully integrated quality of life and economic analysis substudy. For this substudy, 1000 participants from the parent trial will be randomly selected to undergo serial analyses for quality of life, utilities, and health economics that will include the SF-36, the Duke Activity Status, the Seattle Angina Questionnaire, and measurement of utilities by the EuroQol. It was expected that recruitment would be difficult for TACT because chelation therapy is a widely used therapy for which many consumers and physicians have strong—and often opposing—views. In addition, the trial involves substantial participant burden in that 40, 3-hour infusions are required over the course of the study. Therefore, NCCAM implemented a multifaceted recruitment plan including clinical site media training, development of site-specific and national promotional materials by the NCCAM Office of Communications and Public Liaison to be used in all types of paid advertisements, use of earned media (news stories), and centralized national recruitment (http://nccam.nih.gov/chelation) that included both television and newspaper advertising.

SAFETY MONITORING

Since patient safety is of primary importance in this trial, a number of safety cut-off values have been incorporated. For instance, the clinical sites and clinical coordinating center are advised when estimated creatinine clearance is reduced by 25% or more. Infusions are delayed when there is a doubling of serum creatinine, or an increase to a level of 2.5 mg/dL, whichever is lower. Infusions are also delayed in patients whose ALT, AST, alkaline phosphatase, or bilirubin double from baseline, when total white cell count or neutrophils fall below normal limits, or when thrombocytopenia depletes platelets to below 100,000 or 50% below baseline. Since weekly infusions of large fluid volumes may exacerbate existing congestive heart failure, whether previously diagnosed or not, rapid increases in weight between visits will also delay infusions until after a medical evaluation indicates this weight gain is not related to volume overload. Use of conventional medications is monitored to promote the use of best practice guidelines for post-MI medical care. Finally, NCCAM and NHLBI staff, the Data and Safety Monitoring Board (DSMB), the FDA, and Institutional Review Boards review safety data on a regular basis.

Soy protein

BACKGROUND

NCCAM supports a clinical trial to study the effect of isoflavone-enriched soy protein on progression of atherosclerosis in healthy postmenopausal women. Since the findings of the Women's Health Initiative, the continuing concern and discontent with traditional hormone replacement therapy coupled with the growing public interest in natural products has resulted in an escalating use of alternative substances by both women and their physicians alike. A recent survey indicated that up to 45% of postmenopausal Swedish women use some alternative form of hormone replacement therapy,[28] and phytoestrogens are the most sought after alternative. Isoflavones are phytoestrogens of particular interest since soy is the major food source of isoflavones and observational studies have demonstrated that Asian populations who consume soy foods as their dietary staple have a lower incidence of "Western" diseases such as breast, colon, and prostate cancers and CVD.[29]

DESIGN

This 5-year clinical trial, funded in September 2003, is being conducted at the University of Southern California by PI Howard Hodis, MD. It is a randomized, double-blind, placebo-controlled trial of the effect of soy phytoestrogens on the progression of atherosclerosis in healthy postmenopausal women without preexisting CVDs. About 300 participants will be recruited and randomized into two groups. The test group will be given 25 g soy protein enriched with 150 mg of isoflavones, while the control group will be given whey protein. The participants will be followed for 2.5 years to measure the rate of change in the common carotid artery intima-media thickness.

PRODUCT CHOICE AND DOSE

There are many different preparations of soy isoflavone extracts containing different amounts of isoflavones on the market. In addition, it appears that both soy protein and isoflavones are needed for the maximal activity of soy in exerting biological effects. Therefore, it is important to choose a product that has the effective properties. According to epidemiological studies, the consumption of soy protein by Asian population is approximately 30–50 g/d containing 20–200 mg/d isoflavones.[30,31] In that context, the FDA approved a health claim for soy protein (25 g) with naturally occurring isoflavones, not isoflavone isolates.[32]

The typical dietary intake data from Asian population studies, along with an extensive review of the literature concerning the effects of soy protein on atherogenesis, vascular physiology, CVD, and cardiovascular risk factors were used as a guide to determine the intervention formulation and dosage for NCCAM's soy trial. The overall cardiovascular benefits appear to be best expressed with a daily dosage of approximately 25 g soy protein containing 85 mg aglycone weight of naturally occurring isoflavones (or 150 mg total isoflavones) divided as genistein 45 mg aglycone weight (80 mg total weight), daidzein 35 mg aglycone weight (60 mg total weight), and glycitein 5 mg (10 mg total weight) in a 1.3 to 1 to 0.2 ratio, similar to that present in soy beans.[33] Such a preparation, manufactured by The Solae Company and independently analyzed, is used in the trial. The placebo contains total milk protein without any isoflavones.

PATIENT ADHERENCE AND SAFETY

In a trial of a dietary supplement, there is always a concern that patients will not adhere to the protocol. The research team for the soy study created soy isoflavone protein preparations in various forms, such as chocolate bars and powders that can be included in various recipes. The patients are given a recipe and encouraged to come up with new recipes. The procedure has been quite successful and the retention has been over 90%.

DATA FROM COMPLETED NCCAM CLINICAL TRIALS ON CVD

Acupuncture for hypertension

A randomized, placebo controlled, double-blind clinical trial examined whether acupuncture could be used to treat mild to moderate hypertension (Stop Hypertension with the Acupuncture Research Program—SHARP).[34] A total of 192 participants with unmedicated blood pressures of 140/90 to 179/109 (systolic/diastolic in mm Hg) were randomized to one of the three treatments groups: (1) standardized active acupuncture (standardized), (2) individualized acupuncture (individualized), and (3) placebo sham acupuncture (control). All subjects received fully individualized Traditional Chinese Medicine (TCM) acupuncture prescriptions by Chinese-trained acupuncturists, but only individualized subjects were treated according to this prescription. Standardized subjects were needled at a uniform set of TCM points selected *a priori* by an expert panel of TCM acupuncturists. This panel also determined the dosage of treatment for the trial. In control subjects, needles were placed at points not believed to be active according to TCM principles. Subjects were treated for 12 sessions over 6–8 weeks.

Blood pressure was monitored at least every other week out to the primary end point at 10 weeks after randomization and less frequently until 12 months. Blood pressure at each visit was estimated from three to five replicate measurements taken by trained staff using manual mercury sphygmomanometers. Hypertension staff and diagnosing acupuncturists were masked to subject randomizations. Treating acupuncturists were masked to subject blood pressures.

The results showed that mean blood pressure decreased 4.8/4.8 mm Hg from baseline.[35] However, the mean baseline-adjusted decrease in systolic blood pressure at 10 weeks did not differ between subjects randomized to either individualized or standardized acupuncture. Individualized subjects experienced the largest decrease in diastolic blood pressure, but the differences among treatment groups were not significant ($p = 0.46$). A trend toward greater improvement in diastolic blood pressure from 2 to 10 weeks was observed in individualized subjects, suggesting that a longer series of treatments or a large sample size might have revealed greater treatment differences; however, the observed differences in trends were not significant ($p = 0.23$). The lack of difference may be due to the small patient sample, or reflect greater than expected therapeutic activity of the sham intervention, or indicate limited efficacy of TCM acupuncture for treating hypertension.[35] Interestingly, animal mechanistic studies have demonstrated substantial changes in cardiovascular regulation with acupuncture, including modification of blood pressure.[36,37] Data from these groups suggests that acupuncture may have been underdosed in SHARP and that blood pressure monitoring may have been too limited. Further research is needed to test these hypotheses.

Meditation

TRANSCENDENTAL MEDITATION

The Center for Natural Medicine and Prevention, established at the Maharishi University of Management, Fairfield, Iowa, evaluates CAM modalities, including mind-body interventions, for the prevention and treatment of CVD in high-risk older African Americans. Clinical trials conducted at Maharishi include: (1) the effect of transcendental meditation alone on hypertension and CVD; and (2) a controlled study on mechanisms and clinical effects of a traditional herbal antioxidant combined with transcendental meditation, diet, and exercise on carotid atherosclerosis, endothelial function, oxidative stress, CVD risk factors, and quality of life.

Investigators have found that transcendental meditation practice alone results in significantly greater reductions in blood pressure among African Americans with hypertension, relative to either a progressive muscle relaxation or psychoeducation control group, and that these effects are sustained.[38] Initial findings from the investigation of transcendental meditation in combination with a traditional herbal antioxidant, diet, and exercise indicate that, compared with those in a standard care program, patients practicing the multimodal CAM intervention had significantly greater decreases in carotid artery thickness.[39]

These studies had in place many of the essential design features and implementation strategies outlined in our discussion of CAM clinical trial design. For example, these researchers implemented careful blinding strategies where possible, particularly in regard to key outcome variables. In the study of transcendental meditation alone, both the technicians who monitored blood pressure changes in participants, as well as the physicians assessing medication usage, were blinded to participant treatment allocation. In addition, participants randomized to each arm were matched with regard to time spent with instructors, basic structure of the intervention, and level of expectation conveyed for positive results. The dose and dosage of transcendental meditation alone were based on the standard course introduced by Maharishi Mahesh Yogi in the 1950s and practiced widely in the United States. Finally, level of adherence to treatment was assessed in the transcendental meditation alone trial through monthly interviews with the participants; interestingly, those in the meditation group had higher levels of adherence than those in the other groups. This calls into question whether the superiority of the transcendental meditation alone group in previous trials was due to greater adherence only, or also due to greater efficacy. Despite careful attention to these design details, questions regarding the most appropriate dose of transcendental meditation to achieve the specific effects tested are still present, and dose-ranging studies, although uncommon in mind-body intervention studies, are essential for establishing the most effective doses while minimizing participant burden. Finally, the multifaceted treatment offered in the second study illustrates the importance of the choice of control group. Decisions regarding which aspect of the intervention should be controlled will help determine the most appropriate control groups, but this decision becomes more complex as the active treatment increases in complexity. In this instance, the effects of conventional diet and exercise advice were controlled in one group, but the addition of only a standard care control group does not allow the researchers to tease apart the independent effects of social support or attention, nor of any of the components of the intervention, on cardiovascular risk factors.

TAI CHI

Heart failure is an increasing public health issue in the United States and is responsible for significant public health and economic burden. Thus treatments to improve quality of life and functional capacity are especially warranted in heart failure patients. Tai Chi is a gentle, meditative type of exercise that may be ideal for chronic heart failure patients. Researchers at Beth Israel Deaconess Medical Center have investigated the feasibility of incorporating a Tai Chi program into conventional medical care in heart failure patients, and have shown that an intervention combining Tai Chi with standard care resulted in improved self-reported quality of life, increased exercise capacity, and decreased serum B-type natriuretic peptide levels in heart failure patients compared to controls.[40] This is a promising study that suggests that larger efficacy trials are needed, but certain design elements also limit the conclusions that can be drawn. Although participants were randomized to condition, blinding of the experimenters, including those assessing functional outcomes, was not done, allowing the potential for inadvertent bias to influence the results. As the investigators suggest, because the control group was a usual care control, it is not possible to speculate on whether the effects of the intervention were due to exercise in general, or to more specific qualities of Tai Chi exercise. Future trials that incorporate careful design should be performed, and these should specifically characterize the specific improvements that occur with this intervention, identify the duration of the effect and dosing requirements, and test the psychological, metabolic, and neurohormonal mechanisms by which Tai Chi may have its effects. In particular, research is needed to differentiate the meditative effects of Tai Chi from its effects as a low-impact exercise.

CONCLUSION

Clinical trials of CAM interventions face the same general challenges as clinical trials of any intervention, although, in some cases, these challenges may be exacerbated:

1. Identifying an appropriate, reproducible intervention, including production, dose, frequency, and duration—this may be more difficult than in standard drug trials given the variability in practice patterns and training of practitioners.

2. Identifying an appropriate control group(s)—in this regard, the development of valid sham techniques has proven difficult. Control groups should also account for the time and attention paid to trial participants.

3. Randomizing subjects to treatment groups in an unbiased manner—randomization may prove more difficult than in a trial of conventional treatments, since CAM therapies are already available to the public, and thus, it is more likely that participants will have a preexisting preference for a given therapy.

4. Maintaining investigator and subject adherence to the protocol—group contamination may be more problematic than in trials of conventional interventions, since subjects have easy access to CAM therapy providers and products. Conversely, some CAM therapies are associated with substantial treatment burden, which may reduce adherence.

5. Reducing bias by blinding subjects and investigators to group assignment—blinding of subjects and investigators may prove difficult or impossible for certain types of manual therapies. However, the person collecting the outcome data should always be blinded.

For CVD, as for other diseases, it is NCCAM's goal to support the highest quality research possible using the most current and emerging technologies. This commitment is essential since the evaluation of CAM needs to be conducted carefully, using the most rigorous research designs possible. As research clarifies, the role of CAM for CVD and other health conditions, dissemination of this information to health-care practitioners, insurance providers, policy makers, and the general public will allow informed decisions to be made concerning integration of CAM into today's health-care system.

REFERENCES

1. Foster DF, Phillips RS, Hamel MB, Eisenberg DM. Alternative medicine use in older Americans. J Am Geriatr Soc. 2000;48(12):1560–5. [PMID: 11129743]
2. Eisenberg DM, Davis RB, Ettner SL, Appel S, Wilkey S, Van Rompay M, et al. Trends in alternative medicine use in the United States, 1990–1997: results of a follow-up national survey. JAMA. 1998;280(18):1569–75. [PMID: 9820257]

3. Barnes PM, Powell-Griner E, McFann K, Nahin RL. Complementary and alternative medicine use among adults: United States, 2002. Adv Data. 2004;343:1–19. [PMID: 15188733]

4. Agency for Healthcare Research and Quality. Evidence-based report series. Rockville, MD. Available at http://www.ahrq.gov/clinic/epc/epcseries.htm

5. Pittler MH, Thompson CO, Ernst E. Artichoke leaf extract for treating hypercholesterolaemia. Cochrane Database Syst Rev. 2002;3:CD003335. [PMID: 12137691]

6. Atallah AN, Hofmeyr GJ, Duley L. Calcium supplementation during pregnancy for preventing hypertensive disorders and related problems. Cochrane Database Syst Rev. 2002;1:CD001059. [PMID: 11869587]

7. Villarruz MV, Dans A, Tan F. Chelation therapy for atherosclerotic cardiovascular disease. Cochrane Database Syst Rev. 2002;4:CD002785. [PMID: 12519577]

8. Jepson RG, Kleijnen J, Leng GC. Garlic for peripheral arterial occlusive disease. Cochrane Database Syst Rev. 2000;2:CD000095. [PMID: 10796487]

9. Liu JP, Yang M, Du XM. Herbal medicines for viral myocarditis. Cochrane Database Syst Rev. 2004;3:CD003711. [PMID: 15266498]

10. Wu B, Liu M, Zhang S. Dan Shen agents for acute ischaemic stroke. Cochrane Database Syst Rev. 2004;4:CD004295. [PMID: 15495099]

11. Pittler MH, Ernst E. Horse chestnut seed extract for chronic venous insufficiency. Cochrane Database Syst Rev. 2004;2:CD003230. [PMID: 15106197]

12. Hooper L, Thompson RL, Harrison RA, Summerbell CD, Moore H, Worthington HV, et al. Omega 3 fatty acids for prevention and treatment of cardiovascular disease. Cochrane Database Syst Rev. 2004;4:CD003177. [PMID: 15495044]

13. Sommerfield T, Hiatt WR. Omega-3 fatty acids for intermittent claudication. Cochrane Database Syst Rev. 2004;3:CD003833. [PMID: 15266504]

14. Kleijnen J, Mackerras D. Vitamin E for intermittent claudication. Cochrane Database Syst Rev. 2000;2:CD000987. [PMID: 10796571]

15. Wilt T, Ishani A, MacDonald R. Serenoa repens for benign prostatic hyperplasia. Cochrane Database Syst Rev. 2002;3:CD001423. [PMID: 12137626]

16. Hypericum Depression Trial Study Group. Effect of Hypericum perforatum (St John's wort) in major depressive disorder: a randomized controlled trial. JAMA. 2002;287(14):1807–14. [PMID: 11939866]

17. Richardson MA, Post-White J, Singletary SE, Justice B. Recruitment for complementary/alternative medicine trials: who participates after breast cancer. Ann Behav Med. 1998;20(3):190–8. [PMID: 9989326]

18. Ellis PM. Attitudes towards and participation in randomised clinical trials in oncology: a review of the literature. Ann Oncol. 2000;11(8):939–45. [PMID: 11038029]

19. Jenkins V, Fallowfield L. Reasons for accepting or declining to participate in randomized clinical trials for cancer therapy. Br J Cancer. 2000;82(11):1783–8. [PMID: 10839291]

20. Institute of Medicine, National Academies of Science, Committee on the Use of Complementary and Alternative Medicine by the American Public. Complementary and alternative medicine (CAM) in the United States. Washington, DC: National Academies Press; 2005.

21. Multiple Risk Factor Intervention Trial Research Group. Multiple risk factor intervention trial. Risk factor changes and mortality results. JAMA. 1982;248(12):1465–77. [PMID: 7050440]

22. Berman BM, Lao L, Langenberg P, Lee WL, Gilpin AM, Hochberg MC. Effectiveness of acupuncture as adjunctive therapy in osteoarthritis of the knee: a randomized, controlled trial. Ann Intern Med. 2004;141(12):901–10. [PMID: 15611487]

23. Triano JJ, McGregor M, Hondras MA, Brennan PC. Manipulative therapy versus education programs in chronic low back pain. Spine. 1995;20(8):948–55. [PMID: 7644961]

24. Torgerson DJ, Sibbald B. Understanding controlled trials. What is a patient preference trial? BMJ. 1998;316(7128):360. [PMID: 9487173]

25. Schnyer RN, Allen JJ. Bridging the gap in complementary and alternative medicine research: manualization as a means of promoting standardization and flexibility of treatment in clinical trials of acupuncture. J Altern Complement Med. 2002; 8(5):623–34. [PMID: 12470444]

26. Lukito W. Candidate foods in the Asia-Pacific region for cardiovascular protection: nuts, soy, lentils and tempe. Asia Pac J Clin Nutr. 2001;10(2):128–33. [PMID: 11710352]

27. Zhang X, Shu XO, Gao YT, Yang G, Li Q, Li H, et al. Soy food consumption is associated with lower risk of coronary heart disease in Chinese women. J Nutr. 2003;133(9):2874–8. [PMID: 12949380]

28. Stadberg E, Mattsson LA, Milsom I. The prevalence and severity of climacteric symptoms and the use of different treatment regimens in a Swedish population. Acta Obstet Gynecol Scand. 1997;76(5):442–8. [PMID: 9197447]

29. Barnes S. Evolution of the health benefits of soy isoflavones. Proc Soc Exp Biol Med. 1998;217(3):386–92. [PMID: 9492352]

30. Nagata C, Takatsuka N, Kurisu Y, Shimizu H. Decreased serum total cholesterol concentration is associated with high intake of soy products in Japanese men and women. J Nutr. 1998;128(2):209–13. [PMID: 9446845]

31. Arai Y, Uehara M, Sato Y, Kimira M, Eboshida A, Adlercreutz H, et al. Comparison of isoflavones among dietary intake, plasma concentration and urinary excretion for accurate estimation of phytoestrogen intake. J Epidemiol. 2000;10(2):127–35. [PMID: 10778038]

32. Food and Drug Administration, HHS. Food labeling: health claims: soy protein and coronary heart disease. Fed Regist. 1999 Oct 26;64(206 Pt 101):57700–33.

33. Reinli K, Block G. Phytoestrogen content of foods—a compendium of literature values. Nutr Cancer. 1996;26(2):123–48. [PMID: 8875551]

34. Kalish LA, Buczynski B, Connell P, Gemmel A, Goertz C, Macklin EA, et al. Stop Hypertension with the Acupuncture Research Program (SHARP): clinical trial design and screening results. Control Clin Trials. 2004;25(1):76–103. [PMID: 14980754]

35. Macklin EA, Wayne PM, Kalish LA, Valaskatgis P, Thompson J, et al. Stop Hypertension with the Acupuncture Research Program (SHARP): results of a randomized, controlled clinical trial. Hypertension. 2006 Nov;48(5):838–45.

36. Tjen ALS, Li P, Longhurst JC. Medullary substrate and differential cardiovascular responses during stimulation of specific acupoints. Am J Physiol Regul Integr Comp Physiol. 2004;287(4):R852–62. [PMID: 15217791]

37. Zhou WY, Tjen ALS, Longhurst JC. Brain stem mechanisms underlying acupuncture modality-related modulation of cardiovascular responses in rats. J Appl Physiol. 2005;99(3):851–60. [PMID: 15817715]

38. Schneider RH, Alexander CN, Staggers F, Orme-Johnson DW, Rainforth M, Salerno JW, et al. A randomized controlled trial of stress reduction in African Americans treated for hypertension for over one year. Am J Hypertens. 2005;18(1): 88–98. [PMID: 15691622]

39. Fields JZ, Walton KG, Schneider RH, Nidich S, Pomerantz R, Suchdev P, et al. Effect of a multimodality natural medicine program on carotid atherosclerosis in

older subjects: a pilot trial of Maharishi Vedic Medicine. Am J Cardiol. 2002;89(8): 952–8. [PMID: 11950434]

40. Yeh GY, Wood MJ, Lorell BH, Stevenson LW, Eisenberg DM, Wayne PM, et al. Effects of tai chi mind-body movement therapy on functional status and exercise capacity in patients with chronic heart failure: a randomized controlled trial. Am J Med. 2004;117(8):541–8. [PMID: 15465501]

3

CAM TREATMENT MODALITIES: NCCAM CATEGORIES

CHAPTER

6

BIOENERGETIC TECHNIQUES

Brian Olshansky

INTRODUCTION

Since ancient times, and, likely, even in prehistoric times, most cultures and societies and many religious disciplines have considered that an aura, a life force, a radiant energy field can, and does, emanate from and surround, all living things.[1] The quality of this poorly understood energy (a "weak force") has been described as a vital energy (Hindu "prana," Chinese "qi," "chi," and Japanese "ki") or "the source of life" associated with the soul, spirit and mind. This life force impinges on the potential boundaries of modern physics, and involves metaphysical, philosophical, and spiritual concepts that consider the relationship of the mind and consciousness to the physical world.[2-4] Bioenergetic techniques offer the possibility to connect to, and to utilize life force energy for purposes of healing.[5,6]

DEFINITION OF BIOENERGY MEDICINE

Bioenergetics is a loosely collected series of healing "disciplines" that attempt to harness natural, poorly understood, life forces and powers to influence natural healing processes. Bioenergy, a natural harmonious energy manifest as life energy[7] is thought to influence mind/body; mind/mind (person to person) and mind/mind (person to infinite spirit) relationships are thought to alter the course of a disease (Fig. 6-1).[8,9] Bioenergy fields are thought to be altered by conscious and unconscious efforts and events.[8] Bioenergy medicine harnesses what are considered subtle bioenergetic fields that have the potential to evoke a healing response. These may be detectable by some individual[10] and all appear to have some universal properties inherent in all forms of bioenergy healing philosophies.[11]

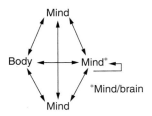

FIGURE 6-1   *The mind and its connections.*

CONSCIOUSNESS, AWARENESS, AND INTENTIONALITY—THE HEART OF BIOENERGETICS

Bioenergy involves the realm of perceptions, self-awareness, intuition, and conscious effort as they interact with mental, spiritual, and physical aspects of health but bioenergy slices to the core of the individual and pervades conscious and subconscious efforts and understanding. A basic underlying concept regarding bioenergy is that it is a link that an individual has to universal spiritual forces.

Bioenergetic techniques involve application of a conscious effort to unravel this link and strengthen it. They may involve a heightened state of awareness and an exquisite and acute sensitivity to what is present in an unhealthy individual. The awareness may involve an intuitive, nonlinear, nonanalytic, and nonscientific grasp of issues critical to the well-being of the patients or the one asking for healing. It requires the ability to connect to the patients in a basic and fundamental way that tends to be ignored in standard medical practices. For these techniques to work, the patient and the healer often need to work in an intensely personal realm that can depend on the patient's social and cultural constraints as it can require a change in the conscious understanding the patient has of the issues related to health. A cultural component can be critical for any specific technique to work but most critical is the relationship of the healer to the patient, as any purported energy transfer must be through open spiritual and psychic channels that help provide meaning to what health really is.

Bioenergy is often taken for granted and may be ignored. In an attempt to develop sterile scientific approaches to health, conscious understanding and interpretation of physical health has been ignored. Even so, it remains a strong part of, if not even the key to, overall health. Separating human potential from health separates us from others, from ourselves, from health, and from the meaning of health. Consciousness itself has been explained away as a meaningless or even irrelevant and powerless response. Modern neurophysiology tends to de-emphasize the importance of consciousness, and has looked upon it as an illusion the brain creates, a person behind the person, which really is not there. On some level, this type of thinking is absurd.

Bioenergetic techniques are in direct apposition to these ideas. The experiences that culminate in heightened state of awareness foster the idea that consciousness has meaning, and the intention has power. For those not initiated to these concepts, any exposure may create an initial fear of what it might mean to be alive rather than a positive and beneficial effect that ultimately can, and will, occur. Spirituality in modern times has been considered an aberration that needs to be avoided but this could lead to terrible results. It removes rather than creates, purpose and meaning in life. This can become manifest or is interpreted as illness. Health requires a connection to a common human spirit that is humane, giving, beneficent, and replete with meaning and answers. Attempting to sterilize these results can be disastrous with a complete demeaning of personal and intimate experiences. Attempt to suppress such experiences are damaging. However, the extent to which tapping into intuitive power unleashes the power of consciousness, through bioenergetic techniques to transform health is not yet shown.

One of the problems working with concepts of consciousness and intentionality is that neither of these can easily be understood and measured. While it is not surprising that the power of intentionality can be underestimated, clearly, conscious intentions can be executed and can have a major impact on understanding of physical reality and on health.[12] Intent can alter outcomes but limits of intent are uncertain. The extent to which consciousness working through concepts of intentionality really affects an individual and health remains obscure. What is clear, however, is that understanding the meaning of a medical condition, having a positive attitude, being compliant and adherent to therapy, and leading a healthy life can affect outcome. These issues can be affected by an individual interpretation of the impact a bioenergetics technical may appear to have. There may be a placebo effect. The placebo effect, whatever that is exactly, does exist and is a manifestation of the effects of consciousness on health and outcomes with regard to disease. Even if much of the effect of bioenergy healing could be ascribed to placebo, the mechanisms responsible can be highly complex.[13,14] Nevertheless, they may help keep individuals from going berserk.[15]

Examples of conditions that may be influenced by conscious intentions and understanding of disease condition include blood pressure abnormalities, myocardial ischemia with angina, memory loss, dyspnea, obesity, diabetes, palpitations, and neurocardiogenic syncope. It is likely that most medical conditions have a "psychosomatic" as well as a physical aspect. Some conditions, likely, the majority of conditions seen by a physician, border on the realm of psychosomatic more than physical in essence. Many of these concepts are incorporated into a recent consensus document developed for cardiologists.[16]

CAN BIOENERGY HEAL? IS THERE POWER IN BELIEF?

Living things do emanate energy. Humans emit weak electromagnetic waves (nerves and heart), chemicals, sounds, heat, and movement that are easily quantitated, evaluated, and measured, but bioenergetic fields, for which there is no conclusive evidence, are not that. Bioenergy affects psychological states and physiological processes of the nervous, endocrine, and immune systems (psychoneuroimmunology). It is likely that consciousness manifest as thought, emotion, memories, fears, and self-concept can create physical changes in the body and this appears modulated by many circulating mediators such as TNF-α, which may reduce or eliminate a reward response in animals and may be manifested by conditions such as myocardial infarction. Blockers of TNF-α restore the reward response.[17,18] The core from which these measured effects emanate is still a matter of dispute. No sound scientific evidence demonstrates the existence of bioenergy fields, but provocative data indicate that such fields can affect physical properties and conditions.

Meditation, concentration, and shaman drumming may influence seed sprouting presumably by nonlocal energy transfer.[19] Experienced external Qi Gong practitioners directing healing intentionality toward normal brain cell cultures may enhance cultured human cell growth. In a study involving 28 experiments, Qi Gong-treated samples showed more colony-forming units than sham samples ($p = 0.036$) but the data could not be replicated.[20] Bioenergy, scientific or not, real or not, is deeply ingrained, has gained popularity, and is an indisputable power to many individuals.

The mind can influence health, life, and death.[21,22] Belief in a therapy can foster a profound effect even if the therapy itself cannot be measured scientifically. Energy that facilitates connectedness, harmony, and health can be as simple as emotional release in the form of mirthful laughter or tears. Mirthful laughter can improve immune system functioning.[23] This form of bioenergy can be harnessed to improve a patient's well-being and outcome.

HOW DOES BIOENERGY WORK?

If bioenergy exists, therapies properly designed to affect bioenergy may be effective. The direct healing effects of bioenergetic techniques have not yet been proven. If these techniques do work, it is not known how that may be. Any measured benefits may be related to the direct conscious intent of the healer, expectations of the patients, the healing relationship (friendship), intense monitoring ("Hawthorn effect"), natural history of the condition, reinterpretation of symptoms, or an otherwise undefined placebo effect.[14]

Belief in the benefit of treatment can improve outcome even if the treatment is a placebo. Placebo effects can be potent in cardiac patients as long as they comply with and adhere to treatment prescribed.[14,24-26] Recently, the benefits of the poorly defined, poorly understood "placebo effect" have been challenged.[27] The issue remains unsettled but new approaches, including functional magnetic resonance imaging (MRI), positron emission tomography (PET) scanning,[28] and quantitative electroencephalogram (EEG) measurements have shown changes in the brain with placebo.[29,30] Improving optimism,[31,32,33] generating anticipation affecting self control[34] and providing understanding to a patient and the family can alter progression, interpretation, severity, manifestation, and mortality of many cardiovascular conditions including: coronary artery disease, heart failure, syncope, hypertension, and hypercholesterolemia.[27,35]

Controlled clinical studies showing benefit of bioenergy approaches over placebo raise the issue that these techniques may have an effect over and above a placebo effect. A functional MRI scan can show blood flow changes during brain mapping. Provocative data indicate that acupuncture in the foot can light up areas in the brain responsible for vision during functional MRI measurements but only at visual acupuncture points. The results depend on the personality type of the individual (Yin vs. Yang).[36] Other bioenergetic techniques may have other effects and work by different mechanisms.

Prayer, a potential bioenergetic technique, may be effective[37,38] but this has been disputed and prayer may even be dangerous.[39,40] Prayer may lead to a relaxation response that is not always advantageous such as can be observed in the face of an acute ischemic event. Similar adverse responses have been shown in a rat myocardial infarction model in which sympathetic output is ablated in the brain at the level of the third ventricle.[41]

The doctor-patient relationship, a classic model of bioenergy transfer, may be a method to foster and strengthen the placebo effect. A doctor affects health in many ways, often unbeknownst by the physician. The act of simply performing more and more tests can affect a health response as has been observed.[42]

Many cardiovascular symptoms are not treated easily with present medical therapy.[43] Functional complaints such as chest pain, palpitations, dyspnea, fatigue and weakness not associated with measurable physical abnormalities are poorly understood and methods to eliminate consequences could greatly improve health. Reinterpretation of symptoms and their severity by the patient (mental energy) may have an influence on outcome. The real benefit of bioenergetic treatments to affect a beneficial response may be as an adjunct to improve patient optimism and outcomes by their psychosocial effects at least in part.[43] No bioenergetic technique alone can cure a disease but it can improve outcomes based on symptoms and can have potentially beneficial adjunctive effects.[31–35]

A sense of peace, serenity, calm, power, or emotional connection can have potent influence on outcomes. Removal of "stress" (still not well defined) by a technique utilizing bioenergy may modify severe disabling symptoms. Even if the therapy has no proven benefit, it can have an apparent benefit. Such an approach can be advocated as long as the approach does not exclude standard proven therapy, does not cause harm to the patient, does not disrupt the doctor-patient relationship but fosters a healing response.

METHODS TO STUDY BIOENERGY

Scientific approaches demonstrating the presence of vital energy are difficult to design. Bioenergy may be immeasurable yet many patients, and therapists, will continue to use bioenergy approaches if they are convinced of its efficacy, no matter the resolve of a specific scientific or medical, community to discount benefits wheneven there is scientific demonstration of inefficacy. Adjusting bioenergy fields through: acupuncture, therapeutic touch, Qi Gong, Johrei, Reiki, crystal therapy, and magnet therapy may improve health but much of the data are too preliminary to recommend any therapy without question[44] (except, perhaps, for acupuncture, which will be discussed in detail in Chap. 7). If they do alter disease processes, the extent of benefit, and the mechanisms responsible are unknown.

Traditional Chinese medicine (TCM) encompasses folk practices based on mysticism and bioenergy.[45,46] A recent analysis of 2938 clinical trials reported in Chinese medical journals showed the Chinese data are inconclusive.[46,47] Chinese trials were qualitative, short term, small, poorly controlled, rarely blinded, and contained inadequate data outcomes can vary by country. Over half did not report baseline characteristics or side effects. The quality of these studies has not been compared to data upon which cardiologists make clinical decisions.

FORMS OF BIOENERGETICS

The techniques share common features: (1) focus on "bioenergy" by practitioners and (2) "energy transfer" leading to beneficial effects. These techniques are often culturally based, intention-based, ritualistic, and regimented even though they may be tailored to the patient.[49,50] They can involve an external healer or the patient himself (such as self-hypnosis). They can involve healing at a distance, nonliving, or inanimate objects to facilitate the response. The response can be taught but it can vary from individual to individual healer.

Psychotherapy

Often not considered a bioenergetic technique, this type of "talk therapy" offers no substantial intervention and may be one of the purest and most acceptable bioenergetic techniques to heal the mind using a series of well-defined, but often disputed, concepts and techniques. This may be one of the purist forms of placebo response seen in medical care and yet is well accepted broadly throughout the medical profession. Recent data on existential psychotherapy support the use of this technique[51] but psychotherapy in general is well grounded in data that show its benefits. For example, recent data show that psychotherapy can affect physical conditions, such as diabetes,[52] and can affect sleep in individuals with fibromyalgia.[53]

Relaxation and meditation

Relaxation therapy in 192 men having two or more risk factors for coronary artery disease was associated with better outcomes compared to a control group.[54] "Type A" persons tend to have a higher incidence of hypertension and death from cardiovascular disease. They may benefit from the relaxation response.[55–59] The relaxation response may affect heart failure the outcomes.[60] Meditation may affect cortical thickness of the brain.[61] Self-hypnosis techniques and meditation may affect anxiety, psychological distress, and influence secondary outcomes.[62–64] Meditation may even be a form of hypnotism.[65]

Hypnotism

Hypnotism has been used with and without other psychological interventions to improve outcomes in patients, reduce pain, reduce anxiety, and have other beneficial effects.[65–73] It may be useful to combine hypnotism with standard analgesic therapy for those in pain.[74] Hypnotism may improve wound healing.[75]

There are several forms of hypnotism. Not all patients can be hypnotized,[76,77] but the effects appear to be real and impressive depending on the condition, the patient, the cause for the condition, and the patient's response to hypnotism. Those individuals who can be hypnotized may be at lower risk for poor cardiovascular outcomes than those who cannot. Therefore, it may be difficult to compare outcomes based on hypnosis when less than proper randomization is undertaken.[78] Patients who can be hypnotized may differ from those who cannot.[79] Hypnosis does appear to have many potential medical uses. It can affect pain, irritable bowel syndrome, autonomic responses, healing responses, and have cardiovascular variables.[75,78,80–87] It may have a beneficial effect in multiple sclerosis.[88] There appears to be specific neurobiological affects of hypnotism that may explain its effect but the data are not robust.

Qi Gong

Practitioners of the external Qi Gong generally claim the ability to emit or direct healing energy to treat patients. Qi Gong has increased dramatically over the past several years. "Qi" is life force energy and "Gong" is "practicing skill." Vital energy is said to circulate through "meridians," connecting all organs. Illness is attributed to an imbalance, or interruption, of qi. Qi Gong is said to rebalance "yin" and "yang".[89] "External Qi Gong" affects things outside one's body. It is performed by masters who claim to cure with energy released from their fingertips.[90] Devotees claim they can control Qi to diagnose and cure various physical conditions.[91,92] Attempts have been made to store the beneficial forms of Qi Gong on paper and other materials.[93] It is said that Qi can bounce off individuals.[94] On the EEG, the peak frequency of alpha activity during a Qi Gong state, occurring predominantly in the anterior regions, is slower than the resting state.[95]

Over 1300 references on Qi Gong suggest benefit to treat hypertension, respiratory diseases, and cancer. For hypertension, lower stroke and mortality rates have been shown in preliminary studies.[96] Qi Gong may benefit some patients with atherosclerotic obstruction of the lower extremities.[97] Breathing approaches may influence patients with mitral valve prolapse.[98] Qi Gong may influence and reduce respiratory rate, heart rate, blood pressure, and accentuate vagal tone demonstrated by changes in heart rate variability.[99–101] Qi Gong has been reported to improve circulation and lower blood pressure, as well as relax spastic muscles[90] and qi training may affect heart rate, respiration rate, and blood pressure.[94] The clinical significance and mechanisms are unclear.[91] External qi energy may affect phagocytic activity of human polymorphonuclear leukocytes.[102] It may facilitate cardiac rehabilitation in the elderly and improve outcomes in trail fibrillation.[104]

Internal Qi Gong involves deep breathing, concentration, and relaxation. It is self-discipline that trains body and mind to alter flow of "vital energy," for self-reliance and adjustment, to cure disease; and to strengthen and prolong life. A form of Qi Gong, using breathing and relaxation instruction in 76 post-myocardial infarction patients, showed improvement in respiratory rate, heart rate, and respiratory sinus arrhythmia.[104] In hypertensive patients, Qi Gong was associated with 6-K-PGF1-α-level increases and a decrease in TXB2/6-K-PGF1-α ratio.[94] While Qi Gong may or may not have benefit it appears harmless.[105a,b,106]

Reiki

Rei is "universal" or "spiritual," and Ki is "life force energy." Reiki uses "healing energy" to enhance vitality, resilience, and health for practitioner and patient.[107] It is another form of laying in the hands.[108] Its most profound effect is deep relaxation, resulting in reduction of stress. It works supposedly, only if the receiver can detect the subtle, personal, unconscious energy. Energy patterns are considered as different "vibrational frequencies." A practitioner "attuned" to the energy places his hands onto or just above the patient's body at strategic points (chakras) to transfer energy. The patient may report a flow of energy, often in places remote from the point at which the practitioner has their hands. Channeling this energy is purported to produce beneficial effects but scientifically demonstrable cardiovascular benefits have not been shown. There do appear to be, however, of Reiki touch healing that may be related to blood pressure and humeral immune function.

There are several stages of Reiki. A first-degree therapist (Reiki I) uses 12-hand positions placed gently on the body to facilitate flow of energy through the practitioner. A second-degree therapist (Reiki II) can send energy to anyone, anywhere (i.e., a form of distance healing). A Reiki Master (Reiki III) can initiate others to all levels of Reiki. Reiki can only enhance natural healing already taking place and it is considered an adjunct to other treatments. It supposedly benefits healer and patients.

No scientific study demonstrates any cardiovascular benefits. There is an ongoing National Center for Complementary and Alternative Medicine (NCCAM) study to evaluate if Reiki can improve glycemic control and dysautonomia in diabetics with autonomic neuropathy. Initial studies suggest that Reiki has an affect on the autonomic nervous system.[109]

Johrei

Johrei, a spiritual energy healing practice, differs from Reiki and Qi Gong. In the latter two disciplines, the therapist is removing negative energy from the individual, who has health problems. With Johrei, it is possible that the giver of energy can obtain a benefit as well as the receiver. In one report, 236 participants rated 21 items related to feelings plus an overall well-being measure, before and after a Johrei session. Receivers experienced a greater decrease in negative emotional state than givers; however, both experienced a positive emotional state and overall well-being. The mechanisms for these effects were unknown.[110]

Music therapy

Music has been used to enhance hypnotic states for millennia. Those who appreciate it know the benefits of music. There are indeed some data to support the use of medicine in the health-care environment[111] and promote relaxation.[112] Music can enhance specific emotions, create both positive and negative affects. It can be enlightening or relaxing dependent upon the type of music, the situation, and the individual experiencing the music. Music may have more of an impact on those who appreciate it and not have a universal effect. Little has been done to evaluate scientifically the benefits of music on mood and outcome with respect to health. Nevertheless, music is frequently used in the health-care environment to benefit outcomes. Further, from a business standpoint, music and Muzak have both been used to enhance shopping and improve the environment in which the customer may feel more comfortable to spend more money.

Art therapy

Similar to music therapy, any form of art therapy, including poetry and literature and visual arts, may have benefits in terms of changing emotional responses to specific adverse medical conditions. While this makes perfect sense, very little scientific data support the use of art therapy to enhance outcomes of patients. Nevertheless, in a medical setting, the presence of a relaxing and artistic environment improves the acceptability of delivering healthcare to those who are in need. While this is not clearly known by the health-care profession, it is also self-evident and used by administrators and those involved in the business of medicine to improve acceptability of health-care environments for patients. Therapies, such as guided imagery, that may tap into artistic endeavors similarly provide accepting environment into which an individual requiring healing or in pain may be more likely to develop a beneficial rather than an adverse response. All of these responses are related to the cultural milieu and the individual.

Healing touch/therapeutic touch

Healing touch is another form of "laying on of the hands." Healing touch has been associated with reduction in a stress response and perceived enhancement that is independent of a placebo effect.[113] A recent review of 30 studies showed no generalizable effect could be found from healing touch.[114]

Some have declared healing touch to be a pseudoscience.[115] Despite these caveats, techniques such as healing touch continue to be used.[116] Studies also continue, some of which show benefit from a gentle touch approach for stress reduction.[117]

In therapeutic touch, hands are used to direct healing energy as well. Healing supposedly results from transfer of "excess energy" from healer to patient. Therapeutic touch was conceived in the 1970s by Dolores Krieger.[118] Therapeutic touch involves "centering" (align the healer to the patient's energy level), "assessment" (hands detect forces from the patient), "unruffling the field" (sweeping stagnant energy downward to prepare for energy transfer), and energy transfer (from practitioner to patient).[119] This technique has been promoted and discussed intensively over years,[120] even though there was little sound scientific data supporting its use and it is clearly not shown to work for every condition.[121] Data are often in the form of case report benefits.[122]

Therapeutic touch may reduce anxiety.[123,124] There may be a relationship between autonomic affects, stress, and therapeutic touch but this relationship may or may not be robust.[125] No sound scientific evidence supports postulated "energy transfer" benefits claimed. Benefits reported may simply be due to literal "laying on of hands." Controlled trials are hard to design.[126] A similar technique, known as "bioterapia," "unifies mind, body and energy dimensions."[127]

Therapeutic touch is based on the concept of a human energy field. In one trial of therapeutic touch, 21 practitioners were tested in blinded fashion to determine if they could identify an individual's correct hand.

Therapeutic touch practitioners identified to correct hand in 123 out of 280 (44%) trials. This is similar to random chance. The investigators were unable to detect any specific energy field. Therefore, data do not suggest that therapeutic touch is based on any true observations. It was stated that "unrefuted evidence that claims of therapeutic touch are groundless and its use is unjustified."[128] It has been suggested that the study showing no benefit of therapeutic touch had an inadequate study design.[129] Eleven other studies using therapeutic touch were also negative. Recent data suggest that therapeutic touch may even benefit patients with dementia.[130]

Distance healing

There is much overlap between therapeutic touch, distance healing, and distance prayer. Beutler showed small but significant changes in diastolic blood pressure in a double-blind controlled study of distance healing.[131] One study has shown benefit of distance (blinded) prayer on autonomic tone based on skin conductance levels and "blood volume pulse."[132]

Astin reviewed the data on distance healing systematically (prayer, mental healing, therapeutic touch, or spiritual healing).[37] Based on a total of 23 trials involving 2774 patients, 5 examined prayer, 11 assessed noncontact therapeutic touch, and 7 examined other forms of distant healing (study heterogeneity precluded a meta-analysis). Thirteen (57%) had statistically significant treatment effects and nine showed no effect over control. One study showed a negative effect.[133,134] While these data made it difficult to draw conclusions, Astin thought the 57% positive treatment effect was remarkable and may be a reason to consider further study.[37] Intercessory prayer, discussed in Chap. 12, may be a form of distance healing.[39,40,133–135]

Meditation

With meditation, the distinctions between unconscious and the conscious mind are presumably removed. The potential psychic, spiritual, emotional, reordering may have consequent physical effects. Meditation, although not universally considered bioenergy therapy, can alter blood distribution in the brain observed by MRI scans and can increase delta wave activity observed on the EEG. Rage behavior decreases. Transcendental meditation has been linked to reduction in cardiovascular mortality.[136–139] It can lower blood pressure and have other beneficial cardiovascular effects.[140–143] Zen meditation has been associated with improved heart rate variability and slowing in respiratory rate.[144,145] Alternatively, even years ago, data did not support anything unique about meditation practice with regard to any specific physiological measurements.[146–148]

Meditation may reduce cardiovascular mortality and improve blood pressure. On the functional MRI, improvements have been seen. Delta wave activity increases on the EEG. Heart rate variability improves and it is a slowing in the heart rate. A recently pilot study compared transcendental meditation with Ayurvedic medicine and dietary interventions to an American Heart Association-based diet and exercise program and assessed atherosclerosis progression by measuring changes in carotid intimal medial thickness at 1 year. There is an ongoing NCCAM trial in patients with coronary artery disease to evaluate vasomotor dysfunction (i.e., brachial artery reactivity), autonomic nervous system imbalance (by heart rate variability), transient myocardial ischemia (by ST-segment depression on the electrocardiogram), psychological stress, and quality of life.

Yoga

Different types of yoga have been developed. Some evolved because of focusing only on physical postures and not on the philosophical basis of the practice. Iyengar yoga is comprehensive and traditional with basis in philosophy and theory. Pranayama is yoga of breathing. Kevala Pranayama means isolated, pure, absolute, and perfect. The master of Kevala Pranayama is in tune with the Infinite. The mind absorbed with Prana is described as free.

Movements and positions in yoga and the breathing exercises can lower the blood pressure and alter breathing patterns. Hatha yoga appears to improve the vital capacity of college students.[149] Breathing techniques can affect and improve ambulatory blood pressure and heart rate.[150] Yoga is described as improving strength and flexibility and helping to control blood pressure, respiration and heart rate, and metabolic rate.[151,152]

Pranic psychotherapy

Application of pranic healing to psychological ailments uses chakras, meridians ("bioplasmic channels"), and an "energy body" that consists of an "inner aura," an "outer aura," and a "health aura." Pranic psychotherapy includes removal and disintegration of "traumatic psychic energy," disintegration of "negative elementals" ("bad spirits"), and creation of a "positive thought entity."

Ho'oponopono

A Hawaiian form of conflict resolution, ho'oponopono, is a method to resolve conflict through culturally appropriate family therapy and maintain dynamics of Hawaiian social relations.[152] This Hawaiian approach alleges to find the divine within oneself to remove stress and release problems. It involves repentance and "transmutation" to provide spiritual freedom, love, peace, and wisdom.

Applied kinesiology

This chiropractic technique is performed by therapists, using acupressure points and a muscle-testing method to diagnose nutritional and glandular "deficiencies," which are then "corrected" by manipulation or nutrition supplements but there is little substantiated supportive data.

Mental physics

Mental Physics is purported to be a practical, holistic, futuristic science that manifests "hidden meaning" of the Bible and involves "astral travel," aura reading, chanting, meditation, pranayama ("deep scientific breathing exercises"), "pranic therapy" (a variant of channeling), reflexology, shiatsu, and individualization of diet according to "chemical type". Its use is not supported by sound data.

Rei-so

Rei-so is based on the concept that consciousness, energy, or vibration from the dead can influence health but there is no proven benefit.

Vibrational medicine

Considers humans as dynamic energy systems ("body/mind/spirit" complexes). The dynamic energy system, the life force, is influenced by subtle emotional, spiritual, nutritional, and environmental energies. The concept is to resonate with these energies. Health and illness originate in "subtle energy systems". Several "therapies" use the concepts of vibrational medicine: aromatherapy, chakra rebalancing, distance healing, flower essence therapy, homeopathy,

Kirlian photography, moxibustion, orthomolecular medicine, past life regression, radionics, and other unfounded approaches.

Magnetotherapy

This is applied with permanent or fluctuant magnetic fields, but there are no proven benefits for the cardiovascular disease.[153–155] Scherlag has been evaluating, in an animal model, low-level gauss fields in the right atrium. He has shown change in sinus rate and interruption in atrial fibrillation in preliminary studies with low-level gauss fields.[156]

Crystal therapy

Crystal therapy uses the power of crystal energy fields to heal. Each crystal is associated with different energy fields or emotions. There is no evidence for this approach.

Homeopathy

This is, in a sense, not bioenergetics but the concept is that water is energized by compounds in extremely dilute amounts. Water is thought to retain the memory of the compounds that existed in it. A recent large meta-analysis of homeopathic treatments in the *Lancet* of over 80 manuscripts indicated, compared to placebo, that homeopathic treatments might be effective but not all agree with this.[158] While the results were significant, concerning any one-disease entity no significant treatment could be discerned but the therapies were not standardized. MRI scanning of water suggests there might be some truth to this but no data have demonstrated health benefits for cardiovascular disease.

BIOENERGY SUMMARY

Bioenergy therapies tap into vital energy. The evidence demonstrating healing properties of bioenergetic techniques is relatively weak.[159a,b] Studies are ongoing but they are difficult to design. A recent review of energy-healing therapies even suggests that there could be potential harm and that energy-healing therapies only have shown evidence of a placebo effect without any additional efficacy.[159a,b] There is now even some evidence to suggest that energy healing may have potentially adverse effects. Despite the lack of any conclusive data, therapies are likely to continue in lieu of any scientific data showing inefficacy. They may continue even if data demonstrated was based on standard scientific approaches.

Apparent benefits may be simply a placebo effect but there are some data to demonstrate that bioenergetic therapies may be more than that. It is difficult to sort out actual effects of the therapies being studied since evaluations are often carried out by individuals strongly biased in favor of the therapy being tested. Potential apparent benefits from bioenergy therapies may be related to other explanations. Patients may undergo "energy healing" and be cured from a condition that they do not even have (a misdiagnosis). A bioenergy practitioner may exaggerate or create an illusion of the benefit of therapy. Biases for, and against, bioenergy healing make it even more difficult to assess the quality of the data.

WHEN TO CONSIDER BIOENERGETICS

Bioenergetic approaches should be considered when the standard medical therapies fail to provide complete efficacious results. Bioenergetic techniques should also be considered for potential functional problems or for symptoms that appear to be extremely difficult to manage. These techniques, however, will most likely work only if affective to the individual who may have a preference for one form or the other. It is unlikely that any one bioenergetic technique will work for all patients.

Nevertheless, there are practitioners who use many of these bioenergetic techniques and know how to apply them to specific patients to get a beneficial response. Most medical problems involve issues that are related to the mind-body interaction and that attempting to address a specific organ system or problem may not achieve complete desirable results. Supplementation with a bioenergetic technique can facilitate better outcomes. Most bioenergetic techniques should not be used in lieu of standard, accepted, and proven medical therapy. It is only when standard therapy does not elicit an optimal symptomatic improvement that a bioenergetic technique should be considered. There is no bioenergetic approach that is fully recommended but then none is fully contraindicated. To date, there have been no specific dangers of bioenergetic techniques that have caused harm to patients unless they avoid medical therapies that could improve their outcome.

CAVEATS

The listed approaches appear safe. Potential adverse influences may be the release of inhibitions causing anger, hostility, or "negative" energy or reduction of needed sympathetic tone. No bioenergy therapy has been shown to alter the natural course of cardiovascular disease.[32,153] These therapeutic approaches may have benefit as an adjunct to standard medial therapies and may be a godsend for patients with severe functional, symptomatic complaints. They could be considered a first-line approach as long as serious cardiovascular conditions are ruled out, but ethics of using unproven approaches are arguable. Bioenergy approaches should not be considered substitutes for standard medical care; they may offer false hope at an expensive price.

Specific benefits from bioenergetic therapies are difficult to measure, and therefore it is difficult to design studies. Practitioners who have developed expertise in these techniques and patients who use them will likely continue to use them even without a scientific foundation. How to determine practitioner qualifications is difficult.[32] The only way is to go by "reputation," essentially, by patient referrals. It would be best to work with bioenergy practitioners who respect standard practices as well and do not turn patients away from accepted care and physicians. Certifications and qualifications are questionable. Studies evaluating benefits of these techniques may be difficult to design as practitioners often have an antiscientific focus.

Controlled trials in bioenergy are difficult to design. Withholding standard medical therapy to assess bioenergy therapies is unethical. "Benefits" may represent the natural course of a disease or the patient's or therapist's interpretation of the condition, and any study demonstrating benefit of a bioenergy therapy must be considered carefully. Positive results may represent experimenter biases not obvious from the study design.

It is important that patients do not expect that bioenergetic techniques alone will provide full healing. False hope given in this regard may be harmful to the patient. There is also the issue of considering the use of an unproven therapy and its ethics. Nevertheless, it appears that as long as the patient is properly treated otherwise and nothing else is overlooked, bioenergetic techniques may be useful in improving outcomes of selected patients.

CHOOSING A PRACTITIONER

There are no specific rules to follow when choosing a bioenergy healer. It is best to consider a committed practitioner with a good reputation, who appears to have good results and is willing to work closely with patients and with other medical professionals. Such an individual is likely to share information with other practitioners to enhance the outcome of the patients. Such an individual is often committed to the best for the patient.

RECOMMENDATIONS

If a bioenergy treatment does not interfere with standard, accepted, and proven therapy, it can be used. If standard therapies do not provide optimal, symptomatic, improvement, or are potentially functional for a condition, it is acceptable to consider a bioenergy approach. No such approach is fully recommended but none is contraindicated. The most data exist for acupuncture. No bioenergy therapy should be considered a substitute for standard, accepted, and approved therapies. If any bioenergy approach is considered, a practitioner who has a good reputation, appears to have good results, and is willing to work with the medical professionals should be chosen and could be recommended.

THE POWER OF BIOENERGY—A LITTLE SECRET

Patients need laying on of hands. All true healers possess that power to do this well. It may not involve science but it is important nevertheless. Every committed healer has the power and this can be manifest. Use the power well for the benefit of the patients.

REFERENCES

1. Benford MS. Radiogenic metabolism: an alternative cellular energy source. Med Hypotheses. 2001;56:33–9.
2. Talbot M. The holographic universe. New York: Harper Perennial; 1991.
3. Pribram K. The holographic paradigm.
4. Bohm D. Phyisics. The perennial philosophy and seth. St. Louis, MO: Living Lake Books; 1994.
5. Seaward BL. Alternative medicine complements standard. Various forms focus on holistic concepts. Health Prog. 1994;75:52–7.
6. Radin D. The conscious universe. San Francisco, CA: Harper; 1997.
7. Patterson EF. The philosophy and physics of holistic health care: spiritual healing as a workable interpretation. J Adv Nurs. 1998;27:287–93.
8. Song LZ, Schwartz GE, Russek LG. Heart-focused attention and heart-brain synchronization: energetic and physiological mechanisms. Altern Ther Health Med. 1998;4:44–52, 54–60, 62.
9. Lin MC, Nahin R, Gershwin ME, Longhurst JC, Wu KK. State of complementary and alternative medicine in cardiovascular, lung, and blood research: executive summary of a workshop. Circulation. 2001;103:2038–41.
10. Nelson LA, Schwartz GE. Human biofield and intention detection: individual differences. J Altern Complement Med. 2005;11:93–101.
11. Warber SL, Cornelio D, Straughn J, Kile G. Biofield energy healing from the inside. J Altern Complement Med. 2004;10:1107–13.
12. Olshansky B, Dossey L. Retroactive prayer: a preposterous hypothesis? BMJ. 2003;327:1465–8.
13. Staats PS, Hekmat H, Staats AW. The psychological behaviorism theory of pain and the placebo: its principles and results of research application. Adv Psychosom Med. 2004;25:28A–40.
14. Olshansky B. Placebo and Nocebo in Cardiovascular Health: Implications for Healthcare, Research and the Doctor-Patient Relationship. J Am Coll Cardiol. 2007;49:415–421.
15. Hoyersten JG. The berserks—what was wrong with them? Tidsskr Nor Laegeforen. 2004;124:3247–50.
16. Vogel JHK, Bolling SF, Costello RB, Guarneri EM, Krucoff MW, Longhurst JC, et al. Integrating complementary medicine into cardiovascular medicine. A report of the American College of Cardiology Foundation Task Force on Clinical Expert Consensus Documents (Writing Committee to Develop an Expert Consensus Document on Complementary and Integrative Medicine). J Am Coll Cardiol. 2005;46:184–221.

17. Grippo AJ, Francis J, Weiss RM, Felder RB, Johnson AK. Cytokine mediation of experimental heart failure-induced anhedonia. Am J Physiol Regul Integr Comp Physiol. 2003;284:R666–73.

18. Grippo AJ, Francis J, Beltz TG, Felder RB, Johnson AK. Neuroendocrine and cytokine profile of chronic mild stress-induced anhedonia. Physiol Behav. 2005;84: 697–706.

19. Haid M, Huprikar S. Modulation of germination and growth of plants by meditation. Am J Chin Med. 2001;29:393–401.

20. Yount G, Solfvin J, Moore D, Schlitz M, Reading M, Aldape K, et al. In vitro test of external Qi Gong. BMC Complement Altern Med. 2004;4:5.

21. Ostendorf GM. Naturopathy and alternative medicine—definition of the concept and delineation. Offentl Gesundheitswes. 1991;53:84–7.

22. Dossey L. Healing words: the power of prayer and the practice of medicine. San Francisco, CA; Harper, 1993.

23. Berk LS, Felten DL, Tan SA, Bittman BB, Westengard J. Modulation of neuroimmune parameters during the eustress of humor-associated mirthful laughter. Altern Ther Health Med. 200;7:62–72, 74–6.

24. Coronary Drug Project Research Group. Influence of adherence to treatment and response of cholesterol on mortality in the coronary drug project. N Engl J Med. 1980;303:1038–41.

25. Horwitz RI, Viscoli CM, Berkman L, Donaldson RM, Horwitz SM, Murray CJ, et al. Treatment adherence and risk of death after a myocardial infarction. Lancet. 1990;336:542–5.

26. Gallagher EJ, Viscoli CM, Horwitz RI. The relationship of treatment adherence to the risk of death after myocardial infarction in women. JAMA. 1993;270:742–4.

27. Hrobjartsson A, Gotzsche PC. Is the placebo powerless? An analysis of clinical trials comparing placebo with no treatment. N Engl J Med. 2001;344:1594–602.

28. Ray WJ, Oathes D. Brain imaging techniques. Int J Clin Exp Hypn. 2003; 51:97–104.

29. Freeman TB, Vawter DE, Leaverton PE, Godbold JH, Hausner RA, Goetz CG, et al. Use of placebo surgery in controlled trials of a cellular-based therapy for Parkinson's disease. N Engl J Med. 1999;341:988–92.

30. Leuchter AF, Cook IA, Witte EA, Morgan M, Abrams M. Changes in brain function of depressed subjects during treatment with placebo. Am J Psychiatry. 2002; 159:122–9.

31. Maruta T, Colligan RC, Malinchoc M, Offorc KP. Optimism-pessimism assessed in the 1960s and self-reported health status 30 years later. Mayo Clin Proc. 2002;77:748–453.

32. Daly J, Elliott D, Cameron Traub E, Salamonson Y, Davidson P, Jackson D, Chin C, Wade V. Health status, perceptions of coping, and social support immediately after discharge of survivors of acute myocardial infarction. Am J Crit Care. 200;9:62–69.

33. Fry PS. Perfectionism, humor, and optimism as moderators of health outcomes and determinants of coping styles of women executives. Genet Soc Gen Psychol Monogr. 1995;121:211–245.

34. Schroder KE, Schwarzer R. Habitual self-control and the management of health behavior among heart patients. Soc Sci Med. 2005;60:859–875.

35. Sears SF, Serber ER, Lewis TS, Walker RL, Conners N, Lee JT, Curtis AB, Conti JB. Do positive health expectations and optimism relate to quality-of-life outcomes for the patients with an implantable cardioverter defibrillator? J Cardiopulm Rehabil. 2004;24:324–331.

36. Cho ZH, Chung SC, Jones JP, Park JB, Park HJ, Lee HJ, et al. New findings of the correlation between acupoints and corresponding brain cortices using functional MRI. Proc Natl Acad Sci USA. 1998;95:2670–3.

37. Astin JA, Harkness E, Ernst E. The efficacy of "distant healing": a systematic review of randomized trials. Ann Intern Med. 2000;132:903–10.

38. Sicher F, Targ E, Moore D, II, Smith HS. A randomized double-blind study of the effect of distant healing in a population with advanced AIDS. Report of a small scale study. West J Med. 1998;169:356–63.

39. Krucoff MW, Crater SW, Gallup D, Blankenship JC, Cuffe M, Guarneri M, et al. Music, imagery, touch, and prayer as adjuncts to interventional cardiac care: the Monitoring and Actualisation of Noetic Trainings (MANTRA) II randomised study. Lancet. 2005;366:211–7.

40. Krucoff MW, Crater SW, Green CL, Maas AC, Seskevich JE, Lane JD, et al. Integrative noetic therapies as adjuncts to percutaneous intervention during unstable coronary syndromes: Monitoring and Actualization of Noetic Training (MANTRA) feasibility pilot. Am Heart J. 2001;142:760–9.

41. Francis J, Wei SG, Weiss RM, Beltz T, Johnson AK, Felder RB. Forebrain-mediated adaptations to myocardial infarction in the rat. Am J Physiol Heart Circ Physiol. 2002;282:H1898–906.

42. Sox HC, Jr., Margulies I, Sox CH. Psychologically mediated effects of diagnostic tests. Ann Intern Med. 1981;95:680–5.

43. Patel C. Psychophysiological coping strategies in the prevention of coronary heart disease. Act Nerv Super (Praha). 1982;Suppl 2:403–21.

44. Shang C. Emerging paradigms in mind-body medicine. J Altern Complement Med. 2001;7:83–91.

45. Yu GP, Gao SW. Quality of clinical trials of Chinese herbal drugs, a review of 314 published papers. Zhongguo Zhong Xi Yi Jie He Za Zhi. 1994;14:50–2.

46. Xie ZF LN. Methodological analysis of clinical articles on therapy evaluation published in Chinese Journal of Integrated Traditional and Western Medicine. Chin J Integrated Tradit West Med. 1995;1:3016.

47. Tang JL, Zhan SY, Ernst E. Review of randomised controlled trials of traditional Chinese medicine. BMJ. 1999;319:160–1.

48. Vickers A, Goyal N, Harland R, Rees R. Do certain countries produce only positive results? A systematic review of controlled trials. Control Clin Trials. 1998;19:159–66.

49. Schwartz GE, Swanick S, Sibert W, Lewis DA, Lewis SE, Nelson L, et al. Biofield detection: role of bioenergy awareness training and individual differences in absorption. J Altern Complement Med. 2004;10:167–9.

50. Schlitz M, Wiseman R. Experimenter effects and the remote detection of staring. J Parapsychol. 1997;61:197–208.

51. Iglesias A. Hypnosis and existential psychotherapy with end-stage terminally ill patients. Am J Clin Hypn. 2004;46:201–13.

52. Ellis DA, Frey MA, Naar-King S, Templin T, Cunningham PB, Cakan N. The effects of multisystemic therapy on diabetes stress among adolescents with chronically poorly controlled type 1 diabetes: findings from a randomized, controlled trial. Pediatrics. 2005;116:e826–32.

53. Edinger JD, Wohlgemuth WK, Krystal AD, Rice JR. Behavioral insomnia therapy for fibromyalgia patients: a randomized clinical trial. Arch Intern Med. 2005;165:2527–35.

54. Patel C, Marmot MG, Terry DJ, Carruthers M, Hunt B, Patel M. Trial of relaxation in reducing coronary risk: four year follow u. Br Med J (Clin Res Ed). 1985;290:1103–1106.

55. Wolsko PM, Eisenberg DM, Davis RB, Phillips RS. Use of mind-body medical therapies. J Gen Intern Med. 2004;19:43–50.
56. Jacobs GD. Clinical applications of the relaxation response and mind-body interventions. J Altern Complement Med. 2001;7(Suppl 1):S93–101.
57. Esch T, Frivvhione GL, Stefano GB. The therapeutic use of the relaxation response in stress-related diseases. Med Sci Monit. 2003;9:RA23–24.
58. Nelson C, Franks S, Brose A, Raven P, Williamson J, Shi X, McGill J, Harrell E. The influence of hostility and family history of cardiovascular disease on automatic activation in response to controllable versus noncontrollable stress, anger imagery induction and relaxation imagery. J Behav Med. 2005;28:213–221.
59. Benson H, Alexander S, Feldman CL. Decreased premature ventricular contractions through use of the relaxation response in patients with stable ischaemic heart-disease. Lanect. 1975;2:380–332.
60. Chang BH, Jones D, Hendricks A, Boehmer U, Locastro JS, Slawsky M. Relaxation response for veterans affairs patients with congestive heart failure: results from a qualitative study within a clinical trial. Prev Cardiol. 2004;7:64–70.
61. Lazar SW, Kerr CE, Wasserman RH, Gray JR, Greve DN, Treadway MT, et al. Meditation experience is associated with increased cortical thickness. Neuroreport. 2005;16:1893–7.
62. Benson H, Frankel FH, Apfel R, Daniels MD, Schniewind HE, Nemiah JC, et al. Treatment of anxiety: a comparison of the usefulness of self-hypnosis and a meditational relaxation technique. An overview. Psychother Psychosom. 1978;30:229–42.
63. Deckro GR, Ballinger KM, Hoyt M, Wilcher M, Dusek J, Myers P, et al. The evaluation of a mind/body intervention to reduce psychological distress and perceived stress in college students. J Am Coll Health. 2002;50:281–7.
64. Lang R, Dehof K, Meurer KA, Kaufmann W. Sympathetic activity and transcendental meditation. J Neural Transm. 1979;44:117–35.
65. Barmark SM, Gaunitz SC. Transcendental meditation and heterohypnosis as altered states of consciousness. Int J Clin Exp Hypn. 1979;27:227–39.
66. Hypnosis: a safe and potent pain reliever. Consum Rep. 2005;70:49.
67. Hypnosis. Deep relaxation can relieve pain and more. Mayo Clin Womens Healthsource. 2002;6:7.
68. Hypnosis. More than a suggestion. Harv Health Lett. 1997;22:4–5.
69. Agargun MY, Tekeoglu I, Kara H, Adak B, Ercan M. Hypnotizability, pain threshold, and dissociative experiences. Biol Psychiatry. 1998;44:69–71.
70. Croft RJ, Williams JD, Haenschel C, Gruzelier JH. Pain perception, hypnosis and 40 Hz oscillations. Int J Psychophysiol. 2002;46:101–8.
71. Crawford HJ, Knebel T, Kaplan L, et al. Hypnotic analgesia: 1. Somatosensory event-related potential changes to noxious stimuli and 2. Transfer learning to reduce chronic low back pain. Int J Clin Exp Hypn. 1998;46:92–132.
72. Chaves JF, Dworkin SF. Hypnotic control of pain: historical perspectives and future prospects. Int J Clin Exp Hypn. 1997;45:356–76.
73. Cadranel JF, Benhamou Y, Zylberberg P, Novello P, Luciani F, Valla D, et al. Hypnotic relaxation: a new sedative tool for colonoscopy? J Clin Gastroenterol. 1994;18:127–9.
74. Faymonville ME, Fissette J, Mambourg PH, Roediger L, Joris J, Lamy M. Hypnosis as adjunct therapy in conscious sedation for plastic surgery. Reg Anesth. 1995;20: 145–51.
75. Ginandes C, Brooks P, Sando W, Jones C, Aker J. Can medical hypnosis accelerate post-surgical wound healing? Results of a clinical trial. Am J Clin Hypn. 2003;45:333–51.
76. Lynn SJ, Shindler K. The role of hypnotizability assessment in treatment. Am J Clin Hypn. 2002;44:185–97.

77. Nash M. Salient findings: a potentially groundbreaking study on the neuroscience of hypnotizability, a critical review of hypnosis' efficacy, and the neurophysiology of conversion disorder. Int J Clin Exp Hypn. 2005;53:87–93.

78. Sebastiani L, Simoni A, Gemignani A, Ghelarducci B, Santarcangelo EL. Autonomic and EEG correlates of emotional imagery in subjects with different hypnotic susceptibility. Brain Res Bull. 2003;60:151–60.

79. Jorgensen MM, Zacharia R. Autonomic reactivity to cognitive and emotional stress of low, medium, and high hypnotizable healthy subjects: testing predictions from the high risk model of threat perception. Int J Clin Exp Hypn. 2002;50:248–75.

80. Forbes A, MacAuley S, Chiotakakou-Faliakou E. Hypnotherapy and therapeutic audiotape: effective in previously unsuccessfully treated irritable bowel syndrome? Int J Colorectal Dis. 2000;15:328–34.

81. Ray WJ, Sabsevitz D, De Pascalis V, Quigley K, Aikins D, Tubbs M. Cardiovascular reactivity during hypnosis and hypnotic susceptibility: three studies of heart rate variability. Int J Clin Exp Hypn. 2000;48:22–31.

82. Ture H, Ture U, Gogus FY, Valavanis A, Yasargil MG. The art of alleviating pain in Greek mythology. Neurosurgery. 2005;56:178–85; discussion 185–6.

83. Tan G, Hammond DC, Joseph G. Hypnosis and irritable bowel syndrome: a review of efficacy and mechanism of action. Am J Clin Hypn. 2005;47:161–78.

84. Butler LD, Symons BK, Henderson SL, Shortliffe LD, Spiegel D. Hypnosis reduces distress and duration of an invasive medical procedure for children. Pediatrics 2005;115:e77–85.

85. Sebastiani L, Simoni A, Gemignani A, Ghelarducci B, Santarcangelo EL. Human hypnosis: autonomic and electroencephalographic correlates of a guided multi-modal cognitive-emotional imagery. Neurosci Lett. 2003;338:41–4.

86. Ray WJ, Keil A, Mikuteit A, Bongartz W, Elbert T. High resolution EEG indicators of pain responses in relation to hypnotic susceptibility and suggestion. Biol Psychol. 2002;60:17–36.

87. Emdin M, Santarcangelo EL, Picano E, Raciti M, Pola S, Macerata A, et al. Hypnosis effect on RR interval and blood pressure variability. Clin Sci (Lond). 1996;91 Suppl:36:36–8.

88. Dane JR. Hypnosis for pain and neuromuscular rehabilitation with multiple sclerosis: case summary, literature review, and analysis of outcomes. Int J Clin Exp Hypn. 1996;44:208–31.

89. Kuang AK, Jiang MD, Wang CX, Zhao GS, Xu DH. Research on the mechanism of "Qi Gong (breathing exercise)". A preliminary study on its effect in balancing "Yin" and "Yang," regulating circulation and promoting flow in the meridian system. J Tradit Chin Med. 1981;1:7–10.

90. Omura Y, Lin TL, Debreceni L, Losco BM, Freed S, Muteki T, et al. Unique changes found on the Qi Gong (Chi Gong) master's and patient's body during Qi Gong treatment; their relationships to certain meridians & acupuncture points and the re-creation of therapeutic Qi Gong states by children & adults. Acupunct Electrother Res. 1989;14:61–89.

91. Sancier KM. Medical applications of Qi Gong. Altern Ther Health Med. 1996;2:40–6.

92. Omura Y, Beckman SL. Application of intensified (+) Qi Gong energy, (-) electrical field, (S) magnetic field, electrical pulses (1–2 pulses/sec), strong Shiatsu massage or acupuncture on the accurate organ representation areas of the hands to improve circulation and enhance drug uptake in pathological organs: clinical applications with special emphasis on the "Chlamydia-(Lyme)-uric acid syndrome" and "Chlamydia-(cytomegalovirus)-uric acid syndrome." Acupunct Electrother Res. 1995;20:21–72.

93. Omura Y. Strong of qi gong energy in various materials and drugs (qigongnization): its clinical application for treatment of pain, circulatory disturbance, bacterial or viral infections, heavy metal deposits, and related intractable medical problems by selectively enhancing circulation and drug uptake. Acupunt Elecrother Res. 1990; 15:37–157.

94. Li W, Xing Z, Pi D, Li X. Influence of qi-gong on plasma TXB2 and 6-keto-PGF1 alpha in two TCM types of essential hypertension. Hunan Yi Ke Da Xue Xue Bao. 1997;22:497–9.

95. Zhang JZ, Zhao J, He QN. EEG findings during special psychical state (Qi Gong state) by means of compressed spectral array and topographic mapping. Comput Biol Med. 1988;18:455–63.

96. Xing ZH, Li W, Pi DR. Effect of qi gong on blood pressure and life quality of essential hypertension patients. Zhongguo Zhong Xi Yi Jie He Za Zhi. 1993;13:413–414, 388–89.

97. Agishi T. Effects of the external Qi Gong on symptoms of arteriosclerotic obstruction in the lower extremities evaluated by modern medical technology. Artif Organs. 1998;22:707–10.

98. DeGuire S, Gevirtz R, Kawahara Y, Maguire W. Hyperventilation syndrome and the assessment of treatment for functional cardiac symptoms. Am J Cardiol. 1992;70:673–7.

99. Lee MS, Kim BG, Huh HJ, Ryu H, Lee HS, Chung HT. Effect of Qi-training on blood pressure, heart rate and respiration rate. Clin Physiol. 2000;20:173–6.

100. Lim YA, Boone T, Flarity JR, Thompson WR. Effects of Qi Gong on cardiorespiratory changes: a preliminary study. Am J Chin Med. 1993;21:1–6.

101. Xu SH. Psychophysiological reactions associated with Qi Gong therapy. Chin Med J (Engl). 1994;107:230–3.

102. Fukushima M, Kataoka T, Hamada C, Matsumoto M. Evidence of Qi-gong energy and its biological effect on the enhancement of the phagocytic activity of human polymorphonuclear leukocytes. Am J Chin Med. 2001;29:1–16.

103. Stenlund T, Lindstrom B, Granlund M, Burell G. Cardiac rehabilitation for the elderly: Qi Gong and group discussions. Eur J Cardiovasc Prev Rehabil. 2005;12:5–11.

104. Pippa L, Manzoli L, Corti I, Congedo G, Romanazzi L, Parruti G. Functional capacity after traditional Chinese medicine (qi gong) training in patients with chronic atrial fibrillation: A randomized controlled trial. Prev Cardiol. 2007;10: 22–25.

105a. Zhang SX, Guo HZ, Jing BS, Wang X, Zhang LM. Experimental verification of effectiveness and harmlessness of the Qi Gong maneuver. Aviat Space Environ Med. 1991;62:46–52.

105b. Consoli SM. Stress and the cardiovascular system. Encephale. 1993;19 Spec No 1: 163–70.

106. Sancier KM. Therapeutic benefits of Qi Gong exercises in combination with drugs. J Altern Complement Med. 1999;5:383–9.

107. Wardell DW, Engebretson J. Biological correlates of Reiki touch(sm) healing. J Adv Nurs. 2001;33:439–45.

108. Wardell DW, Mentgen J. Healing touch—an energy-based approach to healing. Imprint. 1999;46:34–5, 51.

109. Mackay N, Hansen S, McFarlane O. Autonomic nervous system changes during Reiki treatment: a preliminary study. J Altern Complement Med. 2004;10:1077–81.

110. Reece K, Schwartz GE, Brooks AJ, Nangle G. Positive well-being changes associated with giving and receiving Johrei healing. J Altern Complement Med. 2005;11: 455–7.

111. Nilsson U, Rawal N, Enqvist B, Unosson M. Analgesia following music and therapeutic suggestions in the PACU in ambulatory surgery; a randomized controlled trial. Acta Anaesthesiol Scand. 2003;47:278–83.

112. Richards K, Nagel C, Markie M, Elwell J, Barone C. Use of complementary and alternative therapies to promote sleep in critically ill patients. Crit Care Nurs Clin North Am. 2003;15:329–40.

113. Wilkinson DS, Knox PL, Chatman JE, et al. The clinical effectiveness of healing touch. J Altern Complement Med. 2002;8:33–47.

114. Wardell DW, Weymouth KF. Review of studies of healing touch. J Nurs Scholarsh 2004;36:147–54.

115. Henkelman WJ. Healing touch is pseudoscience. J Nurs Scholarsh. 2004;36:288; author reply 288–9.

116. Healing touch: hands-on help for the heart? Touch therapies are reaching growing numbers of patients. Harv Heart Lett. 2005;16:3.

117. Weze C, Leathard HL, Grange J, Tiplady P, Stevens G. Evaluation of healing by gentle touch. Public Health. 2005;119:3–10.

118. Mansour AA, Beuche M, Laing G, Leis A, Nurse J. A study to test the effectiveness of placebo Reiki standardization procedures developed for a planned Reiki efficacy study. J Altern Complement Med. 1999;5:153–64.

119. Umbreit A. Therapeutic touch: energy-based healing. Creat Nurs. 1997;3:6–7.

120. Cox C, Hayes J. Experiences of administering and receiving therapeutic touch in intensive care. Complement Ther Nurs Midwifery. 1998;4:128–32.

121. O'Mathuna DP, Ashford RL. Therapeutic touch for healing acute wounds. Cochrane Database Syst Rev. 2003:CD002766.

122. Smyth PE. Therapeutic touch for a patient after a Whipple procedure. Crit Care Nurs Clin North Am. 2001;13:357–63.

123. Lewis D. A survey of therapeutic touch practitioners. Nurs Stand. 1999;13:33–7.

124. Heidt P. Effect of therapeutic touch on anxiety level of hospitalized patients. Nurs Res. 1981;30:32–7.

125. Sneed NV, Olson M, Bubolz B, Finch N. Influences of a relaxation intervention on perceived stress and power spectral analysis of heart rate variability. Prog Cardiovasc Nurs. 2001;16:57–64, 79.

126. Spence JE, Olson MA. Quantitative research on therapeutic touch. An integrative review of the literature 1985–1995. Scand J Caring Sci. 1997;11:183–90.

127. Rubens D, Gyurkovics D, Hornacek K. The cultural production of Bioterapia: psychic healing and the natural medicine movement in Slovakia. Soc Sci Med. 1995;41: 1261–71.

128. Rosa L, Rosa E, Sarner L, Barrett S. A close look at therapeutic touch. JAMA. 1998; 279:1005–10.

129. Cox T. A nurse-statistician reanalyzes data from the Rosa therapeutic touch study. Altern Ther Health Med. 2003;9:58–64.

130. Woods DL, Craven RF, Whitney J. The effect of therapeutic touch on behavioral symptoms of persons with dementia. Altern Ther Health Med. 2005;11:66–74.

131. Beutler JJ, Attevelt JT, Schouten SA, Faber JA, Dorhout Mees EJ, Geijskes GG. Paranormal healing and hypertension. Br Med J (Clin Res Ed). 1988;296:1491–1494.

132. Wirth DP, Cram JR. The psychophysiology of nontraditional prayer. Int J Psychorom. 1994;41:68–7.

133. Dusek JA, Sherwood JB, Friedman R, Friedman R, Myers P, Bethea CF, et al. Study of the Therapeutic Effects of Intercessory Prayer (STEP): study design and research methods. Am Heart J. 2002;143:577–84.

134. Benson H, Dusek JA, Sherwood JB, Lam P, Bethea CF, Carpenter W, Levitsky S, Hill PC, Clem DW Jr., Jain MK, Drumel D, Kopecky SL, Mueller PS, Marek D, Rollins S, Hibberd PL. Study of the therapeutic effects of intercessory prayer (STEP) in cardiac bypass patients: A mullticenter randomized trial of uncertainty and certainty of receiving intercessory prayer. Am Heart J. 2006;151:934–942.

135. Krucoff MW. Mitchell W. Krucoff, MD. The MANTRA Study Project. Interview by Bonnie Horrigan. Altern Ther Health Med. 1999;5:74–82.

136. MacLean CR, Walton KG, Wenneberg SR, Levitsky DK, Mandarino JP, Waziri R, et al. Effects of the Transcendental Meditation program on adaptive mechanisms: changes in hormone levels and responses to stress after 4 months of practice. Psychoneuroendocrinology. 1997;22:277–95.

137. Bagga OP, Gandhi A. A comparative study of the effect of transcendental meditation (T.M.) and shavasana practice on cardiovascular system. Indian Heart J. 1983;35:39–45.

138. Elson BD, Hauri P, Cunis D. Physiological changes in yoga meditation. Psychophysiology 1977;14:52–7.

139. Schneider RH, Nidich SI, Salerno JW. The Transcendental Meditation program: reducing the risk of heart disease and mortality and improving quality of life in African Americans. Ethn Dis. 2001;11:159–60.

140. Calderon R, Jr., Schneider RH, Alexander CN, Myers HF, Nidich SI, Haney C. Stress, stress reduction and hypercholesterolemia in African Americans: a review. Ethn Dis. 1999;9:451–62.

141. Cauthen NR, Prymak CA. Meditation versus relaxation: an examination of the physiological effects of relaxation training and of different levels of experience with transcendental meditation. J Consult Clin Psychol. 1977;45:496–7.

142a. Castillo-Richmond A, Schneider RH, Alexander CN, Cook R, Myers H, Nidich S, et al. Effects of stress reduction on carotid atherosclerosis in hypertensive African Americans. Stroke. 2000;31:568–73.

142b. Wirth DP, Cram JR. The psychophysiology of nontraditional prayer. Int J Psychosom. 1994;41:68–75.

143. Puente AE, Beiman I. The effects of behavior therapy, self-relaxation, and transcendental meditation on cardiovascular stress response. J Clin Psychol. 1980;36:291–5.

144. Lehrer PM, Woolfolk RL, Rooney AJ, McCann B, Carrington P. Progressive relaxation and meditation. A study of psychophysiological and therapeutic differences between two techniques. Behav Res Ther. 1983;21:651–62.

145. Malec J, Sipprelle CN. Physiological and subjective effects of Zen meditation and demand characteristics. J Consult Clin Psychol. 1977;45:339–40.

146. Delmonte MM. Physiological responses during meditation and rest. Biofeedback Self Regul. 1984;9:181–200.

147. Delmonte MM. Electrocortical activity and related phenomena associated with meditation practice: a literature review. Int J Neurosci. 1984;24:217–31.

148. Delmonte MM. Meditation practice as related to occupational stress, health and productivity. Percept Mot Skills. 1984;59:581–2.

149. Birkel DA, Edgren L. Hatha yoga: improved vital capacity of college students. Altern Ther Health Med. 2000;6:55–63.

150. Lee JS, Lee MS, Lee JY, Cornelissen G, Otsuka K, Halberg F. Effects of diaphragmatic breathing on ambulatory blood pressure and heart rate. Biomed Pharmacother. 2003;57 Suppl 1:87s–91s.

151. Raub JA. Psychophysiologic effects of Hatha Yoga on musculoskeletal and cardiopulmonary function: a literature review. J Altern Complement Med. 2002;8:797–812.

152. Raghuraj P, Ramakrishnan AG, Nagendra HR, Telles S. Effect of two selected yogic breathing techniques of heart rate variability. Indian J Physiol Pharmacol. 1998;42:467–72.

153. Navratil L, Hlavaty V, Landsingerova E. Possible therapeutic applications of pulsed magnetic fields. Cas Lek Cesk. 1993;132:590–4.

154a. Myloslavs'kyi DK, Koval SM, Sheremet MS. The clinico-biochemical, functional, immunological and cellular characteristics of the body reactions in patients with the initial stages of hypertension to the effect of a magnetic field. Lik Sprava. 1996:58–62.

154a. Ito KL. Ho'oponopono, "to make right": Hawaiian conflict resolution and metaphor in the construction of a family therapy. Cult Med Psychiatry. 1985;9:201–17.

155. Vasil'ev IM, Iakovleva SD. Magnetotherapy in cardiology (a review of the literature). Vrach Delo. 1990:42–7.

156. Scherlag BJ, Yamanashi WS, Hou Y, Jacobson JI, Jackman WM, Lazzara R. Magnetism and cardiac arrhythmias. Cardiol Rev. 2004;12:85–96.

157. Linde K, Clausius N, Ramirez G, Melchart D, Eital F, Hedges LV, Jonas WB. Are the clinical effects of homeopathy placebo effects? A meta-analysis of placebo-controlled trials. Lancet. 1997;350:834–843.

158. Scheen A, Lefebvre P. Is homeopathy superior to placebo? Controversy apropos of a meta-analysis of controlled studies. Bull Mem Acad R Med Belg. 1999;154: 295–304, discussion 304–307.

159a. Hankey A. Are we close to a theory of energy medicine? J Altern Complement Med. 2004;10:83–6.

159b. Ernst E. Distant healing—an "update" of a systematic review. Wien Klin Wochenschr. 2003;115:241–5.

CHAPTER 7

ACUPUNCTURE

John C. Longhurst

DESCRIPTION

Acupuncture is a clinical practice that originated in China almost 4000 years ago during the reign of the Yellow Emperor (2697 BC). The first reference to this technique was in the Yellow Emperor's Inner Classic (200 BC).[1] The practice of acupuncture has evolved with technological developments. Early needles were made of wood, bamboo, bone, and more recently available metals. Today, disposable stainless steel needles are used. Most acupuncture technique and practice was shaped empirically and, in fact, even today much teaching of this ancient technique is based on observations of masters and practitioners that were recorded in texts and passed down to students as gospel or dogma. Only in the last 50 years has modern science begun to provide insight into the mechanisms and actions of acupuncture. Since the early 1970s there have been over 500 randomized controlled clinical trials investigating the clinical influence of acupuncture,[2, 3] yet its influence has been proven rigorously for only a few diseases, most notably pain and nausea and vomiting.

TRADITIONAL CHINESE MEDICINE

Like western physicians, practitioners of acupuncture obtain a history from patients, then examine them using inspection, palpation, smell, and listening. There are a number of culturally distinct practices of acupuncture, originating from China, Korea, Japan, and even Europe. For example, Chinese acupuncture typically relies on manual or electrical stimulation of deeper neural pathways while Japanese promote more superficial and delicate manipulation of needles. Even within a given culture, such as Chinese acupuncture, there are many approaches and this variability leads to many inconsistencies and variations in outcome as well as confusion in interpretation of studies. A reasonable suggestion is the call for "manualized" protocols consisting of carefully constructed standardized treatment designs gained from input from practicing acupuncturists and western comple-mentary and alternative medicine (CAM) physicians to achieve consistency between studies.[4]

Acupuncture as a part of traditional Chinese medicine (TCM) is based on a theory of interconnecting meridians or channels through which energy flows. This energy is called Qi (pronounced "chee"), a term that originated in the work of a French scholar in the early nineteenth century.[5] The 12 bilaterally symmet-rical principal meridians are named after specific Chinese organs, such as the heart and pericardium, to which they are connected. Additionally, two extra mid-line meridians have been described. The anatomical designations can be confusing however, since the heart, for example, is represented by the western equivalent of the heart and the brain. Qi is believed to flow through the meridians and the associated Chinese organ in a circular fashion. A series of acupuncture points or acupoints have been identified along the meridians that are used in the treatment of acupuncture. These points are stimulated by needles during acupuncture, by pressure during acupressure, or by heat during moxibustion. Moxibustion incor-porates the use of locally heating an acupoint, commonly by burning a herb on a needle. Once inserted, acupuncture needles can be either left in place, manipu-lated mechanically, or stimulated with a small battery-driven current during elec-troacupuncture (EA). Despite some claims to the contrary, neither meridians nor acupoints along the meridians can be identified anatomically or by any device. Rather, they serve as useful landmarks and guideposts that guide stimulation dur-ing acupuncture. TCM theory postulates that under normal conditions Qi flows in an unimpeded manner through the meridians and the associated Chinese organ. Qi is composed of yin (female essence expressing cold, dark, moist, and calm as descriptors) or yang (male essence including heat, light, dry, and activity) forces that are balanced in health when homeostasis exists. Disease interrupts the flow of Qi and treatment with acupuncture or herbal medicine is used to restore normal flow. Diseases in TCM are classified into those that have an excess or deficiency of either the yin or yang. Despite the fact that TCM theory, including many of its concepts may seem arcane, modern science has provided a framework that helps to explain many of its aspects.

Although many authors suggest there is little correspondence between TCM theory and our modern understanding of biology and physiology, in fact, there are a number of parallels that can be drawn. For example, the balance between yin and yang under normal conditions represents homeostasis, which is disrupted by various diseases. It is clear that acupuncture stimulation involves activation of somatic afferent neural pathways,[6, 7] including both group III finely myelinated[8] and, to a lesser extent, group IV unmyelinated pathways.[8, 9] As such, Qi is really represented by the flow of sensory neural information to the central nervous sys-tem (CNS). Deqi, the sensation patients experience during acupuncture, repre-sents a paresthesia produced by stimulation of a neural pathway underlying the acupoint along a meridian. Finally, it is interesting to note that the heart and pericardial meridians are located on pathways along the middle and inner arms that are virtually identical to the radiating pattern of referred pain in patients with cardiac chest pain, angina pectoris.

TRANSCUTANEOUS ELECTRICAL AND SPINAL CORD STIMULATION

Transcutaneous electrical nerve stimulation or TENS has been employed for a number of years to reduce pain,[10] including ischemic chest pain.[11–13] This technique uses a patch electrode on the surface of the skin to stimulate underlying neural pathways and through a gating mechanism involving cathodal and anodal blockade, first described by Melzack and Wall in 1965,[14] which operates mainly in the dorsal horn of the spinal cord, TENS blocks afferent neural impulses associated with transmission of nociceptive stimuli. A number of studies have used this technique as a surrogate for transcutaneous needling (i.e., acupuncture) since it is noninvasive. Although there are many similarities to classical acupuncture, TENS typically employs higher currents and is spread out over a larger area than needling with acupuncture. TENS therefore likely activates a different profile of sensory nerve fibers in underlying neural pathways. These different patterns of afferent activation may lead to differences in physiological and clinical response. In fact, in contrast to acupuncture, the anti-nociceptive effect of TENS is not reversible by generalized opioid blockade with naloxone.[13]

Other techniques that have been used, more commonly in Europe than in the United States, are spinal cord and deep brain stimulation.[10, 15] Spinal cord stimulation (SCS) with an implanted device stimulates both dorsal roots and dorsal columns, including the spinothalamic tract (a major spinal pathway conducting afferent signals from the heart to the thalamus)[16, 17] in much the same manner as TENS. Both TENS and SCS have been used in patients with refractory angina pectoris.[18, 19] Early concern that these methods would place patients at risk by simply eliminating an important warning system (angina) appears to be unfounded since there is an increase in the angina threshold, perhaps as a result of reduced myocardial oxygen demand.[18, 20] Like TENS, SCS improves exercise tolerance and limits ST depression in patients with ischemic heart disease and angina.[21, 22] Because coronary flow, as measured by positron emission tomography does not change,[23] it is possible that the underlying mechanism may be either reduced pain through a gating mechanism centrally or a decrease in myocardial oxygen demand. Mortality after 2 years of SCS is superior to bypass surgery, while after 5 years it is similar with equivalent symptom relief and quality of life, suggesting that in refractory patients, this modality may be a viable alternative to surgery.[24, 25] Thus, electrical stimulation of many of the same central neural pathways activated by acupuncture, using methods that are considerably more invasive, appears to improve symptoms of angina through physiological mechanisms that reduce myocardial ischemia.

SAFETY

In comparison to most western medical therapies, particularly those used to treat cardiovascular disease, acupuncture is a relatively safe modality, with an incidence of complications ranging between 0.14 and 11.4%.[26–29] Most side effects are mild. For example, it can cause minor pain because needles are inserted either through or in close proximity to major neural pathways. On the other hand, neuralgia expressed as sensations of warmth, tingling, heaviness, mild aching, or pain is essential to the successful outcome of acupuncture and suggests that neural stimulation is an integral component. Chinese physicians call this sensation deqi, which means obtaining Qi. Deqi can be accompanied by a tugging of the needle, presumably as a result of local neuromuscular stimulation around the needle, although there is speculation that collagen may wrap around the needle. Bleeding also can occur occasionally, although because the needles are very small, typically approximately 32 gauge, the extent of bleeding is minimal, even with arterial puncture. Patients can experience relaxation, which actually is an expected result since acupuncture suppresses pain and reduces sympathetic outflow.[30] Less commonly needle retention, syncope, and infections can occur, as a result of poor technique, lowered blood pressure, or contamination. Pneumothorax has been rarely described.[31] Infections are most commonly localized but hepatitis, bacterial endocarditis, and HIV have been described.[28, 32–35] These latter problems occur only rarely, mostly in communities that do not insert disposable needles commonly used in the United States and Europe today. A final complication is induction of labor in late-term pregnant women. This may occur more commonly with certain acupoints, particularly those located in one of the midline meridians. Acupuncture is actually used to promote labor and even reposition late-term breech presentations, since it can stimulate uterine muscle contraction.[36] Overall, although acupuncture, like any other invasive treatment, can be accompanied by side effects and complications, the incidence of serious events is very low. Individuals at particular risk would be those with a bleeding disorder or depressed immune function.

RESEARCH IN ACUPUNCTURE

A consensus conference sponsored by the National Institutes of Health in 1997 suggested that more research needs to be conducted to fully understand the biological actions and the clinical efficacy of acupuncture.[37] This conclusion was reinforced in the executive summary of a special report stemming from a workshop in 2001 examining the state of complementary and alternative medicine in cardiovascular, lung, and blood research.[38] There have been more than 500 randomized controlled clinical trails in acupuncture over the last 30 years.[2] A randomized controlled trial should be hypothesis driven, prospective, blinded (preferably double blinded), adequately powered with sufficient numbers of subjects, well controlled and analyzed using appropriate statistical methodology. Additionally, description of the randomization process and dropouts should be provided. Many of these issues have not been adequately addressed in previous clinical acupuncture research.[26] According to the U.S. public health-care service, Agency for Health Care Research and Quality (AHRQ), clinical trials can be graded according to the following criteria:

1. Well-designed and constructed studies
2. Observational studies, including small clinical trials
3. Expert opinion and consensus panels

When considering the strength of evidence, the AHRQ identified three key elements including quality, quantity, and consistency of evidence.[39] While acupuncture may have beneficial effects on the cardiovascular system,[40] there are a number of considerations regarding clinical trials in acupuncture. First, it is difficult to blind subjects and almost impossible to blind the therapist. If patients have any previous experience with acupuncture, they will expect a sensation of deqi. Interaction between the acupuncturist and the patient during acupuncture cannot be prevented and this interaction, of course, is the basis of many placebo responses, sometimes called the Rosenthal Effect.[41] One solution is to use acupuncture-naive patients and to be sure there is a sensation associated with the needling. In this respect, while subjects who have previously experienced acupuncture demonstrate vasodilation of the radial artery during 20 minutes of acupuncture (acupoints not specified), acupuncture-naive subjects manifest no response.[42] Also, individuals performing data analysis should be blinded to the intervention.

A second and related issue is what constitutes an adequate control. It is this last issue that plagues many studies of acupuncture. Unfortunately, a number of older studies and almost half of the 500 randomized controlled clinical trials did not use adequate controls. The following have been used to control for nonspecific responses to acupuncture, unrelated to the intervention: acupuncture outside a meridian, acupuncture at an inactive acupoint, sham needling involving tapping of the skin without penetration, and tablet placebo. In my view, a tablet placebo would be unacceptable.

Meyer (2000) reviewed a number of acupuncture studies in treatment of pain and nausea and vomiting and made a convincing argument that the strongest control is to perform acupuncture along a meridian at an inactive acupoint.[43] However, this consideration brings up the concept of point specificity. The concept of point specificity states that separate physiological and clinical responses result from stimulation of different acupoints. Clearly, acupuncture's success derives, in part, from a practitioner's ability to stimulate the best single or best combination of acupoints for a particular condition. For example, it has been shown that there is a hierarchy of acupoints that influence cardiovascular function.[44] Thus, it seems very possible that the most active and inactive acupoints for specific clinical conditions, such as hypertension or demand-induced myocardial ischemia, can be identified for intervention and control stimulation.

Recently, another type of control has been identified. Experimental studies have shown that insertion of a needle without manipulation or electrical stimulation does not activate afferent pathways and hence does not provide information to the CNS.[45] In the absence of any information transmitted to the CNS, any response to acupuncture would have to be a placebo effect. However, the absence of suitable controls is one of most serious issues limiting the value of much of the world's literature on acupuncture research today, particularly in the area of clinical application.

The World Health Organization (http://www.who.int/medicines/library/trm/acupuncture/acupuncture_trials.doc) has reviewed clinical trials in acupuncture and grouped them according to the following criteria:

1. Proven through controlled clinical trials to be effective.
2. Therapeutic effect shown but further proof needed.
3. Individual controlled trials (worth trying because conventional and other therapies difficult).
4. Acupuncture may be tried if practitioner has special medical knowledge and adequate monitoring equipment.

With respect to cardiovascular disease, category 1 includes hypertension and stroke, category 2 non-insulin dependent diabetes mellitus, hyperlipidemia, obesity, Raynaud's syndrome, Sjogren's syndrome, tobacco dependence, and vascular dementia, category 3 chronic pulmonary heart disease, and category 4 angina and coronary artery disease. This chapter will concentrate on three clinical conditions, hypertension and stroke, symptomatic coronary artery disease and peripheral vascular disease, and organ dysfunction caused by blood flow abnormalities.

INFLUENCE ON HYPERTENSION AND STROKE

Several investigations have examined the influence of acupuncture in hypertension, including the exaggerated blood pressure responses associated with spinal cord injury. An experimental study has demonstrated in paraplegic and quadriplegic rats that 20 minutes of TENS, using high frequencies (60 Hz) and intensities (~600 mA) over the paraspinal muscles (T_{12}-S_3), can reduce the exaggerated increase in blood pressure associated with colon distension.[46] Sham TENS, involving the same procedure without electrical stimulation did not alter the hypertensive responses. No attempt was made to stimulate with a similar current at a different location. While acupuncture appears to be safe in patients with chronic spinal cord injury, who are at risk for autonomic dysreflexia, and does not precipitate hypertension,[47] further research is required to determine if this modality can be used to limit the exaggerated blood pressure responses.

Acupuncture lowers short-term reflex-induced elevation in blood pressure through a naloxone-sensitive mechanism.[8, 48] Hindlimb acupuncture over the distribution of the sciatic nerve (Zusanli acupoint, ST 36) can lower blood pressure in spontaneously hypertensive rats for up to 12 hours after termination of treatment.[49] The reduction in blood pressure in hypertensive animals appears to be dependent on elevated sympathetic outflow, since hypertensive models without increased sympathetic activity are not influenced by acupuncture.[50] Interestingly, blood pressure in normotensive animals is not altered. The absence of an effect by acupuncture on blood pressure in animals and human subjects with normal blood pressures, as noted below, appears to be a consistent finding.

There are no good published large-scale randomized clinical trials on the efficacy of acupuncture in hypertension or stroke. A small study of 50 patients with essential hypertension found that shortly after 30 minutes of acupuncture, both systolic and diastolic arterial pressures were lowered by 10–20 mm Hg.[51]

One of the more common uses for acupuncture in China is in stroke rehabilitation. However, a review of nine studies in the literature suggests that there is no compelling evidence to conclude that acupuncture is effective in stroke rehabilitation, including range of movement, motor function, balance, and quality of life.[52] In fact, although five studies showed positive outcomes, the two most carefully conducted studies, which provided sham EA[53, 54] showed no improvement. Superficial acupuncture at acupoints was used as a control for one study,[54] while acupuncture outside a meridian was used by another.[53] The outstanding feature of all of these nine studies is their poor design. A more recent meta-analysis incorporating 14 trials of 1213 patients also showed that acupuncture versus no acupuncture has no effect on motor recovery but may have a small influence on disability due to a placebo effect.[55] Again, a finding in common with the other review was the poor quality of most studies. Two recent prospective randomized studies published in *Stroke*[55, 56] of 150 patients in Sweden and 106 patients in Hong Kong confirm earlier reviews by showing neither short (10 week) nor long-term (3 month and 1 year) improvement in functional outcome or life satisfaction.

Thus, while hypertension may respond acupuncture, the most studies suggest that following stroke, there is little objective evidence demonstrating that acupuncture improves the quality of life. Clearly, however, more research in both hypertension and stroke is warranted.

INFLUENCE ON MYOCARDIAL ISCHEMIA, EXERCISE, AND CORONARY ARTERY DISEASE

Early experimental studies involving complete coronary ligation in rats showed that acupuncture for 10 minutes at the Jianshi acupoint (P 6) reduced electrocardiographic (ECG) ST depression during reperfusion.[57] Furthermore, acupuncture at Jianshi-Neiguan (P 5–P 6) may reduce the extent of myocardial infarction and, compared to a poorly defined control group, could lower coronary vascular resistance during prolonged ischemia.[58, 59] Acupuncture at a moderately high frequency (40 Hz) for 60 minutes applied bilaterally at Neiguan (P 6) acupoints, in contrast to control stimulation outside a meridian, promotes recovery of left ventricular function, determined from measurements of end-systolic pressure in a canine model of hemorrhage-induced hypotension. The mechanism in this study may involve vasopressin, the muscle pump, and enhanced venous return since the acupuncture response was abolished by neuromuscular blockade with vecuronium.[60] This study suggests that, when the frequency of acupuncture is increased, there is a muscle component that participates in the acupuncture-related cardiovascular response.

Recent studies have revealed that 30 minutes of low-frequency (2 Hz), low-intensity (2–5 V, 1–2 mA) acupuncture at Jianshi-Neiguan (P 5–P 6) virtually eliminates ischemia in a feline model of demand-induced ischemia.[8, 30, 61] This model was created by partial occlusion of a branch of the left anterior descending coronary artery, which provided adequate flow to meet demand at rest but developed ischemia when blood pressure was elevated during a visceral reflex involving stimulation of the gallbladder with bradykinin. Ischemic regional wall motion abnormality was prevented through a reduction of the reflex-induced increase in arterial blood pressure, which reduced myocardial oxygen demand, rather than through an enhancement in coronary blood flow by a mechanism that was naloxone sensitive.[51, 8] The improvement in regional dysfunction was not mediated by muscle contraction since it was not altered by neuromuscular blockade.

Compared to placebo (electrodes without stimulation), high-frequency TENS (150 Hz, intensity just below pain threshold, electrodes on chest and back) reduces the increase in diastolic blood pressure during static handgrip exercise, but does not alter the hemodynamic responses to the Valsalva maneuver, cold pressor test, or head-up tilt.[62] These responses occur only when electrodes are placed ipsilaterally to the exercising arm, suggesting that the TENS-related reduction in blood pressure occurs when they converge at the same spinal level and that there is no supraspinal component.[63]

Bilateral acupuncture for 30 minutes at either Nieguan-Jianshi (P 5–P 6) or Hegu-Lique (LI 4–L 7), but not at control acupoints Guangming-Xuanzhong (G 37–G 39), can increase maximal workload during bicycle exercise in subjects without cardiovascular disease. Acupuncture also can reduce increases in systolic and mean blood pressure as well as the rate pressure or double product in approximately 70% of patients.[64] Interestingly, acupuncture does not reduce resting (pre-exercise) blood pressure or diastolic blood pressure during exercise. Thus, acupuncture has the potential to reduce myocardial oxygen demand but does not alter baseline blood pressure in normal volunteers. This study suggested that acupuncture may be beneficial in patients experiencing demand-induced ischemia during exercise.

Brief (~15 seconds) unilateral manual acupuncture at Hegu (LI 4), Taichong (LIV 3), and Sanyinjiao (SP 6) with needle retention for 15 minutes reduced the increase in blood pressure but not the increase in muscle sympathetic nerve activity associated with mental stress, in comparison with needle stimulation outside a meridian and no-needle controls.[65] This carefully conducted study indicates that manual acupuncture may alter centrally mediated increases in blood pressure by acting on regions other than the muscle.

In the mid-1980s through the early 1990s, several reports suggested that TENS and acupuncture could reduce ischemia during exercise in patients with angina and ECG evidence of myocardial ischemia.[66, 12, 67, 13, 68–73]

Similar to findings in experimental studies, TENS performed for 60 minutes three times daily for 10 weeks, in comparison to a control group, reduced ECG ST depression and decreased myocardial venous lactate through a mechanism that involved reduced afterload and hence myocardial oxygen demand.[66, 12, 67, 13] However, in contrast to the experimental studies involving acupuncture, TENS also has been found to increase coronary blood flow in both normal subjects and in patients with coronary artery disease. The increase in coronary flow may be through a mechanism that involves the sympathetic nervous system, since this therapy does not alter flow in heart transplant recipients who have been denervated.[74] Augmentation of peripheral flow is consistent with studies on the influence of acupuncture in patients with vascular insufficiency (see below). Differences between these studies and those observed in experimental preparations may be related to anesthesia, acupuncture versus TENS, species. or the model (acute partial ligation vs. chronic coronary artery disease).

An early study from China[75] suggested that, in comparison to sham controls at undefined acupoints, manual acupuncture at Neiguan (P 6), Zusanli (ST 36), and Jiuwei (CV 15) as well as a number of supplementary points every other day for a total of approximately 10 treatments decreased nitroglycerine consumption and resting ECG ST abnormalities. The authors also claimed improved echocardiographic posterior wall motion and systolic time intervals but did not present these data. It is unclear if the subjects were blinded and the acupuncture technique used does not appear to have been standardized between patients, limiting the value of this study.

Ballegaard's group[68, 69] found similar improvements in nitroglycerin consumption and angina attack rate as well as exercise tolerance and the rate-pressure product in a group of well-characterized patients with ischemic heart disease, who had stable angina and in a group of control subjects treated with acupuncture at the same spinal segment outside a meridian. Interestingly, when the entire group of subjects were compared retrospectively to patients who demonstrated local and remote increases in pain threshold and finger skin temperature (suggesting a centrally mediated decrease in sympathetic outflow and an increase in peripheral blood flow), the investigators noted significant improvement in angina and nitroglycerin consumption. The authors suggest that this study was double blinded, but it is likely that a trained acupuncturist would know the difference between stimulation along versus outside a meridian. Acupuncture consisted needle placement without stimulation at unspecified acupoints. Thus, this study is limited methodologically, since, as noted above, experimental evidence indicates that there is no somatic afferent input to the CNS in the absence of needle manipulation. Furthermore, placement of needles outside meridians may not be associated with deqi. It is, perhaps, not surprising that the symptomatic improvement could not be differentiated from the control group.

A more recent small study of 26 patients resistant to medical therapy for angina from Ballegaard's group[76] demonstrated an acupuncture-related increase in rate-pressure product achieved during work but failed to show a significant difference in clinical response of the acupuncture compared to a sham acupuncture group with respect to exercise tolerance, time to maximal ST depression, degree of ST depression, number of anginal attacks, or nitroglycerin consumption. In this study, subjects received seven 20 minutes treatments with acupuncture over a 3-week period with needle placement at Neiguan (P 6), Zusanli (ST 36), and Jueyinshu (BL 14). Although the subjects apparently developed deqi, the needles were not manipulated nor electrically stimulated, suggesting that afferent stimulation required to evoke a clinical response was minimal. Furthermore, sham treatment consisted of needling outside meridians in the same spinal segment, which may not be the strongest control since subjects may be able to note a difference between real and sham acupuncture (see Chap. 19 on Mechanisms of Cardiovascular Action of Acupuncture).

Richter and coworkers[73] used a cross-over design to investigate the influence of 30 minutes of acupuncture three times per week for 4 weeks compared to a tablet placebo control in a small group of patients with angina pectoris and ECG exercise-induced ischemia. They stimulated five main acupoints, including Neiguan (P 5), Zusanli (ST 36), Tongli (HT 5), Xinshu (BL 15), and Pishu (BL 20) and four supplementary acupoints, Shenmen (HT 7), Hegu (LI 4), Quchi (LI 11), and Taichong (LIV 3). They found that, compared to pre-acupuncture and a tablet placebo, acupuncture reduced the number of anginal attacks, the amount of chest pain, and the degree of ST depression. Acupuncture also increased their submaximal workload. In addition to the small number of observations, this study is limited by an inadequate control group.

A small study of 22 patients with angina and angiographically proven coronary disease evaluated the influence of mechanical acupuncture for 30 minutes at Neiguan (P 6) on left ventricular function using radionucleotide angiography.[77] In comparison to a group of 22 normal subjects who showed no response to this intervention, the patients with coronary disease demonstrated short-term improvements in ejection fraction during and for 15 minutes following acupuncture. Acupuncture was not associated with any blood pressure or heart rate changes. The authors comment that the increase was still present 1 week later but did not reach statistical significance. Sham acupuncture nearby but outside the pericardial meridian did not alter ejection fraction. This study was limited by the small sample and the type of control stimulation.

Ballegaard's group has conducted a prospective long-term nonrandomized evaluation of 168 patients with angina pectoris in an integrated rehabilitation study consisting of acupuncture, self-administered acupressure, Chinese health philosophy, stress reduction, and lifestyle modification.[70, 72, 78] Of the 168 patients, 103 were candidates for invasive treatment, yet only 18% still required surgery after 3 years. Furthermore, in-patient hospital days were decreased by 96% and medication was reduced by 78%, while cost savings were $36,000 and $22,000 for surgical and nonsurgical patients, respectively. The accumulated mortality rate for the participants was 2% compared to 6.4% for the Danish population and 5.4% and 8.4%, respectively, for patients who were treated with angioplasty and bypass grafting. These data suggest that an integrative health rehabilitation program, incorporating acupuncture, in addition to several other nonstandard components to reduce stress and conventional risk reduction therapy, may be cost effective and capable of reducing both morbidity and mortality in patients with severe coronary disease. However, this study does not allow determination of the individual contribution of acupuncture.

Overall, good experimental data indicates that acupuncture can reduce myocardial oxygen demand during exercise and mental stress. The question of whether it improves coronary flow is still open. Small trials suggest that acupuncture may improve symptoms and reduce medicine usage and when it is used as part of a comprehensive care program, acupuncture seems to reduce cost and benefit patients. Additional larger randomized controlled clinical trials are warranted to define subgroups of patients with symptomatic coronary disease, who will benefit from needling. Furthermore, the frequency and specific acupoints that are most effective in chronic angina need to be defined, although substantial direction can be taken from information gained in the experimental laboratory.

INFLUENCE ON PERIPHERAL VASCULAR INSUFFICIENCY

TENS (80 Hz, 20 mA) applied for 1 hour each day over a 7-day period, beginning immediately postoperatively increases skin flap survival in rats.[79] Fifteen minutes of low frequency TENS (4 Hz) at intensities above muscle threshold increases local but not distal (remote) cutaneous blood flow as measured by laser Doppler and no change in skin temperature.[80]

Clinically, TENS but not acupuncture has been used in a small trial of 20 patients with ischemic skin flaps after reconstructive surgery with short term follow-up.[81] The investigators noted improved Doppler blood flow with TENS compared to the control group.

A nonrandomized study of SCS in patients with peripheral vascular insufficiency, including 34 patients with atherosclerosis, Berger's disease and vasospasm over a 7-year period demonstrated increased skin temperature and a lower amputation rate in the treated (38%) compared to an untreated group (90%).[82] The same investigative group demonstrated a 91% decrease in rest pain and a 58% improvement in ulcer healing in 32 patients with distal atherosclerotic or diabetic lower limb gangrene with SCS treatment over a 3-year period.[83] Again there was no randomized control group for comparison. A later prospective randomized controlled clinical trial of 41 patients with atherosclerosis and 10 patients with diabetes and inoperable severe leg ischemia experiencing rest pain and/or ischemic ulceration demonstrated improvement in 25 patients randomized to treatment versus 26 treated with analgesic medication.[84] They observed no differences between microcirculatory parameters but better pain relief and less tissue loss in the SCS group and modest, but insignificant, differences in limb salvage rates (62% vs. 45%, SCS vs. control, respectively). These data suggest that SCS reduces pain and tissue loss and may reduce amputation, although a larger study would be required to prove the latter point.

It would be interesting to see if acupuncture improves peripheral blood flow sufficiently to reduce claudication and enhance limb salvage in patients with peripheral arterial disease since it shares many similar physiological responses with SCS. The only data currently available come from several divergent experimental preparations that have examined the effect of needle stimulation on regional flow to a number of organ systems. In this respect, electrical stimulation at low-to-mid frequencies (1–20 Hz) and intensities (>1.5 mA) of the hindpaw (acupoint unspecified) of rats, at an intensity sufficient to recruit both group III and IV somatic afferent nerve fibers, was found to increase blood pressure and muscle (biceps femoris) blood flow but simultaneously reduce renal flow in rats through a sympathetic reflex.[85] Similarly, low-frequency (2 Hz) and moderate-to-high-intensity (2–6 mA) needle stimulation of the biceps femoris (acupoint unspecified) increases ovarian blood flow through a sympathetic reflex in both normal rats and those with steroid-induced polycystic ovaries.[86, 87] High-frequency electrical stimulation of the same region reduces ovarian flow. EA administered once or twice weekly for 10–14 treatments at acupoints in somatic segments common to innervation of the uterus and ovary has been shown to increase ovulation from 0.15 to 0.66 ovulations per month in women with polycystic ovary syndrome.[88]

A study employing indirect measures of blood flow has suggested that acupuncture improves circulatory flow in patients. Thus, 15 minutes of either manual or low-frequency (1 Hz) moderate-intensity (7–15 mA) EA at either the Hegu (LI 4) or Zusanli (ST 36) acupoints causes a generalized increase in skin temperature, which has been interpreted to represent a centrally (CNS, not spinal) mediated cutaneous vasodilation.[89]

In reviewing studies that have employed acupuncture or needle stimulation, it is important to note the simulation parameters. Both the frequency and intensity of somatic sensory nerve stimulation during acupuncture can determine the response. Low currents and frequencies mainly used in clinical acupuncture typically do not alter blood pressure and neither do they influence or increase blood flow. Conversely, high currents and intensities (typically not tolerated by patients) used in some experimental studies cause reflex increases in blood pressure and vasoconstriction (see Chap. 19 on Mechanisms of Cardiovascular Action of Acupuncture).

A clinically oriented experimental study showed that low-frequency EA at the base of a skin flap (outside any meridian), increases Doppler blood flow in a musculocutaneous flap in rats.[90] It is unclear from this study if the acupuncture-related response was locally or centrally mediated. The same group of investigators[91] showed that a similar technique, employing 1 hour of manual or EA (low frequency, high intensity) immediately after surgery and once daily for the next 2 days at the base of a skin flap, increased survival of an ischemic musculocutaneous flap. Superficial acupuncture did not alter survival of the flap.

Deep but not superficial needle stimulation of the Zusanli acupoint (ST 36) overlying the deep peroneal nerve of normal patients increases blood flow in the anterior tibialis muscle measured by photophethysmography in healthy subjects.[92] Both superficial and deep needle insertion and manual stimulation for 5 minutes in a region over the anterior tibia (a non-painful region) related to the Zusanli acupoint, stimulated blood flow in patients with fibromyalgia.[93] Deep stimulation caused the greatest changes in skin and muscle flow (62% and 93%, respectively), although pain was associated with deeper form of stimulation.

Superficial stimulation was not associated with significant alterations in skin or muscle flow in healthy subjects. Although not significant, the responses tended to persist for up to 30 minutes following stimulation. It is uncertain if these blood flow responses were local or systemic in nature.

Another example of a beneficial response of acupuncture is the improvement in low salivary flow associated with xerostomia in patients after radiation or with Sjogren's syndrome following a several week series of 20 minutes bilateral manual acupuncture sessions at Juliao (ST 3), Jiache (ST 6) in the face, Hegu (LI 4) in the hands, and Zusanli (ST 36) and Sanyinjiao (SP 6) acupoints in the legs.[94, 95, 96, 97] The increase in salivary flow may be related to the acupuncture-induced increase in salivary vasoactive intestinal polypeptide, which is known to increase salivary blood flow.[94, 98]

In summary, a number of small studies suggest that in a number of diverse conditions, acupuncture may improve blood flow, reduce organ dysfunction, and hence might be a useful adjunctive therapy. However, because there are numerous limitations in these studies, including small sample size, use of inadequate controls, lack of blinding, and employment of nonstandard techniques, it is premature to conclude that acupuncture can be used as part of a standard therapeutic regimen for treatment of peripheral vascular flow abnormalities and the associated functional abnormality.

CONCLUSIONS

The fact that TCM and acupuncture have existed for several thousand years means that, not only has this intervention stood the test of time, but that there is a lot of truth in its ability to treat a number of conditions including pain, nausea and vomiting, and possibly certain cardiovascular abnormalities. Acupuncture appears to be potentially useful as a therapeutic option that is effective in treating symptoms, including the pathophysiology causing the symptoms, rather than treating the underlying disease process itself. A number of well-constructed experimental studies indicate that acupuncture works through neural-hormonal mechanisms that have the capability of improving disease, for example, reducing blood pressure, decreasing myocardial ischemia, and possibly improving peripheral blood flow when it is limited. Despite the fact that *some* evidence is available for acupuncture in a number of clinical cardiovascular conditions, the design of most studies is not sufficiently rigorous to be considered to be acceptable by conventional standards used for establishing evidence-based medical practice. However, the evidence that is available is very tantalizing and provides a strong rationale for conducting carefully constructed clinical trials. A logical and relatively safe recommendation, therefore, can be made for well-considered RCTs as well as more basic studies of acupuncture and associated techniques like TENS and SCS to help identify mechanisms of action and to assist in the construct of these trials. It will only be through this type of careful hypothesis testing that we will be able to identify the usefulness of acupuncture in clinical cardiology. Such evaluation is correctly demanded by Western scientists and physicians before they will consider acupuncture or any other form of integrative or CAM therapy as acceptable and useful in the treatment of cardiovascular disease.

REFERENCES

1. Ergil KV. China's traditional medicine. In: Micozzi MS, editor. Fundamentals of complementary and alternative medicine. New York: Churchill Livingstone; 1996. p. 185–223.
2. Vickers AJ. Bibliometric analysis of randomized trials in complementary medicine. Complement Ther Med. 1998;6:185–9.
3. Klein L, Trachtenberg AI. Acupuncture. 1997. Current Bibliographies in Medicine.
4. Ahn AC, Kaptchuk TJ. Advancing acupuncture research. Altern Ther Health Med. 2005;11:40–5. [PMID: 15943131]
5. Helms JM. Acupuncture energetics: a clinical approach for physicians. Berkeley (CA): Medical Acupuncture Publishers 1995;3–17.
6. Kline RL, Yeung KY, Calaresu FR. Role of somatic nerves in the cardiovascular responses to stimulation of an acupunture point in anesthetized rabbits. Exp Neurol. 1978;61(3):561–70. [PMID: 710567]
7. Zhou W, Fu L-W, Tjen-A-Looi S, Li P, et al. Afferent mechanisms underlying stimulation modality-related modulation of acupuncture-related cardiovascular responses. J Appl Physiol. 2004;98(3):872–80. [PMID: 15531558]
8. Li P, Pitsillides KF, Rendig SV, et al. Reversal of reflex-induced myocardial ischemia by median nerve stimulation: a feline model of electroacupuncture. Circulation. 1998;97:1186–94. [PMID: 9537345]
9. Tjen-A-Looi S, Fu L-W, Zhou W (Syuu Y), et al. Role of unmyelinated fibers in electroacupuncture cardiovascular responses. Auton Neurosci. 2005;118: 43–50. [PMID: 15881777]
10. Longhurst JC. Alternative approaches to the medical management of cardiovascular disease: acupuncture, electrical nerve and spinal cord stimulation. Heart Dis. 2001;215–6 (Editorial). [PMID: 11975795]
11. Mannheimer C, Carlsson C-A, Eriksson K, et al. Transcutaneous electrical nerve stimulation in severe angina pectoris. Eur Heart J. 1982;3:297–302. [PMID: 6982163]
12. Mannheimer C, Carlsson C-A, Emanuelsson H, et al. The effects of transcutaneous electrical nerve stimulation in patients with severe angina pectoris. Circulation 1985;71(2):308–16 [PMID: 3871177].
13. Mannheimer C, Emanuelsson H, Waagstein F, et al. Influence of naloxone on the effects of high frequency transcutaneous electrical nerve stimulation in angina pectoris induced by atrial pacing. Br Heart J. 1989;62(1):36–42. [PMID: 2788001]
14. Melzack R, Wall PD. Pain mechanisms: a new theory. Science 1965;150:971–9. [PMID: 5320816]
15. Simpson BA. Electrical stimulation and the relief of pain. 1st ed. Amsterdam: Elsevier Science; 2003.
16. Longhurst JC. Neural regulation of the cardiovascular system. In: Squire LR, Bloom FE, McConnel SK, Roberts JL, Spitzer NC, Zigmond MJ, editors. Fundamental Neuroscience. 2nd ed. San Diego (CA): Academic Press; 2003. p. 935–66.

17. Chandler MJ, Brennan TJ, Garrison DW, et al. A mechanism of cardiac pain suppression by spinal cord stimulation: implications for patients with angina pectoris. Eur Heart J. 1993;14:96–105. [PMID: 8432300]

18. Eliasson T, DeJongste MJL, Mannheimer C. Neuromodulation for refractory angina pectoris. In: Simpson BA, editor. Electrical stimulation and the relief of pain. New York: Elsevier; 2003. p. 143–60.

19. Mannheimer C, Camici P, Chester MR, et al. The problem of chronic refractory angina. Report from the ESC Joint Study Group on the Treatment of Refractory Angina. Eur Heart J. 2002;23:355–70. [PMID: 11846493]

20. Mannheimer C, Eliasson T, Andersson B, et al. Effects of spinal cord stimulation in angina pectoris induced by pacing and possible mechanisms of action. Br Med J. 1993;307:447–80. [PMID: 8400930]

21. Sanderson JE, Brooksby P, Waterhouse D, et al. Epidural spinal electrical stimulation for severe angina: a study of its effects on symptoms, exercise tolerance and degree of ischaemia. Eur Heart J. 1992;13:628–33. [PMID: 1618204]

22. DeJongste MJL, Haaksma J, Hautvast RWM, et al. Effect of spinal cord stimulation on myocardial ischemia during daily life in patients with severe coronary artery disease. Br Heart J. 1994;71:413–8. [PMID: 8011403]

23. Landsherre CD, Mannheimer C, Habets A. Effect of spinal cord stimulation on regional myocardial perfusion assessed by positron emission tomography. Am J Cardiol. 1992;69:1143–9. [PMID: 1575182]

24. Andrell P, Ekre OET, Blomstrand C, et al. Cost-effectiveness of spinal cord stimulation vs coronary artery bypass grafting in patients with severe angina pectoris—long term results from the ESBY study. Cardiology 2003;99:20–4. [PMID: 12589118]

25. Ekre O, Eliasson T, Norrsell H, et al. Long term effects of spinal cord stimulation and coronary artery bypass grafting on quality of life and survival in the ESBY study. Eur Heart J. 2002;23:1938–45. [PMID: 12473256]

26. Ernst E, White AR. A review of problems in clinical acupuncture research. Am J Chin Med. 1997;XXV(1):3–11. [PMID: 9166992]

27. Yamashita H, Tsukayama H, Tanno Y, et al. Adverse events in acupucnture and moxibustion treatment: a six-year survey at a national clinic in Japan. J Altern Complement Med. 1999;5(3):229–36. [PMID: 10381246]

28. Ernst E, White AR. Prospective studies of the safety of acupuncture: a systematicreview. Am J Med. 2001;110(6):481–5. [PMID: 11331060]

29. Ernst G, Strzyz H, Hagmeister H. Incidence of adverse effects during acupuncture therapy—a multicentre survey. Complement Ther Med. 2003;11(2):93–7. [PMID: 12801494]

30. Longhurst JC. Central and peripheral neural mechanisms of acupuncture in myocardial ischemia. In: Saito H, Li P, editors. International congress series. 1238 ed. Elsevier Science; 2002. p. 79–87.

31. Wright RS, Kupperman JL, Liebhaber MI. Bilateral tension pneumothoraces after acupuncture. West J Med. 1991;154(1):736–7. [PMID: 2024504]

32. Kent GP, Brondum J, Keenlyside RA, et al. A large outbreak of acupuncture-associated Hepatitis B. Am J Epidemiol. 1988;127(3):591–8. [PMID: 3341362]

33. Lao L. Safety issues in acupuncture. J Altern Complement Med. 1996;2(1):27–31. [PMID: 9395638]

34. Ernst E, White A. Life-threatening adverse reactions after acupuncture? A systematic review. Pain 1997;71:123–6. [PMID: 9211472]

35. Ernst E, Sherman KJ. Is acupuncture a risk factor for hepatitis? Systemic review of epidemiological studies. J Gastroenterol Hepatol. 2003;18(11):1231–6. [PMID: 14535978]

36. Beal MW. Acupuncture and related treatment modalities-part II: applications to antepartal and intrapartal care. J Nurse Midwifery. 1992;37(4):260–8. [PMID: 1403172]

37. NIH Consensus Conference. Acupuncture. JAMA. 1997 Nov 3;15(5):1–34. [PMID: 10228456]

38. Lin MC, Nahin R, Gershwin ME, et al. State of complementary & alternative medicine in cardiovascular, lung and blood. Circulation 2001;103:2038–41. [PMID: 11319191]

39. Systems to rate the strength of scientific evidence. AHRQ Publication 47. 2003

40. Longhurst JC. Acupuncture's beneficial effects on the cardiovascular system. Prev Cardiol. 1998;1(4):21–33.

41. Rosenthal R. Interpersonal expectations: effects of the experimenters hypothesis. In: Rosenthal R, Rosnow RL, editors. Artifact in behavioral research. New York: Academic Press; 1969. p. 182–279.

42. Boutouyrie P, Corvisier R, Azizi M, et al. Effects of acupuncture on radial artery hemodynamics: controlled trials in sensitized and naive subjects. Am J Physiol Heart Circ Physiol. 2001;280(2):H628–33. [PMID: 11158960]

43. Longhurst J. The ancient art of acupuncture meets modern cardiology. Cerebrum: the Dana Forum on brain science 2001;3(4):48–59.

44. Tjen-A-Looi S, Li P, Longhurst JC. Prolonged inhibition of rostral ventral lateral medullary premotor sympathetic neuron by electroacupuncture in cats. Auton Neurosci. 2003;106(2):119–31. [PMID: 12878081]

45. Zhou W, Fu L-W, Tjen-A-Looi S, et al. Afferent mechanisms underlying stimulation modality-related modulation of acupuncture-related cardiovascular responses. J Appl Physiol. 2005;98(3):872–80. [PMID: 15531558]

46. Collins H, DiCarlo S. TENS attenuates response to colon distension in paraplegic and quadriplegic rats. Am J Physiol Heart Circ Physiol. 2002;283:H1734–9. [PMID: 12234830]

47. Averill A, Cotter AC, Nayak S, et al. Blood pressure response to acupuncture in a population at risk for autonomic dysreflexia. Arch Phys Med Rehabil. 2000;81(11):1494–7. [PMID: 11083354]

48. Chao DM, Shen LL, Tjen-A-Looi S, et al. Naloxone reverses inhibitory effect of electroacupuncture on sympathetic cardiovascular reflex responses. Am J Physiol. 1999 Jun;276 (Heart Circulation Physiology 45):H2127–34. [PMID: 10362696]

49. Yao T, Andersson S, Thoren P. Long-lasting cardiovascular depression induced by acupuncture-like stimulation of the sciatic nerve in unanaesthetized spontaneously hypertensive rats. Brain Res. 1982;240:77–85. [PMID: 7201339]

50. Hoffman P, Thoren P. Long-lasting cardiovascular depression induced by acupuncture-like stimulation of the sciatic nerve in unanesthetized rats. Effects of arousal and type of hypertension. Acta Physiol Scand. 1986;127:119–26. [PMID: 3728043]

51. Chiu YJ, Chi A, Reid IA. Cardiovascular and endocrine effects of acupuncture in hypertensive patients. Clin Exp Hypertens. 1997;19(7):1047–63. [PMID: 9310203]

52. Park J, Hopwood V, White AR, et al. Effectiveness of acupuncture for stroke: A systematic review. J Neurophysiol. 2001;248:558–63. [PMID: 11517996]

53. Naeser MA, Alexander M, Stiassny-Eder D, et al. Real versus sham acupuncture in the treatment of paralysis in acute stroke patients: a CT scan lesion site study. Neuro Rehab. 1992;6:163–73.

54. Gosman-Hedstrom G, Claesson L, Klingenstierna U. Effects of acupuncture treatment on daily life activity and quality of life: A controlled, prospective, and randomized study of acute stroke patients. Stroke 1998;29:2100–8. [PMID: 9756589]

55. Sze FK, Wong E, Or KK, et al. Does acupuncture improve motor recovery after stroke? A meta-analysis of randomized controlled trials. Stroke 2002;33(11): 2604–19. [PMID: 12411650]

56. Johansson B, Haker E, von Arbin M, et al. Acupuncture and transcutaneous nerve stimulation in stroke rehabilitation. Stroke 2001;32:707–13. [PMID: 11239191]

57. Cao Q, Wang S, Liu J. Effect of acupuncture on acute myocardial ischemic injury in rabbits. J Tradit Chin Med. 1981;1:83–6.

58. Youmi Y, Ruiting L, Jingbi M, et al. Effects of acupuncture on experimental acute myocardial infarction. Research On Acupuncture, Moxibustion and Acupuncture Anaesthesia.1986;876–82.

59. Meng JB, Fu WX, Cai JH, et al. Effect of electroacupuncture on the oxygen metabolism of myocardium during myocardial ischemic injury. J Trad Chin Med. 1986 Sept; 6(3):201–6. [PMID: 3492636]

60. Syuu Y, Matsubara H, Hosogi S, et al. Pressor effect of electroacupucnture on hemorrhagic hypotension. Am J Physiol Regulatory Integrative Comp Physiol. 2003; 285(6):R1446–52. [PMID: 12893654]

61. Sato A, Li P, Campbell JL (eds.), Acupuncture: is there a physiological a basis? Excerpta Medica; 2002.

62. Sanderson JE, Tomlinson B, Lau MSW, et al. The effect of transcutaneous electrical nerve stimulation (TENS) on autonomic cardiovascular reflexes. Clin Auton Res. 1995;5:81–4. [PMID: 7620297]

63. Hollman JE, Morgan BJ. Effect of transcutaneous electrical nerve stimulation on the pressor response to static handgrip exercise. Phys Ther. 1997;77(1):28–36. [PMID: 8996461]

64. Li P, Ayannusi O, Reed C, et al. Inhibitory effect of electroacupuncture (EA) on the pressor response induced by exercise stress. J Auton Clin Res. 2004;14:182–8. [PMID: 15241647]

65. Middlekauff HR, Yu JL, Hui K. Acupuncture effects on reflex responses to mental stress in humans. Am J Physiol Regulatory Integrative Comp Physiol. 2001;280(5):R1462–8. [PMID: 11294769]

66. Mannheimer C, Carlsson C-A, Emanuelsson H, et al. Transcutaneous electrical nerve stimulation (TENS) in angina pectoris. Pain. 1986;26:291–300. [PMID: 3534690]

67. Emanuelsson H, Mannheimer C, Waagstein F, et al. Catecholamine metabolism during pacing-induced angina pectoris and the effect of transcutaneous electrical nerve stimulation. Am Heart J. 1987;114:1360–6. [PMID: 3500628]

68. Ballegaard S, Pedersen F, Pietersen A, et al. Effects of acupuncture in moderate, stable angina pectoris: a controlled study. J Intern Med. 1990;227:25–30. [PMID: 2105371]

69. Ballegaard S, Meyer CN, Trojaborg W. Acupuncture in angina pectoris: does acupuncture have a specific effect? J Int Med. 1991;229:357–62. [PMID: 2026989]

70. Ballegaard S, Johannessen A, Karpatschof B, et al. Addition of acupuncture and self-care education in the treatment of patients with severe angina pectoris may be cost beneficial: an open, prospective study. J Altern. Complement Med. 1999;5:405–13. [PMID: 10537240]

71. Ballegaard S, Karpatschof B, Holck JA, et al. Acupuncture in angina pectoris. Do psycho-social and neurophysiological factors relate to the effect? Acupunct Electrother Res Int J. 1995;20:101–16. [PMID: 7491848]

72. Ballegaard S, Norrelund S, Smith DF. Cost benefit of combined use of acupuncture, shiatsu and lifestyle adjustment for treatment of patients with severe angina pectoris. Acupuncture and Electro-Therapeutics Res Int J. 1996;21:187–97. [PMID: 9051166]

73. Richter A, Herlitz J, Hjalmarson A: Effect of acupuncture in patients with angina pectoris. Eur Heart J. 1991;12:175–8. [PMID: 2044550]

74. Chauhan A, Mullins PA, Thuraisingham SI, et al. Effect of transcutaneous electrical nerve stimulation on coronary blood flow. Circulation. 1994;89:694–702. [PMID: 8313557]

75. Liu F, Li J, Liu G, et al. Clinical observation of effect of acupuncture on angina pectoris. In: Chang HT, editor. Research on acupuncture, moxibustion and acupuncture anesthesia. Beijing: Science Press and Springer Verlag; 1986. p. 861–75.

76. Ballegaard S, Jensen G, Pedersen F, et al. Acupuncture in severe, stable angina pectoris: a randomized trial. Acta Med Scand. 1986;220:307–13. [PMID: 3541499]

77. Ho F-M, Huang P-J, Lo H-M, et al. Effect of acupuncture at Nei-Kuan on left ventricular function in patients with coronary artery disease. Am J Chin Med. 1999;27: 149–56. [PMID: 10467449]

78. Ballegaard S, Borg E, Karpatschof B, et al. A. Long-term effects of integrated rehabilitation in patients with advanced angina pectoris: a nonrandomized comparative study. J Altern Complement Med. 2004;10:777–83. [PMID: 15650466]

79. Atalay C, Kockaya EA, Cetin B, Kismet K., Akay MT. Efficacy of topical nitroglycerin and transcutaneous electrical nerve stimulation on survival of random-pattern skin flaps in rats. Scand J Plast Reconstr Surg Hand Surg. 2003;37:10–3. [PMID: 12625388]

80. Cramp FL, McCullough GR, Lowe AS, et al. Trancutaneous electric nerve stimulation: the effect of intensity on local and distal cutaneous blood flow and skin temperature in healthy subjects. Arch Phys Med Rehabil. 2002;83:5–9. [PMID: 11782825]

81. Lundeberg T, Kjartansson J, Samuelson U. Effect of electrical nerve stimulation in healing of ischaemic skin flaps. Lancet. 1988;2:712–4. [PMID: 2901569]

82. Augustinsson LE, Carlson CA, Holm J, Jivegard L. Epidural electrical stimulation in severe limb ischemia: pain relief, increased blood flow and possible limb saving effect. Ann Surg. 1985;202:104–10. [PMID: 3874610]

83. Jivegard LD, Augustinsson LE, Carlsson C-A, Risberg B, Ortenwall P. Long-term results by epidural spinal electrical stimulation (ESES) in patients with inoperable severe lower limb ischaemia. Eur J Vasc Surg. 1987;1:345–9. [PMID: 3509725]

84. Jivegard LD, Augustinsson LE, Holm J, et al. Effects of spinal cord stimulation (SCS) in patients with inoperable severe lower limb ischemia: a prospective randomised controlled study. Eur J Vasc Endovasc Surg. 1995;9:421–5. [PMID: 7633987]

85. Noguchi E, Ohsawa H, Kobayashi S, et al. The effect of electro-acupuncture stimulation on the muscle blood flow of the hindlimb in anesthetized rats. J Auton Nerv Syst. 1999;75:78–86. [PMID: 10189107]

86. Stener-Victorin E, Kobayashi R, Kurosawa M. Ovarian blood flow responses to electro-acupuncture stimulation at different frequencies and intensities in anaesthetized rats. Auton Neurosci. 2003;108:50–6. [PMID: 14614964]

87. Stener-Victorin E, Kobayashi R, Wantanabe O, et al. Effect of electro-acupuncture stimulation of different frequencies and intensities on ovarian blood flow in anaesthetized rats with steroid-induced polycystic ovaries. Reprod Biol Endocrinol. 2004;2:16–24. [PMID: 15046638]

88. Stener-Victorin E, Waldenstrom U, Tagnfors U, et al. Effects of electro-acupuncture on anovulation in women with polycystic ovary syndrome. Acta Obstet Gynecol Scand. 2000;79:180–8. [PMID: 10716298]

89. Ernst E, Lee MH. Sympathetic effect of manual and electrical acupuncture of the Tsusanli knee point: comparison with the Hoku hand point sympathetic effects. Exp Neurol. 1986;94(1):10. [PMID: 3758275]

90. Jansen G, Lundeberg T, Kjartansson J, et al. Acupuncture and sensory neuropeptides increase cutaneous blood flow in rats. Neurosci Lett. 1989;97:305–9. [PMID: 2469996]

91. Jansen G, Lundeberg T, Samuelson UE, et al. Increased survival of ischaemic musculocutaneous flaps in rats after acupuncture. Acta Physiol Scand. 1989;135:555–8. [PMID: 2735200]

92. Zhang Q, Lindberg LG, Kadefors R, et al. A non-invasive measure of changes in blood flow in the human anterior tibial muscle. Eur J Appl Physiol. 2001;84(448): 452. [PMID: 11417434]

93. Sandberg M, Lindberg LG, Gerdle B. Peripheral effects of needle stimulation (acupuncture) on skin and muscle blood flow in fibromyalgia. Eur J Pain. 2004;8: 163–71. [PMID: 14987626]

94. Dawidson I, Angmar-Mansson B, Blom M, et al. Sensory stimulation (acupuncture) increases the release of vasoactive intestinal polypeptide in the saliva of xerostomia sufferers. Neuropeptides 1998;32:543–8. [PMID: 9920452]

95. Blom M, Lundeberg T, Dawidson I, et al. Effects on local blood flux of acupuncture stimulation used to treat xerostomia in patients suffering from Sjogren's syndrome. J Oral Rehabil. 1993;20:541–8. [PMID: 10412476]

96. Blom M, Dawidson I, Fernberg JO, et al. Acupuncture treatment of patients with radiation-induced xerostomia. Eur J Cancer B Oral Oncol. 1996;32B:182–90. [PMID: 8762876]

97. Blom M, Dawidson I, Angmar-Mansson B. The effect of acupuncture on salivary flow rates in patients with xerostomia. Oral Surg Oral Med Oral Pathol. 1992;73:293–8. [PMID: 1545961]

98. Larsson O, Duner-Engstrom M, Lundberg JM, et al. Effects of VIP, PHM and substance P on blood vessels and secretory elements of the human submandibular gland. Reg Peptides. 1986;13:319–26. [PMID: 2422707]

8

HERBAL AND DIETARY SUPPLEMENTS IN CARDIOVASCULAR CARE: EFFICACY AND INCORPORATION INTO PRACTICE

Robert Alan Bonakdar, Erminia Guarneri and Rebecca Costello

INTRODUCTION

Herbal and dietary supplements account for more than $20 billion in yearly sales, with cardiovascular conditions being one of the most common reasons for utilization. Unfortunately, the use of supplements is often done without the knowledge, input, or guidance of a health-care professional. This creates a scenario which requires improved patient–clinician discussion regarding the proper utilization of dietary supplementation. In order to optimize patient management, it is imperative for clinicians to take an active role in understanding several key issues surrounding dietary supplementation, including:

1. The current context of use for dietary supplements including prevalence, rationale, and regulation
2. The evidence for cardiovascular benefit, harm, and interaction for selected dietary supplements
3. Incorporation of dietary supplements into practice including strategies for successful discussion and management

DIETARY SUPPLEMENTS IN CONTEXT

Definition

Dietary supplements have various definitions and are typically thought of as herbal products—Hawthorn, feverfew—or nonherbal products—omega-3 fish oils, vitamin B$_6$, D-ribose. However, the definition as listed in the Dietary Supplement Health and Education Act (DSHEA) of 1994 is more encompassing and includes any single or combination ingredient products containing the following (with examples in parentheses):

- A vitamin (folate)
- A mineral (magnesium)
- A herb or other botanical (Hawthorn)
- An amino acid (L-arginine)
- A dietary substance for use by humans to supplement the diet by increasing the total dietary intake (D-ribose)
- A concentrate, metabolite, constituent, or extract (isoflavonoid extract of soy) (Food and Drug Administration, 2002)

The definition effectively incorporates most substances used by consumers or patients outside the realm of prescription or over-the-counter (OTC) medications. Because of the broad definition, clinicians should be clear in asking about all categories of dietary supplements potentially used.

Prevalence and rationale

Dietary supplement sales have grown steadily, at times dramatically, since the early 1990s with an approximate 400% increase since that time.[1,2] Since the late 1990s, supplements have demonstrated a variable picture where certain markets (Internet, catalogs, and health food stores) have increased while others have slowed. Additionally some individual supplements demonstrate stronger (glucosamine) or weaker (Kava) sales based on recent studies, advertising, or government warnings. Overall, the supplement industry continues to demonstrate impressive numbers with approximately $20 billion in total sales by the most recent estimates.[3] Currently, the use of dietary supplements in surveys range from a low of 18% to over 50% of the American population based on the definition utilized and subjects surveyed.[4,5]

The use of dietary supplements is predicted by several demographic characteristics. The typical user of dietary supplement tends to be a female with higher education and income, with potentially more severe and long-standing medical issues than a nonuser.[6–7] The rationale for supplement use is additionally correlated with a number of factors including the type of medical diagnoses as well as patient belief systems. A survey of cardiac patients found that 64% currently used complementary and alternative medicine (CAM), with the most common types used being supplements (40%) and megadose vitamins (35%). Most of the users of CAM (65%) cited their cardiac condition as the main rationale for their use.[8]

The health beliefs and values of the person considering supplements are also quite important and often misinterpreted. Those who are involved in "active coping behaviors," such as greater physical activity, tend to view supplement use in a similar manner. Also, several surveys demonstrate that those with a more "holistic outlook" wish to utilize complementary methods including dietary supplements, which may take this viewpoint into consideration. Although there has been speculation regarding the use of CAM and dietary supplements as secondary to dissatisfaction with conventional care, the more prevalent theme is that of CAM utilization for optimization of care. In fact, dissatisfaction with conventional care did not predict use of CAM in a previous national survey and less than 5% of CAM users did so in isolation from conventional care. Most CAM users state their motivations for CAM incorporation encompass more global control over their health care, with up to 80% reporting substantial benefit from its use.[6] In their pursuit of CAM, users have actually been found to have more frequent relationships with a primary care physician, regular physician follow-up, and compliance with recommended preventative health behaviors such as regular mammography.[9]

Knowledge base

The knowledge base of the average clinician and consumer regarding dietary supplements has been shown to be suboptimal. Physician surveys have found that physicians in training may have a poor general understanding of commonly used supplements as well as their safety, interaction, and regulation profiles. Similarly, consumers and patients tend to receive their information regarding supplements from nonclinical sources including magazines, friends, and family, with clinician consultation occurring rarely. A survey of cardiac patients found that the most common source of information about CAM was a friend or relative.[10] As pointed out by a recent Harris Poll, the outcome of inaccurate or biased supplement information may be overestimation of the regulatory and evidence basis of dietary supplements. The poll demonstrated that 55% of consumers believed that the government does not allow claims of safety without supporting evidence, 59% believed that products must be preapproved by the FDA before sale, and 68% believed the government required labels to have warnings about potential side effects.[5]

Discussion

One of the other key deficiencies in the dietary supplement scenario is the level of clinician–patient discussion. Initial surveys found that in approximately 70% of encounters, there was no discussion of CAM use, including dietary supplements.[1] More recently, the level of discussion appears to be improving and in one survey of cardiac patients, 80% had informed their physician of the dietary supplements they were utilizing.[10] Unfortunately, when a patient is hospitalized by a specialist, at a time when use of CAM and dietary supplements may be most pertinent, it is not identified up to 88% of the time.[10] The importance of identifying, discussing, and charting CAM and supplement use cannot be understated. The immediate motivation for discussing dietary supplements involves identification of any potential interactions or adverse effects of which the patient may not be aware. More importantly, full discussion enables a better understanding of patient rationale for consideration and utilization of supplements. As mentioned previously, supplement users share health behaviors, which, when identified by clinicians, enable improved coordination and guidance of conventional and complementary treatment options.

To help improve discussion, it is important to better understand why patients do not disclose supplement (or other CAM) use. Surveys indicate that factors including anticipation of negative or disinterested clinician response, as well as belief that the clinician will not provide useful information, motivated nondisclosure.[11] However, most important may be clinician inquiry, with patients demonstrating willingness to disclose supplements use, but only if asked by a clinician directly.[12] Unfortunately, a recent survey of physicians found that few of those surveyed felt comfortable discussing CAM with their patients. Of all responders, 84% felt they needed a greater knowledge base in order to adequately counsel patients on CAM topics. It is hypothesized that with improved education about CAM, physicians may be more willing to discuss this topic and counsel patients.[13]

In addition to knowledge base, clinicians often find time an obstacle for effective supplement counseling. First, they do not view counseling as a one-time effort, but an ongoing effort. Initially, clinicians should make patients complete a supplement intake form prior to the visit, which notes brand name and dosage of supplements, start date, source of recommendation, and reason for use. This will help to focus the discussion and also let you know where the patient is receiving recommendation regarding supplements and why they are taking a certain supplement. Each visit can be an opportunity to update and further discuss the items on the intake form in a manner similar to a medication list. If the completed intake form is not available initially, it may be necessary to review this form at a follow-up meeting and focus the initial discussion on supplements that are most relevant (i.e., are there any supplements which may interfere with the patient's warfarin?). Second, the use of ancillary staff and community resources for supplement counseling is highly recommended. Explain to the patient that if additional supplements are considered they should be reviewed prior to initiation. This may mean a call to the nursing staff, who can provide initial information regarding most common supplements inquiries (using some of the resources noted in Table 8-1). Additionally, other clinic and community health professionals (dieticians, pharmacists) are quite helpful for providing unbiased information for the patient and input back to the treating clinicians. With this ongoing, team approach, the sometimes daunting task of supplement discussion and counseling can be made manageable.

There are a number of resources available to clinicians interested in better understanding dietary supplements as a means of increasing and improving patient communication. These resources are listed in Table 8-1 and include print and online information on evidence-based use of supplements, as well as continuing medical education courses available to clinicians.

Regulation

The regulation of dietary supplements in the United States is based on the DSHEA of 1994, which places supplements under the "food umbrella" as

TABLE 8-1

DIETARY SUPPLEMENT RESOURCES AND REFERENCES

Web Sites

- http://NCCAM.NIH.GOV
  - National Institutes of Health (NIH) Center for Complementary and Alternative Medicine. Clearinghouse of articles including *Considering Complementary and Alternative Therapies?* and *herbal fact sheets*
- http://ods.od.nih.gov
  - NIH Office of Dietary Supplements (ODS) with free resources including
  - Dietary supplement fact sheets
  - Annual bibliographies of significant advances in dietary supplement research
- http://www.naturaldatabase.com*
  - Natural Medicines Comprehensive Database. An objective, subscriber-funded database of herb/supplement information and interactions
- http://www.ahrq.gov
  - Agency for HealthCare Quality Research (AHRQ)
- http://herbmed.org
  - A searchable herbal database operated by the Alternative Medicine Foundation
- http://www.ahpa.org
  - The American Herbal Products Association. Publishers of The Botanical Safety Handbook
- http://www.drugfacts.com*
  - Comprehensive database by facts and comparisons
- http://www.micromedex.com*
  - A list of supplement monographs by Micromedex
- http://www.consumerlab.com**
  - Independent testing of supplements since 1999 with listing of qualifying supplements
- http://www.InteractionReport.org**
  - Summary of article dealing with herb-drug interactions provided by Integrated Medical Arts

Texts

- American Herbal Products Association. *Botanical Safety Handbook*
- Barrett, M. *The Handbook of Clinically Tested Remedies.* 2004.
- Blumenthal M, et al. *The ABC Clinical Guide to Herbs.* 2003
- Bone, K. *The Essential Guide to Herbal Safety.* 2005
- Facts and Comparisons. *Review of Natural Products.* Monthly updates
- Gruenwald J, et al. *PDR for Herbal Medicines.* 2nd ed. 2000
- American Botanical Council. *The Complete German Commission E Monographs: Guide to Herbal Medicines*
- Fetrow C, Avila J. *Professional Handbook of Complementary and Alternative Medicines*

(Continued)

TABLE 8-1

DIETARY SUPPLEMENT RESOURCES AND REFERENCES (CONTINUED)

Journals

- *Herbalgram*
- *Alternative Medicine Alert*
- *Journal of Alternative and Complementary Medicine*
- *Alternative Therapies in Health and Medicine*
- *Journal of Herbal Pharmacotherapy*

Continuing medical education

- Botanical Medicine in Modern Clinical Practice
  Sponsored by Columbia University Medical Center
  Yearly in June http://ColumbiaCME.org
- Natural Supplements: An Evidence-Based Update
  Cosponsored by Scripps Center for Integrative Medicine and UCSD
  Yearly in January, http://www.scrippsintegrativemedicine.org

---

*Subscription required for access.
**Subscription required for full access.

opposed to drugs. The key components of this act are important for all practitioners to review to better understand how regulation differs from prescription medications. First, unlike prescription medications that need to proceed through multiphase trials to gain premarketing approval from the FDA, supplements (with established ingredients) are not required to have safety, efficacy, or bioavailability data prior to marketing.[14] Ensuring these important qualities, along with having a clear and truthful label, is solely the responsibility of the manufacturer. Second, because supplements are not required to go through premarketing clearance, they also fall into a different labeling scheme than prescription products. In short, supplements typically have "structure or function" claims that cannot imply prevention, treatment, or cure of a condition. Rarely, such as in the case of folic acid for prevention of neutral pulse defects where the evidence is strong, a health claim may be granted by the FDA after petition stating a supplement may be of benefit in a given health condition.[15] The line can at times be difficult to distinguish with a number of manufacturers being cited for going beyond allowed standards.[16]

The key role of the FDA (and in the case of advertising, the FTC) begins after the supplement is marketed and involves monitoring safety, label claims, and product advertising. Thus, the typical premarketing steps needed for prescription medication approval are replaced with postmarketing surveillance. In this scenario, the FDA must utilize adverse drug reports and product analysis to prove a supplement poses significant health risks. Two recent examples of this are the attempt to ban ephedra secondary to adverse reactions and "PCSPES" (a dietary supplement marketed to patients with prostate cancer) because of product adulteration.[17]

As it currently stands, the supplement regulatory system contrasts greatly to that for prescription medication and will likely see additional scrutiny and amendments in the near future. Although many manufacturers utilize proper standards, the publicity of an adulterated or unsafe supplement tarnishes the standing of well-regulated supplements as well as decreases the confidence of practitioners and consumers wishing to incorporate evidence-based supplements. The incorporation of new good manufacturing practice (GMP) standards will be helpful in standardizing the manufacturing process. Also, greater organizational support for monitoring claims, advertising, and adverse events should improve the enforcement of existing statutes.

External regulation

Several independent agencies now offer testing and monitoring services, allowing manufacturers the opportunity to demonstrate their adherence to regulatory standards. Because no federal standard has been clearly established, these agencies allow manufacturers to identify themselves as meeting various manufacturing standards. Typically, manufacturers submit their product for review, which can take various forms including ingredient verification, manufacturing site monitoring, and random off-the-shelf testing. Those that pass inspection may carry an independent "seal-of-approval" on their label and advertising. These agencies typically charge a fee for the verification process. Several of the federal and independent agencies currently involved in dietary supplement testing, safety, and monitoring are listed in Table 8-2.

Safety and adverse effects

The rate and severity of adverse effects associated with dietary supplements are difficult to estimate. This is due to minimal if any premarketing safety data as well as a suboptimal system of capturing and verifying postmarketing events. The Dietary Supplement and Nonprescription Drug Consumer Protection Act was signed into law December 2006 and will become effective in December 2007.

In accordance with the new law, serious adverse events that are reported to the manufacturer must be reported to the FDA within 15 days. Because this will not capture all adverse effects or potential interactions, it continues to be imperative for clinicians to engage in discussion with their pateints regarding the use and effects of dietary supplements.

Data on the occurrence or potential for herb–drug interactions (HDIs) also are quite preliminary. Broad estimates indicate that approximately 20–43% of patients take dietary supplements along with prescription medications.[2,18] In most cases, this use may pose little actual danger as determined by a recent survey that found a 3–6% occurrence of concomitant use of a medication with a potentially interacting supplement. However, certain scenarios should prompt further discussion, monitoring, or supplement/medication alteration to avoid the potential for negative interactions.

One of the most common scenarios for a clinician is that of a patient on dietary supplements, which have a potential to affect blood clotting. When the

TABLE 8-2

FEDERAL AND INDEPENDENT REGULATORY AGENCIES

Agency	Web Site
Federal	
Food and Drug Administration (FDA) Medwatch Program • Site for collecting adverse reactions to prescription and OTC medications as well as dietary supplements	www.fda.gov/medwatch
Federal Trade Commission (FTC) • Site for submitting complaints on false or misleading advertising	www.ftc.gov/ftc/complaint.htm
American Association of Poison Control Centers • Site for report and management of adverse effects	www.poison.org
Independent Labs/Agencies Providing Supplement Verification	
The Consumerlab Product Review	www.Consumerlab.com
Dietary Supplement Verification Program (DSVP) through the United States Pharmacopeia (USP)	www.uspverified.org
National Sanitation Foundation (NSF)	www.NSF.ORG/consumer/ dietary_supplements
The Natural Products Association good manufacturing practices (GMPs) Certification Program	http://www.naturalproductsassoc.org

supplement is concomitantly used with prescription agents with similar properties or in the setting of surgery, increased caution is advised. In recent surveys, up to 22% of presurgical patients routinely used herbs (8% reported multiple herbs) and 51% routinely used vitamins. Of the products reviewed, 27% of patients used herbs that could potentially interfere with blood clotting.[19,20]

A list of dietary supplements with such a potential is provided in Table 8-3. Although extremely rare, this combination has been implicated in cases of hemorrhage.[21] Overall, the field of HDI identification, monitoring, and management is quite young. Most of the published literature deals with case reports as opposed to clinical trials. Those supplements which have been evaluated in a clinical trial have typically been tested in patients on warfarin therapy to assess effects on coagulation. The full report of the NIH Conference on Dietary Supplements, Coagulation, and Antithrombotic Therapies is available and provides a full bibliography on this important topic.[21] Selected findings of controlled clinical trials

TABLE 8-3

HERBS ASSOCIATED WITH ANTIPLATELET/BLOOD THINNING POTENTIAL

Herb	Name	Herb	Name
Agrimony	(*Agrimonia eupatoria*)	Horse chestnut	(*Aesculus hippocastanum*)
Alfalfa	(*Medicago sativa*)	Horseradish	(*Armoracia rusticana*)
Angelica	(*Angelica archangelica*)	Licorice	(*Glycyrrhiza glabra*)
Anise	(*Pimpinella anisum*)	Northern prickly ash	(*Zanthoxylum americanum*)
Asafoetida	(*Ferula assa-foetida*)	Onion	(*Allium cepa*)
Aspen	(*Populi cortex*)	Papain	(*Carica papaya*)
Bladderwrack	(*Fucus vesiculosis*)	Passionflower	(*Passiflora incarnata*)
Black cohosh	(*Cimicifuga racemosa*)	Pau d'Arco	(*Tabebuia impetiginosa*)
Bogbean	(*Menyanthes trifoliate*)	Plantain	(*Plantago major*)
Dong quai	(*Angelica sinensis*)	Poplar	(*Populus tacamahacca*)
Boldo	(*Peumus boldus*)	Quassia	(*Quassia amara*)
Borage seed oil	(*Borago officinalis*)	Red clover	(*Trifolium pratense*)
Bromelain	(*Ananas comosus*)	Roman chamomile	(*Chamaemelum nobile*)
Capsicum	(*Capsicum frutescen*)	Safflower	(*Carthamus tinctorius*)
Celery	(*Apium graveolens*)	Southern prickly ash	(*Zanthoxylum clava-herculis*)
Clove	(*Syzygium aromaticum*)	Stinging nettle	(*Urtica dioica*)
Danshen	(*Salvia miltiorrhiza*)	Sweet clover	(*Melilotus officinalis*)
Devils claw	(*Harpagophytum procumbens*)	Sweet vernal grass	(*Anthoxanthum odoratum*)
European Mistletoe	(*Viscum album*)	Tonka bean	(*Dipterux odorata*)
Fenugreek	(*Trigonella foenum-graecum*)	Feverfew	(*Tanacetum parthenium*)

(Continued)

TABLE 8-3

HERBS ASSOCIATED WITH ANTIPLATELET/BLOOD THINNING POTENTIAL (*CONTINUED*)

Herb	Name	Herb	Name
Garlic	(*Allium sativum*)	St. John's Wort Turmeric	(*Curcuma longa*)
Ginkgo	(*Ginkgo biloba*)	Wild carrot	(*Daucus carota*)
Ginseng, Panax	(Asian ginseng)	Wild lettuce	(*Lactuca virosa*)
Goldenseal	(*Hydrastis canadensis*)	Yarrow	(*Achillea millefolium*)

Reference: www.NaturalDatabase.com

in this scenario (typically healthy subjects initiated on warfarin therapy with introduction of a dietary supplement) are highlighted below.

- Fish oil supplementation (up to 6 g/day) does not appear to interfere significantly with warfarin therapy ($N = 16$).[22]
- Vitamin E intake did not interfere with warfarin therapy ($N = 21$).[23]
- Coenzyme Q10 (Co-Q10) 100 mg daily and Ginkgo Biloba 100 mg daily did not interfere significantly with warfarin therapy ($N = 14$).[24]
- Use of St. John's Wort, but not ginseng was associated with a significant reduction in the pharmacological effect of warfarin ($N = 12$).[25]
- Use of American Ginseng (Panax Quinquefolius), 500 mg daily for 4 weeks in healthy subjects decreased the peak international normalized ratio (INR) and peak plasma warfarin levels ($N = 20$).[26]
- Recent trial of ginkgo and ginseng did not demonstrate any significant alteration in warfarin parameters in healthy subjects ($N = 12$).[27]
- Over the counter, vitamin K_1 containing multivitamins (containing 25 mcg of vitamin K) decreased INR significantly in those with low-serum vitamin K status. No decrease was seen in subjects with normal vitamin K status ($N = 102$).[28]

These clinical trials should be utilized as a guide and are not absolute in their conclusions. There have been inconsistencies in the characterization of interactions based on the type, brand, and dosage of dietary supplements examined. In addition, these trials do not take into consideration the typical scenario of patients on multiple dietary supplements and/or medications taken concomitantly with their warfarin therapy. Until more is known on the subject, it behooves the clinician to have continued vigilance in discussing and monitoring patients in certain clinical scenarios (such as those on anticoagulation therapy) to minimize potential interactions.

In addition to dietary supplements that affect blood clotting, a number of other categories of supplements that can affect the cardiac patient need to be considered. These include dietary supplements with stimulant and laxative ability as well as those which can cause direct (i.e., cardiac ionotrope) or indirect cardiac toxicity (i.e., alter digoxin metabolism). Stimulants with potential cardiac toxicity are listed in Table 8-4. These agents have various active ingredients or derivates which may act as biostimulants including caffeine, ephedrine, and theophylline among others. These agents may have minimal to no significant cardiac effects when used in dietary form (drinking green tea in moderation) or have significant potential for cardiac toxicity when used in any dose (ephedra). Some of the more potent stimulants have been associated with palpitations, arrythmias, increased heart rate and blood pressure as well as hypertension, myocardial ischemia, and stroke. Therefore all patients, including those without a cardiac history, should be routinely questioned and counseled regarding the use of these dietary supplements.

TABLE 8-4

DIETARY SUPPLEMENTS WITH STIMULATORY EFFECTS

Dietary Supplement with Stimulatory Constituents Effects
Areca nut (alkaloid arecoline)
Bitter orange (*Citrus aurantium*) synephrine
Coffee varies on an average contains 60–120 mg caffeine per 80 g of brewed coffee
Cola nut (1–3.5% caffeine)
Country mallow (Heartleaf) (0.8–1.2% ephedrine)
Ephedra (*Ma huang*) alkaloid constituents contain ephedrine and pseudoephedrine with variable concentration
Guarana (2.5–7% caffeine)
Khat (cathine and cathinone)
Tea (white, green, black) varies on average 15–45 mg caffeine per 80 g serving
Wahoo root bark (*Euonymus atropurpiuretus*) (2–4% caffeine)
Yerba mate (0.2–2.0% caffeine) (contains theophylline and theobromine)

www.naturaldatabase.com
- Klepser TB, Klepser ME. Unsafe and potentially safe herbal therapies. Am J Health-Syst Pharm. 1999;56:125–38.
- Miller LG. Herbal medicinals. Selected clinical considerations focusing on known or potential drug-herb interactions. Arch Intern Med. 1998;158:2200–11.
- Nemecz G. Hawthorn. US pharmacist. 1999 Feb; 52,54:57–8, 60.
- Nykamp DL, Fackih MN, Compton ALl. Possible association of acute lateral-wall myocardial infarction and bitter orange supplement. Ann Pharmacother. 2004;38:812–6 (227).
- Vogel JK et al. ACC complementary medicine expert consensus document. Integrating complementary medicine into cardiovascular medicine. J Am College Cardiol. 2005;46(1):184–221.

There are numerous other supplements that are often listed for possessing either potential intrinsic cardiotoxicity or toxicity based on use with other cardiac agents. Because the level of evidence for most of these listings is either theoretical or anecdotal, the clinician is cautioned to analyze these scenarios carefully before deciding on the appropriateness of continuing or discontinuing supplementation. Table 8-5 provides additional resources for identifying and researching these agents in order to better understand their safety and level of evidence for interaction when utilized in a cardiovascular setting.

TABLE 8-5

RESOURCES FOR IDENTIFYING DIETARY SUPPLEMENT REACTIONS AND INTERACTION

Organization/Product	Web Site
HerbMed by the Alternative Medicine Foundation	http://www.herbmed.org
ePocrates Rx	http://www.epocrates.com
Guide to popular natural products by facts and comparisons	http://www.factsandcomparisons.com
InteractionReport.org sponsored by Integrative Medical Arts	http://www.interactionreport.org
Lexi-Natural products	http://www.lexi.com
Medscape drug interaction checker* druginterchecker	http://www.medscape.com/druginfo/
Micromedex	http://www.micromedex.com
NAPRALERT (**Na**tural **pr**oducts **alert**)	http://www.ag.uiuc.edu/napralert.org/ napra.html
Natural medicine comprehensive database	http://www.naturaldatabase.com
PhytoNet provided by the European Scientific Cooperative on Phytotherapy (ESCOP)	http://www.escop.com/phytonet.htm
Pocket PDR	http://www.PDR.net
Tarascon Pocket Pharmacopoeia	http://www.tarascon.com

*No fee.

DIETARY SUPPLEMENT EVIDENCE-BASED REVIEW

Table 8-6 attempts to summarize the evidence for selected dietary supplements utilized in cardiovascular care. The format of the table is as follows:

1. Name/descriptors
2. Indications
3. Dosage
    - Most common dosage is listed, although this may vary widely between trials and brands.
4. Efficacy
    - The levels of evidence are noted in Table 8-6. These are adapted from those utilized by the Natural Medicine Comprehensive Database (www. naturaldatabase.com).
5. Comments/notes
    - Summary of efficacy if available (i.e., level of improvement in low-density lipoprotein (LDL), systolic blood pressure, etc.).
6. Key references

Although Table 8-7 provides the levels of evidence for various supplements, the clinician must translate the evidence to help patients find supplements that can provide consistent results. As discussed in section "Incorporating Dietary Supplements into Practice" the existence of supportive evidence must be combined with identifying a supplement containing a clinically proven formulation with consistent dosage, purity, and bioavailability. This can at times be a difficult task requiring ongoing utilization of the resources listed in Table 8-1.

INCORPORATING DIETARY SUPPLEMENTS INTO PRACTICE

There are a number of key steps involved in the proper incorporation of dietary supplements in clinical practice. The H-E-R-B-A-L mnemonic is offered in Table 8-8 as a practice tool for alerting clinicians to the most important steps involved in the discussion and management of dietary supplement use.

The steps noted in the H-E-R-B-A-L mnemonic are applied to the three cardiovascular patient scenarios noted below. The majority of scenarios involving the incorporation of dietary supplements in cardiovascular care involve patients presenting in one of two states. The first involves a patient presenting with a borderline status such as borderline cholesterol or hypertension. In most cases, there are clinically defined parameters for the borderline status such as National Cholesterol Education Program (NCEP) Step I defined by total cholesterol between 200 and 240 or LDL between 100 and 130 with less than two risk factors. In this scenario, lifestyle change including exercise and diet, including the incorporation of dietary supplements, may be indicated. In addition, from

T A B L E 8 - 6

SELECTED DIETARY SUPPLEMENTS IN CARDIOVASCULAR DISEASE—A THERAPEUTIC REVIEW

Name	Condition	Dose	Level of Evidence*	Notes/Comments	Ref.
β-Sitosterol (Plant Sterol/Stanols)	Dyslipidemia CHD	800 mg to 2 g daily	Effective	• Approved FDA health claim • Part of NCEP Step II • ↓ LDL by 10% • ↓LDL by 20% when added to a low-fat/cholesterol diet • Adding sterols or stanols to statin medication is more effective than doubling the statin dose • Appears safe and effective in children with familial hypercholesterolemia	1, 2, 3, 4
Calcium	Dyslipidemia	1200 mg calcium carbonate daily	Possibly effective	6 weeks of Tx in combination with a low-fat diet • ↓ LDL 4.4% • ↑ HDL 4.1%	5
	HTN	1–1.5 g daily	Possibly effective	• May decrease systolic BP by 2 mm Hg with potentially more benefit in patients with low calcium intake • May be beneficial in ↑BP in pregnancy • See Chapter 5 and (AHRQ review)	6
Co-Q10	CHF	50–200 mg daily	Possibly effective	• Significant variability in absorption	7
		As above		• May improve subjective measures with variability noted on objective measures	8, 9

	Condition	Dose	Efficacy		References
	HTN	As above	Possibly effective	• May have additive role when used with anti-HTN medication ↓ of 6–17 mm Hg systolic and 3 mm Hg diastolic	10, 11
Fiber (psyllium, guar gum, pectin, whole oats)	Dyslipidemia	15 g daily	Effective	• Approved for FDA Health claim • Part of NCEP Step II • Utilizing psyllium (15 g/day) can be more effective than doubling statin dose • Eating cereal with psyllium can reduce LDL 5–9%	12, 13, 14
Flavanoids Commonly measured as quercetin and found in tea, onion, and apples	CHD Dyslipidemia	Varies based on source	Likely effective	• Flavonoids exist as polyphenolic antioxidants found naturally. • Risk reduction of CHD mortality in highest versus lowest tertile of flavonoid intake 0.42	15, 16
Flaxseed (Linum usitatissimum)	Dyslipidemia	40–50 g daily	Likely effective	• Rich source of soluble fiber and stanols • ↓ LDL 8–18%	17, 18
Garlic (Allium sativum)	Dyslipidemia	Extract 600–1200 mg standardized to 1.3% alliin content	Inconclusive	• Isolated supplement may demonstrate mild benefit with uncertainty regarding long term benefit	19

(Continued)

SELECTED DIETARY SUPPLEMENTS IN CARDIOVASCULAR DISEASE—A THERAPEUTIC REVIEW (CONTINUED)

Name	Condition	Dose	Level of Evidence[*]	Notes/Comments	Ref.
	HTN	As above	Incon-clusive		20
	Peripheral arterial disease	As above	Likely not effective		21
Green Tea (Camellia sinensis)	Dyslipidemia	375 mg daily of a theaflavin-enriched green tea extract	Possibly effective	12 weeks of a theaflavin-enriched green tea extract ↓LDL by 16.4%	22, 23
Guggul Guggulipid (Commiphora mukul)	Dyslipidemia	3–6 g/day	Likely not effective	• No benefit in largest, most controlled trials, which contrasts with previous positive trials from India	24, 25
Hawthorn (Crataegus)	CHF	160–1800 mg of standardized extract (LI 132 or WS 1442 used in trials)	Possibly effective	• May improve ejection fraction, exercise tolerance, and reduce subjective symptoms associated with NYHA stage II heart failure after 6–12 weeks of treatment	26
Horse chestnut (Aesculus hippocastanum)	Chronic venous insufficiency	300-mg extract containing 50 mg aescin	Incon-clusive	• May be as effective as compression therapy in decreasing lower leg volume and leg circumference at the calf and ankle	27

	Condition	Dose	Effectiveness	Comments	References
L-Arginine	Angina		Possibly effective	Utilized as a nitric oxide precursor L-arginine	
				May decrease symptoms and improve exercise tolerance and quality of life in patients with class II, III, and IV angina	28
	CHF		B	Appears to improve perfusion parameters with questionable improvement in exercise capacity	29, 30
	CHD		Possibly ineffective	No benefit noted in chronic CHD and preliminary concern of worsening outcome with chronic use	31, 32
	HTN		Possibly effective but preliminary	Arginine in CHD found beneficial in decreasing HTN in DM II	33, 34
Magnesium	HTN	600–1000 mg daily (10–40 mmol daily)	Possibly effective	Dose-dependent ↓ of 4.3 mm Hg systolic and ↓ 2.3 mm Hg diastolic for each 10 mmol/day increase	35, 36
Niacin (nicotinic acid, nicotinamide, niacinamide)	Dyslipidemia	500 mg to 2 g daily	Effective	• Prescription form approved by FDA • Most effective for increasing HDL (15–35%) and reducing triglycerides (20–50%) • Extended release may decrease side effects including flushing • Periodic check of liver function required	37, 38, 39

(Continued)

TABLE 8 - 6

SELECTED DIETARY SUPPLEMENTS IN CARDIOVASCULAR DISEASE—A THERAPEUTIC REVIEW (CONTINUED)

Name	Condition	Dose	Level of Evidence*	Notes/Comments	Ref.
Nuts (e.g., walnuts and almonds are good sources of folate, magnesium, plant sterols, and soluble fiber)	CHD	5 oz/week	Possibly effective	• In patients with CHD, eating 5 oz of nuts per week associated with a risk reduction of 0.66 • Physicians' Health Study, nut consumption > 2 per week: ↓ risk of sudden cardiac death risk reduction of 0.53 ↓ total CHD deaths risk reduction of 0.70	40, 41, 42
Oils					
Omega-3 oils Fish oils)		Dose range 1–4 g daily with minimum of 360 EPA and 240 DHA per gram			
	Arrythmia prevention		Possibly effective	Posible benefit may depend on type and etiology of arrhythmia	43
	HTN		Incon-clusive	• One preparation ↓ 6 mm Hg systolic BP and ↓ 5 mm Hg diastolic	44
	Cardiac (SP) mortality		Possibly effective	↓ Incidence of death due to MI by 24%	45
	All cause mortality		Possibly effective	↓ All cause mortality by 16%	As above
	Hypertrigly-ceridemia		Possibly effective	• May ↓ TG 20–50% • Available in FDA-approved form • See Chapter 5 and AHRQ	46, 47

Supplement	Condition	Dose	Effectiveness	Notes	Reference
Mono- and polyunsaturated oils: canola, olive, sunflower oil				• Emphasize to patients that these oils should be a replacement for saturated fats in the diet	
	Dyslipidemia		Possibly effective	Possible increased benefit from canola versus other oils	48, 49
	CHD		Possibly effective	• FDA health claim for olive oil and CHD	50, 51
Policosanol	Dyslipidemia	10–20 mg daily	Possibly effective	• ↓ LDL by 21–29%, (HDL 8–15% • Majority of research based in Cuba and not replicated elsewhere. The type of policosanol utilized in supplements may vary considerably from type found in Cuba	52
Potassium	HTN	350 mg daily	Inconclusive	• May ↓ systolic by 2–4 mm Hg and diastolic by 0.5–3.5 mm Hg. Most effective for African Americans and those with low potassium, high sodium intake	53
Acetyl L-carnitine	Angina and	500–3000 mg/day	Likely effective	May provide mild-moderate improvementsin exercise capacity and myocardial ischemia in patients with stable angina	54
					55

(Continued)

TABLE 8-6

SELECTED DIETARY SUPPLEMENTS IN CARDIOVASCULAR DISEASE—A THERAPEUTIC REVIEW (CONTINUED)

Name	Condition	Dose	Level of Evidence*	Notes/Comments	Ref.
	Ischemic heart disease	IV formulation	Likely effective	As above	56
	CHF		Likely effective	May improve left ventricular function and exercise capacity in people with class II or III CHF	57
	PVD		Likely effective	May increase walking distance in patients with more severe PVD	58, 59
Red rice yeast (*Monascus purpureus*)	Dyslipidemia	1.2–2.4 g daily	Likely effective	• Chemical constituents similar to lovastain • 8 weeks of 2.4 g/day ↓ LDL ~20% point • Significant product variability	60, 61
Soy (*Glycine max*)	CHD	20–50 g of soy protein daily	Inconclusive	• Approved FDA health claim for CHD • Does not appear to have a protective effect at low doses	62, 63
	Dyslipidemia	As above	Variable and mild	• AHRQ 2005 meta-analysis less dramatic effects ~50 g/day: ↓ LDL 13%; ↓TG 10.5%; ↑ HDL 2.4%; isolated soy isoflavanoid appear not be as effective	64, 65

HTN	As above	Possibly effective	• Questions regarding optimal dose and formulation protein, isoflavonoid • ↓ 4 mm Hg systolic and 3 mm Hg diastolic • Combined with psyllium ↓ 8 mm Hg systolic and 2 mm Hg diastolic	
Vitamin B[6], B[12], folate	Elevate plasma homocysteine	Possibly effective	• Consistent decrease in Hcy observed with variable results in the ability to decrease cardiovascular events and stent restenosis	66, 67, 68
Vitamin C	CHD, primary prevention	Typically >250 mg daily	Possibly effective Inconclusive	• Ineffective in AHRQ review • See Chapter 5	
Yogurt	Dyslipidemia	125–450 ml yogurt products daily	Possibly effective	• Yogurt with Lactobacillus acidophilus and other probiotic strains can ↓ LDL by 4.4–8.4%	69, 70

*Efficacy ratings broaden review of natural medicines and comprehensive database (www.naturalmedicine.com, www.naturaldatabase.com) and/or systematic reviews AHRQ when available.

CHD: coronary heart disease; CHF: congestive heart failure; DMII: diabetes mellitus, type II; Hcy: homocysteine; HTN: hypertension; LDL: low-density lipoprotein; NCEP: national cholesterol education program; PVD: peripheral vascular disease; Ref.: references; RR: relative risk; NYHA: NEW YORK Heart Association

1. Katan MB, Grundy SM, Jones P, Law M, Miettinen T, Paoletti R (Stresa Workshop Participants). Efficacy and safety of plant stanols and sterols in the management of blood cholesterol levels. Mayo Clin Proc. 2003 Aug;78(8):965–78. (Review)

2. Becker M, Staab D, Von Bergmann K. Treatment of severe familial hypercholesterolemia in childhood with sitosterol and sitostanol. J Pediatr. 1993;122:292–6.

3. Lichtenstein AH, Deckelbaum RJ. Stanol/sterol ester-containing foods and blood cholesterol levels: a statement for healthcare professionals from Nutrition Committee, Council on Nutrition, Physical Activity, Metabolism of American Heart Association. Circulation. 2001;103:1177–9.

4. FDA authorizes new coronary heart disease health claim for plant sterol and plant stanol esters. http://www.fda.gov/bbs/topics/ANSWERS/ ANS01033.html October 10, 2005.

5. Bell L, Halstenson CE, Halstenson CJ, et al. Cholesterol-lowering effects of calcium carbonate in patients with mild to moderate hypercholesterolemia. Arch Intern Med. 1992;152:2441–4.

6. Dwyer JH, Dwyer KM, Scribner RA, et al. Dietary calcium, calcium supplementation, and blood pressure in African American adolescents. Am J Clin Nutr. 1998;68:648–55.

7. Bonakdar RA, Guarneri E. Coenzyme Q10. Am Fam Physician. 2005 Sep 15;72(6):1065–70.

(Continued)

8. Berman M, Erman A, Ben-Gal T, et al. Coenzyme Q10 in patients with end-stage heart failure awaiting cardiac transplantation: a randomized, placebo-controlled study. Clin Cardiol. 2004;27:295–9.

9. Watson PS, Scalia GM, Galbraith A, et al. Lack of effect of coenzyme Q on left ventricular function in patients with congestive heart failure. J Am Coll Cardiol. 1999;33:1549–52.

10. Hodgson JM, Watts GF, Playford DA, et al. Coenzyme Q10 improves blood pressure and glycaemic control: a controlled trial in subjects with type 2 diabetes. Eur J Clin Nutr. 2002;56:1137–42.

11. Burke BE, Neuenschwander R, Olson RD. Randomized, double-blind, placebo-controlled trial of coenzyme Q10 in isolated systolic hypertension. South Med J. 2001;94:1112–7.

12. Moreyra AE, Wilson AC, Koraym A. Effect of combining psyllium fiber with simvastatin in lowering cholesterol. Arch Intern Med. 2005;165:1161–6.

13. Olson BH, Anderson SM, Becker MP, et al. Psyllium-enriched cereals lower blood total cholesterol and LDL cholesterol, but not HDL cholesterol, in hyper-cholesterolemic adults: results of a meta-analysis. J Nutr. 1997;127:1973–80.

14. Staking a claim to good health: FDA and science stand behind health claims on foods. Accessed at http://www.cfsan.fda.gov/~dms/fdhclm.html October 10, 2005.

15. Hertog MG, Feskens EJ, Hollman PC, et al. Dietary antioxidant flavonoids and risk of coronary heart disease: the Zutphen Elderly Study. Lancet. 1993;342:1007–11.

16. Conquer JA, Maiani G, Azzini E, et al. Supplementation with quercetin markedly increases plasma quercetin concentration without effect on selected risk factors for heart disease in healthy subjects. J Nutr. 1998;128:593–7.

17. Jenkins DJ, Kendall CWC, Vidgen E, et al. Health aspects of partially defatted flaxseed, including effects on serum lipids, oxidative measures, and ex vivo androgen and progestin activity: a controlled, crossover trial. Am J Clin Nutr. 1999;69:395–402.

18. Lucas EA, Wild RD, Hammond LJ, et al. Flaxseed improves lipid profile without altering biomarkers of bone metabolism in postmenopausal women. J Clin Endocrinol Metab. 2002;87:1527–32.

19. Stevinson C, Pittler MH, Ernst E. Garlic for treating hypercholesterolemia: a meta-analysis of randomized clinical trials. Ann Intern Med. 2000;133:420–9.

20. Steiner M, Khan AH, Holbert D, Lin RI. A double-blind crossover study in moderately hypercholesterolemic men that compared the effect of aged garlic extract and placebo administration on blood lipids. Am J Clin Nutr. 1996;64:866–70.

21. Jepson RG, Kleijnen J, Leng GC. Garlic for peripheral arterial occlusive disease (Cochrane Review). In: The cochrane library. Issue 2. 2000. Oxford: Update Software.

22. Maron DJ, Lu GP, Cai NS, et al. Cholesterol-lowering effect of a theaflavin-enriched green tea extract: a randomized controlled trial. Arch Intern Med. 2003;163:1448–53.

23. Imai K. Nakachi K. Cross-sectional study of effects of drinking green tea on cardiovascular and liver diseases. BMJ. 1995;310:693–6.

24. Szapary PO, Wolfe ML, Bloedon LT, et al. Guggulipid for treatment of hypercholesterolemia: a randomized controlled trial. JAMA. 2003;290:765–72.

25. Singh RB, Niaz MA, Ghosh S. Hypolipidemic and antioxidant effects of Commiphora mukul as an adjunct to dietary therapy in patients with hypercholesterolemia. Cardiovasc Drugs Ther. 1994;8:659–64.

26. Pittler MH, Schmidt K, Ernst E. Hawthorn extract for treating chronic heart failure: meta-analysis of randomized trials. Am J Med. 2003;114:665–74.

27. Pittler MH, Ernst E. Horse-chestnut seed extract for chronic venous insufficiency. A criteria-based systematic review. Arch Dermatol. 1998;134:1356–60.

28. Maxwell AJ, Zapien MP, Pearce GL, et al. Randomized trial of a medical food for the dietary management of chronic, stable angina. J Am Coll Cardiol. 2002;39:37–45.

29. Rector TS, Bank AJ, Mullen KA, et al. Randomized, double-blind, placebo-controlled study of supplemental oral L-arginine in patients with heart failure. Circulation. 1996;93:2135–41.

30. Kanaya Y, Nakamura M, Kobayashi N, Hiramori K. Effects of L-arginine on lower limb vasodilator reserve and exercise capacity in patients with chronic heart failure. Heart. 1999;81:512–7.

31. Feskens EJM, Oomen CM, Hogendoorn E, et al. Arginine intake and 25-year CHD mortality: the seven countries study (letter). Eur Heart J. 2001;22:611–2.

32. Venho B, Voutilainen S, Valkonen VP, et al. Arginine intake, blood pressure, and the incidence of acute coronary events in men: the Kuopio Ischaemic Heart Disease Risk Factor Study. Am J Clin Nutr. 2002;76:359–64.

33. Siani A, Pagano E, Iacone R, et al. Blood pressure and metabolic changes during dietary L-arginine supplementation in humans. Am J Hypertens. 2000;13:547–51.

34. Huynh NT, Tayek JA. Oral arginine reduces systemic blood pressure in type 2 diabetes: its potential role in nitric oxide generation. J Am Coll Nutr. 2002;21:422–7.

35. Widman L, Wester PO, Stegmayr BK, et al. The dose-dependent reduction in blood pressure through administration of magnesium. A double blind placebo controlled cross-over study. Am J Hypertens. 1993;6:41–5.

36. Jee SH, Miller ER, III, Guallar E, et al. The effect of magnesium supplementation on blood pressure: a meta-analysis of randomized clinical trials. Am J Hypertens. 2002;15:691–6.

37. Wolfe ML, Vartanian SF, Ross JL, et al. Safety and effectiveness of Niaspan when added sequentially to a statin for treatment of dyslipidemia. Am J Cardiol. 2001;87:476–9, A7.

38. McKenney J. New perspectives on the use of niacin in the treatment of lipid disorders. Arch Intern Med. 2004;164(164):697–705.

39. Guyton JR, Blazing MA, Hagar J, et al. Extended-release niacin vs gemfibrozil for the treatment of low levels of high-density lipoprotein cholesterol. Niaspan-Gemfibrozil Study Group. Arch Intern Med. 2000;160:1177–84.

40. Stampfer MJ, Manson JE, et al. Frequent nut consumption and risk of coronary heart disease in women: prospective cohort study. BMJ. 1998;317:1341–5. 93.

41. Fraser GE, Sabate J, Beeson WL, Strahan TM. A possible protective effect of nut consumption on risk of coronary heart disease. The Adventist Health Study. Arch Intern Med. 1992;152:1416–24, 92.

42. Albert CM, Gaziano JM, Willett WC, Manson JE. Nut consumption and decreased risk of sudden cardiac death in the Physicians' Health Study. Arch Intern Med. 2002;162:1382–7.

43. Geelen A, Brouwer IA, Schouten EG, Maan AC, Katan MB, Zock PL. Effects of n-3 fatty acids from fish on premature ventricular complexes and heart rate in humans. Am J Clin Nutr. 2005 Feb;81(2):416–20.

44. Prisco D, Paniccia R, Bandinelli B, et al. Effect of medium-term supplementation with a moderate dose of n-3 polyunsaturated fatty acids on blood pressure in mild hypertensive patients. Thromb Res. 1998;1:105–12.

45. Yzebe D, Lievre M. Fish oils in the care of coronary heart disease patients: a meta-analysis of randomized controlled trials. Fundam Clin Pharmacol. 2004 Oct;18(5):581–92.

46. Marckmann P, Bladbjerg EM, Jespersen J. Dietary fish oil (4 g daily) and cardiovascular risk markers in healthy men. Arterioscler Thromb Vasc Biol. 1997;17:3384–91.

47. Roche HM, Gibney MJ. Effect of long-chain n-3 polyunsaturated fatty acids on fasting and postprandial triacylglycerol metabolism. Am J Clin Nutr. 2000;71:232S–7S.

48. Mata P, Alvarez-Sala LA, Rubio MJ, et al. Effects of long-term monounsaturated- vs polyunsaturated-enriched diets on lipoproteins in healthy men and women. Am J Clin Nutr. 1992;55:846–50.

49. Pedersen A, Baumstark MW, Marckmann P, et al. An olive oil-rich diet results in higher concentrations of LDL cholesterol and a higher number of LDL sub-fraction particles than rapeseed oil and sunflower oil diets. J Lipid Res. 2000;41:1901–11.

50. Brackett RE. Letter responding to health claim petition dated 2003 August 28: Monounsaturated fatty acids from olive oil and coronary heart disease. CFSAN/Office of Nutritional Products, Labeling and Dietary Supplements. Nov 1 2004; Docket No 2003Q-0559. Available at: http://www.fda.gov/ohrms/dockets/dailys/04/nov04/110404/03q-0559-ans0001-01-vol9.pdf

(*Continued*)

51. Fernandez-Jarne E, Martinez-Losa E, Prado-Santamaria M, et al. Risk of first non-fatal myocardial infarction negatively associated with olive oil consumption: a case-control study in Spain. Int J Epidemiol. 2002;31:474–80.

52. Gouni-Berthold I, Berthold HK. Policosanol: clinical pharmacology and therapeutic significance of a new lipid-lowering agent. Am Heart J. 2002;143:356–65.

53. Whelton PK, He J, Cutler JA, et al. Effects of oral potassium on blood pressure. Meta-analysis of randomized controlled clinical trials. JAMA. 1997;277:1624–32.

54. Dickinson HO, Nicolson DJ, Campbell F, Beyer FR, Mason J. Potassium supplementation for the management of primary hypertension in adults. Cochrane Database Syst Rev. 2006 Jul 19;3:CD004641. Review.

55. Bartels GL, Remme WJ, den Hartog FR, et al. Additional anti-ischemic effects of long-term L-propionylcarnitine in anginal patients treated with conventional antianginal therapy. Cardiovasc Drugs Ther. 1995;9:749–53.

56. Chiddo A, Gaglione A, Musci S, et al. Hemodynamic study of intravenous propionyl-L-carnitine in patients with ischemic heart disease and normal left ventricular function. Cardiovasc Drugs Ther. 1991;5 Suppl 1:107–11.

57. Anand I, Chandrashekhan Y, De Giuli F, et al. Acute and chronic effects of propionyl-L-carnitine on the hemodynamics, exercise capacity, and hormones in patients with congestive heart failure. Cardiovasc Drugs Ther. 1998;12:291–9.

58. Hiatt WR, Regensteiner JG, Creager MA, et al. Propionyl-L-carnitine improves exercise performance and functional status in patients with claudication. Am J Med. 2001;110:616–22.

59. Brevetti G, Diehm C, Lambert D, et al. European multicenter study on propionyl-L-carnitine in intermittent claudication. J Am Coll Cardiol. 1999;34:1618–24.

60. Heber D, Yip I, Ashley JM, et al. Cholesterol-lowering effects of a proprietary Chinese red-yeast-rice dietary supplement. Am J Clin Nutr. 1999;69:231–6.

61. Wang J, Lu A, Chi J. Multicenter clinical trial of the serum lipid-lowering effects of a monascus purpureus (red yeast) rice preparation from traditional Chinese medicine. Cur Ther Res. 1997;58:964–78.

62. New health claim proposed for relationship of soy protein and coronary heart disease. http://www.fda.gov/bbs/topics/ANSWERS/ANS00923.html on October 10, 2005.

63. van der Schouw YT, Kreijkamp-Kaspers S, Peeters PH, et al. Prospective study on usual dietary phytoestrogen intake and cardiovascular disease risk in Western women. Circulation. 2005;111:465–71.

64. Anderson JW, Johnstone BM, Cook-Newell ME. Meta-analysis of the effects of soy protein intake on serum lipids. N Engl J Med. 1995;333:276–82.

65. Crouse JR, III, Morgan T, Terry JG, et al. A randomized trial comparing the effect of casein with that of soy protein containing varying amounts of isoflavones on plasma concentrations of lipids and lipoproteins. Arch Intern Med. 1999;159:2070–6.

66. Liem A, Reynierse-Buitenwerf GH, Zwinderman AH, Jukema JW, van Veldhuisen DJ. Secondary prevention with folic acid: effects on clinical outcomes. J Am Coll Cardiol. 2003;41:2105–13.

67. Schnyder G, Roffi M, Flammer Y, Pin R, Hess OM. Effect of homocysteine-lowering therapy with folic acid, vitamin B12, and vitamin B6 on clinical outcome after percutaneous coronary intervention: the Swiss Heart study: a randomized controlled trial. JAMA. 2002;288:973–9.

68. Clarke R, Collins R. Can dietary supplements with folic acid or vitamin B6 reduce cardiovascular risk? Design of clinical trials to test the homocysteine hypothesis of vascular disease. J Cardiovasc Risk. 1998;5:249–55.

69. Schaafsma G, Meuling WJ, van Dokkum W, Bouley C. Effects of a milk product, fermented by Lactobacillus acidophilus and with fructo-oligosaccharides added, on blood lipids in male volunteers. Eur J Clin Nutr. 1998;52:436–40.

70. Agerholm-Larsen L, Raben A, Haulrik N, et al. Effect of 8 week intake of probiotic milk products on risk factors for cardiovascular diseases. Eur J Clin Nutr. 2000;54:288–97.

TABLE 8-7

LEVELS OF EVIDENCE FOR EFFICACY

Evidence Grade	Description of Evidence
Effective	The product has passed a rigorous scientific review equivalent to a review by the FDA, Health Canada, or other governmental authority and has been found to be effective for a specific indication as an OTC drug, orphan drug, or prescription drug product.
Likely effective	Reputable references generally agree that the product is effective for the given indication, based on two or more randomized, controlled, clinical trials involving several hundred to several thousand patients, giving positive results for clinically relevant end points and published in established, refereed journals.
Possibly effective	Reputable references suggest that the product might work for the given indication based on one or more clinical trials giving positive results for clinically relevant end points.
Possibly ineffective	Reputable references suggest that the product might not work for the given indication based on one human study giving negative results for clinically relevant end points.
Likely ineffective	Reputable references generally agree that the product is not effective for the given indication, based on two or more randomized, controlled, clinical trials giving negative results for clinically relevant end points and published in established, refereed journals.
Ineffective	Most reputable references agree that the product is not effective for the given indication, or multiple high-quality studies resulted in negative results; there are no equally reliable human studies offering convincing contradictory data.

Source: The Natural Medicine Comprehensive Database (www.Naturaldatabase.com).

TABLE 8 - 8

THE H-E-R-B-A-L MNEMONIC

H ear the patient out with respect
- The patient often has a fear of ridicule with disclosure
- Ask in a nonjudgmental manner: "Some of my other patients are using herbs and supplements for various conditions. Have you tried any of these?"
- The patient has important personal reasons for choosing supplements:
  - Previous positive experience
  - More time to discuss issues with alternative health practitioner or health food salesperson
  - Anecdotal evidence "It worked for my friend."
- Thank them for taking an active role in their healthcare (discuss other ways they can do this that you can agree on: diet, exercise, stress management, etc)

E ducate the patient
- Supplements are potentially powerful agents that can have serious side effects and interactions, just like prescription medication
- Your job is not to be an expert, but simply to dispel the myths and balance the picture
- Give the patient resources that are objective and reliable (http://NCCAM.NIH.GOV, www.naturaldatabase.com)

R ecord
- Treat supplements like other medications: chart all supplement use in the progress note and medication section for your benefit as well as other practitioners viewing the chart
- Try to record an evaluation date to discuss if the supplement has shown any benefit for treatment. If no benefit is seen, discuss options including changing dosage or brand as well as stopping or switching supplements

B eware of interactions & reactions
- If the patient develops new or worsening side effects or abnormal laboratory values (especially PT/INR) and the usual suspects have been ruled out—THINK SUPPLEMENTS
  - Monitor patients with polypharmacy, especially those on anticoagulants

A gree to discuss
- Forge an agreement that all new supplements will be discussed before commencement
- Gives you a chance to balance most of the anecdotal/testimonial information the patient hears through the media, mailings, and the internet

L earn about new supplements
- Try to keep up with what the patient is hearing about and considering using
- A wide variety of peer-reviewed resources are available to help decipher the increasing amount of information on supplements (see Table 8-1)

a clinician and patient perspective, the ability to prevent the need for long-term prescription medication use is typically the most agreeable choice.

The second general scenario involves the patient refractory to conventional care. Typical conditions that fall into this category include refractory dyslipidemia, angina, or hypertension. In this scenario, the patient is likely on multiple medications and/or may have attempted a number of additional therapies, which may have been ineffective or not well tolerated. The three patient scenarios fall into these two categories and are discussed with the use of the H-E-R-BA-L mnemonic.

In addition to incorporation of dietary supplementation, the need for evidence-based resources for patient and clinician are incredibly important in helping to identify safe and effective supplements on an ongoing basis. There are a number of resources available to clinicians interested in better understanding dietary supplements as a means of increasing and improving patient communication. These resources are listed in Table 8-1 and include print and online information on evidence-based use of supplements as well as continuing medical education courses available to clinicians. Additional resources, which can be offered to patients, are also listed.

I. Incorporating dietary supplements in the borderline setting
    Scenario 1: 46-year-old with borderline cholesterol
    Scenario 2: 41-year-old with borderline HTN
II. Incorporating dietary supplements in the setting of refractory conditions
    Scenario 3: 62-year-old with refractory dyslipidemia

Scenario 1: Borderline Dyslipidemia

Diane is a 46-year-old whose recent lipid panel as part of her yearly check up revealed the following:

- TC = 226 mg/dl
- LDL = 163 mg/dl
- HDL (high-density lipoprotein) of 43 mg/dl
- TG = 158 mg/dl

Her total and LDL cholesterol as well as TG fall into the category of "borderline high" per the National Cholesterol Education Program Adult Treatment Panel (NCEP ATP) III primary guideline. The remainder of Diane is history and physical reveal no other significant past or current medical issues such as obesity, diabetes, hypertension, or cigarette use. Diane states that several members of her family have also been diagnosed with high cholesterol and other male members of her family including her father have suffered heart attack in their 50s and 60s. She describes a recent history of adequate physical activity including walking 30 minutes most days of the week as well as following a low-cholesterol, low-fat diet although she admits that she continues to have difficulty incorporating adequate amounts of fruits and vegetables. She is surprised regarding her lipid panel in light of her recent lifestyle attempts and is hesitant about any medication for her cholesterol because of side effects her relatives have mentioned. She is interested in additional nonpharmacological options at this point and heard that Guggul and Co-Q10 were helpful. (See Table 8-9 for clinical recommendations.)

FOLLOW-UP

Diane is seen in follow-up approximately 12 weeks later. She reports minimal bloating which subsided over the first several weeks of dietary supplement therapy. She has been able to increase fruit and vegetable intake levels to foster these numbers to 6–8 servings per day as well as maintain her activity regimen. Her most recent lipid panel demonstrates the following improvement

- TC = 189 mg/dl ($\downarrow$17%)
- LDL = 126 mg/dl ($\downarrow$ 23%)
- HDL = 45 mg/dl ($\uparrow$ 8%)
- TG = 147 mg/dl ($\downarrow$ 7%)

The patient is congratulated on her results and compliance with the lifestyle change program and asked to continue with plan as discuss with recheck of her lipids in approximately 3 months to confirm maintenance of levels.

Scenario 2: Borderline Hypertension

Joe is a 41-year-old African American male with a history of gastroesophageal reflux disease (GERD) and a family history of hypertension and cardiovascular disease including an uncle who died of MI at age 59. He has been seen on several occasions in the office, including a yearly physical exam and follow-up for his GERD, and blood pressures that have been repeated in the opposite arm. The readings are consistently noted to be between 130–140 systolic and 80–90 diastolic with occasional readings above 140/90 mm Hg. Other than borderline obesity, the remainder of Joe's history and physical reveal no other significant past or current medical issues such as diabetes, hypertension, elevated BMI or cigarette use. Recent screening tests including electrocardiograph (ECG) and standard clinical laboratory testing have demonstrated no endocrine or metabolic abnormalities. Joe admits to struggling with adequate physical activity due to his long hours as an accountant and frequent "fast food" lunches during the work week. Joe states that high blood pressure "runs in my family" and knows many relatives on medications. As per the JNC7 guidelines (JNC7: Joint National Committee on Prevention, Detection, Evaluation, and Treatment of High Blood Pressure), Joe was asked to increase physical activity and initiate dietary approaches to stop hypertension (DASH)* recommendation with a focus on decreasing dietary sodium intake of salt and saturated fats.

TABLE 8-9

THE H-E-R-B-A-L MNEMONIC IN SCENARIO 1

H	After reviewing her numbers and congratulating her on her progress with diet, exercise you proceed to educate the patient on additional steps:
E	• Let Diane know that Guggul and Co-Q10 in isolation has not been shown to improve hyperlipidemia • Education and initiation of NCEP guidelines (http://www.nhlbi.nih.gov/about/ncep/index.htm). Let her know that her 10-year Framingham risk percentage is <10%. Her risk factors (in addition to age >45) are difficult to assess without full family history knowledge but would in the worst case place her at >1 risk factor and establish an LDL goal of <130. In addition, you discuss your desire to decrease her total cholesterol <200, TG <150, and to elevate her HDL. Thus you begin more intense therapeutic lifestyle change (TLC) as recommended by the NCEP • Add soluble fiber at 15 g/day. This is especially helpful as she is not incorporating the recommended quantity of fruits and vegetables • Add plant sterol in the form of β-sitosterol with a goal of 2g/day. You make her aware that this regimen has been shown to decrease LDL by 10–20% and may enable her to reach goal as part of her TLC program.[31] Dietary and dietary supplement options for reaching 2 g/day are recommended as noted below In addition, you mention other lifestyle and dietary supplements recommendations including initiating decaffeinated green tea and 1 oz of nuts during her midday snack as well as strategies for increasing fruit and vegetable intake

R	The start date, brand, and dose of dietary supplements are recorded in the progress note and medication section for your benefit and the benefit of other clinicians using the chart
	• Metamucil 2 tablespoons (15 g soluble fiber)/day
	• Cholest-off 2 tabs (900 mg plant sterols/stanols)/day
	• Diet intervention with fortified sterols:
	  • Butter replacement (Take Control butter replacement spread) 2 tablespoons daily
	  • Fortified juices (Minute Maid Heart Wise) 8 oz daily (plant STEROLS 16 mg per day)

B	Let the patient know the most common adverse reactions such as GI side effects including bloating and report any significant reactions once initiating therapy
A	Diane is asked to call the office to discuss any other dietary supplements she may be considering before initiating
L	Diane is referred to the NCEP program materials for additional information on cholesterol management including the handout "High Blood Cholesterol—What You Need to Know." She is also given patient handouts on the supplements discussed from www.naturaldatabase.com and http://www.nhlbi.nih.gov/health/public/heart/chol/hbc_what.htm

Joe follows up in 6 weeks and is noted to have a blood pressure of 136/86. While incorporating the DASH diet with some success Joe is a bit frustrated and asks if use of vitamin E may help his effort. At this point several steps are discussed. (See Table 8-10.)

FOLLOW-UP

Joe returns after 6 weeks of the intervention and reports difficulty advancing beyond 20 mmol of magnesium per day. He has lost 3 lb with his activity and diet regimen and has a blood pressure of 126/78 with confirmation in the opposite arm during today's visit. He is content with his progress since the last visit and is encouraged to continue his lifestyle change program including continuing with consistent activity, the DASH program as well as his use of soy protein, soluble fiber, and high-dose mineral formula. He will be seen back in 12 weeks for recheck and laboratory testing and is asked to also monitor his blood pressure at home in the interim.

Scenario 3: Refractory Dyslipidemia

Mike is a 62-year-old male with a history of diabetes and dyslipidemia, including elevated LDL and triglycerides. He has had significant improvements with the use of statins (Lipitor tolerated at 40 mg daily) and prescription niacin (Niaspan tolerated at 1500 mg daily). He has attempted higher dosages of both as well as a number of other medications and has had difficulty with tolerance including myalgia and/or flushing. His most recent lipid panel is noted below:

- TC = 194 mg/dl
- LDL = 118 mg/dl
- HDL = 45 mg/dl
- TG = 172 mg/dl

Mike's LDL cholesterol as well as TG is still not in control as per the NCEP ATP III guideline. His diabetes diagnosis is a CHD equivalent and requires an LDL < 100, which he has had great difficultly reaching with the intervention attempted thus far. Also his TG of < 150 has also been difficult to attain. In addition to medication interventions, Mike has incorporated walking several days per week as well attempted dietary intervention by decreasing cholesterol intake. He wishes to try additional interventions although he is frustrated that recent medication have either not been successful or not been well tolerated. (See Table 8-11.)

FOLLOW-UP

Mike returns 12 weeks later and states that he had minimal problems incorporating high dose fish oils and soy at the dose specified. He has decreased saturated fat intake by use of replacement soy protein products. His most recent lipid panel demonstrates:

TABLE 8-10

THE H-E-R-B-A-L MNEMONIC IN SCENARIO 2

H	After reviewing Joe's lifestyle changes you encourage continuation of activity and dietary improvements. You discuss additional therapies which may be of benefit

E	• Let Joe know that vitamin E in isolation has not been shown to improve cholesterol[32]
	• Initiate additional dietary supplement interventions
	  • Soluble fiber at 15 g/day
	  • Soy protein 25–50 g daily
	    • Can ↓ systolic blood pressure by 4 mm Hg and ↓ diastolic blood pressure by 3 mm Hg in patients with prehypertension or mild hypertension[33]
	    • Combining soy protein with psyllium seems to reduce systolic blood pressure by about 8 mm Hg[34]
	• Magnesium: 10–20 mmol/day with increase to 40 mmol/day as tolerated
	  • Each addition of 10 mmol/day magnesium resulted in 4.3 mm Hg systolic BP and of 2.3 mm Hg diastolic BP[35]
	• Calcium: 1–1.5 g elemental calcium daily
	  • Appears to ↓ BP by approximately 1–2 mm mm Hg
	• Potassium: insure atleast 350 mg/day through food and dietary supplementation[36]

R	The start date, brand, and dose of supplement are recorded in the progress note and medication section for your benefit and the benefit of other clinicians using the chart • Metamucil 2 tablespoons (15 g) daily • Calcium carbonate 2 tabs (1 g)/day • Mineral supplement with 150 mg potassium and 20 mmol magnesium (1–2 tabs/day as tolerated) • Soy protein supplement
B	Let Joe know the most common side effects are GI side effects, such as loose stools, especially linked to magnesium
A	Joe is asked to call the office to discuss any other dietary supplements he is considering
L	• Joe is referred to patient materials summarizing recommendation of JNC7 including "Your Guide to Lowering High Blood Pressure" available at http://www.nhlbi.nih.gov/health/public/heart/index.htm • Provide patient handouts on the supplements discussed from www.naturaldatabase.com

TABLE 8-11

THE H-E-R-B-A-L MNEMONIC IN SCENARIO 3

H	After reviewing Mike's situation and difficulty meeting NCEP ATP III goal, you encourage initiation of dietary supplementation to see if they may enable him to reach his targets.

E	• Initiate additional dietary supplement interventions
	  • <Soluble fiber at 15 g/day
	    • Adding soluble fiber can be as effective as doubling statin dose[37]
	  • Plant sterol/stanol with a goal of 2 g/day. This dose has been shown to be as effective as doubling statin dose[38] Dietary and supplement options for reaching 2 g/day are recommended as noted below
	  • Omega-3 fish oils 3–4 g daily
	    • Fish oils have demonstrated up to a 30–50% ↓ in TG when used in high doses
	  • Soy protein 25–50 g daily
	    • Soy can ↓ LDL 13%; ↓ TG 10.5%; ↓ HDL 2.4%[39,40]
	  • Calcium: 1200 mg calcium carbonate daily
	    • 6 weeks of calcium in combination with a low-fat diet can ↓ LDL by 4.4% and ↓ HDL by 4.1%

R	The start date, brand, and dose of dietary supplement are recorded in the progress note and medication section for your benefit and the benefit of other clinicians using the chart
	• Metamucil 2 tablespoons (15 g soluble fiber)/day
	• Cholest-off 2 tabs (900 mg plant sterols/stanols)/day
	• Diet intervention with fortified sterols:
	  • Butter replacement (Take Control butter replacement spread) 2 tablespoons daily
	  • Fortified juices (Minute Maid Heart Wise 8 oz daily)
	• Pro-Omega 4 tabs (2800 mg omega-3) daily
	  • Calcium carbonate (brand specified)

B	Let Mike know the most common side effects including GI side effects, such as loose stools and bloating, especially linked to magnesium and fish oils. Also he should space the use of fibers by supplements/medication by several hours optimally to minimize any loss in absorption
A	Mike is asked to call the office to discuss any other dietary supplements he is considering using before his next visit
L	• Mike is referred to the NCEP for additional information on cholesterol (website or handout) • He is provided with patient handouts on the supplements discussed from www.naturaldatabase.com

- TC = 180 mg/dl ($\downarrow$ 7%)
- LDL = 96 mg/dl ($\downarrow$ 19%)
- HDL = 50 mg/dl($\uparrow$ 12%)
- TG = 140 mg/dl ($\downarrow$ 19%)

Mike is informed of his progress and asked to continue with his lifestyle changes and use of dietary supplements including fish oils, soy, and plant sterol with follow-up including lipid panel and hepatic function testing in 3 months.

CONCLUSION

The field of herbal and dietary supplementation is rapidly evolving in multiple arenas. These include the type, brand, and dosage of supplements utilized, the research on these supplements, as well as their level of regulation. As our patients are being introduced to these supplements for cardiovascular conditions, it is imperative for clinicians to be informed of their efficacy, toxicity, and interaction potential. It is hoped that the H-E-R-B-A-L mnemonic, the reference tables, and case studies will allow a greater level of support in engaging and educating patients in this area. In some cases, dietary supplements may be incorporated in borderline or refractory cases to provide additional therapeutic options. In others, the clinician may need to advise against the use of certain supplements or supplement-medication combination. Overall, the most important aspect of the clinician–patient interaction will be the openness to discussion, which will allow the patient to appreciate the importance of reviewing and managing supplement use on a regular basis.

REFERENCES

1. Eisenberg DM, et al. Unconventional medicine in the United States. Prevalence, costs, and patterns of use. New Engl J Med. 1993;32(4):246–52.
2. Eisenberg DM, et al. Trends in alternative medicine use in the United States, 1990–1997: results of a followup national survey. JAMA. 1998;280:1569–75.
3. Nutrition Business Journal. (2001). 6, 1–3.
4. Barnes P, Powell-Griner E, McFann K, et al. CDC advance data report #343. Complementary and alternative medicine use among adults: United States, 2002. May 27, 2004.
5. Taylor H, Leitman R (eds). Widespread ignorance of regulation and labeling of vitamins, minerals and food supplements. Harris Interactive Health Care News. 2002; 2(23):1–5.
6. Astin JA. Why patients use alternative medicine: results of a national study. JAMA. 1998;279(19):1548–53.
7. Leung JM, et al. The prevalence and predictors of the use of alternative medicine in presurgical patients in five California hospitals. Anesth Analg. 2001;93:1062–8. Matoid arthritis: a randomized, double blind trial. Eur J Clin Invest. 22(10):687–91.

8. Wood MJ, Stewart RL, Merry H, Johnstone DE, Cox JL. Use of complementary and alternative medical therapies in patients with cardiovascular disease. Am Heart J. 2003 May;145(5):806–12.

9. Astin JA, et al. Complementary and alternative medicine use among elderly persons: one-year analysis of a Blue Shield medicare supplement. J Gerontol. Series A. Biol Sci Med Sci. 2000;55(1):M4–9.

10. Azaz-Livshits T, et al. Use of complementary alternative medicine in patients admitted to internal medicine wards. Int J Clin Pharmacol Ther. 2002;40(12): 539–47.

11. Adler SR, et al. Disclosing complementary and alternative medicine use in the medical encounter: a qualitative study in women with breast cancer. J Fam Pract. 1999; 48 (6):453–8.

12. Hansrud DD, et al. Underreporting the use of dietary supplements and nonprescription medication among patients undergoing a periodic health examination. Mayo Clin Proc. 1999;74:443–7.

13. Corbin-Winslow L, et al. Physicians want education about CAM to enhance communication with their patients. Arch Intern Med. 2002;162(10):1176–81.

14. Dietary Supplements: Background Information from the Office of Dietary Supplements, National Institutes of Health. Accessed November 28, 2005 at http://ods.od.nih.gov/factsheets/DietarySupplements.asp

15. Food and Drug Administration Sec. 101.79 Health claims: Folate and neural tube defects. [Revised as of April 1, 2006] http://www.accessdata.fda.gov/scripts/cdrh/cfdocs/cfcfr/CFRSearch.cfm?fr=101.79 accessed 3.21.07

16. Federal Trade Commission for the Consumer Newsletter. FTC and FDA take new actions in fight against deceptive marketing. 2003, June 10. Retrieved May 1, 2004 from http://www.fcc.gov/opa/2003/06/trudeau.htm

17. Federal Drug Administration Press Release. FDA announces plans to prohibit sales of dietary supplements containing Ephedra. December 30, 2003. Accessed at http://www.fda.gov/oc/initiatives/ephedra/december2003/ Accessed on May 1, 2004.

18. Peng C, et al. Incidence and severity of potential drug–dietary supplement interactions in primary care patients. Arch Intern Med. 2004;164:630–6.

19. Norred CL, Zamudio S, Palmer SK. Use of complementary and alternative medicines by surgical patients. AANAJ. 2000;68(1):13–8.

20. Tsen LC, et al. Survey of residency training in preoperative evaluation. Anesthesiology. 2000;93(4):1134–7.

21. An NIH Conference on Dietary Supplements, Coagulation, and Antithrombotic Therapies. January 13–14, 2005. Accessed at http://ods.od.nih.gov/News/Conferences_and_Workshops.asp on February 1, 2006.

22. Bender NK, Effects of marine fish oils on the anticoagulation status of patients receiving chronic warfarin therapy. J Thromb Thrombolysis. 1998 Jul;5(3):257–61.

23. Kim J, White RH. Effect of vitamin E on the anticoagulant response to warfarin. Am J Cardiol.1996 Mar 1;77(7):545–6.

24. Engelsen J, Nielsen JD, Hansen KF. Effect of coenzyme Q10 and Ginkgo biloba on warfarin dosage in patients on long-term warfarin treatment. A randomized, double-blind, placebo-controlled cross-over trial. Thromb Haemost. 2002 Jun;87 (6):1075–6.

25. Jiang X, Williams KM, Liauw WS, Ammit AJ, Roufogalis BD, Duke CC, et al. Effect of St John's wort and ginseng on the pharmacokinetics and pharmacodynamics of warfarin in healthy subjects. Br J Clin Pharmacol. 2004;57(5):592–9.

26. Yuan CS, Wei G, Dey L, Karrison T, Nahlik L, Maleckar S, et al. Brief communication: American ginseng reduces warfarin's effect in healthy patients: a randomized, controlled trial. Ann Intern Med. 2004;141(1):23–7.
27. Jiang X, Williams KM, Liauw WS, Ammit AJ, Roufogalis BD, Duke CC, et al. Effect of ginkgo and ginger on the pharmacokinetics and pharmacodynamics of warfarin in healthy subjects. Br J Clin Pharmacol. 2005 Apr;59(4):425–32.
28. Kurnik D, Loebstein R, Rabinovitz H, Austerweil N, Halkin H, Almog S. Over-the-counter vitamin K1-containing multivitamin supplements disrupt warfarin anticoagulation in vitamin K1-depleted patients. A prospective, controlled trial. Thromb Haemost. 2004 Nov;92(5):1018–24.

THE MODIFIED MEDITERRANEAN DIET

Robert A. Vogel

There are two good places to eat on earth to prevent cardiovascular disease. They are the Mediterranean region and the Pacific Rim, epitomized by southern France, Italy, and Japan. Food in these regions is delicious, plentiful, and heart-healthy. Heart disease in these regions occurs 50–80% less frequently than in the United States at the same cholesterol levels. In each region, heart disease increases with cholesterol level, but the region-specific curves are quite different. This surprising finding was discovered by the Seven Countries Study[1] and is commonly labeled the French paradox. Some of the lower heart disease incidence in France may be due to differences in their reporting of causes of death, but a clear difference in regional heart disease exists. It is not surprising that diet is intricately connected to heart disease. The Russian pathologist, Anitschkow first induced atherosclerosis in rabbits by feeding them high-fat and cholesterol food.[2] The question then arises what components in the Mediterranean Diet are cardioprotective? Additionally, can the Mediterranean Diet be modified to make it more cardioprotective? The answers to these questions and the underlying vascular biology are the subjects of this chapter.

THE MEDITERRANEAN AND MODIFIED MEDITERRANEAN DIETS

The Mediterranean Diet is characterized by:[3]

1. An abundance of fresh fruits and vegetables, including the use of fruit as dessert
2. High content of whole grain, complex carbohydrates eaten as pasta and bread
3. Low use of refined sugar and processed foods
4. Moderate fish and poultry consumption
5. Use of olive oil in contrast to butter and tropical oils

6. Low to moderate dairy products such as cheese and yogurt

7. Rare red meat consumption

8. Moderate wine consumption, usually accompanying meals

Importantly, the Mediterranean Diet does not exist in isolation. It is one component of an entire lifestyle. Smaller food portions and increased physical activity are important aspects of the Mediterranean lifestyle.

In addition to observational data, several studies have demonstrated that a Mediterranean-style diet reduces cardiovascular risk, especially in secondary prevention cohorts. The prototypical trial of the Mediterranean Diet is the Lyon Diet Heart Study.[4-8] This study randomized 605 men and women who had experienced a prior myocardial infarction to either an experimental or prudent diet for 46 months. The experimental diet used:

1. α-Linolenic acid (ALA)-enriched canola oil margarine, and advice to eat:

2. More whole grains

3. More fruits and vegetables

4. More fish

5. Less red meat, and

6. Fewer whole milk products

The use of ALA-enriched canola oil margarine instead of increased olive oil consumption is what defines the Lyon Diet Heart Study experimental diet as "modified Mediterranean." The experimental diet group experienced 72% fewer cardiovascular events, 60% fewer deaths, and 80% fewer late diagnoses of cancer than did the prudent diet group. Importantly, the reduction in cardiovascular risk in the experimental diet group was unaccompanied by any significant changes in weight or serum lipoproteins. Similar to the Seven Countries Study, they had less heart disease at the same cholesterol level. A 67% increase in serum ALA was observed in the experimental diet group.

The results of the Lyon Diet Heart Study are supported by those of the Indo-Mediterranean Diet Heart Study,[9] which also randomized 1000 subjects with prior myocardial infarction, angina pectoris, or coronary risk factors to an experimental versus a National Cholesterol Education Program (NCEP) diet for 2 years. The experimental diet recommended increases in fruits, vegetables, legumes, walnuts, and almonds and resulted in a twofold increase in ALA consumption. Walnuts and almonds are rich in polyunsaturated fatty acids and reduce the absorption of dietary cholesterol. In contrast to the Lyon Diet Heart Study, the experimental diet resulted in 3-kg weight loss, 3/2 mm Hg lower blood pressure, and 19 mg/dL lower low-density lipoprotein (LDL) cholesterol. The experimental diet group experienced 49% fewer cardiovascular events, 62% fewer sudden deaths, and 51% fewer nonfatal myocardial infarctions than the NCEP diet group.

Both the Lyon and Indo-Mediterranean Diet Heart Studies suggest that a major cardioprotective component of the Mediterranean Diet is its high content of polyunsaturated fatty acids and especially omega-3 fatty acids.[10] Omega-3 fatty acids include ALA, eicosapentaenoic acid (EPA), and decosahexaenoic acid (DHA), which contain three, five, and six double bonds, respectively. Fish oil contains EPA and DHA, but ALA is found in plant oils such as canola, walnut, and flaxseed oils. Humans are able to metabolized ALA into EPA and DHA, although very slowly.

The Diet and Reinfarction Trial (DART) provided major support for the cardioprotective efficacy of omega-3 fatty acids.[11] It randomized 2033 men, who had experienced a myocardial infarction to advice versus no advice on three dietary factors, more fish, more fiber, and less fat. The men advised to eat more fish experienced a 29% reduction in 2-year all-cause mortality compared to those not so advised. Significant changes in mortality were not experienced in response to the fat and fiber advice. The GISSI-Prevenzione Trial randomized 11,324 subjects with recent myocardial infarction to 1-mg omega-3 fatty acid (70% DHA) versus placebo and followed them for 3.5 years.[12] Omega-3 fatty acid administration was associated with a significant 10% reduction in death, myocardial infarction, or stroke and a 17% reduction in cardiovascular death. A 41% reduction in mortality was experienced during the trial's first 3 months.[13]

Hu and Wilett reviewed 147 epidemiological and dietary intervention studies to determine the cardioprotective benefit afforded by specific nutrients and food groups.[14] They concluded that three general dietary principles hold for the prevention of coronary heart disease:

1. Increase consumption of omega-3 fatty acids from fish, fish oil supplement, and plant sources.
2. Substitute nonhydrogenated unsaturated fats for saturated and trans fats.
3. Consume a diet high in fruits, vegetables, nuts, and whole grains, and low in sugar and refined grain products.

These recommendations are very much in keeping with the modified Mediterranean Diet. These authors also concluded that simply lowering the total dietary fat was unlikely to reduce heart disease. The value of a moderate fat diet as compared to a low-fat diet for the prevention of coronary heart disease was recognized in the 2003 NCEP recommendations for consumption of about 30% of calories from fat.[15]

The effect of adherence to a Mediterranean Diet on all-cause mortality was studied in 22,043 Greek subjects over 44 months.[16] A point scale was developed to evaluate consumption of beneficial foods (vegetables, fruits, legumes, nuts, cereal, and fish) and avoidance of meat, poultry, and dairy products. Adherence to the general principles of the Mediterranean Diet was inversely associated with less heart disease and mortality, but the consumption of individual food groups did not correlate with outcome. The health effects of a Mediterranean lifestyle were evaluated in 2339 elderly (70–90 years old) subjects from 11 European countries over 10 years.[17] Adherence to a Mediterranean Diet, moderate alcohol use, non-smoking, and physical activity were associated with both less cardiovascular disease and mortality.

DIETARY EFFECTS ON RISK FACTORS AND VASCULAR BIOLOGY

Understanding how the Mediterranean Diet affects cardiovascular risk depends on an appreciation of both tradition coronary risk factors, such as weight and lipoproteins, and more basic dietary vascular biology. Body mass is associated with increased cardiovascular risk, through associations with several risk factors, including:

1. Increased LDL cholesterol
2. Decreased high-density lipoprotein (HDL) cholesterol
3. Increased triglycerides
4. Increased blood pressure
5. Decreased insulin sensitivity
6. Decreased nitric oxide availability
7. Increased inflammation

Although body mass is increasing in the Mediterranean region, it remains less than in the United States. The body-mass index in the experimental diet group of the Lyon Diet Heart Study[8] was 26 kg/m^2 compared to 28 kg/m^2 in the United States. Packaged and restaurant foods in this country come in inappropriately large portions. A recent trial compared restaurant portion sizes in Philadelphia and Paris. Compared to Parisian restaurants, Philadelphian restaurants served:

1. 25% larger average portion sizes
2. 73% larger portion sizes for Chinese food, and
3. 52% larger soft drinks
4. Parisian diners also spent 55% more time eating their smaller meals

The Mediterranean Diet is generally low in saturated fat and high in monounsaturated and polyunsaturated fats, which have important effects on lipoproteins.[18] Dietary saturated and especially trans fats increase LDL cholesterol. The latter also decreases HDL cholesterol. Dietary monounsaturated fats do not decrease HDL cholesterol, but polyunsaturated fats do. This latter effect may not be detrimental to cardiovascular disease risk because of two reasons. Polyunsaturated fats decrease triglycerides more than monounsaturated fats. This results in a shift in LDL particle size toward larger, more buoyant particles, which are less atherogenic. Secondly, the mechanism by which polyunsaturated fatty acids reduce HDL cholesterol appears to be an increase in the SR-B1 receptor (Scavenger receptor class B member 1), which is an integral part of reverse cholesterol transport.

The Nurses' Health Study evaluated the effect of substitutions of dietary fat for an equivalent energy from carbohydrate in 80,082 women followed for at least 14 years.[19] Each substitution of 5% of dietary energy from monounsaturated fat reduced cardiovascular risk 19%, but a 5% substitution of polyunsaturated fat resulted in a 38% risk reduction. This finding that polyunsaturated fat is more cardioprotective than monounsaturated fat is consistent with the Lyon Diet Heart Study, and suggests that polyunsaturated and omega-3 fatty acids from fish and plants in the Mediterranean Diet are more cardioprotective than is olive oil.[20] In a recent study, coronary calcification was found to vary inversely with dietary plant-derived ALA consumption, further supporting the Lyon Diet Heart Study results.[21] The effect of dietary saturated, monounsaturated, and polyunsaturated fats on coronary atherosclerosis was compared in African green monkeys.[22] The addition of dietary polyunsaturated fats resulted in the least development of atherosclerosis.

Dietary fats and sugar have important effects on postprandial vascular biology independent of changes on LDL and HDL cholesterol. Both high-fat and high-sugar diets and single meals reduce endothelium-dependent vasodilation and increase inflammatory markers, such as CRP, interleukin-6, interleukin-8, interleukin-18, and tumor necrosis factor-α (TNF-α). The vascular effects of a high-fat meal last longer than those of a high-sugar meal, but the addition of a large sugar load to a high-fat meal increases the magnitude of the effects.[23,24] A single high-fat meal also increases circulating microparticles, another index of endothelial dysfunction, activates coagulation factor VII, and impairs vascular compliance.[25,26] Several studies have shown that postprandial vascular biological impairment is greater in subjects with diabetes mellitus.

Considerable evidence suggests that high-fat and high-sugar meals induce vascular dysfunction through increases in oxidative stress. Reactive oxygen species are increased following a high-fat meal, especially in diabetic subjects, and increased nitric oxide inactivation has been demonstrated. The addition of direct (e.g., vitamins C and E) and indirect (e.g., folic acid) antioxidants to single meals reduces postprandial endothelial dysfunction. Increased oxidative stress reduces the activity of the redox-sensitive enzyme, dimethylarginine dimethylaminohydrolase (DDAH), increasing levels of asymmetric dimethylarginine (ADMA), which competes with L-arginine for nitric oxide synthase substrate availability. Postprandial oxidative stress increases the expression of intercellular adhesion molecule-1 (ICAM-1) and vascular cell adhesion molecule-1 (VCAM-1), at least in part due to increases in nuclear factor κB, a proinflammatory nuclear regulator.

Testing the vascular effects of single meals has greatly accelerated our understanding of dietary influences on atherosclerosis. The initial single-meal trial compared the effects of a typical American fast food and a low-fat meal.[23] This and subsequent studies have taught us much about diet and vascular biology. In general, endothelium-dependent vasodilation is reduced to the greatest extent by unsaturated fatty acids, especially of the long-chain variety. The oxidation of cooking oil, which occurs during its reuse, also increases its adverse effect. At the other end of the saturation spectrum, highly unsaturated omega-3 fatty acids, such as DHA (six double bonds), found in fish oil, do not impair endothelial function when ingested in a single meal and improves endothelial function when given chronically.[27] Concordant with these observations is the finding that fatty acids inhibit inflammatory markers proportional to how many double bonds they contain.[28] Again, this would suggest dietary superiority for highly unsaturated fatty acids over monounsaturated oleic acid, found in olives.

Foods given together may have different vascular effects than the sum of the individual components. Antioxidant-rich foods, such as fruits, vegetables, red wine, and red wine-based ingredients (e.g., balsamic vinegar) ingested with high-fat foods, reduce subsequent vascular impairment.[29] Given chronically, Mediterranean-style diets following several of these principles have been shown to improve endothelium-mediated vasodilation and reduce markers of inflammation and coagulation.[30,31] These vascular findings may explain the dramatic results of the Lyon Diet Heart and Indo-Mediterranean Diet Heart Studies. The lack of effect on lipoproteins and subject weight in the Lyon study strongly suggests that the direct vascular biological impact was predominately responsible for the experimental diet's efficacy.

ALCOHOL

William Heberden, a pioneering cardiologist, first reported a beneficial effect of alcohol on coronary heart disease in 1786. He observed that heart disease patients experienced less chest pain if they drank alcohol. Since that time, more than 60 observational studies have found 30–60% less heart disease in moderate drinkers compared with abstainers.[32] These studies have found that alcohol use is associated with fewer heart attacks and strokes and less atherosclerosis on autopsy. A reduction in heart disease remains even after adjustments are made for the confounding factors of diet and smoking. The reduction in heart disease risk is confined to middle-aged and older individuals, because heart disease is a much larger factor in these groups. Women derive somewhat less protection from alcohol. Despite the many observational studies, no randomized, controlled trials (RCTs) using alcohol have been performed to verify its beneficial effect on heart disease.

Moderate alcohol consumption is defined as 1–3 drinks per day. One drink is defined as 12 oz of beer, 5 oz of wine ($^1/_6$ bottle), or 1 oz of whiskey ($^2/_3$ jigger). All of these beverage amounts supply $^1/_2$ oz of alcohol. More than two drinks per day reduce heart disease very little because it is associated with increases in blood pressure, arrhythmias such as atrial fibrillation, heart failure, and possibly bleeding strokes. Many diseases increase with more than moderate drinking, including trauma, violence, cirrhosis, pancreatitis, gastrointestinal bleeding, neuropathy, encephalopathy, and cancer (e.g., liver and breast). Based on overall longevity, the best amount to drink is one drink per day, although minimal cardiovascular risk is associated with the consumption of two to three drinks per day.

The best explanation for why alcohol reduces cardiovascular disease risk is that alcohol increases HDL cholesterol.[33] On an average, HDL cholesterol increases about 10–15% for every two drinks per day consumed. Individuals vary in their HDL cholesterol responses to alcohol. The strongest evidence that the health benefit of drinking comes from the alcohol, not the type of beverage, is that people who have reduced alcohol dehydrogenase activity have the greatest reduction in heart disease. Alcohol also decreases procoagulant factors, including platelet aggregation, fibrinogen, lipoprotein A, and von Willebrand factor and increases anticoagulants, such as plasminogen and tissue plasminogen activator (tPA).[34] Alcohol is the only sugar that reduces the incidence of diabetes. Moderate alcohol intake is also associated with reduced inflammation, but C-reactive protein levels increase with heavy consumption.

The Mediterranean Diet is associated with moderate wine consumption, especially in the form of red wine. This has been proposed as an explanation for the "French paradox." Several explanations have been offered.[32] Red wine is higher in complex antioxidant molecules that have experimentally been shown to increase nitric oxide synthase expression. Wine drinkers also tend to be thinner, to exercise more, and to drink with meals. In the Mediterranean lifestyle, wine is usually consumed with meals, which blunts the postprandial reduction in endothelial function associated with fatty meals.

There is no advantage of red wine over other beverages in American studies. In the largest American trial, almost 129,000 Californians, enrolled in a health maintenance organization, were followed for 13 years according to their alcohol consumption.[35] After 8 years, moderate drinkers experienced 30% fewer deaths, mostly due to a reduction in heart disease. Older individuals experienced the greatest reduction in risk. The type of alcohol consumed did not matter. Women who drank heavily had an especially high mortality. After 13 years, beer drinking appeared to be slightly more protective in men and red and white wine more protective in women. There was no evidence for any selective effect of red wine. Men and women together had exactly the same protection from red and white wine.

In contrast to the type of alcohol consumed, drinking patterns appear to affect cardiovascular risk. The Mediterranean pattern of drinking is moderate and daily, as opposed to binge or weekend consumption. This appears to prevent the platelet reactive hyperaggregation that occurs about 48 hours after cessation of drinking.

SUMMARY

In summary, the modified Mediterranean Diet is associated with reduced cardiovascular disease risk in both observational and prospective interventional trials. Important components of the Mediterranean Diet include reduced calorie consumption, increased consumption of fish and plant-derived omega-3 fatty acids, fruits, vegetables, nuts, and whole grains, reduced consumption of red meat and whole milk products, and moderate daily alcohol consumption. This diet favorably affects both traditional coronary risk markers, such as lipoproteins and blood pressure and vascular markers of endothelial function, inflammation, and coagulation. Perhaps, the greatest advantage of the Mediterranean Diet is that on top of its health benefits, it tastes so good.

REFERENCES

1. Vershuren WMM, Jacobs DR, Bloemberg BPM, et al. Serum total cholesterol and long-term coronary heart disease mortality in different cultures. Twenty-five-year follow-up of the Seven Countries Study. JAMA. 1995;274:131–6.
2. Anitschkow M. Experimental atherosclerosis in animals. In: Cowdry EV, editor. Arteriosclerosis: a study of the problem. New York, Macmillan; 1933:271–322.
3. Parikh P, McDaniel MC, Ashen D, et al. Diets and cardiovascular disease. An evidence-based assessment. J Am Coll Cardiol. 2005;45:1379–87.
4. de Longeril M, Renaud S, Mamelle N, et al. Mediterranean alpha-linolenic acid-rich diet in secondary prevention of coronary heart disease. Lancet. 1994;343:1454–9.
5. Renaud S, de Loneril M, delaye J, et al. Cretan Mediterranean diet for prevention of coronary heart disease. Am J Clin Nutr. 1995;61 Suppl:1360S–7S.
6. de Longeril M, Salen P, Martin J-L, et al. Effect of a Mediterranean type diet on the rate of cardiovascular complications in patients with coronary artery disease. Insights into the cardioprotective effect of certain nutrients. J Am Coll Cardiol. 1996;28: 1103–8.
7. de Longeril M, Salen P, Martin J-L, et al. Mediterranean dietary pattern in a randomized trial. Prolonged survival and possibly reduced cancer rate. Arch Intern Med. 1998;158:1181–7.
8. de Longeril M, Salen P, Martin J-L, et al. Mediterranean diet, traditional risk factors, and the rate of cardiovascular complications after myocardial infarction. Final report of the Lyon Diet Heart Study. Circulation. 1999;99:779–85.
9. Singh RB, Dubnov G, Niaz MA, et al. Effect of an Indo-Mediterranean diet on progression of coronary artery disease in high risk patients (Indo-Mediterranean Diet Heart Study): a randomized single-blind trial. Lancet. 2002;360:1455–61.
10. Kris-Etherton PM, Harris WS, Appel LJ (for the Nutrition Committee). Fish consumption, fish oil, omega-3 fatty acids, and cardiovascular disease. Circulation. 2002; 106:2747–57.
11. Burr ML, Gilbert JF, Holliday RM, et al. Effects of changes in fat, fish, and fibre intakes on death and myocardial reinfarction: Diet and Reinfarction Trial (DART). Lancet. 1989;2:757–61.
12. GISSI-Prevenzione Investigators. Dietary supplementation with n-3 polyunsaturated fatty acids and vitamin E after myocardial infarction: results of the GISSI-Prevenzione trial. Lancet. 1999;354:447–55.
13. Marchioli R, Barzi F, Bpmba E, et al. Early protection against sudden death by n-3 polyunsaturated fatty acids after myocardial infarction. Timecourse analysis of the results of the Gruppo Italiano per lo Studio della Sopravvivenza nell'Infarto Miocardico (GISSI)-Prevenzione. Circulation. 2002;105:1897–1903.

14. Hu FB, Wilett WC. Optimal diets for prevention of coronary heart disease. JAMA. 2002;288:2569–78.

15. Executive Summary of The Third Report of The National Cholesterol Education Program (NCEP) Expert Panel on Detection, Evaluation, and treatment of high blood cholesterol in adults (Adult Treatment Panel III). JAMA. 2001;285:2486–97.

16. Trichopoulou A, Costacou T, Barmia C, Trichopoulos D. Adherence to a Mediterranean diet and survival in a Greek population. N Engl J Med. 2003;348: 2599–608.

17. Knoops KTM, de Groot LCPGM, Kromhout D, et al. Mediterranean diet, lifestyle factors, and 10-year mortality in elderly European men and women. The HALE project. JAMA. 2004;292:1433–9.

18. Kris-Etherton PM for the Nutrition Committee. Monounsaturated fatty acids and the risk of cardiovascular disease. Circulation. 1999;100:1253–8.

19. Hu FB, Stampfer MJ, Manson JE, et al. Dietary fat intake and the risk of coronary heart disease in women. N Engl J Med. 1997;337:1491–9.

20. Kris-Etherton P, Daniels SR, Eckel RH, et al. Summary of the scientific conference on dietary fatty acids and cardiovascular health. Conference summary from the Nutrition Committee of the American Heart Association. Circulation. 2001;103:1034–9.

21. Djousse L, Arnett DK, Carr JJ, et al. Dietary linolenic acid is inversely associated with calcified arteriosclerotic plaque in coronary arteries. The National Heart, Lung, and Blood Institute Family Heart Study. Circulation. 2005;111:2921–6.

22. Rudel LL, Parks JS, Sawyer JK. Compared with dietary monounsaturated and saturated fat, polyunsaturated fat protects African green monkeys from coronary artery atherosclerosis. Arterioscler Thromb Vasc Biol. 1995;15:2101–10.

23. Vogel RA, Corretti MC, Plotnick GD. Effect of a single high-fat meal on endothelial function in healthy subjects. Am J Cardiol. 1997;79:350–54.

24. Ceriello A, Assaloni R, Da Ros R, et al. Effect of atorvastatin and irbesartan, alone and in combination, on postprandial endothelial dysfunction, oxidative stress, and inflammation in type 2 diabetic patients. Circulation. 2005;111:2518–24.

25. Nestel PJ, Shige H, Pomeroy S, Cehun M, Chin-Dusting J. Post-prandial remnant lipids impair arterial compliance. J Am Coll Cardiol. 2001;37:1929–35.

26. Ferreira AC, Peter AA, Mendez AJ, et al. Postprandial hypertriglyceridemia increases circulating levels of endothelial cell microparticles. Circulation. 2004;110:3599–603.

27. Goode GK, Garcia S, Heagerty AM. Dietary supplementation with marine fish oil improves in vitro small artery endothelial function in hypercholesterolemic patients. A double-blind placebo-controlled study. Circulation. 1997;96:2802–7.

28. De Caterina R, Bernini W, Carluccio MA, Liao J, Libby P. Structural requirements for inhibition of cytokine-induced endothelial activation by unsaturated fatty acids. J Lipid Res. 1998;39:1062–70.

29. Vogel RA, Plotnick GD, Corretti MC. The postprandial effects of components of the Mediterranean diet on endothelial function. J Am Coll Cardiol. 2000;26: 1455–60.

30. Esposito K, Marfella R, Ciotola M, et al. Effect of a Mediterranean-style diet on endothelial dysfunction and markers of inflammation in the metabolic syndrome. JAMA. 2004;292:1440–6.

31. Chrysohoou C, Panagiotakos DB, Pitsavos C, et al. Adherence to the Mediterranean diet attenuates inflammation and coagulation in healthy adults. The Attica study. J Am Coll Cardiol. 2004;44:152–8.

32. Vogel RA. Vintners and vasodilators: are French wines more cardioprotective? J Am Coll Cardiol. 2003;41:479–81.

33. De Oliveria E, Silva ER, Foster D, et al. Alcohol consumption raises HDL cholesterol levels by increasing the transport rate of apolipoproteins A-I and A-II. Circulation. 2000;102:2347–52.

34. Rimm ER, Williams P, Foster K, et al. Moderate alcohol intake and lower risk of coronary heart disease: meta-analysis of effects on lipids and haemostatic factors. BMJ. 1999;319:1523–8.

35. Klatsky AL, Armstrong MA, Friedman GD. Red wine, white wine, liquor, beer, and risk for coronary artery disease hospitalization. Am J Cardiol. 1997;80:416–20.

10

GUIDED IMAGERY IN INTEGRATIVE CARDIOLOGY

Martin L. Rossman

INTRODUCTORY CASE HISTORY

I was teaching guided imagery to a group of patients in a cardiac rehabilitation program, beginning with a lecture about the nature of imagery in health and self-care, and progressing to a first "mental experiment" for the class to explore. I guided participants to deepen their breathing, and to briefly focus on each major muscle group as they mentally scanned their bodies, inviting each muscle group to relax and then to imagine themselves in a beautiful and safe place. They were then encouraged to notice what they imagined seeing, what sounds or silence they imagined there, and to pay attention to the time of day, season of the year, and temperature and feel of the air.*

Once the group seemed quiet and comfortable, I invited them to imagine their hearts, accepting whatever images came to mind, whether or not they were anatomically correct. They were encouraged to simply observe the image or images that came to mind from whatever perspective they chose to take, and notice what seemed healthy and what, if anything seemed less healthy. They were then invited to imagine that they could "talk with" or communicate to their hearts and "tell" them (silently) that they were here because they wanted to provide what their hearts needed in order to heal as effectively and thoroughly as

---

*Research utilizing functional MRI now tells us that this process of "sensory recruitment," long used in hypnosis, activates the areas of the brain that process these sensory types of information, creating a cortical activation pattern similar to that created by actually being in and perceiving these same stimuli through the sense organs. This relays to the limbic system, hypothalamus, and autonomic nervous system the message that "this looks like a safe place, this sounds like a safe place, smells like a safe pace, and it's ok to relax here." The result in most people is that they find themselves physically and mentally relaxing, eliciting a "relaxation response" in which their physiology shifts from one of sympathetic nervous system dominance to parasympathetic dominance. This in itself offers many benefits to patients with cardiac disease.

possible. Then I asked them to begin imagining that their hearts were getting what they needed and that they were healing or moving toward better health.

Most of these people had severe coronary artery disease (CAD), had numerous diagnostic and therapeutic interventions, and had seen many cardiologists over the years. Most of them imagined that they had blocked coronary vessels and began imaging that in some way they were opening their arteries ("roto-rooting" being a common image) and restoring blood flow to damaged areas of their hearts. They often imagined that their heart tissues were becoming pink, strong, and healthy again. Most of them found this calming and reassuring, though often quite emotional.

After a while, I invited the group to stretch their imaginations a bit further and imagine that their hearts could communicate back to them, and to listen to what they imagined their hearts would say, or ask for if they could communicate. Some imagined their hearts asking for better food, or more exercise or activity, while others imagined that more fun and joy in living was needed. With many the request was for more love and time for the self. Some people fell asleep, and others had difficulty imagining anything at all, but most people found that they could imagine some kind of inner dialogue with an image that represented their heart.

Afterwards we took some time to discuss what people experienced, what questions they have, what they learned, and what they might do with what they learned. On this particular day, one dignified, studious-looking woman in her 60 s stood up and with tears in her eyes, said, "I have had heart disease for over 10 years and I've been to many doctors and cardiologists. I have had every exam and treatment available and have studied heart disease myself over that time. But...(more tears)... this is the first time I have realized that this is *my* heart." There was a stillness in the room and more than a few heads nodded in silent acknowledgment. After a while, she went on to say that realizing that it was her heart opened up the possibility that she could help it to heal.

I take the time to share this story with you because while in this chapter I will review studies that illustrate that guided imagery can be helpful to cardiac patients for relaxation, stress reduction, blood pressure control, smoking cessation, and weight reduction, its most powerful use may be the strengthening of the personal relationship that the patient has to his own health care. Without this sense of personal relationship to health, it's difficult to sustain good self-care. Patients with chronic illnesses who learn and practice better self-care tend to have an increase in "self-efficacy," the sense that you can do something about your situation, and when patients feel that, they are empowered to make changes in their habits, lifestyles, and the way they approach life that often result in health improvement.[1]

As physicians, we are trained to diagnose and treat physically observable manifestations of disease and illness. In some instances, we can provide definitive, even life-saving interventions and both we and our patients are pleased and grateful. In many other situations, we can give the condition a name and provide some symptomatic relief, but can do little or nothing about the underlying disease process unless we can find a way to engage the patient in modifying their lifestyle as it affects their health. This is certainly often true in cardiology, and this aspect of patient management often represents the most challenging and time-consuming facets of our practices.

People with chronic heart and circulatory illnesses have a good deal of depression, anxiety, and suboptimal patterns of dealing with stress and emotions. This complicates their care and may directly affect their physiology, adherence to treatment regimens, and disease outcome. They need not only excellent medical care, but attention to what we might call the invisible, yet important aspects of health care that are only accessible through their own awareness. Guided imagery provides us with tools to help them attend to these unseen dimensions of human illness.

Guided imagery can help patients with heart disease in many ways, from reducing their levels of stress, anxiety, and depression to helping them change health-related lifestyles, to relieving common cardiac symptoms, to reducing anxiety related to cardiac interventions such as angiography and cardiac surgery. It can also help the willing patient become more aware of the roles they can play in better managing their medical conditions, and even help to heal emotional and psychological patterns that lie beneath health-damaging lifestyles.

WHAT IS IMAGERY?

Imagery is a natural form of thinking that uses sensory or quasi-sensory thought forms to create internal representations of personal reality. Images may be concrete and anatomic, or metaphorical and abstract. Most, but not all, have some visual component, but may also have sound, smell, and kinesthetic aspects as well. Not everyone visualizes, but nearly everyone imagines in his or her own way.

Imagery is a natural way the human nervous system stores, accesses, and processes information. It is the coding system in which memories, fantasies, dreams, daydreams, and expectations are stored. It is a way of thinking with sensory attributes and in the absence of competing sensory cues, the body tends to respond to imagery as it would to a genuine external experience. The two most common and familiar examples of this phenomenon are worrying and sexual fantasy, with their attendant physiological, psychological, and behavioral responses. Recalling or imagining the worst thing that ever happened to you is likely to upset you emotionally and physiologically, especially if you focus on the remembered sights, sounds, smells, and feelings of the time. If you are prone to cardiac symptoms, you may even create tachycardia, palpitations, chest pain, or transient hypertension. Conversely, recalling or imaging yourself in a beautiful, serene, and safe place, again noticing all the sensory cues, is likely to produce a pleasant sense of calm and relaxation, and can potentially relieve the same set of signs and symptoms.

Imagery has been shown in dozens of research studies to be able to affect almost all major physiological control systems of the body, including respiration, heart rate, blood pressure, metabolic rates in cells, gastrointestinal mobility and secretion, sexual function, and even immune responsiveness.

Imagery is a rapid way to teach patients to relax and reduce stress, a way to alter physiology, and also a way to access emotional and symbolic information that may affect physiology and the way the patients care for themselves. For instance, a patient with CAD returned from his imaginary conversation with his heart reporting an image of a blue, tired, overburdened heart filled with more grief than he could even imagine. He began talking of old losses and grief that he had kept inside himself for many, many years, and while it brought tears not only to his eyes but the eyes of many of us in the group, it was very relieving to him to finally be able to talk about these things. He felt quite unburdened and by the time he was done, his heart image already looked (in his mind's eye) to be "much lighter and pinker" than it had been for a long time. This is not to say that his severe underlying coronary disease was reversed or cured within that 30-minute time frame, but it did result in being more emotionally aware and accessible to himself and his loved ones through the course of his rehabilitation and afterward. This improved the quality of his life so much that his chronic low-grade depression remitted, making it much easier for him to maintain the healthy lifestyle changes in diet, activity, and approach to life that he learned in the group.

FORMS OF IMAGERY-BASED INTERVENTIONS

Because imagery is the dominant coding language of the unconscious or sub-conscious mind, it is an important aspect of virtually every mind-body approach including most relaxation techniques, hypnosis, biofeedback, autogenic training, and psychotherapies including cognitive behavioral therapy, which include but are not limited to cognitive behavioral therapy (CBT). As we search the litera-ture looking at mind-body approaches, careful reading of the methods used shows that mental imagery is central to their effectiveness. In my later review of relevant research, I will refer to studies that largely use imagery-based methods whether or not they are referred to as "guided imagery studies."

Guided imagery is a term variously used to describe a range of techniques from simple visualization and direct imagery-based suggestion, through metaphor and story telling. Guided imagery is used to help teach psychophysiological relaxation, to relieve symptoms, to stimulate healing responses in the body, and to help people tolerate procedures and treatments more easily.

Interactive Guided Imagery (IGI) is a service-marked term coined by the Academy for Guided Imagery, a professional training academy to represent a process where imagery is used in a highly interactive format to not only modu-late symptoms, illnesses, or responses to illness, but to evoke patient autonomy as well.

In IGI, we find that even if patients have the same clinical diagnosis (CAD, CHF, HT), their personal imagery about their illness and potential for healing can differ tremendously. For some, the images center on eliminating toxic habits like smoking, while others will focus on food, and exercise and getting their blood pressure and lipid values in certain ranges. Many more will find that their imagery focuses them on relaxation and stress reduction, improving their relationships; managing emotions better, resolving internal conflicts, and grieving old losses. What is striking is that these images carry with them an unusual amount of authority and motivational power, perhaps because they arise from the individuals' own personal database of life experience. This gives patients ways to draw on their own inner resources to support healing, to make appropriate adaptations to changes in health, and to better understand what their symptoms may be signaling.

Relaxation techniques are the most widely used, easily learned, and generally useful mind-body techniques because stress is so often a factor in illness and health-related issues. You could say that stress is part of almost any illness, in that it causes the illness, amplifies the distress involved, or is itself caused by the illness. Reducing stress allows the patient to feel better, regain some sense of control, and supports healing in the body. Almost all mind-body approaches begin with teaching the patient to relax body and mind and for many western patients, imagining or daydreaming themselves to a place, real or imaginary, where they experience relaxation is the simplest, quickest, and most effective way to introduce people to relaxation.

Meditation involves concentrating the mind on either a neutral or a meaningful focus—a word, an image, an external object, your breathing, or whatever is occurring at the time. Meditation tends to create a physiologically relaxed state and helps develop peace of mind. There are many forms of meditation, some connected to particular religious belief systems, and others which are nonsecular and compatible with any belief system. Two of the best-researched approaches regarding mind-body effects are transcendental meditation and mindfulness meditation. Images can be the focus of meditation, and conversely, meditation teaches the patient to focus the mind and frees them from the effects of unconscious "runaway" imagery, so common in habitual worriers.

Biofeedback uses sensitive physiological monitors to amplify the reactions the body is having in response to the thoughts in the mind. By being able to see, hear, or otherwise experience the changes the body makes in response to thoughts, patients may be able to gain control over physical functions normally out of their conscious control. Biofeedback is a convincing experience for most patients who explore it, as it is quite startling to see how quickly and sensitively the body responds to various thoughts. While the instrumentation displays the reactions of the body to thoughts, biofeedback therapists generally find that the thoughts that most significantly affect physiology are those that are imagery based.

Hypnosis is often defined as a "relaxed state of focused attention in which suggestibility is enhanced." While there are many studies demonstrating the utility of hypnosis, there is also significant debate about whether a "hypnotic state" exists or whether the effects of hypnosis are due to expectations, suggestions, and desire for improvement. Whether this "trance state" exists is controversial, but it is clear that with or without a trance, there is very little you can do clinically with hypnosis without relying on imagery and imagery-based suggestions. While we use words to create suggestions, the most effective suggestions almost always involve mental imagery. It is crucial to learn to work with imagery to obtain the best results from hypnosis.

Psychotherapy is often useful in cardiac illness, and nearly every form of effective psychotherapy makes significant use of imagery. Freudian and Jungian analyses utilize dream interpretation along with investigation of and reinterpretation of images of self and others, as do therapies based on object relations or control mastery. Gestalt psychotherapy, psychodrama, and related therapies are frankly based on imagery and its modulation, while behavioral therapies like CBT routinely teach relaxation and mood modulation through guided imagery techniques.

Body/Mind therapies like yoga, Tai Chi, and Qi Gong involve physical movements and postures as well as breathing techniques and mental imagery to induce relaxation and physical balance.

WHAT ARE THE APPLICATIONS OF GUIDED IMAGERY IN CARDIOLOGY?

Since imagery is a way of thinking, it has widespread applications in clinical medicine and cardiology, ranging from simple relaxation techniques, through preparation for procedures and surgery, treatment adherence, reducing convalescent time, changing lifestyle behaviors, and finding meaning in illness.

While guided imagery is essentially a way of working with the patient, rather than a way of treating particular disease entities, it is especially effective in the areas listed below:

- Relaxation training and stress reduction
- Reduction of adverse coronary events
- Relief of angina, breathlessness, and anxiety surrounding cardiac conditions
- Blood pressure reduction
- Smoking cessation
- Weight loss and adherence to exercise and healthy lifestyle regimens
- Anxiety reduction prior to angiography, angioplasty, and cardiac surgery, and reduction of postoperative discomfort and complications
- Relief of noncardiac chest pain
- Dealing with issues of meaning in heart disease

Guided imagery in relaxation training and stress reduction

Mental stress is associated with an increased incidence of adverse coronary events in epidemiological studies.[2-3] The links between psychosocial stress, heart disease, and cardiac events have been established for many years, though significantly less attention is paid to them than for other risk factors.[4-5]

Guided imagery, which combines deep relaxation with positive suggestion, is a powerful stress management technique. Studies have shown that groups of smokers, surgical patients, cardiac and cancer patients, and people reporting high stress levels who went through guided imagery sessions had significant reduction in self-reported stress, physiological measures of stress, and state of anxiety relative to control groups. Effects were stronger when patients could practice on their own.[6–7]

Most significantly, a placebo-controlled, randomized study showed that teaching stress reduction techniques to cardiac patients reduced their risk of having further heart problems by a remarkable 75%. Of 107 patients, 40 received standard medical care; 34 additionally engaged in vigorous exercise for 35 minutes, three times a week for 16 weeks; and 33 were also offered weekly group sessions where they learned relaxation and stress reduction techniques (education, progressive muscle relaxation, biofeedback, thought-stopping, anger management). Analysis of results showed 30% of the standard care group had additional heart problems; 21% in the exercise group, and only 10% in the stress management group.[8]

Guided imagery in CAD

The results of Dean Ornish and associates' landmark 1998 study demonstrated that lifestyle changes (diet, exercise, relaxation, and social support) could actually reverse CHD.[9] Other studies have shown that emotions can play a major role in CHD, with fear, grief, anxiety, and anger capable of triggering cardiac events,[10–11] and depression can affect the outcome of long-term survival.[12] Stress also plays a role in the development and progression of CAD both in men and women.[13–14]

Anger, hostility, and other possibly harmful emotional states can be modulated by the inner-focused, relaxed state induced by guided imagery and other mind-body modalities. A sense of emotional well-being can be improved by the use of these mind-body techniques.[15] Guided imagery and relaxation can reduce stress, and lower heart rate and blood pressure.[16–17] Authors of a review of 23 major heart disease studies concluded that when psychosocial approaches were added to standard medical treatments, not only did survival increase but further cardiac event rates were significantly reduced.[18] Mind-body approaches like relaxation training and imagery are so effective that they are routinely used to reduce complications from cardiac surgery at major medical facilities such as Columbia Presbyterian Hospital's Department of Surgery.[19] Relaxation, imagery, and education are important parts of Stanford's Chronic Disease Self-Management Program. Self-management of chronic conditions, including CHD, improves symptom management and reduces medical costs.[20]

According to one lifestyle study, 80% of people who used complementary approaches including relaxation and guided imagery avoided cardiac surgery—a savings of almost $30,000 per patient.[21] Lifestyle change begins in the mind, and guided imagery can be used to reduce stress, lower blood pressure, motivate people to exercise, and help people move toward taking action in improving their nutrition, all of which has a salutary and desirable effect on CAD.

Guided imagery in hypertension

Guided imagery is highly effective in reducing blood pressure using deep relaxation with positive self-suggestion.[22] Centers for Disease Control and Prevention researchers have stated that evidence for the effectiveness of certain nondrug approaches to HNT prevention and control, including guided imagery, is strong.[23] Individual studies and recent reviews of the literature support the effectiveness of imagery, relaxation training, biofeedback with relaxation training, hypnosis, and autogenic training in lowering blood pressure.[24,25]

Astin et al reported in their review that "relaxation techniques (autogenic training, progressive muscular relaxation, behavioral therapy, or biofeedback techniques), can lower elevated blood pressure by an average of 10 mm Hg (systolic) and 5 mm Hg (diastolic). Studies confirm that meditation,[26,27] relaxation, and stress reduction,[28] and even simply breathing techniques[29] can positively affect hypertension. Meditation also appeared to decrease blood pressure among African American women[30] and significantly decreased mortality in hypertensive subjects.[31] Authors of a meta-analysis of 22 biofeedback studies concluded that only the relaxation-assisted biofeedback significantly decreased both systolic and diastolic blood pressures, so its effect may possibly only be from the relaxation component.[32]

Guided imagery and smoking cessation

Cigarette smoking is the largest preventable cause of illness, death, and medical expenditures in the United States, and a major risk factor for cardiovascular disease. While it is typical for smoking cessation programs to achieve short-term success rates of 50–60%, the rate of relapse is often 60–80% in the year following the program.[33] Most widely used smoking cessation programs have long-term success rates under 35%.[34,35]

IMAGERY AND SELF-HYPNOSIS IN SMOKING CESSATION

In two studies, groups who received guided imagery training to encourage relaxation and a sense of personal power had much higher 3-month abstinence rates than a control group that received only counseling.[36] Smokers who practiced imagery at home and continued practicing after the training program ended had abstinence rates over 52% at 3 months.[37] Even a one-session intervention with self-hypnosis resulted in 22% of a group of 226 patients remaining smoke-abstinent after 2 years, a modest result which is still superior to the results of spontaneous efforts to quit.[38] Thus, imagery and self-hypnosis have been at least as effective as other behavioral and psychological approaches, and more effective in patients who found them congenial. A study currently being conducted at Harvard Medical School is investigating the effect of a combined guided imagery and nicotine patch program.

Guided imagery in weight loss

Excessive weight, with or without diabetes, hypertension, or metabolic syndrome, is a significant risk factor for heart disease. Guided imagery can be a significant part of a weight loss, body composition management program.

In a representative study, the effect of adding hypnosis to a behavioral weight-management program on short- and long-term weight change was studied. 109 subjects, ranging in age from 17 to 67, completed a behavioral treatment either with or without the addition of hypnosis. At the end of the 9-week program, both interventions resulted in significant weight reduction. However, at the 8-month and 2-year follow-ups, the hypnosis subjects showed significant additional weight loss, while those in behavioral treatment alone exhibited minimal further change. More of the subjects, who used hypnosis also achieved and maintained their personal weight goals.[39]

A randomized, controlled, parallel study looked at two forms of hypnotherapy—one directed at stress reduction and the other at intake reduction, as compared to dietary advice alone, in 60 obese patients with obstructive sleep apnea. The hypnotherapy group, which focused on stress reduction achieved significantly more weight loss than the other two treatment conditions ($p < 0.003$), which were not significantly different from each other, and at 18 months, only the hypnotherapy group that focused on stress reduction continued to show a significant ($p < 0.02$), mean weight loss (3.8 kg) compared to baseline. The study concludes that stress reduction hypnotherapy, as an adjunct to dietary advice, produces statistically significant weight loss.[40]

Another study investigated the effects of hypnosis in weight loss for 60 females, at least 20% overweight and not involved in other treatment. Hypnosis was more effective than a control group (17 vs. 0.5 lb on follow-up).[41] In subjects with night eating syndrome, progressive muscle relaxation lowered stress, anxiety, fatigue, anger, and depression, with positive shifts in eating and hunger patterns.[42]

A meta-analysis of the relevant research done at the University of Connecticut shows that adding hypnosis/guided imagery to a weight loss program tends to double the weight loss. Averaged across posttreatment and follow-up assessment periods from all the studies, mean weight loss was 6.00 lb. (2.72 kg) without hypnosis and 11.83 lb. (5.37 kg) with hypnosis. In addition, the benefits of hypnosis increased substantially over time.[43]

Guided imagery for arrythmias

As early as 1975, the *Lancet* published a study of the then new "relaxation response," coauthored by lead researcher Herbert Benson. Benson and colleagues found that the relaxation response decreased activity in the sympathetic nervous system activity, decreasing PVCs in 8 of 11 nonmedicated patients; the effect was particularly significant during periods of sleep.[44] A later study conducted at New England Deaconess Hospital of those using the relaxation response before surgery had fewer incidents of supraventricular tachycardia than the control group.[45] Relaxation also enabled patients lower their respiration rates, leading to beneficial effects on both resting heart rate and respiratory sinus arrhythmia. Van Dixhoorn et al. reported better long-term outcomes in post-cardiac events patients who added relaxation to a cardiac exercise rehabilitation program.[46,47]

In a University of Michigan Medical Center study, patients using relaxation and guided imagery had lower resting heart rates, greater number of medication reductions, and lower self-reported tension levels than the control group.[48] A recent study showed that relaxation and hypnosis modulated the stress response of cardiac rhythm in response to stress.[49] The sum of these studies indicates that relaxation training with guided imagery may offer protective benefits to patients vulnerable to certain arrhythmias.

GUIDED IMAGERY FOR ANGIOGRAPHY, ANGIOPLASTY, AND CARDIAC CATHETERIZATION

Patient anxiety can be a significant problem in invasive cardiac procedures. Insufficient treatment of pain and anxiety can cause cardiovascular strain and restlessness, which may jeopardize the success of the procedure. On the other hand, pharmacological oversedation can provoke respiratory and cardiovascular depression, thereby increasing the procedural risks and delaying the patient's recovery.[50] Among the most effective nondrug approaches to reducing patient anxiety are relaxation with guided imagery (self-hypnosis) and preprocedure provision of information.[51] Preprocedure teaching, tailored to each patient's coping style, can reduce tachycardia and other signs of distress during procedures.[52,53] Mind-body approaches, especially those incorporating guided imagery, relaxation, or self-hypnosis, can result in shorter procedures, less need for medication, lower anxiety, and fewer complications. In a study where patients were encouraged to develop their own images ("interactive imagery"), the approach was found to be more effective than prescribed imagery presented to patients.[54] Similar benefits have been found for imagery and self-hypnosis in other procedures including endoscopy and MRI.[55,56]

Guided imagery in cardiac surgery

Surgeons and anesthesiologists have long looked at nonpharmacological ways to reduce presurgical anxiety, since pharmacological sedation often increases the risk of low blood pressure and lack of oxygen. Relaxation with guided imagery (self-hypnosis) and preprocedure education have been the most effective to date.[57,58] Self-hypnosis, or relaxation with guided imagery used prior to and during surgery has resulted in shorter procedures.[59,60] These techniques can also significantly reduce postsurgical pain and the need for postoperative pain medication,[61,62] shorten the time it takes for the return of normal intestinal motility[63] and reduce the length of hospital stay.[64–65] There is evidence that hypnosis and imagery can reduce blood loss[66–67]and speed wound healing.[68] Hypnosis and guided imagery have been used effectively in cardiac bypass to reduce length of hospital stay, decrease use of pain medications, and lower pharmacy costs.[69,70] Bypass patients using these techniques were more relaxed preoperatively and had lower levels of postoperative depression, fatigue, and anger.[71] Anger can be problematic for cardiac patients and has been associated with cardiac events including heart attacks. Anger can also be associated with re-narrowing of heart arteries and the need for coronary artery bypass grafting. A simple mind-body technique like breathing therapy has been shown to reduce anger scores, and cut by 50% the risk of post-PTCA cardiac events.[72]

In sum, this simple, nontoxic and inexpensive method of mental preparation can reduce surgical time, reduce complication rates of ileus, bleeding, and postoperative cardiac events, shorten hospital stays, reduce postoperative pain and narcotic use,[73] and increase patient satisfaction. There are few interventions of any kind, this effective and this safe in all of medicine and we would hope that this becomes standard of care in preoperative and preprocedure preparation in the near future.

WARNINGS, PRECAUTIONS, AND CONTRAINDICATIONS TO GUIDED IMAGERY

While guided imagery, delivered either by a health professional or via audio materials such as tapes or CDs, are generally quite safe, there are some precautions to heed. The first precaution of course is not to use guided imagery in lieu of a more definitive medical or surgical intervention when one is needed. It would be a good idea to reassure the myocardial infarction (MI) patients in the emergency room by letting them know that they are in good hands, and that it will help them to breathe deeply and let themselves relax while people are taking care of them, but it would be foolish to consider that to be complete care. Guided imagery is a helpful adjunct to almost any medical or surgical intervention, but is rarely a substitute.

The second precaution is using guided imagery with patients that have, or have had, serious psychiatric illness, particularly psychotic or dissociative disorders. In these cases, imagery can sometimes be very useful, but it can also precipitate flooding or disorganization. Encouraging these patients to breathe easily, relax their bodies, and imagine themselves somewhere that they love to be is generally safe, but exploratory, interactive forms of imagery like imagery dialogue should only be used by personnel that have training and experience working with patients with these diagnoses.

A third precaution is with physical symptoms that may be precipitated by stress and emotion. Imagery is closely linked to emotion, and patients who are fragile and highly stressed can encounter imagery that is highly charged with emotion. In rare cardiac patients, this can evoke symptoms like chest pain, arrhythmia, and syncope. In one case attended by the author, a workshop participant who was prone to coronary spasm suffered an episode while involved in an inner dialogue with an image of her heart. The practitioner should know that symptoms that can be precipitated by imagery can almost always be relieved by imagery, and that is a useful thing to tell the patient. In this case, the image this woman evoked was a snake wrapped around her coronary artery, squeezing it shut. While waiting for the ambulance to come, we encouraged her to breathe and suggested that she ask the snake to relax and let the artery open. She was able to do this and her chest pain symptoms resolved before she went to the emergency room.

Asthma and unstable epilepsy can also be triggered by imagery, although, again, this is extremely rare. With patients with any of these conditions, practitioners should make sure that measures are available that can treat these occurrences before proceeding with therapeutic imagery.

The health professional should familiarize themselves with any guided imagery self-care products they might consider using, and either identify local professionals qualified to use guided imagery or take sufficient training to ensure that they can use this powerful approach safely and effectively (see Resources).

BILLING AND REIMBURSEMENT

Practitioners usually bill and are reimbursed for their work with imagery in the same way they are for other professional services. The work is usually identified as psychotherapy, counseling, stress reduction training, or medical hypnosis. When applied for medical purposes, medical practitioners may ethically bill for medical services, although insurance companies may challenge this if services are lengthy and repetitious. There are currently no separate billing codes for guided imagery or IGI. Guided imagery CDs can be billed under codes for educational supplies or materials.

ACCEPTANCE AND USE OF GUIDED IMAGERY

Imagery and visualization are increasingly accepted practices with both patients and physicians, and both have significantly penetrated our culture. A recent survey of 2055 Americans showed that 18.9% had used some form of mind-body therapy within the past year, with imagery, yoga, and meditation being the most frequently used, and about 80% of those users used them as self-care techniques.[74]

Responsible mind-body approaches are generally quite acceptable to physicians. Several studies have recently shown that almost 60% of physicians refer to the top five complementary approaches, with stress reduction, imagery, meditation, and hypnosis being the leading modalities. In addition, physicians utilize these services even more frequently for themselves and their families.[75]

By and large, imagery is a potent form of adjunctive treatment for almost any medical or psychological situation. It is a simple, yet profoundly effective, inexpensive, and safe form of care that allows the patient to participate in their own process of healing.

Imagery is rarely used as a sole form of treatment for serious illness, yet it is almost always helpful in combination with nearly any other type of treatment. The highly desirable risk/benefit ratios and cost reductions available through guided imagery make us hope that this empowering form of treatment becomes standard of care in the many clinical arenas in which it is appropriate.

GUIDED IMAGERY RESOURCES

For patients

Guided imagery is a very useful set of tools for patient self-care, and many excellent guided imagery lessons are available on CD and as audio downloads at the following web sites:

www.thehealingmind.org
Guided imagery books, research, CDs, and downloads, including interactive imagery lessons, by Marty Rossman, MD and other leaders in the field.

www.drmiller.com
Self-hypnosis and guided imagery CDs by mind-body pioneer Emmett Miller, MD.

www.healthjourneys.com
Guided imagery CDs and books by Belleruth Naparstek, MSW.

For professionals

www.thehealingmind.org
Along with guided imagery books and CDs, this web site provides research summaries and access to emerging applications of guided imagery in self-care and medicine.

www.academyforguidedimagery.com
Professional postgraduate training and Certification in IGI. Annual meeting in November and searchable Directory of Imagery Practitioners.

REFERENCES

1. Lorig KR, Sobel DS, Stewart AL, Brown Jr. BW, Ritter PL, Gonzalez VM, et al. Evidence suggesting that a chronic disease self-management program can improve health status while reducing utilization and costs: a randomized trial. Med Care. 1999;37(1):5–14.

2. Kaprio J, Kosvenvuo M, et al. Mortality after bereavement: a prospective study of 95,647 widowed persons. Am J Public Health. 1987;77:283–7.

3. Meisel SR, Kutz I, et al. Effects of Iraqi missile war on incidence of acute myocardial infarction and sudden death in Israeli citizens. Lancet. 1991;338:660–1.

4. Anda R, Williamson D, et al. Depressed affect, hopelessness, and the risk of ischemic events in a cohort of U.S. adults. Epidemiology. 1993;4:285–94.

5. Ulmer D. Stress management for the cardiovascular patient: a look at current treatment and trends. Prog Cardiovas Nurs. 1996 winter;11(1):21–9.

6. Crowther JH. Stress management training and relaxation imagery in the treatment of essential hypertension. J Behav Med. 1983;6(2):169–87.

7. Tiller WA, McCraty R, Atkinson M. Alternative therapies in health & medicine. 1996;2(1):52–65.

8. Blumenthal JA. et al. Stress management and exercise training in cardiac patients with myocardial ischemia: effects on prognosis and evaluation of mechanisms. Arch Int Med. 1997;157:2213–23.

9. Ornish D, Scherwitz LW, Billings JH, et al. Intensive lifestyle changes for reversal of coronary heart disease. JAMA. 1998a Dec 16;280(23):2001–7.

10. Verrier RL, Mittelman MA. Cardiovascular consequences of anger and other stress states. Baillieres Clin Neurol. 1997 Jul;6(2):245–59.

11. Verrier RL, Hagestad EL, Lown B. Delayed myocardial ischemia induced by anger. Circulation. 1987;5:249–54.

12. Barefoot JC, Brummett BH, Helms MJ, Mark DB, Siegler IC, et al. Depressive symptoms and survival of patients with coronary artery disease. J Psychosom Med. 2000 Nov–Dec;62(6):790–5.

13. Allison TG, Williams DE, Miller TD, Patten CA, Bailey KR, Squires RW, et al. Medical and economic costs of psychologic distress in patients with coronary artery disease. Mayo Clin Proc. 1995 Aug;70(8):734–42.

14. Sheps DS, McMahon RP, Becker L, Carney RM, Freedland KE, Cohen JD, et al. Mental stress-induced ischemia and all-cause mortality in patients with coronary artery disease: results from the psychophysiological investigations of myocardial ischemia study. Circulation. 2002 Apr 16;105:1780–4.

15. Zamarra JW, Schneider RH, Besseghini I, Robinson DK, Salerno JW. Usefulness of the transcendental meditation program in the treatment of patients with coronary artery disease. Am J Cardiol. 1996 Apr 15;77(10):867–70.

16. Crowther JH. Stress management training and relaxation imagery in the treatment of essential hypertension. J Behav Med. 1983 Jun;6(2):169–87.

17. Sharpley CF. Maintenance and generalizability of laboratory-based heart rate reactivity control training. J Behav Med.1994;17(3):309–329.

18. Linden W, Stossel C, Maurice J. Psychosocial interventions for patients with coronary artery disease: a meta-analysis. Arch Intern Med. 1996 Apr 8; 156(7):745–52.

19. Oz MC, Lemole EJ, Oz LL, Whitworth GC, Lemole GM. Treating CHD with cardiac surgery combined with complementary therapy. Medscape Womens Health. 1996 Oct;1(10):7.

20. Lorig KR, Sobel DS, Stewart AL, Brown Jr. BW, Ritter PL, Gonzalez VM, et al. Evidence suggesting that a chronic disease self-management program can improve health status while reducing utilization and costs: a randomized trial. Med Care. 1999;37(1):5–14.

21. Ornish D. Avoiding revascularization with lifestyle changes: the Multicenter Lifestyle Demonstration Project. Am J Cardiol. 1998c;82:72T–6T.

22. Agras WS. Behavioral approaches to the treatment of essential hypertension. Int J Obes. 1981;5 Suppl 1:173–81.

23. Taylor CB, Farquhar JW, Nelson E, Agras S. Relaxation therapy and high blood pressure. Arch Gen Psychiatry. 1977;34:339–42.

24. Astin JA, Shapiro SL, Eisenberg DM, Forys KL, Shapiro SL, et al. Mind-body medicine: state of the science, implications for practice. J Am Board Fam Pract. 2003 Mar–Apr;16(2):131–47.

25. Stetter F, Kupper S. Autogenic training: a meta-analysis of clinical outcome studies. Appl Psychophysiol Biofeedback. 2002 Mar;27(1):45–98.

26. Barnes VA, Davis HC, Murzynowski JB, Treiber FA. Impact of meditation on resting and ambulatory blood pressure and heart rate in youth. Psychosom Med. 2004a Nov–Dec;66(6):909–14.

27. Barnes VA, Treiber FA, Johnson MH. Impact of transcendental meditation on ambulatory blood pressure in African-American adolescents. Am J Hypertens. 2004b Apr; 17(4):366–9.

28. Kurz RW, Pirker H, Potz H, Dorrscheidt W, Uhlir H. [Evaluation of costs and effectiveness of an integrated training program for hypertensive patients.] [article in German] Wien Klin Wochenschr. 2005 Aug;117(15–16):526–33.

29. Bernardi L, Porta C, Spicuzza L, Sleight P. Cardiorespiratory interactions to external stimuli. Arch Ital Biol. 2005 Sep;143(3–4):215–21.

30. Schneider RH, Alexander CN, Staggers F, Orme-Johnson DW, Rainforth M, Salerno JW, et al. A randomized controlled trial of stress reduction in African Americans treated for hypertension for over one year. Am J Hypertens. 2005 Jan; 18(1):88–98.

31. Schneider RH, Alexander CN, Staggers F, Rainforth M, Salerno JW, Hartz A, et al. Long-term effects of stress reduction on mortality in persons > or = 55 years of age with systemic hypertension. Am J Cardiol. 2005 May 1;95(9):1060–4.

32. Nakao M, Yano E, Nomura S, Kuboki T. Blood pressure-lowering effects of biofeedback treatment in hypertension: a meta-analysis of randomized controlled trials. Hypertens Res. 2003 Jan;26(1):37–46.

33. CDC Report dated 2001. The burden of tobacco use. Accessed January, 2002 at http://www.cdc.gov/tobacco/overview/oshaag.htm

34. Colletti G, Supnick JA, Rizzo AA. Long-term follow-up (3–4 years) of treatment for smoking reduction. Addict Behav. 1982;7(4):429–33.

35. Hensel MR, Cavanagh T, Lanier AP, Gleason T, Bouwens B, Tanttila H, et al. Quit rates at one year follow-up of Alaska Native Medical Center Tobacco Cessation Program. Alaska Med. 1995 Apr–Jun;37(2):43–7.

36. Wynd CA. Relaxation imagery used for stress reduction in the prevention of smoking relapse. J Adv Nurs. 1992 Mar;17(3):294–302.

37. Wynd CA. Personal power imagery and relaxation techniques used in smoking cessation programs. Am J Health Promot. 1992 Jan–Feb;6(3):184–9.

38. Spiegel D, Frischholz EJ, Fleiss JL, Spiegel H. Predictors of smoking abstinence following a single-session restructuring intervention with self-hypnosis. Am J Psychiatry. 1993 Jul;150(7):1090–7.

39. Bolocofsky DN, Spinler D, Coulthard-Morris L. Effectiveness of hypnosis as an adjunct to behavioral weight management. J Clin Psychol. 1985 Jan;41(1): 35–41.

40. Stradling J, Roberts D, Wilson A, Lovelock F. Controlled trial of hypnotherapy for weight loss in patients with obstructive sleep apnea. Int J Obes Relat Metab Disord. 1998 Mar;22(3):278–81.

41. Cochrane G, Friesen J. Hypnotherapy in weight loss treatment. J Consult Clin Psychol. 1986;54:489–92.

42. Pawlow LA, O'Neil PM, Malcolm RJ. Night eating syndrome: effects of brief relaxation training on stress, mood, hunger, and eating patterns. J Hum Nutr Diet. 2005 Feb; 18(1):3–5.

43. Kirsch I. Hypnotic enhancement of cognitive-behavioral weight loss treatments-another meta-reanalysis. J Consult Clin Psychol. 1996 Jun;64(3):517–9.

44. Benson H, Alexander S, Feldman CL. Decreased premature ventricular contractions through use of the relaxation response in patients with stable ischaemic heart-disease. Lancet. 1975 Aug 30;2(7931):380–2.

45. Leserman J, Stuart EM, Mamish ME, Benson H. The efficacy of the relaxation response in preparing for cardiac surgery. Behav Med. 1989 Fall;15(3): 111–7.

46. van Dixhoorn J. [Favorable effects of breathing and relaxation instructions in heart rehabilitation: a randomized 5-year follow-up study.] Ned Tijdschr Geneeskd. 1997 Mar 15;141(11):530–4. [Article in Dutch.]
van Dixhoorn J. Cardiorespiratory effects of breathing and relaxation instruction in myocardial infarction patients. Biol Psychol. 1998 Sep;49(1–2):123–35.

47. van Dixhoorn J, Duivenvoorden HJ, Staal JA, Pool J, Verhage F. Cardiac events after myocardial infarction: possible effect of relaxation therapy. Eur Heart J. 1987 Nov; 8(11):1210–4.

48. Collins JA, Rice VH. Effects of relaxation intervention in phase II cardiac rehabilitation: replication and extension. Heart Lung. 1997 Jan–Feb;26(1):31–44.

49. Taggart P, Sutton P, Redfern C, Batchvarov VN, Hnatkova K, Malik M, et al. The effect of mental stress on the non-dipolar components of the T wave: modulation by hypnosis. Psychosom Med. 2005 MayJun;67(3):376–83.

50. Lang EV, Hamilton D. Anodyne imagery: an alternative to IV. sedation in interventional radiology. AJR Am J Roentgenol. 1994 May;162(5):1221–6.

51. Lang EV, Joyce JS, Spiegel D, Hamilton D, Lee KK. Self-hypnotic relaxation during interventional radiological procedures: effects on pain perception and intravenous drug use. Int J Clin Exp Hypn. 1996 Apr;44(2):106–19.

52. Ludwick-Rosenthal R, Neufeld RW. Preparation for undergoing an invasive medical procedure: interacting effects of information and coping style. J Consult Clin Psychol. 1993 Feb;61(1):156–64.

53. Wilson JF, Moore RW, Randolph S, Hanson BJ. Behavioral preparation of patients for gastrointestinal endoscopy: information, relaxation, and coping style. J Human Stress. 1982 Dec;8(4):13–23.

54. Fick LJ, Lang EV, Logan HL, Lutgendorf S, Benotsch EG. Imagery content during nonpharmacologic analgesia in the procedure suite: where your patients would rather be. Acad Radiol. 1999 Aug;6(8):457–63.

55. Friday PJ, Kubal WS. Magnetic resonance imaging: improved patient tolerance utilizing medical hypnosis. Am J Clin Hypn. 1990 Oct;33(2):80–84.

56. Zimmerman J. Hypnotic technique for sedation of patients during upper gastrointestinal endoscopy. Am J Clin Hyp. 1998;40(4):284–7.

57. Ashton Jr. C, Whitworth GC, Seldomridge JA, Shapiro PA, Weinberg AD, Michler RE, et al. Self-hypnosis reduces anxiety following coronary artery bypass surgery. A prospective, randomized trial. J Cardiovasc Surg (Torino). 1997 Feb;38(1):69–75.

58. Faymonville ME, Fissette J, Mambourg PH, Roediger L, Joris J, Lamy M. Hypnosis as adjunct therapy in conscious sedation for plastic surgery. Reg Anesth. 1995 Mar–Apr; 20(2):145–51.

59. Lang EV, Benotsch EG, Fick LJ, Lutgendorf S, Berbaum ML, Berbaum KS, et al. Adjunctive non-pharmacological analgesia for invasive medical procedures: a randomised trial. Lancet. 2000 Apr 29;355(9214):1486–90.

60. Tusek DL, Church JM, Strong SA, Grass JA, Fazio VW. Guided imagery: a significant advance in the care of patients undergoing elective colorectal surgery. Dis Colon Rectum. 1997 Feb;40(2):172–8.

61. Halpin LS, Speir AM, CapoBianco P, Barnett SD. Guided imagery in cardiac surgery. Outsomes Manag. 2002 JulSep;6(3):132–7.

62. Syrjala KL, Donaldson GW, Davis MW, Kippes ME, Carr JE. Relaxation and imagery and cognitive-behavioral training reduce pain during cancer treatment: a controlled clinical trial. Pain. 1995 Nov;673(2):189–98.

63. Disbrow EA, Bennett, HL, Owings JT. Effect of preoperative suggestion on postoperative gastrointestinal modility. West J Med. 1993 May;158(5):488–92.

64. Rapkin DA, Straubing M, Holroyd JC. Guided imagery, hypnosis and recovery from head and neck cancer surgery: an exploratory study. Int J Clin Exp Hypn. 1991 Oct; 39(4):215–26.

65. Meurisse M, Faymonville ME, Joris J, Nguyen Dang D, Defechereux T, Hamoir E. Endocrine surgery by hypnosis. From fiction to daily clinical application. Service de Chirurgie des Glandes Endocrines et Transplantation, Centre Hospitalier Universitaire de Liege, Belgique. Ann Endocrinol (Paris). 1996;57(6):494–501.

66. Enqvist B, von Konow L, Bystedt H. Pre- and perioperative suggestion in maxillofacial surgery: effects on blood loss and recovery. Int J Clin Exp Hypn. 1995 Jul; 43(3):284–94.

67. Bennet HL, Benson DR, Kuiken DA. Preoperative instructions for decreased bleeding during spine surgery. Anesthesiology, 1986;65:A245.

68. Holden-Lund C. Effects of relaxation with guided imagery on surgical stress and wound healing. Res Nurs Health. 1998 Aug;11:235–44.

69. Whitworth J, Burkhardt A, Oz M. Complementary therapy and cardiac surgery. J Cardiovasc Nurs. 1998 Jul;12(4):87–94.

70. Halpin LS, Speir AM, CapoBianco P, Barnett SD. Guided imagery in cardiac surgery. Outsomes Manag. 2002 Jul–Sep;6(3):132–7.

71. Ashton Jr. C, Whitworth GC, Seldomridge JA, Shapiro PA, Weinberg AD, Michler RE, et al. Self-hypnosis reduces anxiety following coronary artery bypass surgery. A prospective, randomized trial. J Cardiovasc Surg (Torino). 1997 Feb;38(1):69–75.

72. Appels A, Bar F, Lasker J, Flamm U, Kop W. The effect of a psychological intervention program on the risk of a new coronary event after angioplasty: a feasibility study. J Psychosom Res. 1997 Aug;43(2):209–17.

73. Schwab D. Presentation at the 2002 National Managed Health Care Congress (NMHCC). 2002. To be published. Qtd at www.healthjourneys. com/research-archives.asp. Accessed March, 2003.

74. Wolsko PM, Eisenberg DM, Davis RB, Phillips RS. Use of mind-body medical therapies. J Gen Intern Med. 2004 Jan;19(1):43–50.

75. Borkan J. Referrals for alternative therapies. J Fam Pract. 1994 Dec;39 (6):545–50.

11

THE ROLE OF STRESS AND VARIOUS MODALITIES FOR DEALING WITH STRESS AND PREVENTION

Erminia Guarneri, Christopher Suhar and
Rauni Prittinen King

THE ROLE OF STRESS

Stress defined

While stress can be classified into a nebulous of emotions not easily characterized, it has been shown to have an impact on cardiovascular disease risk factors and overall cardiac morbidity and mortality. Although as physicians it is easy to grasp the concept of acid production, blood pressure elevation, and the angiographic narrowing of a coronary artery, it is much more difficult to understand social relationships, isolation, anger, depression, and their manifestation of disease. Essays by Sterling and Eyer[1] have illustrated how the development of modern society is associated with a disruption of human relationships. These disruptions cause chronic, psychological arousal which is defined as stress. The body's physiological mechanisms are altered by chronic psychological arousal and this leads to pathology and disease.

The function of arousal is to help the individual "cope" with environmental demands. "Coping" may be defined as "contending" or "struggling." This behavior frequently requires excess physical or emotional energy to deal with a difficult situation. Studies have shown that patients entering a hospital for diagnostic tests have elevated norepinephrine, epinephrine, cortisol, and growth hormone levels.[2] Because these patients have little control over their situation, there is little effective coping behavior. Under these circumstances, in which little control over the environment is possible, the stress hormones are maximized. Likewise, students during examination periods demonstrate rises in cortisol, epinephrine, serum blood sugar, cholesterol, and blood pressure. Under exam stress, these same students exhibit a fall in white blood cells.[3] This fall in white blood cells in part explains the high rate of physical illness under stressful situations.

Tax accountants have been shown to have large increases in serum cholesterol (independent of diet) and a decrease in blood clotting time during tax season.[4] Arousal, and as a consequence stress, will be high not only among individuals with little control over life circumstances, but also among individuals with a high demand for performance. Arousal that results from lack of control will frequently manifest with anger or fear. Although high demand situations are frequently accompanied by anxiety, they may result in extreme pleasure if the coping style is successful. However, this success in the end does not mean that the metabolic costs to the body are less.

Impact of stress on cardiovascular disease risk factors

Stress has been shown to adversely affect cardiovascular risk factors such as hypertension, diabetes mellitus, and hyperlipidemia. Ongoing research is now revealing how psychoneuroimmunology is playing a large role in cardiovascular disease including acute, episodic, and chronic psychological risk factors.

In the Framingham study,[5] hypertension was involved in over 80% of all cardiovascular deaths. In addition, hypertension was at least twice as strong a predictor of death as smoking or elevated blood cholesterol. Over 50 million Americans are currently hypertensive. In about 5%, a specific pathology such as a renal artery stenosis can be identified. In the remaining 95%, the blood pressure increase is not attributed to a specific pathology. Different mechanisms may contribute to the development of hypertension. Acute arousal leads to sympathetic stimulation and an increase in cardiac output. When arousal is maintained for long periods of time, the elevation in blood pressure remains even if the inciting stimulus is removed. At this stage, the hypertension is not sustained by increased cardiac output but by increased vascular resistance.

Stress may lead to hypertension through repeated blood pressure elevations and by increasing the amount of vasoconstricting hormones. Stress factors leading to hypertension include job strain, social environment, emotional stress, race, and white coat hypertension. Overall, studies conclude that while stress does not directly cause hypertension, it can clearly effect its development. Stress leads to sympathetic nervous system activation with excessive amounts of cortisol, epinephrine, and aldosterone. The combination of increased cardiac output and vasoconstriction may raise blood pressure for 1 hour. Feelings of frustration, exhaustion, and helplessness can activate the pituitary and adrenocortical hormones. Nonpharmacological treatments to manage stress such as meditation, acupressure, biofeedback, music therapy, and pet ownership have been found to be effective in decreasing blood pressure and the development of hypertension.

Although not a substitute for pharmacological therapy, certain nondrug therapies offer support for individuals with hypertension. Steelman[6] conducted the effect of tranquil music on blood pressure and anxiety in surgery patients. The experimental group listened to music during the intraoperative period. The control group received usual care. Music appears to reduce blood pressure in the experimental group. Pender studied the effect of progressive muscle relaxation (PMR) training in hypertensive patients.[7] Those individuals who received PMR training reported less anxiety. Decreased anxiety correlated with decreased systolic blood pressure. Older African-Americans who were taught the transcendental meditation technique had a significant reduction in diastolic and systolic blood pressure.[8]

In conclusion, although there is a definite correlation between anxiety and blood pressure elevation, the repeated elevation of blood pressure which follows stress events act as a path toward hypertension. In addition, stress is frequently coupled with poor lifestyle habits such as alcohol intake, smoking, and lack of exercise, which further lead to the development of hypertension.

Diabetes, like hypertension, remains an important risk factor for the development of cardiovascular disease. Chronic arousal can contribute to diabetes in two ways. With arousal, there is an increase in catabolic hormones, most notably epinephrine, cortisol, growth hormone, and glucagon. These hormones antagonize the actions of insulin by mobilizing glucose, fatty acids, and protein breakdown. Furthermore, glucagon and norepinephrine act to suppress the secretion of insulin. The resulting hyperglycemia, hyperinsulinemia, and hyperlipidemia all accelerate pathology.

In addition to hypertension and diabetes mellitus, studies linking stress and cholesterol date back to the 1950s. One study demonstrates that when 55 men were stressed by cold water immersion, an immediate rise in their serum cholesterol occurred.[9] Many studies have demonstrated a 25% increase in cholesterol in medical students during examinations.[10] In addition, job stress with associated time pressure, repetitive assembly-line work, overwork, and increased responsibility has shown to raise serum cholesterol.[11] The stress associated with chronic depression or anxiety as well as depression caused by loss of employment can also increase cholesterol. Both cortisol and epinephrine have been linked in humans to serum cholesterol elevation. In many animal experiments, stress has accelerated atherosclerosis. Genetically identical rabbits on a high-fat diet when stressed with electrical stimulation over 10 months have an increased number of atheromas in comparison with nonstressed controls. The administration of epinephrine to cholesterol-fed rabbits further intensifies lipid infiltration of the aortic intima. As mentioned previously, accountants show continuous monthly rises in cholesterol, despite maintaining a constant diet, which peaks at the end of the fiscal year.[4]

Research in the area of psychoneuroimmunology is beginning to shed some light on the relationship between psychological risk factors and future coronary syndromes. Enormous literature addresses the role of psychological factors in the progression of coronary artery disease (CAD) and its clinical sequelae. Chronic psychological risk factors may promote the initial stages of CAD by activating the sympathetic nervous system (e.g., catechol-induced hypercoagulopathy, lipid deposition, and inflammation). In addition, patients under chronic psychological stress may exhibit other CAD risk factors such as hypercholesterolemia, tobacco use, and hypertension. Acute psychological risk factors may trigger malignant arrhythmias or ischemia. The psychological risk factors for coronary syndromes may be broken down into these broad categories: (1) chronic psychological risk factors involved in the gradual progression of CAD such as the hostile personality type, (2) episodic psychological risk factors that last from months to years such as depression, and (3) acute psychological risk factors that precipitate coronary events within hours such as outbursts of anger and mental stress. It is now accepted that the duration of psychological distress can influence the immune system. Certain immunologic mediators may now serve to help us understand the pathophysiological mechanisms.

Acute psychological risk factors

A review of epidemiological studies suggests that natural disasters (i.e., Northridge, CA, earthquake) and outbursts of anger can provoke acute coronary syndromes including myocardial infarction (MI).[12] Sudden, severe emotional stress, such as the loss of a loved one or public speaking, has been shown to cause a "stress cardiomyopathy" leading to severe left ventricular dysfunction.[13] Studies have demonstrated that emotions and mental activities are strong triggers of life-threatening arrhythmias and myocardial ischemia.[14] About 30–60% of patients with stable CAD develop ischemia in such settings as anger recall, mental arithmetic, and public speaking.[15]

   Ambulatory ischemia is triggered by both physical and mental activities. Acute mental stimulation shifts toward increased sympathetic and decreased parasympathetic activity. This shift is associated with increased circulating catecholamines which increase blood pressure, heart rate, and myocardial contractility. Markers of decreased coronary supply in response to mental challenges include impaired vasodilatation, decreased plasma volume, and increased platelet activity.[16] The increased demand and decreased coronary blood supply may lead to ischemia. Mental arousal may lead to cardiac arrhythmia as a result of direct influences on the central nervous system, mainly through vagal withdrawal. The hemodynamic responses of acute stress may lead to increased platelet aggregation, plaque rupture, and acute coronary thrombus. Acute mental arousal has important effects on the immune system. Most studies show increases in B-cells and CD8+ T-cells, and decreases in CD4+ T-cells.[17] Cytokines (interleukin [IL]-1 and IL-2) are reported to increase, as do acute phase proteins (CRP and fibrinogen) and adhesion molecules.[18] These immune system changes may be relevant with respect to triggering acute coronary syndromes, in part because enhanced immune activity may lead to plaque rupture. Immune activators promote intimal cell growth and play a role in plaque disruption and thrombus formation. Indirectly, immune activators may enhance myocardial ischemia by affecting endothelial function leading to vasoconstriction.

Chronic psychological risk factors

Personality traits such as hostility and the Type A behavior pattern have extensively been studied in relationship to cardiovascular disease. In 1959, Friedman and Roseman found that individuals who exhibit Type A behavior had a higher risk for MI.[4] Later studies suggested that hostility is actually the risk factor associated with increased cardiovascular risk. Most studies demonstrate an association between hostility/Type A personality and the severity of CAD, as well as first MI.[19] In one large study by Mittleman et al., episodes of anger were shown to be the triggering event for an acute MI. In that study, the risk for MI was increased by greater than twofold in patients, who experienced episodes of anger.[20] When treating patients with ischemic heart disease, high daily levels of stress have been shown to diminish the anti-ischemic pharmacological treatment effects of beta-blockers and calcium channel blockers.[21]

The main pathophysiological mechanism for progression of CAD in individuals with chronic psychological risk appears to be elevated sympathetic nervous system activity and increased vasoreactivity. The direct effect of elevated sympathetic tone includes arterial lipid deposition and increased arterial pressure. In addition to sympathetic hyperreactivity, chronic psychological risk factors further enhance CAD progression as a result of maladaptive behaviors such as lack of exercise and poor nutrition. Increased catechol reactivity to stress in hostile individuals may affect acute physiological responses which lead to vasoconstriction, increased cardiac demand, and hypercoagulability. These individuals, when faced with acute challenges, are at an increased risk for ischemia and arrhythmia.

Very little is known about the association between psychological personality type and immune function in relation to CAD. It is known that in the early stages of plaque development, lipids and macrophages interact. Some evidence exists which demonstrate an association between hostility and increased levels of oxidized lipids. It may be that hostility promotes early CAD progression by increasing the level of oxidized lipids and by affecting macrophage function.

Episodic psychological risk

Episodic psychological risk factors are recurring in nature and limited to 2 years in duration. Depression may be considered to be the major episodic risk factor in cardiovascular disease. Multiple studies have indicated depression as predictive of sudden death, as well as a first and recurrent MI.[22] A large body of literature has addressed the neuroendocrine correlates of depression. Melancholy, for example, is associated with increased corticotropin-releasing hormone and as a result, elevated plasma cortisol.

Depression is associated with several immune markers including increased neutrophils and myocytes, decreased lymphocytes, and elevated cytokines. In addition, depression is associated with lower natural killer cell activity and increased antibody levels of certain viruses such as CMV. Some of the correlates of depression, most notably increased leukocytes and antibody levels, may be associated with an increased risk for acute coronary syndrome. The proinflammatory state in depression may actually promote CAD by enhancing lipid deposition and macrophage activity. Low-grade inflammation may alter plaque stability, particularly of advanced lesions leading to rupture and acute coronary syndromes. The association of depression and heart disease is well observed and at best it is not certain whether the neuroendocrine pathway, adverse health behaviors (smoking, high-lipid diet, etc.), or both are involved in inflammation.

In conclusion, the field of psychoneuroimmunology helps us understand how the immunologic and physiological correlates of psychological risk are involved in the development and progression of CAD. Chronic psychological risk factors lead to the progression of CAD by two pathways: (1) increased adverse behavior (tobacco use, high-fat diet, lack of exercise, etc.), and (2) an exaggerated response to an acute challenge resulting from high sympathetic tone. Hyperactivity is a primary trigger for acute coronary syndromes. Chronic psychological factors are also indirectly related to coronary disease by decreased phagocytosis of macrophages. Macrophages are involved in lipid deposition and the onset of early atherosclerotic lesions.

Depression and the development of cardiovascular disease

A growing body of evidence suggests that depression may predispose to cardio-vascular events.[23] Individuals with mental stress during daily life have twice the risk of myocardial ischemia. In addition, those patients with post-MI depression have higher mortality rates than nondepressed controls. Depression is common after an acute MI and is associated with an increased risk of mortality for at least 18 months. One reason for this higher morbidity and mortality within the first few months following an MI is that depressed patients are less likely to follow recommendations to reduce further cardiac events. These data suggest a psychophysiological mechanism for the susceptibility of depressed individuals to ischemic heart disease. The higher morbidity and mortality in depressed patients may be caused by platelet activation.

Ziegelstein and colleagues[24] found that patients who were identified with at least mild to moderate depression or major depression reported lower adherence to a low-fat diet, regular exercise, and stress management. Individuals with major depression and/or dysrhythmia reported taking their medication less often than prescribed. Those findings, in part, explain why depression in the hospital is related to long-term prognosis in patients recovering from an MI.

In addition, acute MI patients with unstable angina, who were identified as depressed in the hospital were more likely to experience cardiac death or nonfatal MI than other patients.[21] The impact of depression on 430 patients with unstable angina (41.4% depressed) remained after controlling for other prognostic factors such as left ventricular ejection fraction (LVEF) and number of diseased vessels.[25]

In addition to depression, other research suggests that social support may influence prognosis following an acute MI. In a study of 887 post-MI patients, Frasure-Smith and colleagues[26] found that 32% had mild to moderate depression. After 1-year, follow-up interviews were conducted and demonstrated that elevated Beck depression scores were related to cardiac mortality. The relationship between depression and cardiac morality decreased with increasing support. Furthermore, of those 1-year survivors who were depressed at baseline, higher baseline social support was related to greater than expected improvement in depression symptoms.

In conclusion, although post-MI depression is a predictor of 1-year cardiac mortality, high levels of social support appear to decrease the magnitude of depression. High levels of social support also predict improvement in depression over the first post-MI year in those individuals with baseline depression and may protect patients from the negative prognostic consequences of depression.[26]

DEALING WITH STRESS AND PREVENTION

In a recent survey of primary care physicians and cardiologists, discussing and affecting lifestyle including exercise, diet, and stress continues to be poorly addressed.[27] Fortunately, there are various modalities for dealing with and preventing stress. Multiple studies have demonstrated the effectiveness of various nonpharmacological modalities for stress reduction. The different modalities can be implemented in both the inpatient and outpatient care settings. Many stress management techniques can be taught to patients and self-administered.

Everyone reacts to stress differently and therefore treatment should be tailored to the individual. Centers across the country are now offering multiple therapies for stress reduction and prevention, which include both structured, institutional programs and patient-implemented home therapies. These therapies can be as simple as addressing diet and exercise coupled with pet ownership and/or support groups to a multidisciplinary lifestyle change program utilizing multiple modalities such as group support, music therapy, specialized meditation, guided imagery, and/or healing touch. Some patients suffering from psychological stress will undoubtedly benefit from psychological counseling.

Evidence-based stress management therapies

PET OWNERSHIP

Pet ownership will not only provide medical benefits associated with stress reduction, but also can convey a sense of companionship and purpose. Social science research studies via surveys have shown a self-reported benefit of both physical and psychological health[28,29] leading to fewer doctor visits. In an effort to have a more direct medical correlation, studies were performed linking pet ownership to lower blood pressure ultimately resulting in lower cardiovascular risk.[30] Also, while reduced heart rate variability (HRV) has been associated with increased cardiac disease and mortality, pet ownership was shown to be associated with increased HRV in patients with cardiovascular disease.[31]

Mindfulness-based stress reduction

Mindfulness-based stress reduction (MBSR) is a structured group program that is a moment-to-moment awareness that is designed to help guide a person toward mobilizing their inner resources of mind and body. While this may sound esoteric, it employs the techniques of mindfulness meditation, gentle yoga, and coordinated deep breathing to decrease pain and anxiety. MBSR has not only been used for stress reduction, but can be used for other conditions such as: CAD, chronic pain, hypertension, anxiety, cancer, sleep disturbance, job and family stress, AIDS, Type A behavior, fatigue, or skin disorders. Most programs are nonreligious and nonesoteric and are based upon a systematic procedure.

In a meta-analysis looking at MBSR used for a wide spectrum of clinical populations, it was shown that MBSR may help individuals alleviate stress and suffering associated with these various conditions.[32] Numerous studies have shown perceived improvement in quality of life, mood, symptoms of stress, and quality of sleep.[33,34,35] There was also a trend toward a decrease in stress hormones such as cortisol.[33,35]

Guided imagery

Guided imagery uses the power of thought to influence psychological and physiological states. Guided imagery is a therapeutic technique that allows a person to use his or her own imagination to connect their body and mind to achieve desirable outcomes such as decreased pain perception and reduced anxiety.

Guided imagery has been studied for patients with both pre- and postsurgical intervention. A recent study of cardiothoracic surgery patients demonstrated that both pain and anxiety decreased significantly with guided imagery.[36] By augmenting pain treatment, guided imagery decreased the length of hospitalization by 2 days. Interim data from an ongoing trial at Scripps Clinic utilizing guided imagery and healing touch pre- and postcardiothoracic surgery has demonstrated a 50% reduction in pain and anxiety in the treatment group.

Transcendental meditation

Transcendental meditation (TM) offers a unique technique for meditation and relaxation. It is one of the most-studied CAM therapies with research dating back to the 1970s. TM is practiced for 20 minutes twice daily. Multiple studies have demonstrated improvement in hypertension and cardiovascular morbidity and mortality in patients taught TM. More recently, TM has been shown to not only improve blood pressure, but also the insulin resistance components of the metabolic syndrome as well as cardiac autonomic nervous system tone.[37,38] This form of meditation can be quickly learned and performed in almost all clinical situations.

Biofeedback

Biofeedback is a technique to train people to change habitual reactions to stress. It measures physiological markers such as blood pressure, heart rate, skin temperature, and muscle tension to convey visual or auditory feedback to raise a patient's awareness and conscience control of related physiological activities. Lehrer et al.[39] demonstrated that training subjects to maximize peak heart rate differences via biofeedback can increase homeostatic reflexes, lower blood pressure, and improve lung function.

In cardiovascular patients, biofeedback has been used for stress reduction, blood pressure control, and increase in HRV. Biofeedback has been studied in patients with essential hypertension and shown to effectively lower both systolic and diastolic blood pressure.[40,41] Where low HRV is an independent risk factor for sudden cardiac death, all-cause death, and cardiac event recurrence, studies support the use of biofeedback and breathing retraining as a treatment to reverse the decrease in HRV that occurs with heart disease.[42,43] Guarneri et al.[44] examined the use of biofeedback in patients with CAD and found that this technique increases HRV in this patient population supporting biofeedback as an integral tool for improving cardiac morbidity and mortality rates.

REFERENCES

1. Sterling P, Eyer J. Biological basis of stress-related mortality. Soc Sci Med [E]. 1981 Feb;15(1):3–42.
2. Mason JW. A review of psychoendocrine research on the sympathetic-adrenal medullary system. Psychosom Med. 1968;30:631; Mason JW. A review of psychoendocrine research on the pituitary-adrenal cortical system. Psychosom Med. 1968;30:576; Greene WA, Conron G, Schalch DS, Schreiner BF. Psycologic correlates of growth hormone and adrenal secretory responses in patients undergoing cardiac catheterization. Psychosom Med. 1970;32: 599; Brown GM, Reichlin S. Psycologic and neural regulation of growth hormone secretion. Psychosom Med. 1972;34:45.
3. Mason JW, *op cit*; Mason JW, *op cit*; Brown GM, et al, *op cit*; Westlake PT, Wilcox AA, Haley MI, Peterson JE. Relationship of mental and emotional stress to serum cholesterol levels. Proc Sci Exp Biol Med. 1958;97:163; Thomas CB, Murphy EA. Further studies on cholesterol levels in the Johns Hopkins medical students: the effects of stress at examination. J Chron Dis. 1958;8:661; Grundy SM, Griffin AC. Relationship of periodic mental stress to serum cholesterol levels. Circulation. 1959;19:496; Grundy SM, Griffin AC. Relationship of periodic mental stress to serum lipoprotein and cholesterol levels. JAMA. 1959;171:1794.
4. Friedman M, Rosenman, R.
5. Kannel WB, Dawber TR, Kagan A, Revotskie J. Factors of risk in the development of coronary heart disease—six-year follow-up experience. The Framingham Study. Ann Intern Med. 1961;55:33–50.
6. Steelman VM. Intraoperative music therapy: effects on anxiety, blood pressure. AORN J. 1990 Nov;52(5):1026–34.
7. Pender NJ. Effects of progressive muscle relaxation training on anxiety and health locus of control among hypertensive adults. Res Nurs Health. 1895 Mar;8(1):67–72.
8. Zamarra JW, Schneider RH, Besseghini I, Robinson DK, Salerno JW. Usefulness of the transcendental mediotation program in the treatment of patients with coronary artery disease. Am J Cardiol. 1996 Apr 15;77(10):867–70.
9. van Doornen LJ, Orlebeke KF. Stress, personality and serum-cholesterol level. J Human Stress. 1982 Dec;8(4):24–9.
10. Dreyfuss F, et al. Blood cholesterol and. uric acid of healthy medical students under stress of examination. Arch Int Med. 1959;103:708.
11. Theorell T, Floderus-Myrhed B. "Workload" and risk of myocardial infarction—a prospective psychosocial analysis. Int J Epidemiol. 1977 Mar;6(1):17–21.

12. Mittleman MA, Maclure M, Sherwood JB, Mulry RP, Tofler GH, Jacobs SC, et al. Triggering of acute myocardial infarction onset by episodes of anger. Determinants of myocardial infarction onset study investigators. Circulation. 1995 Oct 1;92(7):1720–5.

13. Wittstein IS, Thiemann DR, Lima JAC, Baughma KL, Schulman SP, Gerstenblith G, et al. Neurohumoral features of myocardial stunning due to sudden emotional stress. NEJM. 2005;352(6):540–8.

14. Verrier RL. Mechanisms of behaviorally induced arrhythmias. Circulation. 1987 Jul; 76(1 Pt 2):148–56.

15. Krantz DS, Kop WJ, Santiago HT, Gottdiener JS. Mental stress as a trigger of myocardial ischemia and infarction. Cardiol Clin. 1996 May;14(2):271–87.

16. Patterson SM, Krantz DS, Gottdiener JS, Hecht G, Vargot S, Goldstein DS. Prothrombotic effects of environmental stress: changes in platelet function, hematocrit, and total plasma protein. Psychosom Med. 1995 Nov-Dec;57(6):592–9.

17. Ader R, Cohen N, Felten D. Psychoneuroimmunology: interactions between the nervous system and the immune system. Lancet. 1995 Jan 14;345(8942):99–103.

18. Dugue B, Leppanen EA, Teppo AM, Fyhrquist F, Grasbeck, R. Effects of psychological stress on plasma interleukins-1 beta and 6, c-reative protein, tumor necrosis factor alpha, anti-diuretic hormone and serum cortisol. Scand J Clin Lab Invest. 1993 Oct;53(6):555–61.

19. Miller TQ, Smith TW, Turner CW, Guijarro ML, Hallet AJ. A meta-analytic review of research on hostility and physical health. Psychol Bull. 1996 Mar;119(2):322–48.

20. Mittleman MA, Maclure M, Sherwood JB, Mulry RP, Tofler GH, Jacobs SC, et al. Triggering of acute myocardial infarction onset by episodes of anger. Circulation. 1995;92:1720–5.

21. Rutledge T, Linden W, Davies RF. Psychological risk factors may moderate pharmacological treatment effects among ischemic heart disease patients. Psychosomatic Med. 1999;61:834–41.

22. Appels, A. Depression and coronary heart disease: observations and questions. J Psychosom Res. 1997 Nov; 43(5):443–52. Review.

23. Frasure-Smith N, Lesperance F, Talajic M. Depression and 18-month prognosis after myocardial infarction. Circulation. 1995 Apr;91:999–1005.

24. Ziegelstein RC, Fauerbach JA, Stevens SS, Romanelli J, Richter DP, Bush DE. Patients with depression are less likely to follow recommendations to reduce cardiac risk during recovery from a myocardial infarction. Arch Intern Med. 2000 Jun 26; 160(12):818–23.

25. Lesperance F, Frasure-Smith N, Juneau M, Theroux P. Depression and 1-year prognosis in unstable angina. Arch Intern Med. 2000 May 8;160(9):1354–60.

26. Frasure-Smith N, Lesperance F, Talajic M. Depression and 18-month prognosis after myocardial infarction. Circulation. 1995 Feb 15;91(4):999–1005.

27. Mosca L, Linfante AH, Benjamin EJ, Berra K, Hayes SN, Walsh BW, et al. National study of physician awareness and adherence to cardiovascular disease prevention guidelines, Circ. 2005:111:499–510.

28. Siegel JM. Stressful life events and use of physician services among the elderly: the moderating effects of pet ownership. J Pers Soc Psychol. 1990;58:1081–6.

29. Headey B. Health benefits and health cost savings due to pets: preliminary results from an Australian national survey. Soc Indicators Res. 1999;47:233–43.

30. Anderson WP, Reid CM, Jennings GL. Pet ownership and risk factors for cardiovascular disease. Med J Aust. 1992;157:298–301.

31. Friedman E, Thomas SA, Stein P, Kleiger R. Relation between pet ownership and heart rate variability in patients with healed myocardial infarcts. JACC. 2003;91:718–21.

32. Grossman P, Niemann L, Schmidt S, Walach H. Mindfulness-based stress reduction and health benefits. A meta-analysis. J Psychosom Res. 2004;57(1):35–43.

33. Carlson LE, Speca M, Patel KD, Goodey E. Mindfulness-based stress reduction in relation to quality of life, mood, symptoms of stress and levels of cortisol, dehydroepiandrosterone sulfate (DHEAS) and melatonin in breast and prostate cancer outpatients. Psychoneruoendocrinology. 2004;29(4):448–74.

34. Tacon AM, McComb J, Caldera Y, Randolph P. Mindfulness meditation, anxiety reduction, and heart disease: a pilot study. Fam Community Health. 2003;26(1):25–33.

35. Robert McComb JJ, Tacon A, Randolph P, Caldera Y. A pilot study to examine the effects of a mindfulness-based stress-reduction and relaxation program on levels of stress hormones, physical functioning, and submaximal exercise responses. J Altern Complement Med. 2004;10(5):819–27.

36. Kshettry VR, Carole LF, Henly SJ, Sendelbach S, Kummer B. Complementary alternative medical therapies for heart surgery patients: feasibility, safety, and impact. Ann Thorac Surg. 2006;81(1):201–5.

37. Schneider RH, Alexander CN, Staggers F, Rainforth M, Salerno J, Hartz A, et al. Long-term effects of stress reduction on mortality in persons >55 years of age with systemic hypertension. Am J Cardiol. 2005;95:1060–4.

38. Paul-Labrador M, Polk D, Dwyer JH, Velasquez I, Nidich S, Rainforth M, et al. Effects of a randomized controlled trial of transcendental meditation on components of the metabolic syndrome in subjects with coronary heart disease. Arch Intern Med. 2006;166:1218–24.

39. Lehrer PM, Vaschillo E, Vaschillo B. Resonant frequency biofeedback training to increase cardiac variability: rationale and manual for training. Appl Psychophysiol Biofeedback. 2000;25:177–91.

40. Nakao M, Nomura S, Shimosawa T, Fujita T, Kuboki T. Blood pressure biofeedback treatment of white-coat hypertension. J Psychosom Res. 2000;48(2):161–9.

41. Nakao M, Nomura S, Shimosawa T, Yoshiuchi K, Kumano H, Kuboki T, et al. Clinical effects of blood pressure biofeedback treatment on hypertension by autoshaping. Psychosom Med. 1997;59(3)331–8.

42. Bigger JT, Fleiss JL, Rolnitzky LM, et al. The ability of several short-term measures of RR variability to predict mortality after myocardial infarction. Circulation. 1993;88:927–34.

43. Kleiger RE, Miller JP, Bigger JT, et al. and the Multicenter Post-Infarction Research Group. Decreased heart rate variability and its association with increased mortality after acute myocardial infarction. Am J Cardiol. 1987;59:256–62.

44. Del Pozo JM, Gevirtz RN, Scher B, Guarneri E. Biofeedback treatment increases heart rate variability in patients with known coronary artery disease. Am Heart J. 2004;147:e11.

12

NOETIC THERAPY, SPIRITUALITY, AND PRAYER

Mitchell W. Krucoff, Suzanne W. Crater and Michael Cuffe

Historically one is inclined to look upon science and religion as irreconcilable antagonists.... I maintain that cosmic religious feeling is the strongest and noblest incitement to scientific research...The fairest thing we can experience is the mysterious. It is the fundamental emotion which stands at the cradle of true art and true science.... In my view, it is the most important function of art and science to awaken this feeling and keep it alive.

Einstein, A. *The World As I See It*

INTRODUCTION: MODERN CARDIOLOGY AND THE HUMAN SPIRIT

Across the spectrum of care, patients with heart disorders are faced with the very proximate and personal reality of their mortality, as both the disease state and complications from the procedures and therapies used to treat it may be associated with hospitalization, severe debility, and death. In addition to concerns about palliation of the organic disorder, emotional states and concerns related to death and dying constitute a range of mind-body-spirit issues central to the patient and family's experience of cardiovascular care. It is less clear, however, how central such concerns are to modern Western "high tech" care strategies or cardiovascular health-care training.

Anecdotally every practitioner in cardiology has cared for a patient admitted to hospital in such advanced multisystem failure that it seems inevitable that they are going to die, but they don't. In that setting it is frequently the case that the health caretaker is left with the impression that in this individual patient there was some other force at work—some kind of vital link, to life, to family, to God, or to some other source—that supported survival when medical therapies otherwise appeared inadequate. While more somatic mechanistic explanations can always be forwarded, this shared experience among practitioners reminds our professional community that in heart disease intangible elements and human capacities may be at work that, if better understood, could promote better outcomes, and offer opportunities to advance new paradigms for modern health care.

Heart disease is the most epidemic source of morbidity and mortality in the Western world, and with epidemic advance in the East as well, development of new cardiovascular therapeutics is one of the largest, most active arenas of human clinical research and new technology application. From a historical infatuation with technology and an allopathic conviction that mechanistic science could provide a complete armamentarium of prevention and cures, more recent, more enlightened views of the real advance of clinical science and medical care recognize the importance of seeking more systematic understanding of the roles of intangible human capacities such as the mind-body connections and the human spirit in the context of high-tech cardiovascular care.[1,2] In fact, with indigenous healers around the world suggesting that tangible medical interventions targeting the body effect only about 20% of the overall healing process,[3] open-minded professionals may contend that the most important new paradigm of medicine may be to understand high-tech cardiovascular care in the context of the human spirit, rather than vice versa.[4]

CULTURAL VERSUS HEALTH CARE SCIENCE PRACTICES

To approach a health care paradigm involving the human spirit requires careful separation between issues of a philosophical or theological nature that are part of the fabric of cultural practices, from scientific issues more relevant to systematic health care (Table 12-1). Cultural practices with healing intention are promulgated through community beliefs and symbolic metaphor, including prayers for the sick that use specific words, capture a "subtle" or magical energy or power, or pray to a specific deity. In their cultural context, such practices and their results may be considered "self evident" without need for proof, may be supported by testimonials or anecdotes, and may be perceived as intrinsically good and free of toxicity for all healing applications.

Conversely, in a progressively data-driven health care environment, "noetic" or intangible therapeutics such as spiritual interventions require a different kind and weight of evidence than is required for cultural practices. Methodologic definition of any noetic intervention must be sufficient to: (1) support interpretations and comparisons of clinical trial results defining safety and effectiveness in defined populations and conditions of use, (2) define reproducible methods and skill sets

TABLE 12-1

ELEMENTS CHARACTERIZING CULTURAL VERSUS MEDICAL HEALING PRACTICES

Condition	Cultural Practice	Medical Practice
Basis of activity	Community tradition	Evidence-based practice
Currency of evidence	Cultural literature Testimonials Personal experience Faith	Clinical data and clinical experience
Methodological definition	Liturgical and philosophical teachings Symbolic metaphor	Defined methodologies with reproducible safety/effectiveness in specific patient cohorts
Tools of integration	Cultural education Family/community participation	Clinical research Curriculum development Practitioner accreditation Practice guidelines
Other interests	Inclusion of others	Health-care role definition Mechanistic research

sufficiently to incorporate them into core curricula or training programs for medical professionals, and (3) to understand and optimize roles for medical staff and resource allocations to address intangible human capacities.

Both methodologic definition and robust safety and effectiveness data are required to support professional society recognition and recommendations for practice standards and guidelines. Mechanistic insight into how intangible therapeutics actually exert their effects could facilitate many aspects of acceptance or use, but is not necessary a priori. Lack of mechanistic knowledge must be accommodated in rigorous clinical trial designs, examples of which have been advanced in the study of depression and noetic intervention.[5,6] A corollary is the challenge to researchers to design studies that can produce informative data without being so intrinsically reductionist that the holistic nature of the therapy itself is lost.

While spiritual healing practices are well ingrained into cultural practices, current scientific knowledge and data in this area are still quite limited, and do not support any specific treatment guidelines at this time.[1] Spiritual interventions such as prayer and other noetic therapies are among the most ancient and most widely applied of healing practices, yet reliable scientific literature on these techniques is notably juvenile. In this chapter, we will first present an overview of published randomized studies of spiritual intervention and prayer, and then examine some of the conceptual frameworks and assumptions involved in the clinical and research approaches to spirituality in cardiovascular care as a means of highlighting opportunities for future work.

PROSPECTIVE RANDOMIZED CLINICAL TRIALS

In an overview of the clinical literature on use of "supraphysical energy," "spiritual healing," and "distant healing" Astin et al[7] reviewed 23 studies with mean methodologic Jadad scores of 3.6.[8] Nomenclature, prayer methodologies, patient populations, and study designs were so heterogeneous, the authors reported, that a classical meta-analysis was not feasible. A Cohen's d effect weighted for sample size was calculated for the primary endpoint from each study.[9] With 57% of studies showing treatment benefit, they concurred with a previous review of the Cochrane Database[10] that "the evidence thus far warrants further study...additional studies of distant healing that address the methodologic issues outlined...are now called for... to shed further light on the potential efficacy of these approaches."[7] In a follow-up to this review, however, Ernst less systematically supplemented these studies with an additional, more recent eight nonrandomized and nine randomized studies of distant healing, concluding that "they shift the weight of evidence against the notion that distant healing is more than a placebo."[11]

The literature specific to cardiovascular patients treated in randomized studies of prayer and otherwise intangible interventions is equally heterogeneous, varying in populations studied, outcomes endpoints measured, and prayer methods used. In addition, certain key descriptors, such as religious proclivities of patients, expectations and beliefs in the setting of double blind therapy (i.e., placebo effects), and the incidence of prayer use off protocol are variously reported, if at all.

From 1988 to 2006, six prospective, randomised trials have been published in patients with heart disease, studying the healing effects of off-site intercessory prayer, in a total of 4905 patients. In three studies, a total of 2205 cardiac care unit (CCU) patients have been reported, each with different primary endpoints. Byrd randomized 393 CCU patients to off-site prayer or not at San Francisco General Hospital, rating hospital course as "good, intermediate, or bad," ultimately reporting a 36% reduction in "bad" ratings ($p < 0.01$).[12] Harris et al randomized 1013 CCU patients at the Mid-America Heart Institute (MAHI), reporting an 11% reduction in a unique MAHI CCU course index ($p = 0.04$) but showing no difference in hospital course when he applied the Byrd outcome score.[13] In both of these studies, the use of independent indices of severity of hospital course as the primary endpoint made the clinical relevance of the treatment effects uninterpretable.

At the Mayo Clinic, Aviles et al studied 799 CCU survivors, who were randomized to double blind distant prayer at the time of discharge from hospital.[14] This study followed a primary composite endpoint of more classical clinical outcomes, including death, cardiac arrest, coronary revascularization, rehospitalization for cardiovascular disease, or an emergency department visit for cardiac disease at 26 weeks. Patients were stratified according to risk of disease progression. Odds ratios for the primary endpoint in the group overall, the "high risk of progression," and the "low risk of progression" strata were 0.83 ($p = 0.25$), 0.90 ($p = 0.90$), and 0.65 ($p = 0.12$), respectively. While some possible trends were documented, the study was interpreted as negative for demonstration of treatment benefit.

In two studies coordinated through Duke University's Clinical Research Institute, the Monitoring & Actualization of Noetic TRAinings (MANTRA) pilot study and the follow-up MANTRA II study, Krucoff et al examined both distant double-blinded and bedside open label intangible or "noetic" therapies, prospectively randomizing cohorts of patients undergoing percutaneous coronary intervention (PCI).[2,15] In the MANTRA pilot study performed at the Durham VA Medical Center, 150 patients with acute coronary syndromes were randomized to one of five treatment arms: double-blinded off-site prayer or standard care, or open label bedside healing touch, imagery, or stress relaxation. Standard clinical endpoints were used, including index hospitalization combined major adverse cardiovascular events (MACE, defined as in-hospital death, new heart failure, myocardial (re-)infarction, or urgent revascularization) and/or continuous ECG monitoring ischemia read by blinded core laboratory. Odds ratio for the 30 patients given standard care versus the 30 patients treated with prayer was 0.48 ($p = 0.32$). In MANTRA II, the first published multicenter study of prayer and of noetic therapies, 748 patients undergoing elective PCI were randomized in a 2×2 factorial design that assigned patients to double blind off-site prayer or not, and also to open label bedside music-imagery-touch (MIT) or not, with the primary endpoint of 6-month death, all cause rehospitalization or index hospitalization MACE (defined as death, new heart failure, myocardial infarction, or urgent revascularization). For the primary composite outcome in patients treated with distant prayer versus not, hazard ratio was 0.97 (0.77–1.24), $p =$ NS. The primary composite endpoint was also negative for MIT versus no MIT, and for combined MIT and off-site prayer versus standard care. Use of the open label, bedside MIT was associated with a reduction of preidentified secondary endpoint 6-month mortality, with a hazard ratio of 0.35 (0.15–0.82) $p = 0.0156$.

In the multicenter Study of Therapeutic Effects of Intercessory Prayer (STEP) study coordinated at Harvard, Benson and colleagues randomized 1,802 patients undergoing elective coronary artery bypass surgery (CABG) to three treatment arms: double-blinded off-site prayer (uncertain, with prayer), double-blinded placebo (uncertain, no prayer), and unblinded off-site prayer (certain, with prayer).[16] Using a primary outcome endpoint of 30-day complication rates based on Society of Thoracic Surgery (STS) criteria for post-CABG adverse events and a prespecified definition of "major complications" over the same time period, comparisons were made between the groups with prayer, blinded versus standard care, blinded, and between the groups with prayer, blinded versus with prayer, unblinded (Fig. 12-1).

Overall complication rates in patients who were blinded were no different between patients treated with standard care versus with off-site prayer, with relative

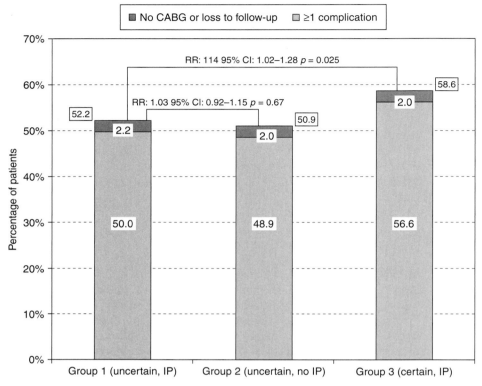

Legend: IP = intercessory prayer, CABG = coronary artery bypass graft surgery, ITT = intent to treat, RR = relative risk, CI = confidence interval

FIGURE 12-1   *All 30-day complications post-CABG. From Benson et al. Study of the therapeutic effects of intercessory prayer (STEP) in cardiac bypass patients—a multicenter randomized trial of uncertainty and certainty of receiving intercessory prayer. Am Heart J. 2006 April;151(4):943–42. (Mosby, Inc. Reprinted with permission from Elsevier.)*

risk 1.02, 95% confidence interval (CI) 0.92–1.15, p = NS. Major events, however, were more frequent in patients receiving off-site prayer in the comparison of blinded groups, with a relative risk of 1.18, 95% CI 1.03–1.35, p = 0.027.

In the comparison of the two groups receiving off-site prayer who were blinded and unblinded, also seen in Figure 12-1, patients who received off-site prayer and were certain of it fared worse over the 30 days following CABG, with the primary endpoint relative risk 1.14, 95% CI 1.02–1.28, p = 0.025. Major event rates in this comparison were no different. The authors did not plan or perform a comparison between the standard care group and the unblinded group receiving prayer; however, it is notable that the absolute rates of all adverse events and of major adverse events were higher in the group receiving protocol prayer. While the STEP authors considered all comparisons to be the play of chance or otherwise uninterpretable, an accompanying editorial high-lighted the importance of recognizing potential safety issues based on these data.[17]

Across all six of these studies, there is noteworthy variation in the prayer methods used, including what religions were included, what prayers were said, how many persons prayed, how long prayers were said for study patients, and what information the prayer groups received about the patients. Comparisons of study results are thus further limited by concerns regarding the "dose" of prayer studied. As in all six studies, off-protocol prayer was not prohibited, and in all but two studies off-protocol prayer was not accounted for, the impact of varia-tions in "dose" also vary depending on whether the treatment effect in each study was more "incremental" versus more "absolute."

Byrd, Harris, Aviles used 3–7 individuals praying, while Benson used 3 prayer groups, all within a range of exclusively Christian traditions.[12,13,16] The MANTRA studies used multiple denominations of Christian groups as well as Buddhist, Muslim, and Jewish groups.[2,15] In the MANTRA pilot study, 10 con-gregations were involved with hundreds of individuals praying. In the MANTRA II study, 12 prayer groups were used through the first two-thirds of the study, and in the final year of enrolment, another 12 groups were engaged as a second "tier" that prayed for the prayers of the first 12 groups.

Duration of prayer across these six studies ranged from enrolment to hos-pital discharge,[12] from enrolment for 14 days[14] from enrolment to 30 days after discharge,[2,13,16] and from discharge for 26 weeks[2,15] with varying frequencies. In four published studies, the content of prayer was left to the practice of the indi-vidual or congregational practice. In the Harris study, those who prayed were instructed to pray for "a speedy recovery with no complications" and "anything else that seemed appropriate to them."[13] In the STEP study, the prayer groups were required to add the phrase "for a successful surgery with a quick, healthy recovery and no complications" to their "usual" prayers.[16]

All published distant prayer studies provided specific patient information to the off-site intercessors, including information such as name or initials, age, and diagnosis. In the MANTRA II study,[15] an additional prayer methods fea-ture was added in the final study year of enrolment, as had been reported by Cha et al.[18] In this "second tier" of prayer groups, the name of the patient was not specified. These groups were asked to pray for the prayers of the congre-gations praying for the individual patients, as a less deterministic "amplifier"[18] of those prayers. Interestingly, in the MANTRA II study as shown in Fig. 12-2 (prayer vs. not, two tiered prayer vs. not for 6 month death and rehospitalization), while there was no difference in any prespecified endpoint for the prayed for group overall, there was a 32% relative reduction in 6-month death and rehos-pitalization in the subgroup receiving two-tiered prayer compared to standard care patients.[15]

As is evident from the above, published studies in cardiology to date help more to clarify questions for future research than to provide guidelines for cur-rent patient care. In the remainder of this chapter, we will explore some of the issues tied to these questions.

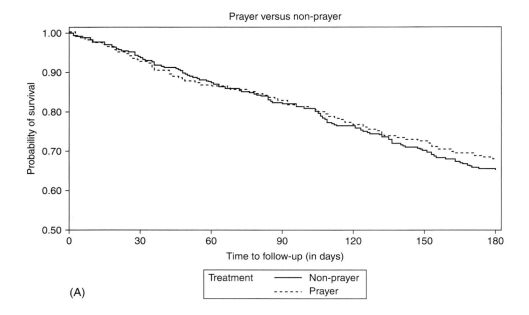

(A)

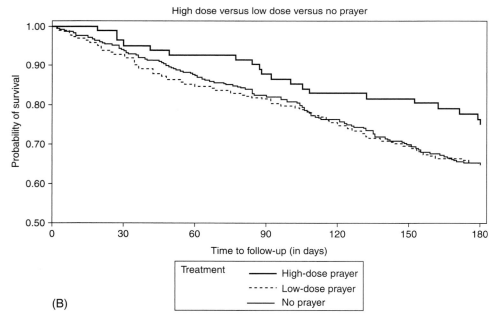

(B)

FIGURE 12-2   *MANTRA II study: six-month death and rehospitalization (Modified from reference 15 with permission).*

SPIRITUAL SUPPORT VERSUS SPIRITUAL THERAPY

Like the differentiation between cultural practices and health care science, it is critical to clearly distinguish between the concepts of spiritual "support" versus spiritual "therapy."[1] *Spiritual support* constitutes the readiness of the health care system to respond to the self-perceived needs of patient and family. This relates to issues such as "do you have a chaplain on site" or "do you have a chapel on site," as well as a spiritual and spiritual needs assessment at nursing intake, currently considered a standard of care by the Joint Commission on Accreditation of Healthcare Organizations (JCAHO). Adequacy and advance of spiritual support services in cardiovascular care is best suited to the quality assessment/quality improvement process, is not considered research per se, and does not require informed consent.

Spiritual therapy constitutes the directed application of an intangible treatment to patients with therapeutic intent. Such interventions are investigational and their application and study in human subjects should be considered research with a full consideration of possible safety issues. The use or study of spiritual or other intangible therapies should be fully subject to Institutional Review Board (IRB) scientific and ethical oversight. In the absence of known safety profiles, all such research should be conducted using informed consent process and good clinical practice standards for experimentation in human subjects.

Other terminology and nomenclature

One of the most immediate challenges to health care in the realm of spiritual therapies is the wide array of largely metaphorical terminologies used, in

TABLE 12-2

SPIRITUAL SUPPORT VERSUS SPIRITUAL THERAPY

Feature	Spiritual Support	Spiritual Therapy
Objective	Provide comfort	Gain knowledge Create data
Impetus	Response to patient, family needs	Pursue hypotheses to advance medicine
Safety considerations	Yes	Yes
IRB review	No	Yes
Informed consent	No	Yes
Process for improvement	Quality Assurance/ Quality Improvement	Research

conjunction with a healing research literature that is historically characterized by indistinct or ambiguous definitions of methods, patient populations,
and outcome endpoints. Consensus recommendations for scientific study of
spiritual interventions have emphasized the need to advance more standardized nomenclature in this area.[1,19]

Apparently subtle differences may have important connotations specifically
for health care applications. A working definition proposed for religion as "an
organized system of beliefs, practices, rituals, and symbols designed (a) to facilitate
closeness to the sacred or transcendent (God, higher power, or ultimate
truth/reality) and (b) to foster an understanding of one's relationship and responsibility to others in living together in a community"[20] might be contrasted to one
proposed for spirituality, defined as "the personal quest for understanding answers
to ultimate questions about life, about meaning, and about relationship to the
sacred or transcendent, which may (or may not) lead to or arise from the development of religious rituals and the formation of community."[20] Implicit for health
care applications are the relatively concrete ethnic, historical, geographical, and
even genetic dimensions of particular religions in modern human civilization,
compared to the more universally human implications of spirituality or human
spiritual healing capacities per se.

A key to clear definitions, particularly of such qualitative aspects of human
mind-body-spirit health and well being, is the ability to develop metrics or instruments for consistent characterization. Measurement tools currently used for
health-related evaluations include the Duke University Religion Index (DUREL),
which characterizes community-based religiosity, personal religiosity, and intrinsic
religiosity.[2,15] the Index of Core Spiritual Orientation (INSPIRIT), and the FACIT
Spiritual Well-Being Scale, among others, are currently available examples of
established instruments.[21-24]

Many obvious conundrums remain. To what degree qualitative characteriza-
tions can be sufficient is unclear. Both patients and health-care practitioners include
a broad range from highly religious to highly secular lifestyles and belief systems,
and what constitutes a "spiritual" therapy demands careful scrutiny. Certain relatively definable elements are implied, including the intangible or "noetic" charac-
teristic of the therapy that facilitates healing, mediated to some degree through a
human role or activity, with some degree of universal access as a capacity of human
beings not necessarily delimited by geography, ethnicity, or such. On the other
hand, many aspects remain fundamentally undefined, if nonetheless included,
under an umbrella terminology such as "noetic" or "spiritual" therapeutics.
Whether terms or constructs such as love, compassion, intention, prayer, energy
healing, Qi Gong, Reiki, and the like are actually agencies of the human "spirit"
insofar as they affect healing, or whether they are importantly different as "energy"
therapies that may each work differently in unique patient populations must be
included at the head of a long list of such poorly understood, and hence poorly or
ambiguously defined arrays of terminology. Thus in even the most basic approaches
to epidemiologic or causal clinical trials in the area of spiritual intervention and
healing, careful attention to nomenclature along the way is critical to the real
advance of knowledge in this area.

ETHICAL ISSUES AND SPIRITUAL HEALING

Perhaps nowhere in medicine are personal sensitivities more important than with regard to spiritual issues in cardiovascular care. Patients with heart disease range from relatively well to acutely ill, but in all cases the sheer presence of heart disease itself touches on issues of mortality, death, and dying. Thus emotional or spiritual crisis may develop concomitantly with exacerbations of the somatic disease, or may develop independently in their timing and/or intensity.

In a progressively global human community, health care systems are more likely to see patients and families from a wide range of ethnic communities and spiritual belief systems, particularly in eclectic societies such as the United States. In optimizing the provision of spiritual support, care must also be taken to avoid unintended discourtesy or insult at both literal and symbolic levels. Spiritual assessments on nursing intake may help understand whether a patient has special dietary needs, or whether a patient might care to be seen, or not be seen, by a chaplain on call. Chaplain training to provide support for patients of other faiths than their own personal religion, or a chapel where color, space, and light can create a sacred or meditative space without the use of symbolic icons from any single religion are all areas where spiritual support must incorporate personal patient/family sensitivities.

Caution must be emphasized as certain "well intended" staff behaviors may become profoundly insensitive and inappropriate. Medical staff with strong personal religious beliefs, who proselytize the tenets of their religion to patients suffering with heart disease are clearly operating outside the ethical boundaries of medical care. Less clear might be offers by staff to pray with patients in their care. For such practice, the concern must be the balance between spiritual support vs. perceived coercion or intrusion. It is conceivable that patient-specific assessment might be used to help understand the impact of or need for such practices.

Even the informal or personal use of prayer by staff presents potential ethical issues. If a nurse or physician cares to pray silently on behalf of a patient, are they obliged to ask the patient's permission, or is the very conversation inappropriately burdensome to both patients and health care staff? If a patient expressly does not want staff to pray, are such prayers unethical? Should a clinician, who considers silent personal prayer as integral to their ability to deliver health care, alter their behavior based on an individual patient's preferences? Would it be unethical to train staff to defer praying unless they specifically have obtained the patient's permission?

Spiritual interventions prescribed by health-care professionals must currently be considered investigational therapy. The primary ethical issues in such research settings are institutional ethical oversight and the provision of informed consent process for patients. In the Harris study, the investigators approached their IRB to waive the informed consent process.[13] Their theoretical concern was that if patients were even aware that a prayer study was being conducted, it would change the spiritual "landscape" being studied. The IRB allowed the study team to waive the consent process on the rationale that distant prayer "could not possibly do harm." While this assumption was controversial even at the time, with the publication of the STEP study showing significant adverse effects in the treatment arms, this assumption currently is untenable.

In addition to the fundamental issues of protection of human subjects participating in clinical research, clinical research in spiritual interventions must also accommodate certain special sensitivities. For instance, if a patient is approached to participate in a prayer study, it is critical that misinterpretations that could upset the patient, such as "you mean I am so sick that I need to be in a prayer study?" be actively avoided. Following the publication of the STEP study, for instance, one explanation advanced for the outcomes findings was that patients who were certain they had been assigned to receive prayer believed it was because they were sicker, and that the anxiety of this belief contributed to the higher incidence of post-CABG atrial fibrillation.

METHODOLOGIC ISSUES AND HEALING PRAYER

Four related yet independent classical methodologic areas can be emphasized for consideration in clinical research using spiritual interventions such as prayer, background therapy, modes of therapy, dose response, and placebo/nocebo effect.

Background therapy: Surveys examining the use of complementary therapies in the Western world report 90–96% of respondents believe in a Higher Power, 40% participate in a spiritual community or attended religious services once a week or more, and 35% include prayer in their response to personal health concerns.[25-27] In MANTRA studies of distant prayer in patients undergoing PCI, 39% of patients reported awareness of someone (family, community, chaplain) praying for their benefit off-protocol prior to urgent PCI,[2] while 89% reported awareness of such healing prayer prior to elective PCI.[15]

With such ubiquitous cultural use of spiritual tools as background therapy, investigators must recognize that there is no scientifically valid means to absolutely examine the healing effects of therapies such as prayer. Most investigators would not only consider it unethical to ask families not to pray for loved ones, or to ask patients not to pray for themselves, but would consider it futile to try to construct "prayer proof" environments for clinical research.

While the study of absolute benefit is prohibited by the ubiquity of background use, incremental benefit tested as the systematic addition of spiritual interventions over and above the background therapy available in the routine clinical care environment can be approached scientifically. In fact, the question of incremental benefit is most closely aligned to the actual question of spiritual intervention for organized health care: with healing prayer so widely used at a cultural level, what is the role for health care systems to systematically add or integrate such practices at all?

Testing incremental benefit importantly affects power calculations for sample size in clinical trials, as the measurable treatment effect is likely to be smaller. With widespread background use, randomized studies and double blinding when possible may be important study design features. In addition, efforts to document the use of background therapy as an uncontrolled variable may also provide important insights.

Placebo/nocebo and the locus of spiritual healing effects: As an intangible therapy without quantitative metrics, the locus of spiritual healing must also be thoughtfully approached in the clinical trials. References to healing through touch, laying on of hands, through the distant prayers of others, or via Divine miracles are all ultimately metaphorical constructs. Whether the healing effects of spiritual therapies actually originate or are importantly mediated through external agencies such as loved ones, healers, congregations or a Divine being at all, or whether such phenomena are predominantly mediated through the awareness, autonomic nervous system, endorphins, or spiritual mechanisms internal to the patient per se are completely unknown.

Culturally and epidemiologically, it is remarkable that interpersonal and social connectivity are perceived of as facilitating the spiritual landscape in important ways, including for healing. In many religions, for instance, certain prayers, including certain healing prayers and prayers for the dead or dying, can ritually only be said by a congregation, not by a single individual. A related yet independent issue regarding connectivity comes from psi phenomenology, where transpersonal connections are consistently reported as more significant between individuals who know one another or who love one another than between strangers.[28]

To what degree such socially based indicators relate to any individual patient's spiritual self-healing capacities, or to what degree an individual human can use intangible capabilities to produce physiologic or psychological/emotional healing effects independent of such social connectivity is unknown. From a cardiovascular perspective, it is well known that stress physiology promotes catecholamine surges with resultant tachycardia, increased inotropy, systemic vasoconstriction, and platelet activation.[29] It has also been shown that skilled meditators can produce vasodilatation, lower blood pressure, and lower heart rate.[30] In a cardiovascular population, significant antianginal effects with placebo pills have been reported.[31] These observations could be taken to suggest that at least part of the locus of healing using intangible therapies originates within the individual patient, potentially independent of connectivity to others.

Other widespread, if metaphorical, observations suggest that the individual patient may have limits to their own intangible healing capacities and that these limits may be overcome through connection to external agencies. For instance, it is generally perceived that a healer treating a patient is more effective than when patients treat themselves. In one context, this perception seems intuitively obvious—if a patient is so sick, so weak, or in so much pain, they simply may not be able to concentrate, to generate the energy, or to conduct a physical manipulation necessary to the therapy. In this construct, the healer may be in a position to "deliver" the energy or facilitate the intervention in some way that reaches beyond the capacities of the individual patient. In a different metaphor, however, it may be that the spiritual posture of "surrender," where the patient gives their well being over to a healer or to a Higher force or some "other" with deep trust and faith, is actually an internal mediator which facilitates somatic re-equilibration, vital energy flow, and healing. From this perspective, the quality of the interconnection between the patient, the healer, and the healing environment could all be considered as defining the true locus of noetic healing.

Considering the locus of noetic healing has both practical and scientific implications. If a family or community or staff are trying to heal a patient, or if a patient is being prayed for, does it matter whether the patient is unconscious, or if conscious whether the patient is aware of these healing prayers? If others are praying for healing, does it matter beyond the ethical issues whether a patient wants to be prayed for, or whether a patient wants to be healed—can one locus of healing actually counteract or otherwise influence another?

In clinical studies of intangible therapies, underlying assumptions with regard to the locus of healing must be delineated and tested as far as possible. Certain study designs may provide unique opportunities to gain insight into this area if appropriate data is collected. In double blind randomized study of distant intercessory prayer, all patients through informed consent would know that they had a 50%-50% chance of actually receiving the protocol therapy. Some patients may believe that they know they were assigned the therapy, even if they were not, potentially generating a placebo effect. Conversely, some patients may feel certain that they did not receive the therapy, even though they did, potentially generating a nocebo effect. In a multicenter, double blind, randomized study of patients undergoing elective PCI, 66% of patients who did not actually receive distant prayer therapy believed that they did.[15] Whether such placebo effect achieves a measurable impact on clinical outcomes can only be examined if data on what patients believe they were assigned is actually gathered. In the primary analysis plan for the STEP study, power calculations were based on the assumption that treatment benefit would be seen in uncertain (blinded) patients who received prayer compared to uncertain patients who did not, and that further treatment benefit would be seen in patients who received prayer and who were unblinded compared to those who were blinded.[16] The actual study data showed exactly the opposite, emphasizing the importance of assumptions and bias in study design for these purposes.

Prayer Modalities: In addition to the distinction between individual and congregational prayers alluded to above, there are many other metaphorical and ritualistic features to spiritual healing modalities, any or all of which might be of consequence to systematic health care applications as methodological variables. While from a cultural perspective, these features may seem self-evident as prescribed through long-standing cultural tradition, and as such be considered beyond further inquiry, from the perspective of health care science the modalities of spiritual therapeutics are aspects as fundamental as what medication is being given, what is the route of administration, and what is the duration and total dose of therapy needed to be effective. Interestingly, even as every spiritual community includes prayers for the sick, so does every spiritual community prescribe a "dosing regimen," that is, the words that are said, how many times a day or a week they are said, and for how long the prayers are to be continued over time. Prayer structures or models of prayer also vary greatly in their form, content, and objectives. From the "prayer warrior" model using prayer as a "spear" to be cast against forces of evil, to the "satellite" model where a personal prayer in one location may reach the heavens and then be reflected in the clinical outcome of the a patient in some distant location, to the "surrender" model where all causal intentions are replaced by faith in terms such as "Thy will be done," to "transcendent" models where articulate words are superceded by a musical tone or simply silence, healing prayer models run a spectrum from very detailed supplication for specific results to very undirected openness or attempts to reach harmony with purposes whose specifics are beyond human understanding. More directed or "intercessory" prayers, defined as calling "for aid to others"[20] and distant-healing models "that purport to heal through some exchange or channeling of supraphysical energy"[20] independent of physical distance have been most widely used in published clinical studies of healing with prayer. On the one hand these models have been used due to their concordance with cultural concepts of therapy—most spiritual communities will pray for a member who is in hospital, regardless of how physically distant the hospital may be. In addition, distant-healing models have logistical utility for double-blinded and for multicenter study designs.[2,12–16]

Skepticism about the study of distant prayer has been voiced,[32–34] with the concerns ranging from the absence of any plausible mechanism for such phenomena to concerns about mixing issues of religion with medical practice. While beyond the scope of this chapter to fully explore, many of these issues have recently been addressed in detail.[35] In addition, the very concepts of quantum physics, such as distant particle entanglement, which concerned Einstein as a science of "spooky actions at a distance" at least provide some conceptual, if still highly theoretical, frameworks for a mechanistic consideration of distant-healing interventions.[36]

The content and focus of spiritual interventions studied in cardiology cohorts is also notable. In all six randomized studies of cardiology patients, petitionary prayers by strangers have been specifically focused on clinical outcomes for patients identified by name, age, and/or illness.[2,12–16] In the MANTRA II study, in addition, less directed praying for the prayers of others have also been included, with some suggestion of greater therapeutic benefit.[15] Whether or not any claims for therapeutic benefit, or differences in therapeutic benefit can be confirmed, awareness of variations of prayer modalities across clinical studies is a key feature of interpretation and future study planning.

Another important feature in spiritual therapies is the import of training, experience, skill levels, and ultimately certification. Culturally, the perception is widespread that spiritual "masters" have healing skills that may be inborn or that may be developed through rigorous training. Though currently there are few instruments with which to meaningfully quantify such features, clinical trials may seek to define certain minimum criteria or document professional certifications for healers delivering intangible therapies.[37]

On a cultural basis, many spiritual healing practices are perceived as most effective for patients when they are most comfortable for patients, for instance when they are affiliated with an ethnic religion that is meaningful to the patient and/or family's traditions. Recitations of prayers that are familiar, in a language that is familiar, in a philosophical context that is familiar, including a shared vision of the meaning of death and dying, at a minimum may provide a unique level of reassurance to patients with cardiovascular disease. How much more or less effective bedside compassion or the prayers of a chaplain whose religious background differs from that of the patient is completely unknown. It is also unknown whether or not this kind of familial, social, and ethnic fabric or alignment might be more important for a patient who is awake or in a more elective or chronic circumstance, compared to a patient who is acutely ill or even unconscious. Finally, it is unknown whether health-care staff training, or a patient's "surrender" of their well being to appropriately trained health-care staff, might present unique opportunities for spiritual intervention even when staff and patient are otherwise strangers to one another.

SAFETY AND EFFECTIVENESS OF SPIRITUAL INTERVENTIONS: IMPORTANCE OF ENDPOINT SELECTION

In cultural use, the benefits of healing intention through spiritual means are widely considered self-evident and intrinsically nontoxic. For health-care applications, especially in vulnerable populations such as patients with cardiovascular disease, however, the safety and effectiveness of spiritual interventions requires actual documentation like any novel therapeutic.

As credible scientific research using spiritual interventions in cardiovascular patients is still in early development, and in the absence of any real mechanistic insight into how spiritual interventions may affect healing, the use of meaningful, well-defined patient descriptors and clinical endpoints seems warranted. At the same time, the elaboration of unique baseline patient descriptors or endpoints above and beyond those already well known to influence cardiovascular outcomes may be informative and of substantial interest to the advance of cardiovascular care that integrates high-tech medicine with intangible human capacities.

The role of assumptions in the construct of noetic therapies research must be carefully considered. For instance, the assumption that a given spiritual intervention might primarily affect mood, customer satisfaction, or peace of mind might select very different primary endpoints than speculation that a spiritual intervention might affect stress-mediated inflammatory reactivity and vascular events.[38–40]

In addition to qualitative or clinical outcomes, addressing certain mechanistic questions is both conceivable and of interest for research documenting effects of intangible therapeutics. For instance, if trainable meditative states or prayerfulness are hypothesized to produce vasodilatation, increase vagal tone, or alter perception of pain, physiologic monitoring of heart rate and blood pressure, documentation of medication needs, or other surrogate measures could serve as effectiveness endpoints for mechanistic observations. Whether or not such practices and their attendant physiologic changes produce clinically meaningful benefit would, as with any surrogate measures, require broader confirmation.[41]

The importance of context for defining appropriate outcomes measures is equally important. At the end of life, when curing the disease, extending the length of life, or reducing mortality are no longer therapeutic objectives, spiritual interventions may well have a role in promoting comfort, acceptance, peace of mind, or other therapeutic objectives.[42] For primary or secondary prevention of cardiovascular events, or as adjuncts to therapeutic procedures, more classical outcomes measures such as mortality rate, disease progression, or major adverse cardiovascular endpoints (MACE) may be appropriate endpoint measures.

From a broader perspective, cardiovascular disorders involving rhythm control, ischemic heart disease, and heart failure represent acute-on-chronic disorders that patients experience both as settings for palliative "cure"-oriented interventions and as confrontations with end-of-life-like issues of peace of mind in the face of death and dying. Work with spiritual interventions in this setting may provide a unique opportunity to gain insights into ameliorating somatic disease expressions and into healing whole human beings, across a wide range of quality and quantity of life measures, and so reach a better definition of optimal modern cardiovascular care.

Safety issues with therapeutic spiritual interventions constitute an area where cultural and health care science practices have critically different concerns. From the cultural perspective, harm from prayer is generally related to prayer with negative intentions—voodoo, black magic, spells, praying for harm to come to others. Many culturally based practitioners do not perceive an ability to do harm with their own healing intention and practices. Ironically, across ethnic boundaries such perceptions may open—that is, one religion may see the healing prayers of another religion as "opening the door to the Devil" or inadvertently promoting some other outcome deleterious to their view of some other patient's best interests. Overall, however, few cultural or ethnic traditions deeply consider whether with a loving, heartfelt prayer for the sick you might actually inadvertently kill someone.

In health-care sciences, intentional harming with voodoo is simply not relevant, as such practices are literally outside the healing paradigm. Safety issues in noetic healing have to do with unintentional harm, relating to the fundamental concerns across all therapeutics with unexpected side effects, distress, overstimulation or other toxicities that produce morbidity and mortality.

For health care sciences, assumptions that spiritual therapies of unknown mechanism would invariably result in restoration of health are inconsistent with all known medical therapeutics. While faith in the Divine nature of healing from prayer may be sufficient for cultural community practice, medical practitioners must begin from the perspective that in the entire history of medicine, every treatment that has actually been shown to have beneficial effect has also been shown, in some one at some time at some dose, to have toxic or side effects relative to its intended therapeutic purpose, and the use of undefined vital "energy" or other intangible human capacities should be regarded no differently. For instance, for an anxious patient presenting with a heart failure exacerbation, a nonpharmacologic meditative or spiritual intervention that promotes peripheral vasodilatation and afterload reduction could be envisioned as likely to be quite beneficial. A similar intervention, however, in an anxious patient on the edge of cardiogenic shock might be life threatening. In another example, patients prior to PCI procedures are generally perceived as worried and anxious, contributing to the pain sensitivity, tachycardia, increased inotropy, vasoconstriction, and platelet activation that are routinely dealt with pharmacologically with sedatives, narcotics, beta blockers, vasodilators, and antiplatelet agents prior to stent implantation. In this setting, relief of worry could significantly be achieved above and beyond all such standard medications with the bedside use of intangible "noetic" therapies prior to PCI.[43] However, when correlated with clinical outcomes, relief of worry was found to be a predictor of higher mortality rates over the 6 months following the index PCI.[44] While these reports come from tightly fit retrospective models that are currently unconfirmed, in an independent report from a larger multicenter study of females surviving myocardial infarctions, randomized to stress-relaxation training versus not, a significantly higher mortality rate was observed in the treatment group compared to controls.[6]

While definitive interpretation of these observations is not yet feasible, the range of considerations regarding safety and spiritual interventions is a broad one. Is it possible that Type A behavior's obsessive qualities are important to a secondary prevention population such as women after myocardial infraction (MI), to keep them focused on their well being, on taking their medications, on reporting symptoms, and maintaining follow-up schedules? Is it possible that relaxation training in such a cohort counteracts such "survival" behaviors? In patients prior to PCI, is it conceivable that worry does more than just promote a cascade of catecholamines and their deleterious effects on cardiac physiology? For instance, shifting from such a Western paradigm, is it important for practitioners and researchers to be aware that in a Chinese medical paradigm, "worry" is a vital energy that emerges from the spleen during stress, and that therapies that eliminate worry at key moments could in fact be life threatening?[44]

Harming the somatic body may also result from states of overexcitation mediated through spiritual practices. From the Biblical exhortation that "those who look directly into the face of God will be destroyed" to anecdotal observations of sudden deaths and acute infarctions during spirited religious ceremonies, the concept that in selected settings "too much" spiritual energy could be unsafe simply cannot be dismissed.

The importance of roles and training in the delivery of spiritual interventions is another key element of safety considerations. At a fundamental level, what constitutes training or certification for health-care staff in the delivery of intangible therapies such as prayer remains completely undefined. Beyond the potential ineffectiveness of mal-conducted spiritual therapies, however, are a whole array of unique safety concerns. For instance, as with medical therapeutics, most spiritual communities have both prayers for the sick and prayers for the dying. The former may be more focused on curing of or recovery from illness, while the latter may be more focused on easing the final release of the spirit from the body. Well-intentioned "dabblers" who utilize prayers in sacred languages whose specifics they do not understand could, at least metaphorically, unintentionally facilitate death in a patient setting where death might not be considered the optimal clinical outcome.

The cultural assumption that well-intentioned spiritual healing methods are intrinsically safe is insufficient for medical practice, health care, or clinical research with these tools.[17] In the absence of mechanistic or methodologic definition, role and training definition, or credible data on safety, research interested in advancing knowledge through the use of human experimentation absolutely must consider these therapeutics investigational, and protect the rights and safety of human subjects who participate in such research with informed consent, data safety monitoring, and thoughtful examination of assumptions and available data in the conduct of such work. In a cardiovascular patient population in particular, the safety of noetic therapies must be demonstrated, not assumed.

Safety for practitioners: Similar to concerns with safety for patients, healthcare science must also be concerned with the safety of practitioners in the use of intangible forces whose mechanistic, electromagnetic, or other qualities are currently unknown. Largely metaphorical warnings to shamans, spiritual and energy healers, and other healing practitioners using intangible tools characterize energy depletion, absorption of large amounts of dark, sticky, foul, and poisonous negative energy, and other such phases of spiritual healing interactions with ailing patients through which the practitioner may promote the recovery of the patient by putting themselves at some risk. In conjunction with such metaphorical observations, many mystical traditions through which spiritual resources and mind-body-spirit healing intersect also prescribe exercises through which the practitioner may restore their own energy or chi, or through which the toxic energy extracted from the patient may be cleansed from the practitioner for their own protection. In the cardiovascular community where health care systematically limits exposure to X-ray, β- and γ-radiation, or other invisible, odorless energies that augment high-tech patient care, attention to the safety of practitioners in the conduct of spiritual therapy at least bears consideration.

CONCLUSION

Heart disorders intrinsically and simultaneously address physical conditions, emotional states, and mortality related belief systems of a spiritual nature. Cardiovascular care has successfully and phenomenally advanced technologies capable of beneficial impact on the somatic domain of cardiovascular physiology. As more data demonstrating the impact of immune system reactivity, depression, hostility, and other social connectivity on cardiovascular outcomes emerge, cardiology practitioners and researchers may recognize that, in addition to our best technology, other intangible human capacities may be an important source of novel and even powerful adjunctive therapeutics. Much more and more systematic data will need to be developed, however, to take these concepts beyond cultural applications and make them integral to best medical practices. Little question remains; however, that noetic therapies such as spiritual interventions are "proper subjects for science, even while transcending its known bounds."[45]

REFERENCES

1. Vogel JHK, Bolling SF, Costello RB, Guarneri EM, Krucoff MW, Longhurst JC, Olshansky B, Pelletier KR, Tracy CM, Vogel RA. Integrating complementary medicine into cardiovascular medicine: a report of the American College of Cardiology Foundation Task Force on Clinical Expert Consensus Documents (Writing Committee to Develop an Expert Consensus Document on Complementary and Integrative Medicine). J Am Coll Cardiol. 2005;46:184–221.

2. Krucoff MW, Crater SW, Green CL, Maas AC, Seskevich JE, Lane JD, et al. Integrative noetic therapies as adjuncts to percutaneous intervention during unstable coronary syndromes: monitoring and actualization of noetic training (MANTRA) feasibility pilot. Am Heart Journal. 2001;142:760–7.

3. Auwae H. Papa Henry Auwae po'okela la'au lapa'au: master of Hawaiian medicine. (Interview by Bonnie Horrigan.) Altern Ther Health Med. 2000;6:82–8.

4. Dossey L. Reinventing medicine. San Francisco (CA): Harper Collins; 1999.

5. Rutledge T, Reis VA, Linke SE, Greenberg BH, Mills PJ. Depression in heart failure: a meta-analytic review of prevalence, intervention effects, and associations with clinical outcomes. J Am Coll Cardiol. 2006;48:1527–37.

6. Frasure-Smith N, Lesperance F, Prince RH, et al. Randomised trial of home-based psychosocial nursing intervention for patients recovering from myocardial infarction. Lancet. 1997;350:473–9.

7. Astin JA, Harkness E, Ernst E. The efficacy of "distant healing": a systematic review of randomized trials. Ann Intern Med. 2000;132:903–10.

8. Jadad AR, Moore RA, Carroll D, et al. Assessing the quality of reports of randomized clinical trials: is blinding necessary? Control Clin Trials. 1996;17:1–12.

9. Cohen J. Statistical power analysis for the behavioural sciences. Hillsdale (NJ): Erlbaum Press; 1988.

10. Roberts L, Ahmed I, Hall S, Sargent C. Intercessory prayer for the alleviation of ill health. Cochrane Database Syst Rev. 1999;2.

11. Ernst E. Distant healing—an "update" of a systematic review. Wien Klin Wochenschr. 2003;115:241–45.

12. Byrd RC. Positive therapeutic effects of intercessory prayer in a coronary care unit population. Southern Med J. 1988;81:826–9.

13. Harris WS, Gowda M, Kolb JW, Strychacz CP, Vacek JL, Jones PG, et al. A randomized, controlled trial of the effects of remote, intercessory prayer on outcomes in patients admitted to the coronary care unit. Arch Intern Med. 1999,159:2273–78.

14. Aviles JM, Whelan E, Hernke DA, Williams BA, Kenny KE, O'Fallon WM, et al. Intercessory prayer and cardiovascular disease progression in a coronary care unit population: a randomized controlled trial. Mayo Clin Proc. 2001;76:1192–8.

15. Krucoff MW, Crater SW, Gallup D, et al. Imagery, touch and prayer as adjuncts to interventional cardiac care: the Monitoring and Actualization of Noetic TRAinings (MANTRA) II randomized study. Lancet. 2005;366:211–17.

16. Benson H. et al. Study of the Therapeutic Effects of Intercessory Prayer (STEP) in cardiac bypass patients: a multicenter randomized trial of uncertainty and certainty of receiving intercessory prayer. Am Heart J. 2006;151:934–42.

17. Krucoff MW, Crater SW, Lee KL. From efficacy to safety concerns: a STEP forward or a step back for clinical research and intercessory prayer? The Study of Therapeutic Effects of Intercessory Prayer (STEP). Am Heart J. 2006;151(4):762–4.

18. Cha KY, Wirth DP, Lobo RA, et al. Does prayer influence the success of in vitro fertilization-embryo transfer? Report of a masked, randomized trial. J Reprod Med. 2001;46:781–7.

19. Dusek JA, Astin JA, Hibberd PL, Krucoff MW. Healing prayer outcomes studies: consensus recommendations. Alt Ther Health Med. 2003;9:A44–53.

20. Koenig HG, McCullough ME, Larson DB. Handbook of religion and health. USA: Oxford University Press, 2001.

21. Hay MW. Principles in building spiritual assessment tools. Am J Hosp Care. 1989;6:25–31.

22. Kass J, Friedman R. Health outcomes and a new index of spiritual experience. J Sci Study Relig. 1991;30:203–11.

23. Brown C. Spirituality in a general practice: a quality of life questionnaire to measure outcome. Complement Ther Med. 2003;3:230–3.

24. King M, Speck P, Thomas A. The royal free interview for religious and spiritual beliefs: development and standardization. Psychol Med. 1995;25:1125–34.

25. King DE, Bushwick B. Beliefs and attitudes of hospital inpatients about faith healing and prayer. J Fam Pract. 1994;39:349–52.

26. Maugans TA, Wadland WC. Religion and family medicine: a survey of physicians and patients. J Fam Pract, 1991;32:210–3.

27. Eisenberg DM, Davis RB, Ettner SL, Appel S, Wilkey S, Van Rompay M, et al. Trends in alternative medicine use in the United States, 1990–1997: results of a follow-up national survey. JAMA. 998:280:1569–75.

28. Radin D. Entangled minds. New York (NY): Paraview; 2006.

29. Rozanski A, Bairey CN, Krantz DS, et al. Mental stress and the induction of silent myocardial ischemia in patients with coronary artery disease. N Engl J Med. 1988;318:1005–12.

30. Benson H, Klipper MZ. The relaxation response. New York: Avon Books; 1990.

31. Benson H, McCallie DP, Jr. Angina pectoris and the placebo effect. N Engl J Med. 1979;300:1424–9.

32. Sloan RP, Bagiella E, Powell, et al. Religion, spirituality, and medicine. Lancet. 1999;353:664–7.

33. Chibnall JT, Jeral JM, Cerullo MA. Experiments on distant intercessory prayer. Arch Intern Med. 2001;161:2529–36.

34. Halperin EC. Should academic medical centers conduct clinical trials of the efficacy of intercessory prayer? Acad Med. 2001;76:791–7.

35. Dossey L, Hufford DB. Are prayer experiments legitimate? Twenty criticisms. Explore. 2005;1(2):109–17.

36. Leder D. Spooky actions at a distance: Physics, psi, and distant healing. J Altern Complement Med. 2005;11(5) 923–30.

37. Dusek JA, Sherwood JB, Friedman R, et al. Study of the therapeutic effects of intercessory prayer (STEP): study design and research methods. Am Heart J. 2002;143:577–84.

38. Warner CD, Peebles BU, Miller J, Reed R, Rodriquez S, Martin-Lewis E. The effectiveness of teaching a relaxation technique to patients undergoing elective cardiac catheterization. J Cardiovasc Nurs. 1992;6:66–75.

39. Tusek DL, Cwynar R, Cosgrove DM. Effect of guided imagery on length of stay, pain and anxiety in cardiac surgery patients. J Cardiovasc Manag. 1999;10:22–8.

40. Luskin F. Review of the effect of spiritual and religious factors on mortality and morbidity with a focus on cardiovascular and pulmonary disease. J Cardiopulm Rehabil. 2000;20:8–15.

41. Koenig HG, George LK, Hays JC, Larson DB, Cohen HJ, Blazer DG. The relationship between religious activities and blood pressure in older adults. Int J Psychiatry Med. 1998;28:189–213.

42. Steinhauser KE, Christakis NA, Clipp EC, McNeilly M, McIntyre L, Tulsky JA. Factors considered at the end of life by patients, family, physicians and other care providers. JAMA. 2000;284:2476–82.

43. Seskevich JE, Crater SW, Lane JD, Krucoff MW. Beneficial effects of noetic therapies on mood before percutaneous intervention for unstable coronary syndromes. Nur Res. March/April 2004;53(2):116–21.

44. Grunberg GE, Crater SW, Green CL, Seskevich J, Lane JD, Koenig HG, Bashore TM, Morris KG, Mark DB, Krucoff MW. Correlations between preprocedure mood and clinical outcome in patients undergoing coronary angioplasty. Cardiology in Review. 2003;11:1–9.

45. MANTRA II: measuring the unmeasurable? Editorial The Lancet. 2005;366:178.

CHAPTER

13

TAI CHI AND QI GONG FOR HEART HEALTH

Victor S. Sierpina, M. Kay Garcia and Gloria Y. Yeh

INTRODUCTION

Tai Chi and Qi Gong are essential elements of traditional Chinese medicine (TCM). As part of that system of care, these graceful, slow-motion movements and breathing exercises are used extensively for health promotion and disease prevention. In this chapter, we will examine the applicability of these techniques to cardiovascular disease. Both Tai Chi and Qi Gong have been shown to have measurable impacts on the autonomic system, plasma catecholamines, cortisol, lipids, and blood pressure. In addition, measurements of oxygen uptake (maximum) (VO_2max), pulmonary capacity, plasma lactate levels, walking speeds, and muscle strength have all been positively affected. The slow, diaphragmatic breathing used in both Tai Chi and Qi Gong, similar to that used in yogic breathwork, has been found to be a stress mitigator and aid to improved oxygenation in multiple studies in cardiovascular and pulmonary health. Finally, the gentle activity of Tai Chi and Qi Gong have surprisingly been found to impact aerobic and fitness capacity, improve flexibility, reduce falls and fears of falling, and enhance general conditioning. By increasing activity levels, Tai Chi and Qi Gong can be a part of useful approaches to cardiac rehabilitation and heart failure.

In this chapter, we will examine the historical health context of Tai Chi and Qi Gong, indications for their use in cardiovascular health, review the scientific studies and evidence for their benefit, and provide useful information on how and when to refer for Tai Chi and Qi Gong practice as well as resources for training.

DESCRIPTION AND BACKGROUND

Foundations of TCM

A meaningful discussion of Tai Chi and Qi Gong must first begin with an overview of the foundations of TCM. Many different models and approaches, ranging from a metaphysical paradigm to strictly neurophysiologic explanations, have been used to describe the mechanisms underlying TCM. In this chapter, we will attempt to integrate biomedical and basic metaphysical perspectives.

A complete system of healthcare that has been practiced in China for thousands of years, TCM is based on the fundamental concept that an animating life-force or energy exists giving us the power to walk, talk, think, and achieve our goals. In India, this life-force is called Prana. In Japan, it is called Ki. In China, it is called Chi or Qi (pronounced chee). Along with acupuncture, herbs, food therapy, and Tui Na (Chinese bodywork), Tai Chi and Qi Qong are primary components of TCM.

The concept of Qi has been discussed by Chinese philosophers throughout time. The term "Qi" may be defined narrowly (i.e., bioelectromagnetic energy existing within the human body) or broadly (i.e., universal energy existing within and between all things). In the Chinese language, the symbol representing Qi indicates something that is simultaneously material and immaterial, and some authors have described Qi as "matter + energy" or "mattergy." Another definition of Qi is that it is "matter on the verge of becoming energy; energy at the point of materializing." Note the dynamic, operational descriptions of Qi.

In ancient Chinese thought, Qi was believed to be a fundamental, vital substance of the universe and necessary for the human body to function. It was believed that all phenomena were produced by its changes. There are many different types of Qi that help maintain normal activities. They are categorized according to source, function, and distribution. According to classical TCM theory, Qi flows along organized pathways known as channels or meridians, and balanced, unobstructed flow throughout the system is necessary for a state of good health.

Ancient Chinese scholars viewed humans as a microcosmic reflection of the universe. A state of mental, physical, emotional, and spiritual good health, known as Wu Chi, is achieved when one becomes aware that all things are connected and that not only do we exist within the world, but the world exists within us. Daily practice of Qi Gong and/or Tai Chi over a number of years can lead one to achieve a state of Wu Chi.

Also fundamental to TCM is yin-yang theory. Yin and yang are relative opposing, positive and negative forces that can be applied to all things, including the human body. Hot/cold, internal/external, male/female are examples of yin and yang. Yin always possesses some characteristics or seeds of yang, and yang always possesses characteristics or seeds of yin. Yin and yang forces are interdependent, support each other, and may be simultaneously opposite and yet complementary. Yin and yang also consume each other and may, under certain circumstances, transform into each other. According to TCM, health problems

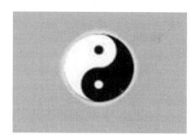

FIGURE 13-1 *Yin-yang symbol.*

develop when there is an imbalance in yin and yang forces. Yin conditions result when there is a Qi deficiency, and yang conditions result when there is excess Qi that needs to be reduced (see Fig. 13-1).

In TCM, it is said that, "The Heart governs Blood and the Lungs govern Qi."* The relationship between Heart and Lungs is thus the relationship between Blood and Qi. Blood is considered yin in comparison to Qi (i.e., denser and more material). Qi has more yang characteristics than blood and is the energetic force behind blood circulation (i.e., relatively immaterial to Blood). It is important to note that the terms Heart, Lung, and Blood have broader meanings in TCM than in Western biomedicine. "Heart" not only refers to the organ, but to additional functional relationships as well. For example, it is said in TCM that "the Heart houses the mind." Interestingly, recent research[1] has confirmed the link between cardiovascular risk factors and Alzheimer's disease.

Similarly, the concept of Blood is much broader in TCM than in biomedicine. Blood is more dense and therefore considered a yin form of Qi. It circulates continuously through blood vessels as well as the meridian pathways, although the latter carries relatively more Qi while the former carries relatively more Blood. The major functions of Blood in TCM are to nourish, maintain, and moisten various parts of the body and to provide the material foundation for mental, emotional, and spiritual activities. Qi and Blood are inseparable. Without Qi, Blood would merely be an inert fluid.

QI GONG

Practiced in China for thousands of years, Qi Gong is mentioned in ancient Chinese books such as the *I Ching* (Book of Changes) and the *Huang Di Nei Jing* (The Yellow Emperor's Classic of Medicine). The *I Ching* was written in 2852 BCE and the *Huang Di Nei Jing* around 2697–2597 BCE. These books provide the accumulated knowledge of many generations underlying the philosophy and foundation of acupuncture, Qi Gong, and Tai Chi and are used in colleges and universities of TCM even today.

---

*Terms such as "Heart," "Blood," and "Lungs" are capitalized here to denote their broad and unique meaning in TCM.

The term "Qi," meaning vital energy or life force, combined with the term "Gong," meaning diligent practice, leads to a general definition of Qi Gong as: "the cultivation of one's life energy through skill and diligent practice." Qi Gong masters claim that improvement of the techniques and skill achievement continues throughout life.

A growing body of literature reveals the potential health benefits of regular Qi Gong practice. Although there are many styles and forms of Qi Gong, the three major categories are martial Qi Gong, spiritual Qi Gong, and medical Qi Gong. Even though these are considered separate categories, they are interrelated. For example, the goal of martial Qi Gong is to enhance fighting skills, but significant improvement in health or enlightenment may be achieved. Initially, emphasis is placed on physical health. As training progresses, however, the focus is turned to the mind, emotions, and spirit. The specific techniques may involve both internal and external Qi Gong exercises. In internal Qi Gong, the individual directs his or her own Qi throughout the body. External Qi Gong requires treatment by a master.

For the purposes of this chapter, our discussion will be limited to internal medical Qi Gong. Easily done, even by deconditioned patients and those not able to participate in aerobic conditioning programs, Qi Gong for general health maintenance may be practiced for as little as 20 minutes a day. For more serious disease, exercises may be done for several hours per day. A typical daily session consists of meditation, deep breathing and relaxation exercises, guided imagery, mindful focus, and physical exercise which may involve either dynamic or static postures. The purpose is to achieve a more balanced (homeostatic) state between yin and yang both within the body and between the body and external environment. Qi Gong exercises should be practiced in a quiet place with fresh air and good ventilation. Direct wind or fan should be avoided, and it is not recommended that one practice Qi Gong during a thunderstorm or under adverse climactic conditions. It is said in Chinese medicine that wind disperses Qi, and although there are no specific data investigating Qi Gong performed under adverse weather conditions, many masters claim the electric charge created during a thunderstorm may interfere with practice outcomes and may cause "chaotic" Qi flow. Some individuals are reported to be hypersensitive to such conditions.

Three key elements of Qi Gong practice are physical relaxation, regulation of the breathing, and mindful concentration. Initially, the focus is placed on the lower abdomen (also called lower Dantian). The practice should begin with several slow deep breaths and progressive relaxation from head to toes followed by various mental and physical exercises. These exercises can vary from small postural and limb movements to meditative walking and larger body movements, all done slowly, gently, deliberately. Occasionally, vivid images or even hallucinations may occur. Although Qi Gong is a safe form of exercise for most people, it may be contraindicated for patients with certain psychiatric or severe neurobiological disorders, therefore, guidance by a trained teacher is recommended. For anyone experiencing acute fever or severe infection, medical advice should be obtained prior to initiating any type of Qi Gong exercise Again, although no specific data are available, any severe infection impacts one's available energy stores. Some masters/teachers report that an exacerbation of signs and symptoms may occur if Qi Gong is practiced during an acute illness.

TAI CHI

Tai Chi (also called Tai Chi Chuan) combines similar meditation and breathing exercises used in Qi Gong with slow, smooth, soft movements that promote the free flow of energy and enhance health. Qi Gong is the more ancient therapy, and Tai Chi is often considered a subtype of Qi Gong. Like Qi Gong, Tai Chi is richly embedded in Chinese culture, history, and philosophical thought. Many Tai Chi movements are modeled after the behavior of animals and the natural world, and although the postures and movements appear to be simple, they are quite precise. Many years of training are required to "master" the techniques.

The Chinese characters for Tai Chi Chuan can be translated as the "Supreme Ultimate Force." The concept of "supreme ultimate" is often associated with yin-yang theory and the notion that one can see a dynamic duality in all things. "Force" (or, more literally translated, "fist") represents the martial arts origins of Tai Chi and can be thought of as the means or way of achieving this yin-yang, or "supreme-ultimate" discipline.

Historically, Tai Chi has its roots in both dance and the martial arts. Chang San Feng, a famous martial artist born in AD 1247, combined his knowledge of Qi Gong with his practice of martial arts in order to improve his health while training. Eventually, he developed the essential principles into 12 movement sequences called the 12 Qi Disruption Forms. Chang lived in the Wu Dang mountain range, and this form eventually became known as Wu Dang Mountain Tai Chi. During the 19th century, the system was studied by other martial artists, and several "family" styles, including Yang and Chen styles, were developed.

The focus and forms for each style of Tai Chi are slightly different. When choosing a master/teacher, it is important to know which style s/he teaches. Some styles are more suited for martial artists while others, such as Yang style, are less aggressive and may be more appropriate for the general public. However, most practitioners would agree that almost any style can be modified to suit a wide range of physical capacities.

Health benefits such as improved circulation, reduced fatigue, enhanced balance and body awareness, improved muscle tone, improved posture, and less joint stiffness or less pain are reported by those who regularly practice Tai Chi. A feeling of warmth during practice is also commonly reported. Initially, mild shaking, a sensation of tingling, slight tension, or tightness may be noticed in areas of Qi blockage. A sense of calmness and well-being or spiritual experiences often occur with continued practice.

Daily practice, ideally performed in loose comfortable clothing, barefoot or in soft flat-soled shoes; practicing on grass, under or near a tree at sunrise is considered optimum. According to TCM theory, sunrise is the best time of day to tonify the Lung meridian. Practicing outside in a park or quiet peaceful area is recommended to enhance relaxation and provide clean, oxygenated air. If it is raining or the weather is damp, cold, or windy, patients should be instructed to practice indoors.

The promise of Qi Gong and Tai Chi in health promotion and prevention provides new avenues for exploring and understanding the natural inclination of human life to seek balance. Modern research into the medical benefits of these ancient practices leads to new thinking about physical, mental, emotional, and spiritual health. Using today's technology to explore functional relationships between systems long emphasized in TCM may help promote health and longevity and reduce the overall costs of healthcare.

INDICATIONS

Tai Chi and Qi Gong practice have been utilized and studied for a variety of health enhancements both traditionally and in contemporary clinical science. Current indications for including them as part of a cardiovascular fitness prescription are as described below. (See Table 13-1)[2-7]

The literature supports the acceptability of Tai Chi/Qi Gong exercises in cardiac patients and particularly in the elderly. Hogan emphasizes the multiple layers of benefit from improvements in cognition, resilience, stress reduction, motivation, and compliance with a sustained exercise program.[8,9] Additional studies have revealed positive impacts on hypertension, lipids, heart rate variability, and on fear of falling, as well as fall prevention.[10-12] Multiple other studies support reduction of stress-related hormones, improved cardiopulmonary efficacy, and musculoskeletal function, which are detailed in the following sections.

As we look across the spectrum of indications for recommending Tai Chi and Qi Gong to our patients, the goals for application are multifaceted, and we need to acknowledge that these are exercises that can be done at practically every level of conditioning, from ambulatory to bedridden. Standard medical care encourages a young patient with a strong family history of hypertension, dyslipidemia, or heart disease to participate in an aerobic fitness program. A more completely dimensioned exercise program would include strength, balance, and flexibility training. These can improve resilience, metabolism, and general fitness in ways that complement aerobic training. Likewise, someone with borderline hypertension or dyslipidemia might find that in addition to dietary modification, such as the Mediterranean diet, and a regular exercise and weight loss program, some of the stress-reducing elements of Tai Chi/Qi Gong practice might positively affect these conditions by downregulating the sympathetic nervous system (SNS).

An important aspect of prescribing Tai Chi and Qi Gong programs to patients is their acceptability and high rates of compliance with sustained participation. Since a prime goal in chronic illness and in wellness promotion is to maintain positive changes contributing to a healthy lifestyle, any program that is sustainable is preferable to others which the patient abandons.

Perhaps the greatest opportunities for implementation of Tai Chi/Qi Gong training and practice is in those with established or advanced cardiovascular disease (CVD). Since 60% or more of our population gets little or no regular

TABLE 13-1

CURRENT INDICATIONS FOR INCLUDING TAI CHI AND QI GONG PRACTICE AS PART OF A CARDIOVASCULAR FITNESS PRESCRIPTION

Primary Prevention/Health and Wellness Promotion	Treatment of Early and Mild Cardiovascular Disease	Cardiac Rehabilitation and Secondary Prevention	Treatment for Advanced Cardiac Disease
Stress reduction, cognitive enhancement, self-efficacy	Hypertension, dyslipidemia, anxiety, depression, stress reduction	Post-myocardial infarction, post coronary bypass, angioplasty/stent—adjunctive to aerobic training	Chronic heart failure—adjunctive to standard medical treatment and fitness prescription
Body awareness	Falling and fear of falling	Improved blood pressure and lipid profile, stress reduction	Low-intensity easily achievable cardiac demand
Improved lipid profile, general conditioning	Improved general conditioning	Improved cardiopulmonary function and musculoskeletal conditioning	Treatment of cardiopulmonary and musculoskeletal deconditioning
Flexibility, balance, leg strength	Reduction in epinephrine, norepinephrine, cortisol	Increased confidence in physical function, self-efficacy, and acceptable for sustained physical activity	Increased sense of self-efficacy, physical capability, balance, leg strength

exercise, essential hypertension, dyslipidemia, angina, myocardial infarction, peripheral vascular disease, and congestive heart failure are highly prevalent in overweight, inactive, deconditioned persons. In the immediate post-cardiac event period, motivation to exercise may be high. Sustainability of such activity is vital. Thus, Tai Chi and Qi Gong may serve as an easy entry point into more active conditioning programs. While there is clearly an aerobic component to Tai Chi and Qi Gong[13,14] after cardiovascular disease is established, getting patients moving regularly is a major achievement. Because Tai Chi and Qi Gong are low impact, even those with minimal exercise capacity can get started and as it has been shown in more than one study, it is an enjoyable and sustainable exercise program.[8]

As their musculoskeletal and cardiopulmonary conditioning improves, more intense aerobic activity can be undertaken with less impairment from stiffness, injury, falls, cardiopulmonary impairment, and other sequelae of a newly established fitness regime in deconditioned, out-of-shape patients. Clearly, the best evidence for cardiac rehabilitation is still for active aerobic exercise which increases cardiac output and oxygen consumption. However, a number of studies have shown that Tai Chi is equivalent to low-moderate aerobic activity (3-5 metabolic equivalents MET) and that it may have other benefits in cardiac fitness by improving balance between sympathetic and parasympathetic tone. Thus, Tai Chi and Qi Gong are still to be considered adjunctive to aerobic conditioning though they may easily substitute for primary training in those unable or unwilling to participate in traditional aerobic, cardiac rehabilitation.

In conclusion, regarding indications for Tai Chi/Qi Gong practice, a number of lines of evidence and reasoning help us to recommend such therapies with confidence to our patients with cardiovascular conditions. Guidelines by the most recent JNC 7 Group on Hypertension continue to emphasize the importance of lifestyle changes to the treatment of borderline and mild hypertension prior to initiating pharmacological treatment. Clearly, hypertension is a major risk factor for cardiovascular disease, stroke, and congestive heart failure though its very name "essential hypertension," reveals our limited understanding of its root causes. Certainly some of the data on Tai Chi and Qi Gong in reducing blood pressure, correlated with reductions in catecholamines and cortisol, indicate a downregulation of the stress response. Increased heart-rate variability is likewise a factor showing improved parasympathetic nervous system (PNS) and SNS balance. Our modern lives are often burdened with ongoing demands on the SNS. Daily news, work and commuting stress, environmental challenges, media and noise pollution, caffeinism, smoking, alcohol, fast foods, and of course, social and financial rewards for being a "Type-A" personality all create a high level of demand on the SNS. In order to survive in modern society, it seems that this limb of our autonomic system gets little relief but very high demands.

Meditation and relaxation are intrinsic to the focused awareness and attention of Tai Chi and Qi Gong practices, which help to rebalance this stress by providing some time for PNS dominance, if even for a short period per day. In TCM, the "yin-yang" balance between PNS and SNS is represented in the meridians of the Master of the Heart and the Triple Heater. The former is commonly referred to as the "Heart Protector." As we can tell from the modern epidemic of cardiovascular disease, our hearts often need such protection. Established risk factors such as cholesterol, homocysteine, smoking, stress, obesity, inactivity, inflammation are all mitigated by attention to our Heart Protector or the "yin" PNS. Thus, Tai Chi and Qi Gong practices may be considered intrinsic to a heart-healthy lifestyle since they contribute so significantly to helping redress the stress on our system engendered by modern life.

EVIDENCE/CLINICAL OUTCOMES RESEARCH

The literature investigating Tai Chi and Qi Gong has dramatically increased in recent years (see Table 13-2). Not only are these therapies becoming popular among the general public, but there is also growing interest from clinicians, academicians, and government-funding agencies. In fact, mind-body exercise, such as Tai Chi, for cardiovascular disease was recently cited as an area of funding priority by the National Institute of Health (NIH) National Center for Complementary and Alternative Medicine.[15]

There has long been a body of evidence supporting the role of stress reduction/management in cardiac disease. However, only recently have these ideas been implemented formally in, for example, cardiac rehabilitation programs. Some programs are just beginning to explore the use of relaxation therapies as part of their curriculum, including meditative exercises like Tai Chi and Qi Gong. Current research will help to define the role of meditative exercise in cardiac health and disease management.

The interconnected relationship between Tai Chi and Qi Gong has been discussed previously but is worth noting here in the context of labeling an intervention trial as one or the other. Most studies labeled as Tai Chi trials, in fact, involve a Tai Chi intervention that includes Qi Gong. Most trials of Qi Gong, however, do not implicitly contain Tai Chi movements. Nonetheless, the two are closely related and share many key components, such as meditation, a focus on breathing, and general mind-body awareness.

There have been several recent reviews of the Tai Chi literature that include cardiovascular effects.[9,16–19] A much smaller body of literature (in peer-reviewed English-language journals) examines cardiovascular effects of Qi Gong alone. Several cardiovascular studies of Qi Gong, however, have been cited as abstracts in the Qi Gong Institute's Qi Gong Database (www.qigonginstitute.org). These abstracts appear in the proceedings from various international Qi Gong conferences, however, have not been published in peer-reviewed journals and are not included here.

The literature on Tai Chi and Qi Gong relevant to cardiovascular effects can be broadly divided into two categories: (1) studies that describe cardiovascular effects in patients with noncardiac conditions or in "healthy" volunteers and (2) disease-specific effects in populations with cardiovascular conditions. The bulk of studies remain in the first category. The most commonly reported cardiovascular

T A B L E 1 3 - 2

SELECTED STUDIES OF TAI CHI/QI GONG

Hypertension +/− Lipid Abnormality

Reference (Author, Year, Country)	Study Design	Population (Mean Age)	N*	Intervention/Control	Relevant Outcomes	Results
				(A) In Individuals with Cardiovascular Disease		
Young 1999 US	RCT	High-normal BP and Stage I hypertension (67)	60	12 weeks Yang style Tai Chi 2×/week vs. walking and aerobic dance	Resting BP Exercise capacity Physical activity	• ↓ SBP, DBP in both groups, but no between group differences • No change in VO_2max • Higher compliance with home exercise c/w aerobics
Tsai 2003 Taiwan	RCT	Stage I (borderline) hypertension (51)	76	12 weeks Yang style Tai Chi 3×/week vs. usual care	BP, Lipid profile Anxiety	• ↓ in SBP, DBP • ↓ in total cholesterol, LDL, ↑ in HDL compared to baseline • ↓ in state and trait anxiety scores c/w baseline • No changes seen in control group
Lee 2004 Korea	RCT	Essential hypertension (53)	36	8 weeks Qi Gong "Shuxinpingxuegong" vs. usual activity	BP, Lipid profile	• ↓ in SBP, DBP • ↓ in total cholesterol, triglycerides • ↑ in HDL, Apo-A1 c/w controls

Coronary Heart Disease

Lee 2003 Korea	RCT	Essential hypertension (56)	58	10 weeks Qi Gong "Shuxinpingxuegong" vs. usual activity	BP, Catecholamines, ventilatory function	• ↓ in SBP and DBP on Qi Gong group (↓ in control) • ↓ in epinephrine, norepinephrine • Improvement in FVC and FEV1
Channer 1996 UK	RCT	Post-acute myocardial infarction (56)	126	8 weeks Wu style short form Tai Chi plus Qi Gong 1–2×/week vs. Exercise to music vs. support group	BP, HR	• ↓ SBP, DBP • TC group had ↓ resting HR after 8 weeks c/w conventional exercise • Greater compliance with TC class than conventional exercise
Lan 1999 Taiwan	NRS	Post-coronary artery bypass, men (57)	20	1 year Yang style Tai Chi 7×/week vs. walking	Exercise capacity Exercise intensity	• ↓VO$_2$peak c/w control • Greater compliance with TC • TC exercise intensity 48–57% HR$_{max}$ reserve
Stenlund 2005 Sweden	RCT	Coronary artery disease (78)	95	12 weeks Qi Gong plus group education 1×/week vs. usual care	Physical activity level Fear of falling Balance and coordination	• ↑activity level • ↑balance and coordination (Single-leg stance, box-climb test) • No change in fear of falling (low level of fear at baseline)

TABLE 13-2

SELECTED STUDIES OF TAI CHI/QI GONG (CONTINUED)

Reference (Author, Year, Country)	Study Design	Population (Mean Age)	N*	Intervention/Control	Relevant Outcomes	Results
(A) In Individuals with Cardiovascular Disease						
Congestive Heart Failure						
Yeh 2004 US	RCT	Heart failure (64)	30	12 weeks modified Yang style Tai Chi 2×/week vs. usual care	Exercise capacity Serum biomarkers Catecholamines Quality-of-life	• ↓ 6 minutes walk, ↑ Disease specific QOL c/w control • ↓ serum B-type natriuretic peptide c/w control • Trend toward ↑ in VO_2peak • No differences in catecholamines
Fontana 2000 US	NRS	Heart Failure (65)	5	12 weeks modified Tai Chi 2×/wk	Quality-of-life Exercise capacity Health status	• ↓ disease specific QOL, ↓ symptoms (dyspnea) • ↓ 6 minutes walk • Improved vigor and physical function score on SF-36 questionnaire • Maintenance of TC practice after 3 months

(B) In the "Healthy Volunteers" or in Individuals with Noncardiac Conditions

Exercise Physiology

Study	Design	Population	N	Intervention	Outcomes	Results
Lan 1998 Taiwan	NRS	Community seniors (66)	38	12 months Yang style Tai Chi 5×/week vs. usual activity	Exercise capacity Exercise intensity Strength, flexibility, body fat	• ↑ VO_2max, strength and flexibility c/w control • TC exercise intensity 52–63% HR_{max} reserve • No change in body fat
Lai 1995 Taiwan	NRS	TC practitioners (63) vs. non-TC practitioner	84	2 years Yang style Tai Chi 5×/week vs. usual activity	Exercise capacity Exercise intensity	• ↓ rate of decline in VO_2max c/w control • TC exercise intensity 53–57% HR_{max} reserve
Wang 2001 Taiwan	OBS w/control	TC practitioners, men (69) vs. non-TC practitioners	20	Classical Yang style Tai Chi vs. usual activity	Exercise capacity cutaneous blood flow, vascular conductance, skin temperature plasma nitric oxide metabolites	• ↑ VO_2peak in TC c/w control • ↑ cutaneous blood flow, vascular conductance, temperature during exercise • ↑ nitric oxide metabolites (endothelium-dependent vasodilator)
Wang 2002 Taiwan	OBS w/control	TC practitioners, men (69) vs. non-TC practitioners	32	Classical Yang style Tai Chi vs. usual activity	Exercise capacity Arterial and venous blood flow Cutaneous microvascular perfusion	• ↑ VO_2peak c/w control • ↑ cutaneous, arterial, and venous blood c/w control

TABLE 13-2

SELECTED STUDIES OF TAI CHI/QI GONG (CONTINUED)

(B) In the "Healthy Volunteers" or in Individuals with Noncardiac Conditions

Reference (Author, Year, Country)	Study Design	Population (Mean Age)	N*	Intervention/Control	Relevant Outcomes	Results
Blood Pressure						
Thornton 2004 Hong Kong	NRS	Community women (48)	34	12 weeks Yang style Tai Chi 3×/week vs. usual activity	BP Balance/functional reach	• ↓ SBP, DBP • Functional reach improved in TC group, no change in control
Schaller 1996 US	NRS	Community seniors (70)	46	10 weeks modified Tai Chi 1×/week vs. usual activity	BP Balance, flexibility, Mood, health status	• ↓ SBP, DBP • Improved balance (single-leg stance) • No changes in trunk or hamstring flexibility, mood or health status
Heart Rate Variability						
Lu 2003 Taiwan	OBS w/ control	TC practitioners (54) vs. non-TC practitioners	40	Classical Yang style Tai Chi One 40 minute session vs. usual activity	HRV (time and frequency domain measures) BP	• Within TC group comparison: ↓ BP 30 and 60 minute after TC; acute ↑ HRV • Baseline comparison with controls: TC practitioners had ↑ HRV

Author, Year, Country	Type	Population	N	Intervention	Outcome measures	Results
Väänänen 2002 China	OBS	TC practitioners men older: (64) younger: (21)	29	Intervention not well described Two 5 minutes Tai Chi sessions performed in series	HRV (time and frequency domain measures)	• Acute ↑ in HRV (more prominent in young) ↑ in RRI (interval between heart beats, SDNN [Std Dev N to N], TV (total variance)
Lee 2002 Korea	NRS	Qi Gong practitioners (25) vs. non-Qi Gong practitioners	40	ChunDoSunBup (Korean) Qi-training Three 1 hour sessions on separate days	HRV (frequency domain measures)	• Acute ↑ in HRV (↑ HF high frequency, ↓ LF/HF low frequency/high frequency ratio) during Qi-training in both groups • Enhanced effects in Qi Gong practitioners

Balance, Strength, Flexibility

Author, Year, Country	Type	Population	N	Intervention	Outcome measures	Results
Wolf 2003 US	RCT	Community seniors (76)	200	15 weeks Yang style Tai Chi 1×/week vs. computerized balance training vs. education	Strength, flexibility Body mass index Psychosocial well-being Systolic blood pressure	• ↓ fear of falling • Less loss of hand group strength c/w education • ↓ SBP • No changes in body mass index, perceived sleep, depression
McGibbon 2005 US	RCT	Vestibulopathy (inner ear balance disorder)	36	10 weeks Yang style Tai Chi 1×/wk vs. conventional vestibular rehabilitation	Truncal kinematics (sway) Gait speed Step length/width Stance duration	• ↑ gait function in both groups, with TC group improving lower extremity stability and faster gait, VR group improving upper body stability

SELECTED STUDIES OF TAI CHI/QI GONG (CONTINUED)

Reference (Author, Year, Country)	Study Design	Population (Mean Age)	N*	Intervention/Control	Relevant Outcomes	Results
				(B) In the "Healthy Volunteers" or in Individuals with Noncardiac Conditions		
Balance, Strength, Flexibility						
Sattin 2005 US	RCT	Transitionally frail older adults (80)	311	48 weeks simplified Tai Chi 2×/week vs. wellness education	Fall events Fear of falling	• ↓ fall rates in those without previous • ↓ fear of falling (activities-specific balance confidence scale) in TC group c/w control
Li 2005 US	RCT	Physically inactive older adults (77)	256	6 months Tai Chi 3×/week vs. stretching	Fall events, fear of falling Functional balance Physical performance	• ↓ fall rates, ↓ fear of falling • ↑ functional balance (Berg Balance Scale, Dynamic Gait Index, functional reach, single-leg stand) and physical performance (50-feet speed walk, up and go)

*N = number of study participants (including intervention and control groups)

RCT = randomized controlled trial; NRS = non-randomized study; OBS = observational study

SBP = systolic blood pressure; DBP = diastolic blood pressure; HR = heart rate; LDL = low-density lipoprotein; HDL = high-density lipoprotein; VO_2 = oxygen uptake; HRV = heart rate variability

TC = Tai Chi; BP = blood pressure; Apo-A1 = apolipoprotein 1

QOL = quality-of-life; FEV_1 = forced expiratory volume in 1 second

FVC = functional residual capacity; VR = vestibular rehabilitation outcome is blood pressure +/– heart rate (both acute and long-term effects of Tai Chi/ Qi Gong). A few studies have measured lipids, and a few have explored heart rate variability (as a measure of autonomic tone). There is also a large literature available on Tai Chi's effect on balance, strength, and flexibility, which can be relevant in terms of facilitating exercise and rehabilitation. A large proportion of the literature in healthy volunteers was designed to better understand Tai Chi exercise physiology (with estimates of energy expenditure and exercise intensity as a percent of maximal heart rate). Other reported outcomes include microvascular perfusion, pulmonary function, cardiac hemodynamic indices, and blood viscosity. The specific cardiac populations that have been studied include coronary heart disease, congestive heart failure, and hypertension. Important outcomes in these cardiac condition studies also include disease-specific quality of life, mood/psychosocial indices, functional measures, exercise self-efficacy, and compliance.

EFFECTS IN SPECIFIC CARDIOVASCULAR CONDITIONS

Hypertension

Although blood pressure is a commonly measured outcome in many Tai Chi/ Qi Gong studies, few published studies examine patients with hypertension.

An older, frequently cited study by Young compared a 12-week Tai Chi intervention to a moderate-intensity conventional exercise program (walking and aerobic dance) in patients with Stage I hypertension. Investigators reported decreases in blood pressure in both groups (systolic/diastolic: change of –7.0/–2.4 with Tai Chi versus –8.4/–3.2 mm Hg with conventional exercise). There were no significant differences between groups, suggesting comparable effects of each intervention. Although class attendance was comparable among the two groups, the home exercise frequency was greater in the Tai Chi group.

A few studies in patients with hypertension also measured lipid profile. Tsai et al randomized 76 individuals with Stage I hypertension to either 12 weeks of Tai Chi or to usual care. In addition to decreases in systolic blood pressure (–15 vs. +6 mm Hg, p <.001) and diastolic blood pressure (–9 vs. +3 mm Hg, p <.05), investigators reported decrease in total cholesterol (–15 vs. +4 mg/dL, p <.01), triglyceride (TG) (–24 vs. +9 mg/dL, p <.001), and low-density lipoprotein (LDL) (–20 vs. +3 mg/dL, p ≤.01), and increases in high-density lipoprotein (HDL) (+4 vs. –1 mg/dL, p <.05) compared to controls. In addition, authors reported improvements in anxiety scores in those who practiced Tai Chi.[10]

Similarly, Lee studied the effects of Shuxinpingxuegong, a particular style of Qi Gong developed in China specifically for circulatory system disease. About 36 individuals with essential hypertension (mean age 53, mean BP approximately 150/95, mean total cholesterol approximately 190 mg/dL) were randomized to either 8 weeks of Qi Gong or to usual care. Investigators reported significant decreases in blood pressure (–15/–12 mm Hg with Qi Gong vs. +1/+2 mm Hg with usual care, p <.01), decreases in total cholesterol (–10 vs. +1 mg/dL, p <.05), increases in HDL (+4 vs. 0 mg/dL, p <.01) and increases in apolipoprotein 1 (Apo-A1) (+27 vs. +2 mg/dL, p <.05).[20]

In a review article of Qi Gong and hypertension by Mayer, 70 studies were found examining Qi Gong for hypertension. Most, as mentioned above, came from conference proceedings, book excerpts, or informal reports. Many studies were incompletely described with varied levels of methodological detail, and most were not subject to peer-review. Of the 30 "representative" articles reviewed, 5 did report a randomized design. Reported improvements included blood pressure, microcirculation, blood flow, blood viscosity, platelet aggregation, left ventricular function, and lipid profile.[21]

Coronary heart disease

As with hypertension, relatively few studies are available specifically in patients with known coronary disease. However, the existing literature suggests that Tai Chi/Qi Gong may be a viable option for cardiac rehabilitation. Two older, yet classic studies investigated patients after cardiac ischemic events.

Channer randomized 126 patients 3 weeks after discharge following an acute myocardial infarction to one of three groups: Tai Chi/Qi Gong, a conventional aerobic "exercise to music" group, or a nonexercise cardiac support group. Patients attended Tai Chi/Qi Gong class twice a week for 3 weeks, then once a week for the remaining 5 weeks. Mean baseline blood pressure was approximately 133/84. At the end of 8 weeks, investigators reported significant within group decreases in systolic blood pressure similarly in both exercise groups, and decreases in diastolic blood pressure only with Tai Chi (each p <.01). In addition, the Tai Chi group showed a trend in decreasing resting HR. Compliance was higher with Tai Chi compared to aerobic exercise (82% vs. 73%), while attendance at support groups was poor (8%).

In a smaller study of 20 patients, Lan examined individuals after coronary artery bypass graft surgery that had completed a postoperative Phase II conventional cardiac rehabilitation program. They were then assigned to either a 1-year Tai Chi program or a home-based exercise program that included walking at a nearby park. After 1 year of training, the Tai Chi group showed significant improvements in cardiorespiratory function, with 10.3% increase in peak VO_2 (p <.05), 11% increase in peak Work rate (p <.05), while the control group had no change or slight decreases in function. Compliance was greater with Tai Chi.

More recently, in Stenlund's study, 95 elder patients with documented coronary artery disease were randomized to either a 12-week Qi Gong and group education class or to usual care. Classes consisted of 1 hour Qi Gong and 2 hours of group discussion on various topics related to cardiac disease in the elderly. At the end of 12 weeks, patients increased their self-reported activity levels (p =.01) and showed improvements in the right-sided one leg stance (p = .03), box climb test (p = .04), stand and flex tests (p = .02), as measures of balance and coordination. Fear of falling did not change, although most reported never or very seldom having fear at baseline. Unfortunately, this study is unable to discern effects from group education from that of Qi Gong.[22]

Congestive heart failure

There have only been a handful of studies of Tai Chi/Qi Gong specifically in patients with heart failure. The most promising evidence comes from a recent report by Yeh.[8] In this study, 30 patients with chronic stable heart failure were randomized to either 12 weeks Tai Chi class as adjunct to usual care, or to usual care alone (per American College of Cardiology guidelines). Patients attended class twice a week and received a videotape for home practice. Classes taught Qi Gong warm-up exercises as well as five classical Tai Chi movements. At the end of 12 weeks, investigators reported statistically significant improvements in exercise capacity (+85 vs. −51 m change in 6-minute walk distance, $p = .001$) and disease specific quality of life (−17 vs. +8 change in Minnesota Living with Heart Failure score, lower is better, $p = .001$) in the Tai Chi group as compared to controls. In addition, improvements were seen in serum B-type natriuretic peptide (−48 vs. +90 pg/mL change, $p = .03$), suggesting a beneficial decrease in cardiac filling pressures. Trends were seen in improvement of peak VO_2, although the study was not sufficiently powered to detect statistically significant differences. Importantly, compliance was very good, with 83% attendance, and most patients intended to continue with Tai Chi after the study was over. This trial extends the earlier work of Fontana who reported similar improvements in quality of life and exercise capacity with a 12-week intervention in a prospective cohort of five heart failure patients.[23]

Research in other mind-body therapies lends support that meditative practices, even without the physical component, can have beneficial effects in this population. For example, in a small study by Curiati, patients with heart failure were randomized to group meetings plus instruction in meditation (audiotape for home practice), or group meetings alone. At the end of 8 weeks, those in the meditation group had improvements in norepinephrine (678–387 pg/mL, $p = .008$), Minnesota Living with Heart Failure score (33–22 points, lower is better, $p = .02$), minute ventilation-carbon dioxide slope (31–28, $p = .04$), while those in the control group had no change. No between group differences, however, were seen in left ventricular ejection fraction, left ventricular end-diastolic volume index, and VO_2.[24]

CARDIOVASCULAR EFFECTS IN THE GENERAL POPULATION

Exercise testing, exercise physiology

Several nonrandomized or observational studies have compared seasoned Tai Chi practitioners to their non-Tai Chi age-matched counterparts, finding improved exercise physiology (e.g., increased peak VO_2 on treadmill or bicycle stress testing). Other studies have measured VO_2 and hemodynamics during Tai Chi to quantify exercise intensity. Studies have estimated Tai Chi to be about 2.6–4.6 metabolic equivalents (or low-moderate intensity aerobic exercise) and between 50 and 74% maximal heart rate reserve.

In a classic, but nonrandomized study conducted in Taiwan, Lai followed those who had practiced Tai Chi for about 6 years to an age and body-size matched non-Tai Chi control group. After 2 years, investigators showed that those who practiced Tai Chi had a statistically significant decreased rate of "age-related" decline in exercise capacity (2.8% vs. 6.6% decrease in VO_2max in men, 2.9% vs. 7.4% decrease in women, both comparisons $p < .05$).

In another nonrandomized study conducted in Taiwan, Lan studied 38 community-dwelling seniors who had not engaged in any regular exercise for at least 5 years. Half participated in a 1-hour early morning Tai Chi program held in Taipei parks for 1 year. The other half served as a usual activity control group. At the end of the study, those who practiced Tai Chi had a significant improvement in VO_2max, oxygen pulse and work rate (all measures of exercise capacity on cardiopulmonary stress testing, each $p < .05$), knee flexor-extensor muscle strength ($p < .05$), and thoracolumbar flexibility (+10 vs. −1.0 degrees, $p < .05$), as compared to the controls.

A recent meta-analysis by Taylor-Piliae (the only meta-analysis in the Tai Chi literature) included seven clinical trials. Using peak VO_2 as the common outcome variable, this study concluded that Tai Chi may improve aerobic exercise capacity. The greatest benefit was seen from classical Yang style when performed for 1 year by otherwise sedentary adults.[25]

Blood pressure and heart rate

A few studies have measured the longitudinal effects of Tai Chi/Qi Gong on blood pressure in normotensive individuals. For example, Thornton studied 34 relatively inactive middle-aged Chinese women assigned to either 12 weeks of Tai Chi or to usual activity, reporting decreases in both systolic and diastolic blood pressure (−9.7 and 7.5 mm Hg, respectively) and improvements in functional reach and flexibility. Baseline blood pressure in these women was in the normal range (mean 122/80 mm Hg). Authors suggest that Tai Chi may be a viable option for healthy aging, given prognostic significance of elevated blood pressure in later life.[26] The immediate clinical significance of the blood pressure changes in normotensive individuals, however, is unclear.

Other studies have examined the acute effects of Tai Chi on blood pressure and heart rate. Perhaps not surprisingly, most effects reported are what one would expect with conventional exercise. Heart rate increases steadily with Tai Chi until a "maximal" steady state is achieved (usually 50–74% of maximal heart rate on bicycle or treadmill stress test). Blood pressure also may increase acutely in response to the physical aerobic activity. A few studies have reported that Tai Chi practitioners have a more rapid return to baseline resting values after exercise.

On the other hand, Lee has reported acute effects of Qi Gong training that is more similar to what one would expect with quiet, motionless meditation. In a small observational trial, 12 healthy volunteers were studied during Korean Qi-training (ChunDoSunBup). The session involved 10 minutes of sound exercise (reciting "meaningless words"), 10 minutes of movement, and

40 minutes of sitting meditation. Investigators reported significant decreases in blood pressure, heart rate, and respiratory rate during training and 10 minutes after training.[27]

Heart rate variability

Recently, power spectral analysis of heart rate variability has emerged as a primary outcome measure in several studies, with growing interest in modulation of autonomic tone as a potential mechanism of mind-body therapies. As discussed previously, healthy states are associated with sympathovagal balance, whereas states of stress trigger sympathetic overactivation and dominance. In cardiac conditions, such as heart failure, this sympathetic overdrive is at the root of disease. Increased heart rate variability suggests an increase in vagal (or parasympathetic) tone, and shift toward a more healthy autonomic balance.

In an observational trial by Väänänen, electrocardiographic recordings were taken while older and younger Tai Chi practitioners performed two sessions of Tai Chi. Acute increases in time domain measures of heart rate variability were seen in both groups (5% increase in R-R interval [RRI] in older group, p <.01; 61% increase in standard deviation of N-N intervals (SDNN) in younger group, p <.001; 143% increase in total variance of N-N intervals (TV) in younger group, p <.001). More prominent changes were seen in the young.

In Lee's trial, both Qi Gong practitioners and non-Qi Gong practitioners performed "Qi training" (meditation with frequency-controlled respiration of 7.5 breaths/minute). Frequency domain measures of heart rate variability acutely increased in both groups (increase in high-frequency (HF) component, p <.01; decrease in low-frequency/high-frequency (LF/HF) ratio, p <.001), although effects in Qi Gong practitioners were enhanced. The results in non-Qi Gong practitioners suggest that certain Qi Gong techniques may have powerful and immediate effects even in those with minimal training.[27]

Balance, strength, flexibility

Much evidence is available for Tai Chi's beneficial effects on measures of balance, strength, and flexibility. Several trials have examined risk and frequency of falls and fear of falling in community elders. In one of the largest and classic Tai Chi studies by Wolf, 200 seniors >70 years of age were randomized to receive either Tai Chi classes, a computerized balance training program, or education classes. At the end of 15 weeks, investigators reported lowered systolic blood pressure, improvements in grip strength and lower extremity range of motion, increased psychosocial well-being, decreased fear of falling, and decreased risk of multiple falls by 48% (p = .01). Interestingly, many Tai Chi participants provided anecdotal testimony of aborted fall events, citing newly acquired awareness of environment and compensatory body maneuvers during unexpected disturbances.[28]

A more recent trial by Li compared Tai Chi to non-meditative stretching exercises in 256 older adults >70 years of age. Participants attended class three times a week. At the end of 6 months, investigators, as in the Wolf study, reported fewer falls (38 vs. 73, $p = .007$), reduced fear of falling ($p < .001$), and decreased risk of multiple falls by 55% (RR = .45, 95% CI 0.3–0.7) in the Tai Chi group as compared to control. Investigators also reported Tai Chi-related improvements in functional balance (Berg Balance Scale, Dynamic Gait Index, functional reach, single-leg stand, each $p < .001$) and physical performance (50-foot speed walk, Up and Go test, each $p < .001$).[29]

HOW TO REFER PATIENTS TO TAI CHI/QI GONG

By now, we hope to have established the general rationale for how, when, and why Tai Chi/Qi Gong may be useful in the holistic plan of treatment of patients with CVD and the evidence supporting such a referral. So if you have decided to refer a patient for such an intervention, how do you go about finding a reliable and competently trained practitioner?

Such a person may not necessarily be a health-care professional. He or she may be a Tai Chi martial arts instructor with many years of experience in the physical movement aspect of Tai Chi, which at the master level, also includes Qi Gong. He or she may also have come about their training in a variety of ways but most typically by serving as a student of a Tai Chi master for a minimum of 5–7 years or longer.

Although there are many excellent books and videos available, some aspects of Tai Chi or Qi Gong may be harmful if practiced incorrectly. Thus, it is wise, at least initially, to seek help from a qualified master/teacher who can provide guidance. Finding a qualified teacher is an important decision that can be challenging, however. Currently in the United States, there is no formal or standardized credentialing of Tai Chi/Qi Gong masters. One must therefore sometimes rely on word of mouth or other sources such as local TCM colleges or universities (A list of accredited programs may be found at: www. aomalliance.org).

Practitioners of TCM also study Tai Chi/Qi Gong in their 3–4 year course of training and certification. This professional degree program also includes acupuncture, Chinese herbal medicine, massage, and other elements of traditional practice. Many of these practitioners include classes or Tai Chi/Qi Gong as a complement to their clinical practices and patients may find this a suitable locale for training. Specific requirements for credentialing TCM providers vary from state to state. Even though an individual licensed TCM practitioner may not be a fully trained Qi Gong or Tai Chi master, they are often excellent sources of information and may be instrumental in helping patients locate a qualified teacher. TCM training programs in the United States have a standardized, clinically based curriculum and are formally accredited by the Accreditation Commission for Acupuncture and Oriental Medicine.[30] In addition, a nonprofit organization, the National Certification Commission for Acupuncture and Oriental Medicine,[31] was established in 1982 to promote nationally recognized standards of competence and safety. A list of questions patients should ask when trying to locate an appropriate Tai Chi or Qi Gong master/teacher is provided in Table 13-3.

Some practitioners may request an initial consultation with the patient prior to starting classes, which is an excellent idea. In patients with established or advanced CVD, it is prudent that either the referring clinician or the patient have a conversation with the instructor prior to initiating a program. In some cases, this should detail the person's condition, any limitations, and goals of therapy, and expectations, much as would be done in a physical therapy or other rehabilitation prescription. This is advisable even though Tai Chi/Qi Gong activities are low in cardiac stress, some susceptible patients may develop symptoms or even ECG changes with active practice.

Many senior centers, YMCA's, community centers, fitness clubs, and rehabilitation programs incorporate Tai Chi classes into their panel of services. While the quality and training of their instructors may vary, for general purposes, accessibility, and low cost, such programs are highly useful, increasingly popular, and widely available. If such a program does not exist in your hospital or community, consider recruiting a qualified Tai Chi/Qi Gong-trained instructor to start one. For public classes, support of the teacher and provision of space by a hospital or clinic can facilitate enrollment and access by keeping tuition minimal. This may be especially important for seniors, who are most likely to benefit from tuition support. As with many other aspects of medical practice and referral, you will soon determine the quality and acceptability of the instructor to your community and patients.

Another route to consider is the wide availability of videotapes, DVDs, and books offering Tai Chi/Qi Gong instruction. These have the benefit of providing

TABLE 13-3

QUESTIONS TO ASK WHEN CHOOSING A MASTER/TEACHER IN TAI CHI/ QI GONG

- What are the credentials of the person and/or organization(s) supporting the training? Is the teacher a recognized Master of Tai Chi/Qi Gong? How long has s/he been practicing?
- What form or style of Tai Chi/Qi Gong is taught? Can s/he explain the applications of each form?
- What is the recommended training schedule?
- What are the costs of the training?
- What is the teacher's background/experience with cardiovascular disorders? Will s/he work with your primary physician to integrate your Tai Chi/ Qi Gong training into an overall treatment regimen?

low-cost instruction in the privacy of a patient's home. The absence of the social support and feedback to correct postures and breathing techniques by the instructor may affect compliance and motivation however. It is difficult for most patients to learn the movements of Tai Chi from a series of still pictures in a book as they rarely can capture the graceful fluidity of the movements. On the other hand, these electronic and print resources may be a good starter for some patients and the only resource in rural or remote areas where an instructor is not available. A useful catalog for such materials is Redwing Books (www.redwing-books.com).

Finally, for personal and professional reasons, you may wish to invest the time and effort in Tai Chi/Qi Gong training yourself. Our best advice is to find a reputable Tai Chi master and to commit yourself to regular daily practice over a period of several years. While you probably can start teaching some basics to patients within a few months, in-depth training, and significant impact on your own physical and mental well-being will take some years. Be patient. It is well worth the effort.

CONCLUSION

As we have seen, there is a growing body of literature on Tai Chi and Qi Gong in cardiovascular health. The best support for its cardiovascular effects has been found on blood pressure, heart rate, heart rate variability and autonomic tone, exercise physiology, and lipids. Additionally, benefits on balance, strength, and flexibility are all relevant to cardiac rehabilitation.

There is also a more limited but growing literature on Tai Chi use in specific cardiac populations such as chronic heart failure (CHF) examining not only cardiac parameters, but also disease-specific quality of life measures such as mood. Furthermore, the benefits of compliance and exercise self-efficacy are important as studies have consistently shown that maintenance of an exercise program is essential to maintaining beneficial effects. Tai Chi and Qi Gong appear to be enjoyable activities that people will continue to do.

The mechanisms of action are increasingly better understood and plausible. Afferent effects on the hypothalamic-pituitary-adrenal axis by mediation of stress through the mind-body, relaxation component are clearly a factor. Efferent effects on sympathovagal tone are demonstrated by changes in blood pressure and heart rate variability. Improvement in oxygen consumption and respiratory efficiency through breathing exercises and general conditioning through Tai Chi movements parallel benefits in other forms of mild to moderate aerobic exercise.

In summary, Tai Chi and Qi Gong have promising benefits across the spectrum of cardiovascular disease from primary prevention to rehabilitation. They should be considered by physicians and other providers who are informed of the scientific support as presented here. Such referrals must be coupled with the usually high degree of patient acceptability. They are most likely to be beneficial when Tai Chi/Qi Gong methods are taught by well-trained teachers.

REFERENCES

1. Whitmer RA, et al. Midlife cardiovascular risk factors and risk of dementia in late life. Neurology. 2005;64:277–81. [PMID: 15668425.]

2. Taylor-Pilae RE, Haskell WL, Stotts NA, Froelicher ES. Improvement in balance, strength, and flexibility after 12 weeks of Tai Chi exercise in ethnic Chinese adults with cardiovascular disease risk factors. Altern Ther Health Med. 2006 Mar–Apr; 12(2):50–8.

3. Motivala, Sarosh J. Tai Chi Chih acutely decreases sympathetic nervous system activity in older adults. The journals of gerontology. Series A, Biological sciences and medical sciences. 2006;61(11):1177.

4. Audette, Joseph F. Tai Chi versus brisk walking in elderly women. Age and ageing. 2006;35(4):388.

5. Wolf, Steven L. The influence of intense Tai Chi training on physical performance and hemodynamic outcomes in transitionally frail, older adults. The journals of gerontology. Series A, Biological sciences and medical sciences. 2006;61(2):184.

6. Arthur, Heather M. The role of complementary and alternative therapies in cardiac rehabilitation: a systematic evaluation. European journal of cardiovascular prevention and rehabilitation. 2006;13(1):3.

7. Taylor-Piliae, Ruth E. Hemodynamic responses to a community-based Tai Chi exercise intervention in ethnic Chinese adults with cardiovascular disease risk factors. European journal of cardiovascular nursing: journal of the Working Group on Cardiovascular Nursing of the European Society of Cardiology. 2006;5(2):165.

8. Hogan M. Physical and cognitive activity and exercise for older adults: a review. Int J Aging Human Dev. 2005;60(2):95–126. [PMID: 15801385.]

9. Li F, et al. Tai Chi, self-efficacy, and physical function in the elderly. Prev Sci. 2001;2:229–39. [PMID: 11833926.]

10. Tsai JC, Wang WH, Chan P, et al. The beneficial effects of Tai Chi Chuan on blood pressure and lipid profile and anxiety status in a randomized controlled trial. J Altern Complement Med. 2003;9:747–54. [PMID: 14629852.]

11. Väänänen J, et al. Taiqiquan acutely increases heart rate variability. Clin Physiol Func Im. 2002;22:2–3. [PMID: 12003094.]

12. Wu G. Evaluation of the effectiveness of Tai Chi for improving balance and preventing falls in the older population—a review. J Am Geriat Soc. 2002;50(4):746–54. [PMID: 11982679.]

13. Chao YF, et al. The cardiorespiratory response and energy expenditure of Tai-Chi-Qui-Gong. Am J Chinese Med. 2002;3(4):451–61. [PMID: 12568273.]

14. Yeh GY, et al. Effects of Tai Chi mind-body movement therapy on functional status and exercise capacity in patients with chronic heart failure: a randomized controlled trial. Am J Med. 2004;117:541–8. [PMID: 15465501.]

15. Wong SS, et al. National center for complementary and alternative medicine perspectives for complementary and alternative medicine research in cardiovascular diseases. Cardiol Rev. 2003;11:94–8. [PMID: 12620133.]

16. Klein P, et al. Comprehensive therapeutic benefits of Taiji: a critical review. Am J Phys Med Rehabil. 2004;83:735–45. [PMID: 15314540.]

17. Taylor-Piliae RE. Tai Chi as an adjunct to cardiac rehabilitation exercise training. J Cardiopulm Rehabil. 2003;23:90–6. [PMID: 12668929.]

18. Verhagen AP, et al. The efficacy of Tai Chi Chuan in older adults: a systematic review. Fam Pract. 2004;21:107–13. [PMID: 14760055.]

19. Wang C, et al. The effect of Tai Chi on health outcomes in patients with chronic conditions: a systematic review. Arch Intern Med. 2004;164:493–501. [PMID: 15006825.]
20. Lee MS, et al. Effects of Qi Gong on blood pressure, high-density lipoprotein cholesterol and other lipid levels in essential hypertension patients. Int J Neurosci. 2004;114:777–86. [PMID: 15204043.]
21. Mayer M. Qi Gong and hypertension: a critique of research. J Altern Complement Med. 1999;5:371–82. [PMID: 10471018.]
22. Stenlund T, et al. Cardiac rehabilitation for the elderly: Qi Gong and group discussions. Eur J Cardiovasc Prev Rehabil. 2005;12:5–11. [PMID: 15703500.]
23. Fontana JA, et al. Tai Chi chih as an intervention for heart failure. Nurs Clin North Am. 2000;35:1031–461. [PMID: 11072287.]
24. Curiati JA, et al. Meditation reduces sympathetic activation and improves the quality of life in elderly patients with optimally treated heart failure: a prospective randomized study. J Altern Complement Med. 2005;11:465–72. [PMID: 15992231.]
25. Taylor-Piliae RE, et al. Effectiveness of Tai Chi exercise in improving aerobic capacity: a meta-analysis. J Cardiovasc Nurs. 2004;19:48–57. [PMID: 14994782.]
26. Thornton EW, et al. Health benefits of Tai Chi exercise: improved balance and blood pressure in middle-aged women. Health Promot Int. 2004;19:33–8. [PMID: 14976170.]
27. Lee MS, et al. Effects of Qi-training on heart rate variability. Am J Chin Med. 2002;30:463–70. [PMID: 12568274.]
28. Wolf SL, et al; Atlanta FICSIT Group (Selected as the best paper in the 1990s). Reducing frailty and falls in older persons: an investigation of tai chi and computerized balance training. J Am Geriatr Soc. 2003;5:1794–1803. [PMID: 14687360.]
29. Li F. Tai Chi and fall reductions in older adults: a randomized controlled trial. J Gerontol A Biol Sci Med Sci. 2005;60:187–94. [PMID: 15814861.]
30. Accreditation Commission for Acupuncture and Oriental Medicine 2005 Handbook (2005). Greenbelt, MD. Accessed at http://acaom.org/handbook.htm.
31. National Certification Commission for Acupuncture and Oriental Medicine. (2004). General information brochure. NCCAOM. Accessed at http://www.nccaom.org/om_ first.htm on Oct. 11, 2005.

14

AN AYURVEDIC APPROACH TO CARDIOVASCULAR DISEASE

Shahla J. Modir and David C. Leopold

Ayurveda is the oldest system of natural medicine in the world. Originating over 4000 years ago, it is the root of the later Chinese and Greek medical systems. As the traditional healing system of India, it is the medical aspect of the Vedic spiritual traditions of India. The term *ayurveda* means knowledge or "science of life". It stems from the Sanskrit word *veda* meaning knowledge or science, and *ayus* meaning life, or life span. Ayurveda follows the principle that living in harmony with the universal elements is important across the life span, and there is a "logical and scientific" aspect to creating and maintaining this balance. When a person is not living in synchronization with the season, time of day, and dietary considerations, then disease can occur.[1–3]

On a more subtle level, Ayurveda views the body, mind, and soul (*atman*) of a person as interdependently connected to the universe. A disruption in the flow of life force or *prana* can create disease or imbalance. A state of *svastha*, a Sanskrit term for health, is not merely the absence of disease. Ayurveda believes that individuals in *svastha* will be connecting to their "higher" self-awareness and will make choices that create balance.[2]

HISTORY OF AYURVEDA

The Vedic texts are among the oldest recorded philosophy. They establish much of the philosophical and spiritual foundation of the religions of India. The *Caraka Samhita*, based on the fourth Vedic text, the *Arthava Veda*, is the foundation of Ayurvedic medicine. It describes the origins of disease, symptoms, physical findings, and treatment prescriptions that include diet, herbs, lifestyle, and disease prevention.[4] (See Table 14-1.)

TABLE 14-1

EIGHT LIMBS OF AYURVEDA

Internal medicine *Kaya chikitsa*	Head and neck disease *Shalakya tantra*
Surgery *Shalya*	Treatment of poisoning *Agada tantra*
Pediatrics *Kaumara bhritya*	Rejuvenation *Rasayana*
Aphrodisiacs (reproduction) *Vajikarana*	Psychology *Bhutavidya*

The first surgical text, the *Sushruta Samhita*, was written around 700 BC. It contains detailed information on operative procedures, surgical instruments and techniques. Over 700 herbal medicinal botanicals are mentioned, along with essential oils used in conjunction with massage and *marma* points which are similar to acupuncture points.[1-3] Over the last decade, several Ayurvedic training programs have emerged in the United States and Europe. Organizations such as the National Ayurvedic Medical Association are working to create regulation in the education provided to participants of these courses. As Ayurveda has become more popular in the West, the need for quality research has become imperative. However, research in Ayurveda is difficult for a number of reasons, including the fact that at basic level, the scientific principle of standardization of care goes against the fundamental belief of Ayurveda, which treats each person as unique and requiring individualized treatments.

CAUSE OF DISEASE

On a gross level, disease manifests in the individual as a state of mind-body discord called *doshic imbalance*. In Ayurveda, each person has a unique physical and mental makeup that is a microcosmic representation of the five universal elements. The quantity of each element or aggregated elements differs in each person. As a result, the psychological temperament, body structure, and predisposition to disease and treatment will be according to a person's individual constitution. Thus, prescribing the same treatment for a particular disease can be medicinal for one individual and have no response or may even cause worsening in another person. Specific dietary, lifestyle, and herbal prescriptions based on the mind-body constitutions, called *doshas* are essential to aligning the inner intelligence and natural healing ability of the individual.[1,2,5]

Pancha Maha Bhuti: the five element theory

The relationship of the microcosmic human to the universe is reflected through the five basic elements of air (*vayu*), fire (*teja*), water (*jala*), earth (*prithivi*), and ether or space (*akasha*). Each element has particular qualities inherent in its nature that manifest in the body. Air represents a cold, gaseous, mobile, unstable state. Fire represents heat, light, mobility, instability, and transformation. Water is cool, liquid, and mobile and earth is dense, thick, and stable. Ether is representative of space and is cold, light, unstable, and mobile.[2,3,5]

As an energetically dense expression, the five elements represent the seven tissues of the body called *dhatus*. The seven tissues or *dhatus* are *rasa* (plasma-like fluids), *rakta* (red blood cells), *mamsa* (muscle, ligaments), *medas* (fat, lubrication), *asthi* (bone), *majja* (nervous system), and *shukra* (sperm, ovaries). *Ojas* is the vital essence of all tissues, and is often considered the eighth dhatu.[6] When a disease occurs at a particular tissue level, it means that this disease has already affected all of the levels preceding it. It may become necessary to treat the disease at another dhatu levels to restore balance.[1]

Tridosha theory

In Ayurveda, the physiology of the human body is ruled by three forces known as the *doshas*. The three doshas, known as *vata*, *pitta*, and *kapha*, are three specific combinations of the five basic elements that create the psychophysiological characteristics of an individual based on their attributes.[2] *Vata* is made up of air and ether. *Pitta* is created from fire and water, and *kapha* is the combination of the elements water and earth. Each person has a unique "fingerprint" combination of the three doshas, called their *prakruti* or constitution. The prakruti is determined from the relative predominance of the doshas of the parents at the time of conception. The prakruti also predicts the types of diseases to which an individual will have a predisposition, as well as the treatments. One can have a prakruti with a relative dominance of any one dosha: vata, pitta, or kapha. It is also common to have a predominance of two doshas: vata-pitta, vata-kapha, or pitta-kapha. Rarely, there may be an equal distribution of all three doshas. All of the doshas have strengths and weakness inherent in their qualities, and there is no best dosha type. As individuals interface with the five elements in the universe through their five senses, this may lead to either harmony or disease. Increase and decrease of each dosha is also affected by diurnal, seasonal variations, and stage of life.[3,6] (See Fig. 14-1.)

The *vikruti* of an individual represents the current state of the three doshas.[5] If the vikruit is the same as the prakruti, then the person is balanced and healthy. When there is disease, the vikruti reflects a relative imbalance in the doshas and may illustrate how diet, lifestyle, emotions, age, and environment have impacted on the prakruti. The goal in Ayurveda is to maintain one's prakruti, as it is the most balanced expression of the doshas in the individual. Vata regulates all activity in the body and mind such as circulation, respiration, digestion, elimination, and physical movement. Vata is the primary force in the

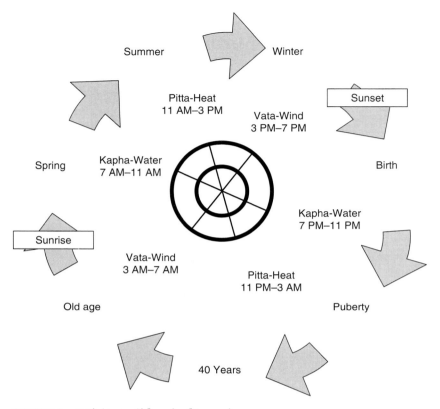

FIGURE 14-1   *Daily/season/life cycle of Ayurveda.*

nervous system, governing sensory and motor function. It controls the expulsion of feces, urine, sweat, menstrual fluid, semen, and the fetus. Individuals with vata predominance are easily excited and can be impulsive or fickle. They are prone to emotions of fear, insecurity, doubt, and worry when vata is in excess. Vata predominant individuals are often light weight with thin and dry tissues, skin, and hair. They may have small, dry eyes and irregular appetite and thirst. Although vata is present throughout the body and mind, its root is in the colon. Conditions of vata imbalance are arthritis, tremors, anxiety, constipation, flatulence, and insomnia.[1,2,4,5]

    The qualities of pitta are hot, sharp, light, liquid, mobile, and slightly oily, and it represents the principle of fire in the body. Pitta is responsible for the digestion and assimilation of physical and mental phenomenon in the body and mind through the metabolic activities of anabolism and catabolism. It is responsible for all the secretions of the gastrointestinal tract, the enzymes and hormones from the ductless glands, and for controlling body temperature. Individuals with pitta predominance have strong intellect, courage, confidence, articulation, organizing capacity, and natural leadership qualities. Emotions such as anger, jealousy, and hatred are signs of excess pitta in the mind, as is being judgmental and perfectionistic. In the physical body, pitta types will have a sensitive and reactive body with a medium frame and weight which is stable. Since pitta is sour and associated with red and yellow color, pitta individuals may have yellowing of teeth, and pungent odor to their bodily fluids. Pitta dosha is primarily located in the small intestine. Pitta is increased in the body/mind during middle age, late spring and summer season, and by consuming spicy "hot" foods, such as chili peppers. Conditions of pitta excess reflect an inflammatory or feverish quality such as heartburn, skin rashes, fevers, infections, and ulcers.[1,2,4,5]

The attributes of kapha are heavy, slow, dull, cold, oily, smooth, dense, sticky, and cloudy. It is responsible for all of the activities pertaining to growth, stability, moisture, and storage in the body. It is the principle of cohesion, structure, and lubrication. The physical structures of kapha are connective tissues, the myelin sheath, and senses of taste and smell. It also protects the digestive tract, respiratory tract, and lubricates the joints. Kapha also regulates water and fat, builds tissues, and aids in wound healing. Individuals with predominant kapha have a strong long-term memory, are tranquil, loyal, faithful, and have a natural capacity for forgiveness. Excess kapha in the mind leads to attachment, lethargy, depression, and greed. Kapha's primary location is in the lungs and upper stomach. It has maximum influence during childhood, and during winter and early spring. It can be increased during those vulnerable periods, but also with the intake of heavy, moist foods such as ice cream. Conditions caused by an imbalanced kapha dosha are obesity, lethargy, diabetes, swelling, and excessive mucus production.[1,2,4,5] (See Table 14-2.)

The activity of the body is governed by the doshas, and this is mediated onto the dhatus or tissues in part through an individual's *agni*. Agni refers to "biofire," or the digestive power of the body and mind to metabolize inputs from emotional and sensory impressions to food. As tissues interact with the doshas through the biofire of agni, metabolic waste is generated. This waste is called *mala*, and each tissue level has a specific waste product associated. Unprocessed waste products can become *ama*, energetic, toxic "sludge" that can obstruct the flow through the communicating dosha channels or *srotas* and cause disease.[2,5] Ama and mala build-up in the body will cause disease through slowing or obstructing the movement of the doshas to the tissues or dhatus. In Ayurveda, a balanced state of health is when the doshas, dhatus, and mala are in harmony.[6]

Six stages of disease: Kriyakala

There are six stages in the pathophysiology of disease in Ayurveda that develop according to the build-up and movement of the doshas. The first two stages of disease are called accumulation and aggravation.[2,5] They represent an increase of the dosha in its respective home sites; vata in the colon, pitta in the small intestine, and kapha in the lungs. This will lead to symptoms in these organs and the corresponding tissues according to which dosha is increased. If preventative lifestyle behaviors and purification interventions are performed, the disease can be eliminated at the aggravation stage.

TABLE 14-2

DAILY/SEASON/LIFE CYCLE OF AYURVEDA

	Vata	Pitta	Kapha
Elements	Space and air	Fire and water	Earth and water
Attributes	Dry, cold, unstable, quick, light	Hot, fluid, moist, sharp, intense	Heavy, cold, wet, slow, smooth, oily
Mental	Creative, imagination, indecisive	Intelligent, confident, leader	Memory, tranquil, devotion
Emotions	Exhilaration, fear, insecure	Excitement, anger, jealous	Love, patience, greed
Physical imbalance	Emaciation, decrease energy Severe acute pains, LBP, arthritis Chapped lips, skin Constipated, gas IBS HTN Intolerance to wind and cold, dysmenorrheal	Increased hunger, thirst GERD Ulcers Heat intolerance Hot flashes Skin inflammation Rash, acne Sour body odor Halitosis Rectal burn Sunburn Bloodshot eyes	Congested chest, throat Nasal congestion Mucous cough Pharyngitis Colds Poor cold tolerance, dampness Allergy, asthma Obesity Hypercholesterolemia Edema Pale cold skin Cysts Diabetes
Mental imbalances	Mind too active Poor relaxation Anxious Worry Restless Impatient Depressed Insomnia Fatigue Anorexia	Hostile Irritable Anger Rage Impatient Self-other critical Arrogant Aggressive and domineering	Lethargy Dull Oversleep Daytime sleepy Depressed Complacent Procrastination Over attachment Greed Possessiveness

(Continued)

TABLE 14-2

DAILY/SEASON/LIFE CYCLE OF AYURVEDA (*CONTINUED*)

	Vata	Pitta	Kapha
Foods to avoid	Dried fruits Raw fruits Dried, froze, raw veggies Barley Granola Dried grains	Sour fruits Pungent veggies Hot peppers Yeast Dry oats	Sweet and sour fruits Sweet and juicy veggies Cooked oats
Foods to use	Sweet fruits Soaked raisins, prunes Cooked veggies Cooked oats Quinoa	Sweet fruits Sweet and bitter veggies Cooked oats Basmati rice Barley	Apples Dry figs Prunes Raisins Pungent and bitter veggies Barley Buckwheat Dry oats Corn Quinoa

However, if no alleviating procedures are followed, these aggravated doshas will overflow and relocate in a weak tissue, organ, or channel and begin to amalgamate. The doshas may settle in a site that has been injured previously or one that is constitutionally prone to weakness by the qualities inherent within the overflowing dosha. In the manifestation stage, symptoms of a specific disease appear. As the doshic disturbance moves into the deeper stages, it becomes harder to manage and more difficult to treat. As the disease process continues untreated, the manifested disease begins to diversify and differentiate. This can lead to the final stage of chronicity and convalescence and that is why prevention is such an important part of Ayurveda.[1,2,5]

Diagnosis

Diagnosis in Ayurveda includes a detailed history and an eightfold physical exam or *ashtavidha pariksha*. It is important to first determine the individual constitution or prakruti before looking for the vikruti or state of current imbalance.[2] This requires taking a history of the long-term patterns of appetite, digestion, urination, sweat, menstruation, sexual function, and general energy level. Examining the *nadi* (pulse), *jihva* (tongue), *shabda* (speech), *sparsha* (touch), *drig* (eyes), and *akruti* (general form) is also completed.[5] It is essential to inquire as to whether these physical and historical traits are a long or short-term tendency to tease out the prakruti from the vikruti. The mental and emotional nature with respect to memory, mood, and sleep should be assessed.

The pulse is an essential component to the Ayurvedic assessment. There are seven levels of pulse that can be palpated. The superficial level expresses the present, imbalanced condition of the doshas or vikruti, and the second, deeper palpation, conveys disturbances in the mental doshas. The third level shows the condition of the subtypes of the doshas, and the fourth level expresses the condition of the subtle, refined essences of the dhatus (tissues). The general condition of the seven dhatus or tissues can be determined at the fifth. The sixth level can reveal the baseline, mental constitution, and the seventh, deepest level of the pulse expresses prakruti, the individual's overall basic constitution.[5] Thus, the original state of the doshas can be read from the pulse, as well as the vikruti. However, the pulse can be affected by many external factors, such as diet, time of day, and season, and it important to have the ability to integrate a reading with respect to many factors.[2]

The tongue is another important site for a practitioner to read the condition of the organs in body and digestive system. Vata, pitta, and kapha will have differing qualities in their tongue according to each respective dosha that can be useful for both prakruti and vikruti. A vata tongue is thin, small, brownish, and may be a little dry, with a fine tremor or twitching. A pitta tongue is broad at the base and tapered at the apex with a red tip and margins that are distinct and sharp. It may have a yellowish or reddish discoloration. A kapha tongue is moist, large, round, glossy, thick, and relatively pale, and it occupies the whole oral cavity.[2,5]

Treatment

After assessing the prakruti and the current state of doshic imbalance, the vikruti, a unique treatment plan is designed to return the individual back to their natural state of balance (*prakruti*). Ayurvedic treatments have the effect of bringing the five elements into the body in a way that will counterbalance the doshic state of excess by prescribing remedies that possess the opposite qualities. For example, if vata dosha is increased in the digestive tract, causing gas and constipation due to its light and dry qualities, then substances that have the inherent qualities of being warm and moist will be prescribed.

The treatment in Ayurveda consists of two main types. One form is called *shamana chikitsa* or palliation, used to subdue the vitiated or excess doshas.[2] Shamana uses a multilevel approach including a dosha-specific diet, medicinal herb-mineral preparations, bodywork, and physical exercise. Mind-body exercises such as the breathing technique called pranayama, meditation, and yoga, along with daily/seasonal routines are also emphasized. When doshas are *vitiated* (agitated) they give rise to various toxins (ama), that accumulate in the body. To purify the build up, a second type of treatment, *shodhana chikitsa* or cleansing therapy, is indicated.[2] The process of panchakarma will pull the excess doshas and ama out of the body by means of the sweat glands, urinary tract, and intestines and into their sites of origin for elimination. The five cleansing therapies are preceded by a preparation period called *purvakarma* and followed up by a rejuvenation treatment. The five cleansing therapies include:

1. *Vamana*: therapeutic vomiting or emesis
2. *Virechana*: purgation through laxatives
3. *Basti*: enemas; detoxifying and nutritive
4. *Nasya*: elimination of toxins through the nose
5. *Rakta moksha*: detoxification of the blood through blood letting

Diet is an important preventative and treatment strategy in Ayurveda. There are six distinct tastes sweet, sour, pungent, bitter, salty, and astringent that are composed of the five elements.[1,5] Based on the intake of the six tastes, the doshas, agni (digestive fire), and dhatus will be increased or decreased. The dietary prescriptions in Ayurveda use this concept to help alleviate imbalanced doshas, returning an individual to an improved state of health, and enabling them to maintain it. Optimum health is obtained through counterbalancing the excess or deficiency with tastes that have an opposite or similar quality. There are several books on Ayurveda containing lists of foods for particular doshas emphasizing the qualities of different types of foods. Thus, if any dosha is increased in the body, it can be reduced by taking in substances with the opposite qualities. If any of the dosha attributes are deficient, they can be supplemented by taking in substances having similar properties. (See Table 14-3.)

Psycho-spiritual treatment

In Ayurveda, the body and mind are interconnected through a subtle energetic matrix. There are several forms of pranayama, yoga, and meditation that are used for different doshas to activate or dissipate the energy. An Ayurvedic specialist can assist in creating this prescription and teaching the techniques.

Pranayama is translated as "prana" or "breathe control."[5] In the Yoga Sutras, the practices of pranayama and yoga postures called *asanas* are considered to be the highest form of purification and self-discipline for the mind and the body. (See Table 14-4.)

TABLE 14-3

BALANCING TASTES FOR EACH DOSHA

Vata	Pitta	Kapha
Heavy/sweet	Cold/sweet	Light/pungent
Oily/sour	Heavy/bitter	Dry/bitter
Hot/salt	Dry/astringent	Hot/astringent

TABLE 4-4

TYPES OF YOGA

Type	Description	Patient Type
Ashtanga or power yoga	A flowing yoga with continuous physical postures or exercises, known as asanas that can be physically demanding. It is best suited for kapha types, however pitta types will be the people most drawn to the challenge.	Hypertension (mild) Dyslipidemia Obesity Diabetes (controlled and stable)
Bikram yoga	Contains a series of 26 asanas (postures) practiced in a 105 degree room in order to warm and stretch the muscles, ligaments, and tendons and to detoxify the body through sweat. This yoga is not suited for pitta disorders, but most beneficial for vata.	Not recommended for cardiovascular patients due to heat. May be considered in mild-moderate and hypertension and dyslipdemia
Hatha yoga	Most commonly practiced form of yoga in the United States today that emphasizes balancing the opposites in one's life. During *Hatha yoga* sessions, flexing is followed by extension, a rounded back is followed by an arched back, and physical exercises are followed by mental meditations. This yoga is best suited for vata and pitta types due to its grounding nature.	Hypertension (mild–severe) Recent and post-MI CHF NYHA I–IV Diabetes mellitus Anxiety and GAD Hostility and anger Depressive disorders
Iyengar yoga	This yoga often requires the use of props such as blocks and belts while performing postures and emphasizes great attention to detail and precise alignment.	HTN mild–moderate Recent and post-MI Hostility amd anger Diabetes mellitus

Specific cardiac disorders

In the classical Ayurvedic text, the *Caraka Samhita*, heart disease is known as *hrdro-ga*, and it has five causes: vata, pitta, kapha, sannipatika (tri-doshic disturbance), and parasites.[4,7] Some of the disorders will require panchakarma and referral to an Ayurvedic specialist will help to determine if this is necessary. It is best to refer to centers that have physician supervision to ensure the safety of the cardiac patient.

VATA-TYPE HRDROGA

The *nidana* or etiology of vata-type hrdroga includes emotional grief, excessive fasting, excessive exercise, failure to regularly void, and persistent, high intake of dry and light foods. From the Ayurvedic perspective, grief creates excess space in heart, which can be filled with vata.

Patients may describe feelings of a "heart that feels torn" or describe a "tearing" type of chest pain. Patients may present with trembling, cramping, syncope, or describe feelings of emotional emptiness. The pulse may be weak, rapid, and irregularly irregular, indicative of a disturbance of the vata dosha.[7]

The *chikitsa* or treatment includes warm, moist, and oily treatments both internally and externally. This may include the use of oleation followed by fomentation. *Oleation* or *snehan* involves the use of herbal medicated oils applied externally through a variety of different massage techniques and/or oils taken internally to help loosen and liquefy toxins from the body. After oleation, *fomentation* or sweating therapy will help to expel excess vata. This is done most commonly by the use of a sweat box where steam made from a boiling medicinal decoction is pumped into a box in which the patient is sitting.[1] Another form of steam therapy may be the use of a herbal wrap. An individual should also be placed on a vata-reducing diet, emphasizing warm, moist, cooked foods.[7]

The Ayurvedic herbs *bala* (*Sida cordifola*) and *arjuna* (*Terminalia arjuna*) may be given alone or in combination. In the United States, *Sida cordifola* known as Country Mallow has been banned due to ephedrine components. Herbs may be mixed with medicated oils or ghee (clarified butter). Further recommendations depend on the overall strength of the patient, and may include *bastis* (enemas) that contain dosha-specific oil that has been decocted with herbs, called *anuvasana basti*.[7] The goal of this treatment is to help to decrease vata at its origin in the colon.

Lifestyle considerations are also significant. Vata disorders may reflect a lifestyle of constant change with a variable pattern in the daily routine, and a diet of light and dry foods. Balancing through consistent daily routines surrounding sleep, hygiene, and eating can be beneficial, as is the self-observation and contemplation on issues of self-love, and practicing self-nourishing behaviors. Transcendental meditation and hatha yoga will help to calm the mind of the vata person.

PITTA-TYPE HRDROGA

According to Ayurveda, the pitta-type hrdroga occurs in patients with a high intake of hot, sour, salty, strongly alkaline or acidic, and heavy foods. Excessive intake of alcohol, regular feelings of hostility, and an intense and stressful lifestyle can also result in pitta-type hrdroga.[7] Patients will often complain of a bitter taste in the mouth, excessive thirst, feelings of exhaustion, burning chest pains, and excessive perspiration.[1,4,7]

In accordance with the treatment of opposite qualities, the ingestion and application of cool substances, such as medicated ghee with arjuna, is recommended. Additional herbs that may be added are utpala (*Saussurea lappa*), madhuka (*Basia latifolia*), pundarika (*Vangueria sponosa*), and kuvalaya (*Beinicasa cerifera*).[8] Traditional recommendation included the ingestion of small amounts of metal *bhasmas*, medicinal preparations of fine metals, but these are unavailable for use in the United States.

Further treatment will include following a pitta-reducing diet, decreasing intensity and perfectionism in the lifestyle, and meditation. Herbs to reduce irritability and critical emotions that may be part of the pitta hrdroga include Gotu kola (*Centella asiatica*) and brahmi (*Bacopa monneri*). Self-observation and reflection for pitta will include the contemplation of "why am I angry, and, what am I striving for?" In addition, working on forgiveness, compassion, and surrender of control are deeper psycho-spiritual issues for pitta hrdroga. Practicing transcendental meditation, lunar pranayama, and hatha yoga will all serve to decrease the excess pitta called *tejas* in the mind.[7]

KAPHA-TYPE HRDROGA

The nidana of kapha heart disease is excessive intake of heavy and oily foods. A sedentary lifestyle, excess sleep, and inadequate mental stimulation may also predispose to kapha heart disease.[1,4,7]

Rupa or symptoms include feelings of heaviness in the chest and sluggishness. Patients may present as bradycardic and complain of stiffness, drowsiness, and anorexia. Treatments include using dry, light, and warm substances. The herbs arjuna and triphala are usually prepared as a powder to improve circulation. Other herbs added to the formula may include *hing* (asafeotida), *lavana* (salt), *ela* (cardamom), and *nagara* (ginger).[3,7] Also recommended are the prepared multi-herb formulations *prabhakara vati, hridayarnava rasa, shilajitwadi loha, dashmoola khada*.[7]

A kapha-reducing lifestyle prescription will include vigorous exercise, a decrease in the amount of time spent sleeping and/or sedentary lifestyle, and dry massage. A kapha-reducing diet should be followed. The psycho-spiritual contemplation for kapha "to what am I over-attached?" with an emphasis on mentally releasing holdings will help to balance the mind of a kapha person. Alternate nostril breathing pranayama, *vinyasa* flow, or *Ashtanga* yoga will increase the sluggish movement of the doshas through the body and help the kapha individual to release mental obstructions. Transcendental meditation will raise awareness and help to clear the heavy elements from their mind.[7]

Atherosclerosis

Atherosclerosis is described as an imbalance of vata and kapha. Vata causes a drying and hardening of the endothelium. Kapha causes lipid deposition into arterial walls and results in thrombus formation.[7]

The vata type is a result of vata exacerbating habits, including ingestion of light, cold, and dry foods. Emotions of distrust tend to harden the body and the mind. Treatment may include the use of rock salt, hawthorn berry, and cinnamon to soften the tissue and increase the flow through the channel. Patients are encouraged to discontinue vata unbalancing activities including smoking.

Recommendations also include avoiding drinks with a diuretic effect such as alcohol and coffee. Oil massage treatments like *abhyanga* and *shirodhara* may be of benefit. The lifestyle and dietary recommendations for vata will also apply.[1,7] Kapha-type atherosclerotic disease is a result of kapha-provoking habits including regular and/or excessive intake of cold, heavy, oily, or fatty foods with a sedentary lifestyle.[1,4,7] An emotionally blocked or repressed person may be prone to this type of disease.

The treatment includes kapha-reducing activities such as exercise and mental activity. If patient is in good physical condition, pancha karma may be utilized to removes excess dosha and ama. Herbs used for this include cinnamon, hawthorn berry, guggul, and turmeric.[8,9] Kapha-reducing lifestyle routines and diet, as mentioned earlier will also be part of the treatment plan.[7]

Hypertension

Primary hypertension has multiple causes and each should be addressed specifically. Vata-type hypertension is due to the typical vata-provoking conditions. Persons with vata-type hypertension are frequently people with worry, nervousness, and feelings of anxiety. The symptoms associated with vata-type hypertension include a sudden rise and fall of blood pressure with nervous tension, irregular or erratic pulse both in rhythm and strength, and possibly vasospasm. It can also relocate to the mind causing anxiety and worry. Treatment may include the use of hawthorn berry, garlic, and arjuna. For the mind, *ashwaganda*, *Gotu kola*, and *jatamansi* may be used in equal parts taken as 1–3 g of the powdered herbs with warm water or ghee. Meditation is advised to treat dysfunction of the nervous system. Yoga *asanas* (postures) also help by increasing flexibility of the physical body including the arteries and also flexibility of the mind.[1,6,9]

Further recommendations include a vata-pacifying diet and self-massage with warm sesame oil. Relaxing aroma therapy including sandalwood and lavender is also beneficial. As described previously, the vata-reducing lifestyle routine, hatha yoga, and meditation are helpful.[1,7] Pitta type of hypertension is usually seen in conjunction with vata and/or kapha. Pitta types are often angry and intense, and will have raised blood pressure associated with stress and aggravation. Pitta types may have a complexion that is ruddy and flushed, complain of burning sensations, and have a wiry and tight pulse.[7]

The treatment of pitta hypertension is to decrease tension and stressors with less focus on achievement. The emotional stress and intensity can be relieved with herbal nervine tonics and sedatives such as gotu kola (*C. asiatica*) and skullcap (*Sculltelaria lateirflora*) in equal parts, combined with rose and chrysanthemum. The herbal formulations *Brahama Rasayana* and *Saraswati* powder can be helpful. In addition, using cool and calming aromas like rose and sandalwood will help to balance the mind. The pitta-reducing lifestyle, lunar pranayama, hatha yoga, and meditation will also aid in reducing pitta in the mind.[7,9]

Causes of kapha hypertension are the result of kapha-increasing behaviors such as the intake of cold, heavy, and oily foods; a lethargic daily routine; and excess body weight.

Kapha hypertension is often continually high without the fluctuations seen in vata and pitta. There is often concomitant obesity, fatigue, edema, and high cholesterol.

Treatment may include the use of cayenne, myrrh, garlic, and hawthorn berry. In addition, incorporating hot spices, such as mustard and onions, into the diet and avoiding dairy, butter, eggs, and high fat foods is recommended. For high cholesterol, *guggul*, turmeric, and garlic may be used with *gurmar* added if weight control is desired. Triphala will aide in proper digestion and elimination. If the patient is strong enough, consider panchakarma to detoxify and rejuvenate the patient at a deeper level. The kapha-reducing lifestyle and yoga recommendations are also important.[1,7,9]

Valvular heart disease

Valvular heart disease is a complex Ayurvedic disorder of vata and pitta. If the origin is rheumatic heart disease, then the likely agent is long-term pitta imbalance. The valve damage itself is due low ojas in combination with imbalanced doshas.

Treatment involves building the rakta dhatu through the use of hawthorn berry and arjuna, either alone or in combination. Triphala may be added to help rebuild ojas. The treatment for emboli can be augmented with turmeric and/or willow bark, which both have mild anti-coagulative properties.[8] For palpitations due to vata, valerian root can be beneficial in combination with hawthorn berry and cinnamon. Lifestyle and dietary recommendations based on constitution and to raise ojas will be beneficial and preventative.[7]

Evidence base for ayurvedic medicine

Most Ayurvedic treatments are not evaluated as a whole system of care in the research literature, but rather individual herbs and therapies such as yoga and pranayama have preclinical and clinical studies performed to evaluate their mechanism and efficacy. There has not been a study using Ayurveda as a complete care system to determine its efficacy for heart disease.

ARJUNA

The bark of *Terminalia arjuna* contains several active alkaloid constituents, and has been used in India for more than 3000 years, primarily as a heart remedy. Pharmacological studies have provided mixed results, and its role in heart disease still remains unclear, with a need for increased research. Nevertheless, *T. arjuna* is used in many Ayurvedic formulations. It has been shown in mammalian studies and clinical trials to have cardiotonic, antihypertensive, anti-hyperlipidemic, and anticoagulant properties. In addition, positive effects to LV function, positive effects on ST changes and T-wave depressions in ischemic heart disease (IHD) have been observed. Toxicity studies have shown it to be safe, although only short-term studies have been examined.

A 1-week, double-blind, placebo-controlled crossover trial of approximately 60 people, evaluated the effectiveness of an extract of *T. arjuna* at 500-mg TID in patients with stable angina and provocable ischemia. *T. arjuna* was compared with placebo and isosorbide mononitrate (40 mg/day). Significant improvement in clinical and treadmill exercise parameters was observed indicating that *T. arjuna* is more effective than placebo, with benefits similar to those observed with isosorbide mononitrate therapy. In addition the extract was well tolerated.[10]

TRIPHALA

Triphala is a combination of *Emblica officinalis, Terminalia chebula, Terminalia bellirica*. *E. officinalis* (Indian gooseberry), is used for lowering cholesterol, treating atherosclerosis, and diabetes. It is also used orally for treatment of obesity. Preliminary evidence suggests it may lower total serum cholesterol, LDL, triglycerides, without affecting HDL levels. It may have positive effects on atherosclerosis. *T. chebula, T. bellirica* are in the same family as *T. arjuna*, however, there is a paucity of specific evidence for their use in cardiac disease.[11]

CINNAMON

There is preliminary research that suggests the cinnamon bark constituent methylhydroxychalcone polymer (MHCP), might improve insulin sensitivity.[12] Biologically active components of cinnamon seem to mimic the activity of insulin, stimulating glucose metabolism. It also appears to work synergistically with insulin, possibly by improving insulin-signaling pathways resulting in an increase of cellular glucose uptake.[13] Cinnamon has been shown to decrease blood glucose levels. A study in people with type II diabetes demonstrated that intake of 1, 3, or 6 g of cinnamon daily reduced serum glucose, triglyceride, LDL cholesterol, and total cholesterol.[14] This suggests that the inclusion of cinnamon in the diet, or frank supplementation for people with type II diabetes, may reduce risk factors associated with diabetes and subsequent cardiovascular disease.

GUGGUL

Guggul (*Commiphora mukul*) was cited for the treatment of atherosclerosis in the Ayurvedic texts dating back to 600 BC. Multiple well-done studies performed in India found evidence that guggul reduced cholesterol levels including reductions in total cholesterol, LDL, and triglycerides with improved total cholesterol:HDL ratios. Combined changes of guggul and diet equaled effects of major statins. Of possibly more significance, measurements of lipid peroxides (an index of oxidative stress) decreased with guggul.[15] A purported mechanism of action for the hypolipidemic properties of guggul has been attributed to the bioactive components, guggulsterones, which have been shown to be powerful antagonists of the hormone receptors involved in the metabolism of cholesterol, thus prompting further investigation. However, the only U.S. trial, a double-blind, placebo-controlled study of 103 people, failed to find guggul effective at a dose of 75 or 150 mg of guggulsterones daily when patients continued on a standard Western diet.[16]

Guggulsterones induce CYP 450 3A enzymes in experimental models, therefore close observation should be utilized in persons using medications metabolized by CYP 450 3A pathways.[17] Guggul may cause a hypersensitivity-type rash in some people.

GURMAR

Gurmar (*Gymnema sylvester*) is known as the sugar destroyer. The entire plant is made into powder or decoction with an alcohol extract. Animal studies show potential monoamineoxidase (MAO) stimulation of insulin release and regeneration of islet cells. Of significant interest is a study showing that genetically modified diabetic rats treated with gurmar lived longer than untreated genetically identical rats. Improved glucose utilization and inhibition of glucose absorption from intestine was also observed.

Gurmar contains gymnemic acids which seem to reduce intestinal absorption of glucose and may stimulate pancreatic β-cell growth. Other research suggests that constituents of gymnema have a direct effect on β-cell function, increasing the release of insulin. Gymnema can increase serum C-peptide levels, suggesting an increase in endogenous insulin secretion. Gymnemic acid and gurmarin inhibit the ability to taste bitter or sweet without affecting the ability to taste sour, astringent, or pungent flavors, and this may decrease the cravings for sweets.[18]

HAWTHORN BERRY

Hawthorn is used to increase cardiac output for congestive heart failure (CHF). It also has been used to treat hypertension, atherosclerosis, dyslipidemia, angina, and arrhythmias. Current studies have not extended past 16 weeks, but hawthorn preparations appear safe within this time frame. Hawthorn increases contractility and lengthens refractory period and may cause peripheral vasodilatation and induce endothelium-dependent arterial relaxation. Preliminary research suggests hawthorn can lower serum cholesterol, LDL, and triglycerides.[19,20] Clinical studies in people with New York Heart Association (NYHA) II heart failure showed improved ejection fraction, exercise tolerance, and decreased subjective symptoms. Maximum effect was seen at 240–600 mg/day and usually requires 6–12 weeks of treatment. In patients with NYHA III heart failure, hawthorn extract combined with pre-existing diuretic therapy also improved exercise tolerance and reduced subjective symptoms. Maximum effect is usually seen after 16 weeks of combined diuretic therapy and 1800 mg/day standardized hawthorn extract.[21,22]

Orally, hawthorn is generally well tolerated with vertigo and dizziness as the most common adverse effects. However, palpitations, headache, and circulatory disturbances have been observed. Care should be used when using in conjunction with digoxin, nitrates, β-blockers, calcium channel blockers, or PDE-5 inhibitors.

A note on botanical formulations

A lack of complete understanding of many pharmacologically active components of individual herbs continues to exist. Often there are multiple active components in any given botanical product, and this is further compounded by products which utilize multiple botanicals per preparation.

As with standard drug-drug interactions, cardiological implications are potentially serious, and the potential for herb-drug interaction (HDI) must be respected. Use of caution when dealing with pharmacological agents with a narrow therapeutic or toxic window, or with significant cost of pharmacological failure is warranted. This would certainly include, but may not be limited to, the use of cardiac glycosides, anticoagulants, and antiarrhythmics. Patients should be informed that, though "natural," herbal products have true pharmacological effects, and should be instructed to report any new side effects immediately to the treating physician. We would refer readers to the section on herbal medications in this text for a more extensive discussion of the use of herbal products and HDI.

Our recommendation for accurate and more extensive information on the botanical and herbal medicines discussed above is www.naturaldatabase.com.

Another subject that warrants at least brief discussion is that of product contamination. A select sample of Ayurvedic herbal remedies manufactured in India and Pakistan were found to be contaminated with high levels of the heavy metals such as lead, mercury, and arsenic in stores in the Boston region.[23] It is imperative that all herbal and natural supplements, not only Ayurvedic products, be obtained through reputable manufacturers with strict standards and quality control, in accordance with accepted U.S. standards.[24]

YOGA

Yoga focuses attention to the mind, breath, and the physical body. Studies have found that yoga has diverse and extensive beneficial physiological and psychological effects. Some observed outcomes include improved blood pressure and decreased heart rate, sympathetic tone, and oxygen requirements. Yoga and meditation improve lipid profiles and carotid atherosclerosis. Yoga trains the cardiovascular system to function more efficiently, enhancing measures of endurance, aerobic power, and circulation, while lowering systolic, diastolic blood pressure, and heart rate.[25]

In 1983, Ornish showed that yoga training plus dietary changes were associated with a reduction of 14 points in cholesterol levels at 3 weeks with increased cardiac work efficiency.[26] Additional documented physiological changes that occur after practicing yoga include improved stress adaptation, decreased serum cortisol, and increasing levels of brain α-wave activity.[27]

Regular yoga practitioners have decreased markers of neuroendocrine stress activity by measure of urinary epinephrine, norepinephrine, dopamine, and aldosterone. A study looking at yoga-based relaxation showed decreased sympathetic activity by decreased heart rate, skin conductance, oxygen consumption, and increased respiratory volumes.[28,29] A randomized clinical trial assessed angiographic evidence of coronary artery disease (CAD) in patients practicing yoga. At 1 year, there were decreased number of anginal events per week, improvement of exercise capacity, and decreased body weight. Improvements were also noted in serum cholesterol (total cholesterol, LDL, triglycerides). Patients practicing yoga required decreased revascularization procedures. Follow-up angiography at 1 year showed a diminished number of overall lesions, a regression of existing lesions, and decreased progression of lesions.[30]

Quality of life (QOL) issues are significant in persons with cardiovascular disease. QOL issues may compound and exacerbate CVD and often account for significant barriers to healing in the cardiac patient. Yoga was found to have significant impact and improvement on subjective well being inventory (SUBI) scores and QOL in people doing yoga for 4 months and may help patients decrease stress and improve QOL.[31] Participation in yogic activity is easy to implement and does not require special equipment. It is enjoyable, social, and rewarding for the patient. Because it directly involves the patient, the patient is vested in their health care, and this may globally increase compliance to the overall treatment and rehabilitative protocol. We recommend the augmentative use of yoga in addition to rehabilitation methods that have been validated as effective. Specific yogic practice type is best done by the yoga instructors themselves, based on information provided by the physician and the patient.

Even the utilization of basic yoga maneuvers shows benefit in post myocardial infraction (MI) patients. Teaching these cardiac patients relaxation, simple postures, and respiratory control along with standard pharmacological intervention and rehabilitation has been shown to yield significant improvement versus standard therapy alone, including improvements in exercise tolerance and illness perception.

We advise monitoring a patient's program via reports from the yoga teacher, similar to reports one would expect from a physical therapist. Patients should be periodically evaluated at 4-week intervals for the first 60–90 days and at 6-month intervals thereafter. While there are many qualified yoga instructors, when using one for the purpose of co-medical care, we strongly encourage working with those who have acceptable cross training in medicine, or those who have successfully worked with physicians in a medical model in the past. BLS Certification should be expected.

MEDITATION

Transcendental Meditation has been found to decrease blood pressure, heart rate, oxygen consumption, plasma cortisol, and heart rate and to increase alpha brain waves associated with relaxation.[32] Meditation lowers cholesterol and improves cardiac ischemia. In a study done on elderly patients with optimally treated CHF, meditation further reduced the ventilation-carbon dioxide production (VE/VCO_2) slope, reduced norpinephrine (NE), and improved QOL.[33] Meditation has a modest effect on decreasing the risk of sudden death due to ventricular fibrillation in high-risk patients.

Depression increases overall risk post-MI and predisposes to poorer outcomes and results in higher costs. Mindfulness based stress reduction (MBSR), based on *vipassana* meditation, has been shown to significantly decrease Hamilton and Beck Anxiety and Depression scores post-intervention, and at 3-month follow-up. It can be a useful adjunct to other, traditional therapies in the cardiac patient.

A complete discussion of meditation goes beyond the scope of this chapter, but meditation is effective for decreasing overall stress levels prior to, and post-cardiac events, and is associated with patients' improved sense of well being. Meditation is safe and beneficial to the body and mind when done with appropriate instruction. We would recommend guidelines similar to those recommended for yoga instruction.

CONCLUSION

Through harmonizing the body, mind, and consciousness of an individual with the environment using the five element theory (*pancha maha bhuti*), Ayurveda provides a unique and complementary approach to cardiovascular healthcare. The core principals of Ayurvedic medicine emphasize and support the optimization of all aspects of the patient's health, and are applicable to both prevention and treatment of cardiovascular disease. Identification of the *prakruti* (mind-body constitution) and the *vikruti* (current state of *doshas*) allows the practitioner to formulate a treatment plan that addresses the distinctiveness of each patient, incorporating yoga, meditation, herbs, and massage/energy medicine, along with dietary and lifestyle recommendations. By providing a complete system of care, Ayurveda forms a solid bridge, bringing a traditional medical paradigm into the cardiovascular prescription of the future.

REFERENCES

1. Frawley D. The principles of ayurveda correspondence course for health care professionals Vol. I–IV. Santa Fe (NM): American Institute of Vedic Studies; 2002.
2. Halpern M. Principles of ayurvedic medicine, Part one. Grass Valley, CA: California College of Ayurveda; 2002.
3. Lad V. An introduction to Ayurveda. Altern Ther Health Med. 1995;1:57–63.
4. Acharya G. The caraka samhita. Vol. V. Jamnagar, India: Shree Gulabkunverba Ayurvedic Society; 1949.
5. Lad V. Textbook of ayurveda, fundamental principles. Albuquerque (NM): Ayurvedic Press; 2002.
6. Ranade Su, Ranade Sun, Qutab A, Deshpande R. Health and disease in ayurveda and yoga. Pune, India: MD Nandurkar; 1997.
7. Halpern M. Principles of ayurvedic medicine, part two. Grass Valley (CA): California College of Ayurveda; 2002.
8 Materia Medica of Indo-Tibetan Medicine. Delhi, India: MDIA Classics India; 1987.

9. Kapoor LD. CRC Handbook of Ayurvedic Medicinal Plants. Boca Raton, FL: CRC Press; 1990.

10. Bharani A, Ganguli A, Mathur LK, Jamra Y, Raman PG. Efficacy of Terminalia arjuna in chronic stable angina: a double-blind, placebo-controlled, crossover study comparing Terminalia arjuna with isosorbide mononitrate. Indian Heart J, 2002 Mar–Apr;54(2):170–5. [PMID: 12086380, PubMed—indexed for MEDLINE.]

11. Anila L, Vijayalakshmi NR. Beneficial effects of flavonoids from Sesamum indicum, Emblica officinalis and Momordica charantia. Phytother Res. 2000;14:592–5. [PMID: 11113993, PubMed—indexed for MEDLINE.]

12. Jarvill-Taylor KJ, Anderson RA, Graves DJ. A hydroxychalcone derived from cinnamon functions as a mimetic for insulin in 3T3-L1 adipocytes. J Am Coll Nutr. 2001;20:327–36.

13. Anderson RA, Broadhurst CL, Polansky MM, et al. Isolation and characterization of polyphenol type-A polymers from cinnamon with insulin-like biological activity. J Agric Food Chem. 2004;52:65–70.

14. Khan A, Safdar M, Ali Khan M, et al. Cinnamon improves glucose and lipids of people with type 2 diabetes. Diabetes Care. 2003;26:3215–8. [PMID: 14633804, PubMed—indexed for MEDLINE.]

15. Wang X, et al. The hypolipidemic natural product Commiphora mukul and its component guggulsterone inhibit oxidative modification of LDL. Atherosclerosis. 2004 Feb;172(2):239–46. [PMID: 15019533, PubMed—indexed for MEDLINE.]

16. Szapary PO, Wolfe ML, Bloedon LT, et al. Guggulipid for the treatment of hypercholesterolemia: a randomized controlled trial. JAMA. 2003;290:765–72. [PMID: 12915429, PubMed—indexed for MEDLINE.]

17. Brobst DE, et al. Guggulsterone activates multiple nuclear receptors and induces CYP3A gene expression through the pregnane X receptor. J Pharmacol Exp Ther. 2004 Aug;310(2):528–35. Epub 2004 Apr 1. [PMID: 15075359, PubMed—indexed for MEDLINE.]

18. Yeh GY, Eisenberg DM, Kaptchuk TJ, Phillips RS. Systematic review of herbs and dietary supplements for glycemic control in diabetes. Diabetes Care. 2003; 26:1277–94. [PMID: 12663610, PubMed—indexed for MEDLINE.]

19. Schwinger RH, Pietsch M, Frank K, Brixius K. Crataegus special extract WS 1442 increases force of contraction in human myocardium cAMP-independently. J Cardiovasc Pharmacol. 2000;35:700–7. [PMID: 10813370, PubMed–indexed for MEDLINE.]

20. Chang Q, Zuo Z, Harrison F, Chow MS. Hawthorn. J Clin Pharmacol. 2002;42:605–12.

21. Tauchert M. Efficacy and safety of crataegus extract WS 1442 in comparison with placebo in patients with chronic stable New York Heart Association class-III heart failure. Am Heart J. 2002;143:910–5. [PMID: 12040357; PubMed—indexed for MEDLINE.]

22. Pittler MH, Schmidt K, Ernst E. Hawthorn extract for treating chronic heart failure: meta-analysis of randomized trials. Am J Med. 2003;114:665–74. [PMID: 12798455, PubMed—indexed for MEDLINE.]

23. Saper RB, et al. Heavy metal content of Ayurvedic herbal medicine products. JAMA. 2004;292:2868–73. [PMID: 15598918, PubMed—indexed for MEDLINE.]

24. Ernst E. Heavy metals in traditional Indian remedies. Eur J Clin Pharmacol. 2002;57:891–6. [PMID: 11936709; PubMed—indexed for MEDLINE.]

25. Pandya DP, Vyas VH, Vyas SH. Mind-body therapy in the management and prevention of coronary disease. Compr Ther. 1999 May;25(5):283–93. [PMID: 10390658; PubMed—indexed for MEDLINE.]

26. Ornish D, et al. Effects of stress management training and dietary changes in treating ischemic heart disease. JAMA. 1983 Jan 7;249(1):54–9. [PMID: 6336794, PubMed—indexed for MEDLINE.]

27. Kamei T, et al. Decrease in serum cortisol during yoga exercise is correlated with alpha wave activation. Percept Mot Skills. 2000 Jun;90(3):1027–32. [PMID: 10883793, PubMed—indexed for MEDLINE.]

28. Mishra L, Singh BB, Dagenais S. Ayurveda: a historical perspective and principles of the traditional healthcare system in India. Altern Ther Health Med. 2001 Mar;7(2):36–42. [PMID:11253415, PubMed—indexed for MEDLINE.]

29. Vempati RP, Telles S. Yoga based guided relaxation reduces sympathetic activity judged from baseline levels. Psychol Rep. 2000;90:487–94. [PMID: 12061588, PubMed—indexed for MEDLINE.]

30. Manchanda SC, et al. Retardation of coronary atherosclerosis with yoga lifestyle intervention. J Assoc Physicians India. 2000; 48:687–694. [PMID: 11273502, PubMed—indexed for MEDLINE.]

31. Malathi A, Damodaran A, Shah N, Patil N, Maratha S. Effect of yogic practices on subjective well being. Indian J Physiol Pharmacol. 2000;44:202–206. [PMID: 10846636, PubMed—indexed for MEDLINE.]

32. Barnes VA, Treiber FA, Johnson MH. Impact of transcendental meditation on ambulatory blood pressure in African-American adolescents. Am J Hypertens. 2004 Apr;17(4):366–9. [PMID: 15062892, PubMed—indexed for MEDLINE.]

33. Curiati JA, et al. Meditation reduces sympathetic activation and improves the quality of life in elderly patients with optimally treated heart failure: a prospective randomized study. J Altern Complement Med. 2005 Jun;11(3):465–72. [PMID: 15992231, PubMed—in process.]

15

APPLICATIONS OF MUSIC THERAPY IN THE CONTINUUM OF CARE FOR THE CARDIAC PATIENT

Cheryl Dileo and Barbara Reuer

INTRODUCTION TO MUSIC THERAPY

Music therapy has a long history, but a short past. Since the beginning of recorded history, music has been used to calm fears and anxieties and stir feelings of hope, love, and unity; its use to affect health and behavior predates the writings of Aristotle and Plato. Throughout the centuries, people have turned to music for comfort and palliation in overcoming the effects of disorders of mind and body.

The discipline of music therapy, however, began following World War I, when both amateur and professional musicians of all types visited veterans' hospitals to perform for the thousands suffering physical and emotional traumas from war. Patients' striking responses to the music led doctors and nurses to request the hiring of musicians. Hospitals soon realized that musicians required more specialized training to perform this work, and the first academic music therapy training program began in 1944. In addition, music therapy's first professional organization was established in 1950.

The undergraduate curriculum, now standardized, requires coursework in the biological, behavioral, and social sciences. Today the discipline has 73 approved baccalaureate programs, approximately 150 clinical training sites, as well as 30 graduate programs offering advanced training. Of these graduate programs, 7 offer PhD studies in related areas with an emphasis in music therapy, and one offers a full PhD program in Music Therapy).

Students are trained to use music therapy with persons exhibiting a wide variety of clinical conditions. Following an extended internship of 900–1040 hours, students are eligible to sit for the national examination (administered by the Certification Board for Music Therapy, Inc.).[1] With successful completion of this exam, the "MT-BC" credential is awarded. Graduate work in music therapy is strongly encouraged if individuals are to specialize, conduct research, or use more in-depth methods of music therapy, including its applications in medicine. In some states, music therapists with advanced degrees are eligible for licensure under several professional titles, for example, Licensed Professional Counselor, Creative Arts Therapist, etc. Besides being employed in a variety of health-care facilities, some music therapists work in private practice.

Credentialed music therapists administer music therapy according to the Standards of Clinical Practice and Code of Ethics of the American Music Therapy Association, Inc. (AMTA).[2] The standards require professional referral, assessment, program planning, implementation, documentation, and termination. The AMTA has more than 5000 members, and the World Federation of Music Therapy, Inc. is the official international organization in the profession.

CLASSIFICATION OF APPROACHES INVOLVING MUSIC IN MEDICAL SETTINGS

The uses of sound and music for healing/therapeutic purposes are numerous, however, three uses of music are most commonly found in medical settings: (a) music therapy, (b) music medicine, and (c) hospital musicians. These practices are differentiated in the following paragraphs.

Music therapy

AMTA (2005)[2] defines music therapy as the clinical and evidence-based use of music interventions to accomplish individualized goals within a therapeutic relationship by a credentialed professional who has completed an approved music therapy program. Music therapists are trained to systematically effect nonmusical outcomes in all of the human domains (physiological, psychological, cognitive, social, spiritual, and behavioral). Music therapy is clearly distinguishable from other practices involving the use of music in hospital settings. Specifically, music therapy always involves the following: (1) a board-certified music therapy professional; (2) a process that includes individualized assessment, treatment, and evaluation; (3) the use of the range of experiences possible within music (e.g., listening to, creating, and improvising music); and (4) a relationship between therapist and patient that develops through the music.[3]

Music medicine

Dileo (1999)[4] refers to the use of music by medical or health-care professionals as "music medicine." In this practice, taped music listening is used, for example, to reduce anxiety or pain or to enhance mood in medical settings. Specifically, prerecorded music *alone* is used as the intervention, and there is no therapeutic process (assessment, treatment, evaluation). Moreover, there is no client-therapist relationship that evolves through shared musical experiences. It is important to note that music medicine, as implemented by medical staff, is often referred to as "music therapy" in the medical literature. Thus, the reader is cautioned to be aware of this misnomer in practice.

Hospital musicians

In some hospital settings, live music is provided by professional musicians (often harpists) in public areas or at patients' bedsides for entertainment purposes. This practice is distinguished from music therapy, as this use of music does not involve: patient assessment, goal-oriented treatment, evaluation, a therapeutic relationship, and a trained music therapist. Although such entertainment can enhance the hospital ambience and improve patients' moods in general, the specialized training of the music therapist is required to design and implement music treatment that focuses on the individual needs of patients and to address the many complex reactions that result from music experiences, especially in medically vulnerable patients.

Other distinctions

Finally, music therapy is neither sound therapy (wherein a person's response to a single frequency may be examined), nor is it limited to the use of a single musical work such as Mozart's Sonata for Two Pianos in D Major (K. 448), which is the focus of the Mozart effect research.

In addition, music therapy is not a self-help procedure. Although there appears to be a widespread use of music for self-help purposes, and many music tapes and CDs with claims to assist an individual in achieving relaxation are available in the marketplace, there is little research that documents the effectiveness of these mass-market products.

The therapist-client relationship in music therapy

A supportive therapist-client relationship, characterized by empathy, trust and safety, is an essential requisite of music therapy interventions. In music therapy, the personal qualities of the therapist and the relationship developed with the client through the music may each and in combination effect change.[4] The ability of the music therapist to be "present" and "resonate" with the client's experience both within and outside of the music is vital, as these are considered essential elements in healing. The music therapist, because of the medium used, is able to focus on "healthy" or creative parts of the individual, rather than on aspects of the illness. Clients associate music therapy with pleasure and relaxation rather than discomfort and stress. Because music is pervasive in everyday life, it may be less threatening to clients than other forms of therapy.[3]

CLINICAL INDICATIONS FOR MUSIC THERAPY

Where music therapy is used

Music therapy is used within many clinical specializations in medicine. In cardiology specifically, it is with all age groups of cardiac patients who receive treatment: (1) in hospital medical/surgical units, (2) in cardiac testing laboratories, (3) in presurgical holding areas and post-anesthesia care units, (4) in cardiac care/intensive care units, (5) in outpatient settings, (6) in cardiac rehabilitation facilities, and (7) through various support groups. In addition, music therapy services aimed at prevention are numerous and are provided through many different sources. Music therapy is offered individually at bedside or in private sessions and/or in groups involving other patients or families.

Because music has the potential to affect all human domains simultaneously (i.e., cognitive, emotional, physical, spiritual, social, behavioral), a wide range of clinical issues can be addressed through music therapy treatment. Also, because participation in music therapy can be either active or passive, it can be adapted to meet the varying physical and psychological capabilities and limitations of the individual receiving treatment.

What music therapy entails

The music therapy process begins with a detailed assessment that identifies the patient's needs, musical preferences and history, medical and social history, and physical and emotional capabilities. Based on this information physical, psychological, cognitive, social, spiritual, and/or behavioral goals are identified, and music therapy interventions to meet these goals are planned (this may also be done in collaboration with the patient's treatment team where relevant). Evaluation of the patient's progress toward the established goals is ongoing throughout treatment and documented in the patient's records. A final summary of progress is documented at the termination of music therapy services.

Music therapy treatment approaches

Music therapy treatment approaches used may be categorized as follows: (1) receptive, (2) creative, (3) recreative, and (4) combined, and within these approaches, all types, styles, and genres of music are included.

RECEPTIVE

The music used in listening approaches may vary considerably and may be precomposed, specially composed by therapist and/or patient or improvised by the therapist. The elements of the music may be matched to the patient's condition, and then gradually changed in the desired direction. Receptive approaches include but are not limited to: music listening, song choices, music and imagery or music visualization, music-assisted relaxation, lyric analysis, and entrainment.

In music listening experiences, the client assumes a relatively passive role with regard to the music that is presented: with or without verbal instructions from the therapist and with or without low-frequency stimulation (vibroacoustic or vibrotactile stimulation).[5] Music is selected by the therapist according to the inherent qualities of its elements (rhythm, harmony, melody, instrumentation, tempo, etc., as well as its gestalt), and its intended therapeutic purposes. Special consideration is given to the patient's familiarity with and preference for the music. The therapist must ascertain that the music used does not stimulate memories, associations or images in the patient that are inconsistent with therapeutic goals.

In addition, the therapist may match elements of the music (e.g., pulse) to a physiological parameter of the patient (e.g., respiration rate). Once matched and sustained for a short period of time, the therapist will gradually decrease the pulse of the music to encourage a slowing down of the breath. The therapist may also improvise music based on a physiological parameter that is being monitored (e.g., heart rate).

The use of song choice involves the patient's selection of a piece of music either freely or according to criteria suggested by the therapist, for example, how he or she is feeling. The therapist often performs this music live for the patient. The song choice method is used in both assessment and treatment, as it may reveal undiscovered aspects of the patient, for example to represent how he or she is feeling. Song choice most often includes verbal processing of the patient's reactions to or feelings about the music following the listening experience.

Music and imagery or music visualization approaches may be quite varied and used for a range of clinical goals, for example, stress reduction, pain management, and transcendence of circumstances, and appropriate music is selected to support the clinical goal. A specific starting point for the imagery may or may not be suggested by the therapist. Patients may image freely to the music, or the therapists may direct the imagery verbally. Generally, there is discussion and processing of the patient's imagery and reactions following the music, or these may be processed using other creative media, for example, drawing.

Music-assisted relaxation is the use of music and the relationship between patient and therapist to induce a relaxed state in the mind and/or body. The music itself serves as the relaxation agent with the patient passively listening to music performed live by the therapist or through pre-recorded music. Additional relaxation techniques may be combined with the music, including progressive muscle relaxation, autogenic suggestions, breathing techniques, and visual imagery.

Lyric analysis is an approach wherein songs are selected by the therapist and/or patient, and their words are the focal point of a verbal discussion following music listening. Lyrics of songs may be used to identify and/or validate patient experiences, provide alternate strategies for coping, facilitate emotional expression, process cognitive/emotional crises, and so forth.

Music therapy entrainment is a process that uses improvised music to match the patient's reported experience of pain, as well as sounds that might alleviate the pain. Once the music has been identified, the therapist provides this music for the patient. An essential component of entrainment is the presence of the therapist and his or her resonance with the patient's pain.[6]

CREATIVE APPROACHES

Creative approaches comprise those methods where music/songs are created spontaneously on voice or instruments, or where music and/or lyrics are purposefully composed by the therapist and patient. These approaches include: songwriting and instrumental and/or vocal improvisation.

Songwriting is the most common type of compositional method used in music therapy wherein patients substitute words to existing melodies or write original words and music; clients without musical training are often assisted in the process by the music therapist who provides appropriate structure for the experience as well as assistance with musical aspects of the piece.[7]

In instrumental and/or vocal improvisation approaches, the therapist engages the patient in spontaneous music-making utilizing the voice (singing, chanting, toning), body movement to music, or musical instruments (e.g., drums, percussion, marimbas). Music improvisation, solo, in a dyad with the therapist or another, or within a group, facilitates self-awareness and encourages exploration of personal and life options and new ways of being. Goals are achieved as the client actively makes music or responds to the music in some fashion. The emphasis shifts from the results of active music-making to the unfolding of therapeutic insights and the intrapersonal and interpersonal processes involved. The musical product achieved is less important than the unfolding experiences with the music or evoked by the music.[8]

In vocal or song improvisation approaches, benefits may derive from the act of singing, musically chanting and/or toning.[9] In toning, the patient experiments with different pitches and observes how these pitches vibrate within the body. Based on these sensations, he or she will select a pitch to sustain using repeated long breaths. No words are used, only the vowel sounds that best support the production of the tones. The client is encouraged to continue toning until the therapeutic goal is achieved (often relaxation), and this may occur quite rapidly. Chanting may involve a similar process although words (that often hold meaning for the patient) are selected to accompany tone. Chanting may be designed by the therapist to progress from faster to slower tempi, thus entraining with the client's physical process of moving from a state of arousal to a state of relaxation. Thus, toning, chanting, and singing provide a means for structuring the breath in a therapeutic manner by facilitating deep and sustained breathing. In addition, toning and chanting stimulate a sensation of internal vibration, the location of which can be controlled by the client according to need.

Song improvisations involve the spontaneous creation of melody and lyrics by the patient while the therapist provides musical (instrumental and/or vocal) support. Song improvisations may take the form of a solo patient creation, a "call and response" between therapist and client, or a musical dialogue between/among therapist and family members.

RECREATIVE APPROACHES

Recreative approaches involve performing previously composed music on an instrument, singing precomposed songs, conducting music, or learning to play an instrument. Performing composed music is suitable for both trained and untrained musicians alike. For clients who have not had musical training, music therapists often utilize specialized music instruction methods, designed to minimize the learning curve in playing an instrument. At the same time, most individuals are able to use their voices for singing favorite songs on or off pitch, and without judgment by the therapist regarding vocal quality. Emphasis is always on the *process* of performing, rather than on the musical product. When words are used in singing, they may enhance the meaning of the experience, as lyrics can also provide messages of significance to the client.

Patients who are confined within stressful circumstances may use learning or practicing an instrument as an effective means of coping with boredom and stress. As hospitalization may be for extended periods of time, some patients may choose to learn to play an instrument or maintain their skills on an instrument during their hospital stays.

COMBINED APPROACHES

Combined approaches are those that involve the use of music therapy approaches in conjunction with non–music therapy approaches, with the assumption that music will enhance the effectiveness of the method used. Combined approaches include: music and meditation, music and touch/massage, music and movement, and music and other arts experiences.

PHYSICAL ENVIRONMENT AND EQUIPMENT

A range of musical instruments is used in music therapy treatment, and these most often include a keyboard, guitar, and a variety of percussion instruments. Simple wind instruments (i.e., recorders) are sometimes available. In addition, CD/cassette players and recording devices are common.

In music therapy, a great deal of attention is given to the sound environment of the space being used, and every effort is made to limit extraneous sounds/noises during sessions. Furthermore, all attempts are made to contain the sounds of the session within the space used, so that patient confidentiality is protected, and other patients or staff members are not disturbed by the music. However, control over these factors varies according to the setting.

Common indications for music therapy treatment

Anxiety is a special concern in patients with cardiac disease. Because anxiety activates the hypothalamic-pituitary-adrenal axis, and because this is manifested by increases in heart rate, blood pressure, and cardiac output, its effects exert an additional workload on the already compromised cardiovascular system in patients with heart disease.[10] Further, anxiety may provoke transient myocardial ischemia.[11]

A host of other, interrelated psychological, social, spiritual, and behavioral factors have also been implicated in one's propensity for heart disease as well as one's recovery from a major cardiac event and/or surgery. Although it is not the purpose of this chapter to review the literature for all of these factors, several are mentioned here, as they pertain to music therapy treatment.

Depression is ubiquitous in cardiac patients and is a major risk factor in prevention and treatment. Meaningful social support and effective coping skills have also been associated with optimal recovery from cardiac illness. Spiritual beliefs along with the identification of the meaning and purpose of one's life are often seen as critical factors in coping with life's major challenges. Lastly, the motivation for making and sustaining healthful, behavioral/lifestyle changes and in acquiring the capacity to self-regulate physiological systems are seen as essential in preventing heart disease and in optimizing future physical functioning after a cardiac event. Music therapy can be used to address many of these salient issues in treatment. The common indications for music therapy treatment are presented in Table 15-1.

INDICATIONS FOR MUSIC THERAPY TREATMENT

Physical	Emotional	Cognitive	Social	Spiritual	Behavioral
Accelerated heart rate	Anxiety	Lack of sensory stimulation	Social isolation	Existential confusion and suffering	Noncompliance with treatment
Elevated blood pressure	Depression, dysphoria, pessimism	Lack of cognitive stimulation; Boredom	Lack of social support	Impaired life satisfaction	Lack of motivation for exercise
Accelerated or shallow respiration	Need to feel safe and trust caregivers	Cognitive deficits	Need for intimacy	Hopelessness	Need for normalized environment
Pain	Emotional expression	Impaired decision-making	Lack of social skills	Need for spiritual comfort	Lethargy
Heightened autonomic arousal	Anger/hostility management	Confusion	Interpersonal conflict	Despair	Lack of leisure skills
Diminished heart rate variability	Impaired self-esteem	Lack of orientation	Withdrawal	Unresolved grief	Need to modify health risk factors
Side effects of pain medications	Helplessness	Lack of self-awareness	Loneliness	Need for solace	Agitation

Side effects of sedatives	Lack of coping mechanisms	Need for diversion	Lack of communication skills	Need for peace	Loss of independence
Difficulties with medical tests	Denial	Depersonalization	Dysfunctional relationships	Need for existential reorganization	Time urgency; impatience
Difficulties with medical procedures	Impaired identity	Negative thinking		Guilt	Sleep difficulties
Masking of unpleasant sounds	Disempowerment	Need for cognitive focus		Victimization	Need for self-management skills
	Fear/Panic	Cognitive distortion in situation appraisal		Need to forgive and/or be forgiven	Need for increased movement
Need for creative outlet				Need for life review	

Although musical experiences and the relationship between client and therapist are considered the essential elements for change in music therapy, patients do not need to have any prior music training or experience to participate successfully in music therapy. Moreover, there are few contraindications for music therapy, and those that exist in the literature are rare in occurrence (i.e., musicogenic epilepsy). Hearing loss does not preclude music therapy treatment, as musical stimuli and vibrations can be "felt" even by those with profound hearing loss. However, a patient's willingness to participate in music therapy and ability to focus on the music are considered necessary.

HOW MUSIC THERAPY IS USED

In this section, the authors provide clinical examples of some of the many ways that music therapy can be used in the continuum of care for cardiac patients. However, these clinical examples are not intended to represent an exhaustive list of the music therapy approaches that may be used.

Overall, the music therapy approaches employed with cardiac patients are simple and direct. In the authors' own work, they have found that music has the capacity of accessing patients' feelings, issues, needs, and concerns rapidly. The experience of "being in the music together" often facilitates the formation of a positive and trusting therapeutic relationship within a short amount of time. Music therapists attempt to meet patients musically "where they are" emotionally, cognitively, socially, physically, and spiritually with care and compassion. Once patients' issues are validated through music, the therapist may provide support for coping and for therapeutic change.

Three levels of intervention have been identified by the first author in her music therapy work with heart failure patients awaiting a transplant.[12] These levels reflect the metaphors often expressed by cardiac patients, that is, of having "closed hearts," and serve as a way of understanding the developmental process of music therapy with these individuals; however, these levels are not intended to portray a universality of practice among music therapists (Table 15-2).

TABLE 15-2

LEVELS OF MUSIC THERAPY INTERVENTION WITH CARDIAC PATIENTS

Level 1: Opening the heart to music
Level 2: Opening the heart to self
Level 3: Opening the heart to others

In level 1, the patient becomes engaged in active and/or passive experiences in music, and the music is selected to reflect and/or meet the patient's current state. As the patient achieves an awareness of the music and can relate to it in one or more ways, physiological processes may be positively altered. This may lead to level 2, wherein the person achieves an awareness of self in relationship to the music. At this level, mood may be enhanced, cognitions stimulated, and behavioral patterns examined and modified. This increased self-awareness may lead to level 3, wherein the person is motivated to make and sustain connections and relationships with other persons and/or a higher power. At this level, emotional, social, and spiritual transformations are possible.

Music therapy in medical/surgical units

Working bedside, music therapists bring live music and their presence to accomplish an array of clinical goals for patients and their families: reduced autonomic reactivity, expression of feelings, distraction, emotional, spiritual, and social support, mood enhancement, pain reduction, and empowerment. In general, they attempt to create a nurturing, personalized, and more "normal" atmosphere within the hospital setting.

Music therapists may ask patients to select a song that describes how they are feeling or what they might need at the moment. The therapist may also select a song that mirrors the clinical issues he/she observes in the patient; in either case, the music is performed live and patients/families are asked to join in singing. In this way, the patient's experience is often validated, and verbal discussion is used, if indicated, to process the patient's/ family members' reactions. The therapist may also use a less structured approach, and ask patients simply to choose a favorite song that might have meaning for them (lists of songs from many styles and genres are often used to assist the patient), and verbal discussion of why this song is important may follow.

When family members are present for example, therapists may ask couples to select "their special love song." While the music therapist provides this song live, powerful memories are often evoked, and love and support are reaffirmed. Therapists may also ask the patient and family members to select music that represents their feelings for each other as intentional "song dedications." Thus, expressions of these feelings transcend words and provide moments of great intimacy.

Of significance is the ability of song lyrics to evoke powerful images of the heart; and these images are ubiquitous in popular music. As such, the use of songs offers patients opportunities to explore a range of clinical issues in an indirect and nonthreatening way, and songs often serve as a springboard for unexpressed feelings.

Music therapy in cardiac testing laboratories and in surgery

Prior to, during, and/or following invasive medical tests and surgical procedures, especially when potential outcomes may prove traumatic for patients, music therapy can be used to reduce anxiety and calm fears, offer a more positive focus, reduce pain, facilitate transcendence of the situation, increase patient compliance and tolerance, and provide emotional and spiritual support.

Using live music, therapists may direct and support imagery experiences, asking patients to "go to a favorite place" in their minds, far away from the immediate situation. The music therapist may improvise music to match the patient's imagined journey, using an instrument and/or singing. The music therapist will often attempt to match the tempo of the music to the patient's heart rate or respiration rate, and then gradually decrease the tempo of the music to effect changes in the physiological parameters.

Music therapists may also provide spiritual support, offering spiritual music requested by the patient, or improvising music to correspond with a patient's prayers.

These music therapy approaches may also be used for pain management. In addition, the therapist may provide a mood-enhancing musical distraction for the patient, or may engage and support the patient in chanting or toning. Furthermore, live music used in combination with a variety of traditional relaxation techniques (progressive muscle relaxation, autogenic suggestions) may be provided for the patient.

Following procedures involving anesthesia, the music therapist may provide live, stimulating music, preferred by the patient, to ease him/her into a gradual state of awareness and to counteract effects of anesthesia.

With pediatric patients undergoing invasive medical procedures, creative and/or recreative approaches are often used to actively engage the children in music experiences. In this way, music serves as a distraction from the anxiety-provoking experience, normalizes the environment, and encourages feelings of comfort and safety. It is not uncommon for music therapists to involve the medical staff directly in these experiences, for example, having them sing along.

Music therapy in cardiac/intensive care

Music therapy may be used to address a number of clinical issues in these critical care settings: anxiety reduction, sensory stimulation, normalization of the environment (e.g., by masking stressful sounds), social, emotional, and spiritual support, sleep enhancement, safety, pain reduction, and so forth, and a corresponding range of music therapy approaches may be implemented depending on the patient's most salient needs. For example, lullabies created and sung by the therapist may help patients sleep and provide feelings of comfort and safety, or therapists may improvise music to match and subsequently alter physiological responses (displayed through various monitoring devices). Therapists may also design personalized listening tapes for patients based on the results of patient assessment.

For patients at the end of life, music therapy may provide opportunities for reminiscence, life review, and for final expression of feelings to loved ones. Live music may be used to help patients and families cope with the process of dying, providing physical and spiritual support for the transition.[13]

In these settings, music therapists may also implement music therapy programs for pretransplant inpatients in heart failure. As hospital stays may be lengthy and survival uncertain, music therapy may play a unique role in facilitating emotional and spiritual support, in creating and sustaining bonds among patients and staff, in allowing expression of intense feelings, and in helping patients to sustain an identity apart from the illness. For example, in the first author's work with these patients, group and individual music therapy (using recreative and receptive methods) supported patients in complying with demanding treatment regimens (and even impacting on patients' decisions to continue to wait for a heart donor), enhanced existential reorganization and meaning, and helped patients prepare for both life beyond the transplant and death. Moreover, musical instruction on piano or guitar assisted patients in structuring their time meaningfully, and in summoning hope for the future.[12]

Music therapy in outpatient and rehabilitations settings

In these settings, music therapy may address numerous biopsychosocial clinical needs, included, but not limited to: treatment compliance, coping skills, lifestyle modification, anxiety reduction, mood enhancement, cognitive restructuring, self-esteem, leisure skill enhancement, as well as emotional, social, and spiritual support. For example, lyric analysis may be used to uncover patients' coping styles, and provide alternate options for doing so. Music therapists may instruct patients in individualized stress reduction approaches and create personal musical programs to enhance their implementation. Music may be used to structure and increase motivation for exercise regimens. Music improvisation may be used in group settings to facilitate the expression of feelings nonverbally and to facilitate social connectedness. Musical performance groups, such as choirs (involving patients, families, and/or staff) may be established to provide opportunities for wider social networks and collaboration. Songwriting may be used to create personal "theme songs" that can motivate and provide hope. Songwriting may also be used to counter irrational beliefs and thinking.

Music therapy may be used in various outpatient and work settings as a means for prevention, that is, in providing a means to control anxiety and to enhance healthy lifestyles.

EVIDENCE: CLINICAL RESEARCH OUTCOMES

Foundational research

There are a number of studies in the literature that provide foundational information to support the use of music medicine or music therapy in effecting physiological or psychological benefits in cardiac patients.

Several studies have supported the potential effectiveness of music listening for stress reduction in cardiac and noncardiac patients. One study[14] compared physiological and mood responses to several musical selections between patients with CAD or arterial hypertension and healthy subjects. Results revealed significant reductions in systolic blood pressure, cortisol levels, and adrenaline levels in cardiac patients; these varied according to the specific music selections used. Similar effects were found in healthy subjects (i.e., significant reductions in systolic and diastolic blood pressure) who listened to their preferred music.[15] In addition, significant alterations in monocyte opiate receptor expression changes as well as increases in Interleukin-6 were found in experimental subjects.[15,16]

Chafin et al (2004)[17] investigated the effects of music on blood pressure recovery from an induced stressor in college students. Results revealed that subjects, who listened to classical music had significantly lower post-task systolic blood pressure levels than controls or those listening to jazz or pop music. The authors conclude that music listening may improve cardiovascular recovery from stress.

In addition to these investigations, there are a number of studies that indicate the positive effects of music listening or music therapy on stress reduction in nonmedical populations. In a recent meta-analysis of this literature (39 studies; 2510 subjects), significant, moderate-effect sizes were found for the following outcome variables: anxiety, tension, mood, and secretory immunoglobulin A (IgA). In addition, smaller but significant effects were found for relaxation and heart rate.[2]

Several pioneering studies have pointed to the potential influence of passive music classical listening or rhythmic chanting in increasing heart rate variability.[9,18] In one of these studies,[9] findings suggest that active, structured methods (recitation of prayer or mantras) that facilitate the slowing of breathing to six cycles per minute result in significant synchronous increases in existing cardiovascular rhythms and significant increases in baroreflex sensitivity.

Meta-analysis results

A recent meta-analysis of 184 studies conducted within 11 medical specialties has detailed the size effects of music medicine or music therapy interventions according to 40 categories of outcome variables.[19] Studies included in the meta-analytic review were limited to pretest–posttest control group designs and within-subjects designs (if a no-treatment control condition was used). Effects of music medicine or music therapy interventions were calculated: (1) for each medical specialization overall, including cardiology/intensive care unit (ICU) (14 studies) and surgery (various surgical procedures including cardiac surgery) (51 studies) and (2) for a range of outcome variables in these two specializations. The r statistic was used in data analysis, and moderator variable analysis was applied when results were not found to be homogeneous across studies.[19] Relevant data across all 11 medical specializations, as well as across cardiology/ ICU and surgery specializations are presented in Table 15-3.

Thus, across all medical specializations, music medicine or music therapy interventions achieved a significant, moderate-effect size, and moderate to approaching moderate significant effect sizes for surgery and cardiology/ICU

TABLE 15-3

OVERALL SAMPLE-LEVEL EFFECT SIZES

Medical Specialty	K[a]	N[b]	r_u^c	95% c.i.[d]	P[e]	Q[f]
Across 11 medical specialties	184	7934	.31	+.26 to +.35	.00	640.48*
Across 11 medical specialties (outliers removed)	180	7794	.29	+.25 to +.33	.00	469.34*
Surgery	51	2779	.26	+.18 to +.35	.00	246.86*
Surgery (outliers removed)	49	2689	.22	+.16 to +.28	.00	114.23*
Cardiology/ICU	14	666	.27	+.14 to +.40	.00	36.50*
Cardiology/ICU (outliers removed)	13	631	.21	+.10 to +.31	.00	20.36

[a]Number of studies.
[b]Total sample size.
[c]Weighted, unbiased effect size: .10 = small; .25 = moderate; .40 = large effect size.
[d]Confidence interval: $p = .05$.
[e]Level of significance.
[f]Homogeneity statistic.
$p < .05$, indicates that the sample is not homogeneous.

specializations. Further moderator analysis revealed that music therapy interventions were significantly more effective than music medicine interventions across all specializations; however, no moderator variables could be identified for the cardiology/ICU and surgery specializations.[19]

In addition, moderator analyses revealed that the use of patient-preferred music yielded significantly greater effects than non-preferred music on heart rate and diastolic blood pressure. Also, music therapy interventions were significantly more effective than music medicine interventions in reducing pain across all specializations.[19]

Significant outcome effects for music medicine or music therapy interventions in the cardiology/ICU and surgery specializations are presented in Table 15-4. For music medicine or music therapy interventions with surgical patients, significant but small effects sizes were found for the outcome variables of respiration rate, analgesic intake and pain, and effect sizes approaching moderate to moderate were found for: heart rate, diastolic blood pressure, systolic blood pressure, sedative intake, and anxiety. A large-effect size was found for depression.[19]

SIGNIFICANT OUTCOME VARIABLES FOR SURGERY AND CARDIOLOGY/ICU

Medical Specialty	K[a]	N[b]	r_u[c]	95% CI[d]	P[e]	Q[f]
Heart Rate						
Surgery	16	803	.34	+.12 to +.53	.00	153.68*
Surgery (outlier removed)[2]	15	763	.24	+.07 to +.38	.00	63.93*
Cardiology/ICU	12	606	.21	+.05 to +.36	.00	39.86*
Cardiology/ICU (outliers removed)[3]	11	579	.13	.00 to +.25	.04	18.76*
Respiration Rate						
Surgery	6	241	.19	+.06 to +.31	.00	4.82
Cardiology/ICU	7	301	.50	+.21 to +.71	.00	39.74*
Cardiology/ICU (outliers removed)	5	274	.37	+.22 to +.51	.00	5.51
Diastolic Blood Pressure						
Surgery	11	541	.44	+.13 to +.67	.01	139.24*
Surgery (outliers removed)	9	491	.23	+.08 to +.38	.00	21.96*
Cardiology/ICU	8	475	.10	+.01 to +.19	.04	5.27
Systolic Blood Pressure						
Surgery	12	550	.44	+.10 to +.69	.01	190.82*
Surgery (outliers removed)	9	450	.26	+.16 to +.35	.00	8.93
Cardiology/ICU	9	505	.12	+.001 to +.24	.05	12.61

	Studies[a]	Sample size[b]	Effect size[c]	Confidence interval[d]	Significance[e]	Homogeneity[f]
Analgesic Intake						
Surgery	9	499	.19	+.06 to +.32	.01	15.73*
Surgery (outlier removed)	8	481	.16	+.04 to +.28	.01	11.81
Sedative Intake						
Surgery (outliers removed)	5	355	.35	+.20 to +.49	.00	8.77
Pain						
Surgery	22	1318	.15	+.08 to +.23	.00	33.01*
Anxiety-measured by STAI						
Surgery	22	1053	.31	+.16 to +.43	.00	106.92*
Cardiology/ICU	8	413	.35	+.17 to +.50	.00	25.25*
Depression						
Surgery	3	70	.41	+.18 to +.59	.00	.14

[a]Adapted from: Dileo C, Bradt J. Music therapy: applications to stress management. In: Lehrer P, Woolfolk R, editors. Principles and practice of stress management. 3rd ed. New York: Guilford Publishers (in press). With permission.
[a]Number of studies.
[b]Total sample size.
[c]Weighted, unbiased effect size: .10 = small; .25 = moderate; .40 = large effect size.
[d]Confidence interval: $p = .05$.
[e]Level of significance.
[f]Homogeneity statistic.
$p < .05$, indicates that the sample is not homogeneous.

For music medicine or music therapy interventions with cardiac or ICU patients, small but significant effects were found for heart rate, diastolic blood pressure, and systolic blood pressure, whereas moderate- to large-effect sizes were found for respiration rate and anxiety.[19] Although there are a number of possible explanations offered in the literature regarding the biopsychosocial mechanisms involved in music's effects (e.g., in anxiety reduction, mood enhancement, and pain reduction), there are currently no overarching theories to guide research and practice. For example, music's effects on pain are often explained in a number of different ways: (1) as an auditory stimulus, it suppresses pain signals directly (Gate Control theory), (2) it stimulates the release of endorphins, (3) it functions as a cognitive distraction, and/or (4) it enhances mood. Any or all of these explanations may account for music's effects, and further research is warranted.

ADDITIONAL RESEARCH EVIDENCE

Cardiac testing

Several studies that investigated the effectiveness of music listening in reducing anxiety and autonomic responsivity in patients awaiting cardiac catheterization have yielded conflicting results. Significant differences between experimental and control subjects in State Trait Anxiety Inventory (STAI) scores were found as result of music listening (experimenter-selected music), and significant increases in blood pressure for the control group (but not the experimental group) were found.[20] No significant differences in anxiety or pain were found between control and experimental subjects who listened to a self-selected audiocassette before, during, and after a catheterization procedure.[21] Similarly, another study[22] found no differences in anxiety, mood, uncertainty, heart rates, or respiratory rates between experimental and control Chinese patients undergoing cardiac catheterization. In contrast, Thorgaard et al (2004)[23] found high levels of patient satisfaction and self-reported well-being associated with the use of music in the sound environment of the cardiac catheterization laboratory. Noteworthy in these studies is the lack of attention to: subjects' musical preferences for the music selections used, the confounding influence of medications, limited sample sizes, and cultural influences.

Surgical procedures

Patients' visitors who listen to music in waiting areas have reported less stress and increased relaxation when compared to controls.[24] In addition, 43% of respondents to a survey of patients' family members in surgical waiting areas rated the availability of soft music as a high priority.[25] In a similar manner, a survey of presurgical patients revealed that the highest percentage of respondents preferred listening to their own choice of music pre-surgically.[26]

Voss et al (2004)[27] found significantly lower anxiety, pain sensation, and pain distress in subjects on chair rest following open-heart surgery. Positive results of this study can be attributed to: the careful preselection of the musical pieces used in this study (done through consultation with a music therapist), attention to potential musical preferences according to subjects' ages and cultures, allowing patients to listen to possible selections before selecting a preferred musical style, and prerecorded instructions for how to use the music. Schwartz et al (2003)[28] studied the benefits of headphone music in the ICU for patients who had undergone CABG surgery. Results revealed significantly shorter lengths of stay in the ICU for patients listening to music as compared to controls.

Combined music and guided imagery procedures

Several studies have examined the effects of interventions that combine the two approaches of guided imagery with music and music listening (without guided imagery) on a variety of parameters. In one study, cardiac surgery patients listened to the guided imagery and music tapes the week prior to surgery and then the music portions only during anesthesia induction and recovery. Subjects again listened to the combined guided imagery and music tapes for 2 weeks postoperatively. Results revealed that subjects receiving guided imagery and music had significantly shorter hospital stays and significantly lower pharmacy direct costs as compared to controls. There was also a tendency for greater patient satisfaction for the experimental group.[29] A similar treatment protocol was tested for patients undergoing cardiac surgery. Results indicated significantly shorter hospital stays and significantly lower pre- and postoperative pain and anxiety scores.[30]

CCU/POST-MI

White (1999)[31] examined the influence of music listening on physiological and psychological outcomes of patients who had had a myocardial infarction within the past 72 hours and who were in a CCU unit. Results indicated immediate and short-term (1 hour) reductions in heart rate, respiration rate, myocardial oxygen demand, and state of anxiety following the implementation of music (as compared to control and resting groups). In addition, significant increases in high-frequency heart rate variability were observed at the onset of the music. Similar results (i.e., significant reductions in blood pressure, respiration rate, and psychological distress in comparison to controls) were found for cardiac patients on bed rest (due to procedural sheaths or IABPs), who listened to experimenter-selected music.[32]

Based on a recent survey of nurses working in acute inpatient facilities in the Midwest,[33] there is fairly widespread knowledge of music therapy (85%), and approximately 70% use it in practice most commonly to reduce anxiety. In addition, music therapy was listed as the independent therapeutic nursing intervention used most frequently to enhance patient sleep and reduce distraction, agitation, aggression, and depression. In a similar survey of 138 critical care nurses in the Midwest[34] regarding complementary and alternative medicine practices, more than three-fourths of the respondents viewed music therapy as a "legitimate" practice, and almost all respondents rated its potential benefits as "neutral to beneficial."

More than half (63%) of the nurses indicated that they had some or a lot of knowledge and training in music therapy, and of this number, 93% have used music therapy or would consider its use in their work. Several points need to be highlighted in these two studies: (1) only nurses in the Midwest were surveyed in these studies, and no other studies for surveys of nurses in other demographic areas could be located; and (2) the use of the term, "music therapy," in these studies is inconsistent with its official professional definition (as discussed previously in this chapter). Specifically, music therapy is not a nursing intervention.

VENTILATOR DEPENDENCY

A number of studies have examined the influence of music listening on a variety of outcomes for patients receiving mechanical ventilation. Wong, et al. (2001)[35] investigated the influence of a music listening session of patient-selected music on anxiety, heart rate, and blood pressure. Significantly lower anxiety scores were found during the music condition (as compared to a rest condition), and significantly lower measures were found between treatment conditions posttest in heart rate and blood pressure. Other researchers[36] have found significant decreases in systolic and diastolic blood pressure during music listening in ventilator-dependent patients, and a significant increase in these measures and heart rate following treatment. In addition, qualitative interviews conducted following hospitalization revealed that patients remembered little of their ICU experience, including the music listening.[36]

In a series of articles and studies, Chlan[37–40] and colleagues[41,42] have reported findings that support the positive effects of music listening with ventilator-dependent patients. In one study, this author found significant differences in anxiety scores, heart rate, and respiratory rates for experimental subjects who listened to music as compared to controls.[38] In a previous study,[37] this author had similar findings, with the addition of improved mood scores for patients having music. In a third study,[40] it is suggested that patient-initiated music, as similar to patient-controlled analgesia, is a feasible intervention for patients on ventilators as well as for their nurses.

CARDIAC REHABILITATION

Exercise to music is ubiquitous, and its use may influence a variety of factors, including perceived exertion, mood, physiological measures, and time compression.[43,44] A recent study also found significant improvements in cognitive performance (verbal fluency) among cardiac rehabilitation subjects who exercised with music.[45]

CONCLUSIONS

There is evidence that music has been used as a healing agent for as long as we have recorded history. Technological advances in measuring the human response (physiological, biological, neurological, etc.) have shown that music as a stimulus is quite complex, as are the individual responses to music. Because the range of experiences possible within music is very broad, it has become apparent that therapists need specialized training to address the nonmusical outcomes in all of the human domains (physiological, psychological, cognitive, social, spiritual, and behavioral).

An attempt has been made in this chapter to describe the wide range of clinical uses of music therapy for cardiac patients, its effectiveness, and the qualifications of its practitioners. As music therapy approaches for these patients continue to evolve, it is hoped that future research will continue to document its benefits—for the patients themselves, for their families, and for their medical professionals.

REFERENCES

1. http://www.cbmt.org (Certification board for misic therapists)
2. http://www.musictherapy.org (American music therapy association)
3. Dileo C, Bradt J. Music therapy: applications to stress management. In: Lehrer P, Woolfolk R, editors. Principles and practice of stress management. 3rd ed. New York: Guilford Publishers (in press).
4. Dileo C. Introduction. In: Dileo C, editor. Music therapy and medicine: theoretical and clinical applications. Silver Spring (MD): American Music Therapy Association; 1999. p. 1–10.
5. Wigram T, Dileo C. Music vibration and health. Cherry Hill (NJ): Jeffrey Books; 1997.
6. Dileo C, Bradt J. Entrainment, resonance and pain-related suffering. In: Dileo C, editor. Music therapy and medicine: theoretical and clinical applications. Silver Spring (MD): American Music Therapy Association. 1999. p. 181–8.
7. O'Callaghan C. Song writing in threatened lives. In: Dileo C, Loewy J, editors. Music therapy at the end of life. Cherry Hill (NJ): Jeffrey Books; 2005. p. 117–28.
8. Crowe B. Music and soul-making: toward a new theory of music therapy. Oxford, England: Scarecrow Press; 2004.
9. Bernardi L, Sleight P, Bandinelli G, Cencetti S, Fattorini L, Wdowczyc-Szulc Lagi A. Effect of rosary prayer and yoga mantras on autonomic cardiovascular rhythms: a comparative study. BMJ. 2001;22:1446–9. [PMID: 11751348.]
10. Bally K, Campbell D, Chesnick K, Tranmer JE. Effects of patient-controlled music therapy during coronary angiography on procedural pain and anxiety distress syndrome. Crit Care Nurse. 2003;23:50–8. [PMID: 1272519.]
11. Taylor-Piliae RE, Chair SY. The use of nursing interventions utilizing music therapy or sensory information on Chinese patients' anxiety prior to cardiac catheterization. Eur J Cardiovasc Nurs. 2002;1:203–11. [PMID: 14622675.]
12. Dileo C, Zanders M. In-between: music therapy with patients awaiting a heart transplant. In: Dileo C, Loewy J, editors. Music therapy at the end of life. Cherry Hill (NJ): Jeffrey Books; 2005. p. 65–76.
13. Dileo C, Loewy J, editors. Music therapy at the end of life. Cherry Hill (NJ): Jeffrey Books. p. 2005
14. Vollert JO, Stork T, Rose M, Rocker L, Klapp BF, Heller G, et al. Reception of music in patients with systemic arterial hypertension and coronary artery disease: endocrine changes, hemodynamics and actual mood. Perfusion. 2002;15:142–52.
15. Salamon E, Bernstein SR, Kim SA, et al. The effects of auditory perception and musical preference on anxiety in naïve human subjects. Med Sci Monit. 2003;9:CR396–9. [PMID: 12960929.]

16. Stefano GB, Zhu W, Cadet P, Salamon E, Mantione KJ. Music alters constitutively expressed opiate and cytokine processes in listeners. Med Sci Monit. 2004;10: MS18–27. [PMID: 15173680.]

17. Chafin S, Roy M, Gerin W, Christenfeld N. Music can facilitate blood pressure recovery from stress. Brit J Health Psychol. 2004;9:393–403. [PMID: 15296685.]

18. Umemura M, Honda K. Influence of music on heart rate variability and comfort: a consideration through comparison of music and noise. J. Human Ergol. 1998;27: 30–8. [PMID: 11579697]

19. Dileo C. Bradt J. Medical music therapy: a meta-analysis and agenda for future research. Cherry Hill (NJ): Jeffrey Books; 2005.

20. Hamel RJ. The effects of music interventions on anxiety in the patient waiting for cardiac catheterization. Intensive Crit Care Nurs. 2001;17:279–85.

21. Bally K, Campbell D, Chesnick K, Tranmer JE. Effects of patient-controlled music therapy during coronary angiography on procedural pain and anxiety distress syndrome. Crit Care Nurse. 2003;23:50–8. [PMID: 1272519.]

22. Taylor-Piliae RE, Chair SY. The use of nursing interventions utilizing music therapy or sensory information on Chinese patients' anxiety prior to cardiac catheterization. Eur J Cardiovasc Nurs. 2002;1:203–11. [PMID: 14622675.]

23. Thorgaard B, Henriksen BB, Pedersbaek G, Thomsen I. Specially selected music in the cardiac laboratory—an important tool for improvement of the wellbeing of patients. Eur J Cardiovasc Nurs. 2004;3:21–6. [PMID: 15053885.]

24. Routhieaux RL, Tansik D. The benefits of music in hospital waiting rooms. Health Care Superv. 1997;16:31–40. [PMID: 10174442.]

25. Carmichael JM, Agre P. Preferences in surgical waiting area amenities. AORN J. 2002;75:1077–83. [PMID: 12085400.]

26. Hyde R, Bryden F, Asbury AJ. How would patients prefer to spend the waiting time before their operations? Anaesthesia. 1998;53:192–200. [PMID: 9534647.]

27. Voss JA, Good M, Yates B, Baun MM, Thompson A, Hertzog M. Sedative music reduces anxiety and pain during chair rest after open-heart surgery. Pain. 2004; 112:197–203. [PMID: 15494201.]

28. Schwartz FJ, Ramey GA, Pawli S. Benefits of headphone music on the ICU postoperative recovery of CABG patients, 2001. Paper presented at the Conference of the International Society for Music in Medicine, Hamburg, Germany, June.

29. Halpin LS, Speir AM, CapoBlanco P, Barnett SD. Guided imagery in cardiac surgery. Outcomes Management. 2002;6:132–7. [PMID: 12134377.]

30. Tusek DL, Cwynar R, Cosgrove DM. Effect of guided imagery on length of stay, pain and anxiety in cardiac surgery patients. J Cardiovasc Manag. 1999 March/April;22–28. [PMID: 10557909.]

31. White JM. Effects of relaxing music on cardiac autonomic balance and anxiety after acute myocardial infarction. Am J Crit Care. 1999;8:220–7. [PMID: 10392221.]

32. Cadigan ME, Caruso NE, Haldeman SM, McNamara ME, Noyes DA, Spadafora MA, et al. The effects of music on cardiac patients on bed rest. Prog Cardiovasc Nurs. 2001 Winter;5–13. [PMID: 11252881.]

33. Gagner-Tjellesen D, Yurkovich EE, Gragert M. Use of music therapy and other ITNIs in acute care. Psychosocial Nurs. 2001;39:27–37. [PMID: 11697072.]

34. Tracy MF, Lindquist R, Watanuki S, Sendelbach S, Kreitzer MJ, Berman B, et al. Nurse attitudes towards the use of complementary and alternative therapies in crucial care. Heart Lung. 2003;32:197–209. [PMID: 12827105.]

35. Wong HIC, Lopez-Nahas V, Molassiotis A. Effects of music therapy on anxiety in ventilator-dependent patients. Heart Lung. 2001;30:376–87. [PMID: 11604980.]

36. Almerud S, Petersson K. Music therapy—complementary treatment for mechanically ventilated intensive care patients. Int Crit Care Nurs. 2003;19:21–30. [PMID: 12590891.]
37. Chlan LL. Psychophysiologic responses of mechanically ventilated patients to music: a pilot study. Am J Crit Care. 1995;4:233–8. [PMID: 7787918.]
38. Chlan LL. Effectiveness of a music therapy intervention on relaxation and anxiety for patients receiving ventilatory assistance. Heart Lung. 1998;27:160–76. [PMID: 9622403.]
39. Chlan LL. Music therapy as a nursing intervention for patients supported by mechanical ventilation. AACN Clin Issues. 2000;11:128–38. [PMID: 11040559.]
40. Chlan LL. Integrating nonpharmacological, adjunctive interventions into critical care practice: a means to humanize care? Am J Crit Care. 2002;11:14–6. [PMID: 11785552.]
41. Chlan LL, Tracy M. Music therapy in critical care: indications and guidelines for intervention. Crit Care Nurs. 1999;19:35–41. [PMID: 10661090.]
42. Chlan LL, Tracy MF, Nelson B, Walker J. Feasibility if a music intervention protocol for patients receiving ventilatory support. Altern Ther. 2001;7:80–3. [PMID: 11712475.]
43. Macnay SK. The influence of preferred music on the perceived exertion, mood and time estimation scores of patients participating in a cardiac rehabilitation exercise program. Music Ther Perspect. 1995;13:91–6.
44. Metzger K. Assessment of use of music by patients participating in cardiac rehabilitation. J Music Ther. 2004;41:55–69.
45. Emery CF, Hsiao ET, Hill SM, Frid DJ. Short-term effects of exercise and music on cognitive performance among participants in a cardiac rehabilitation program. Heart Lung. 2003;32:368–73. [PMID: 14652528.]

16

NATUROPATHIC MEDICINE

Michael Traub

INTRODUCTION

This survey chapter should reveal valuable approaches that naturopathic physicians have learned over the past 25 years or more in the treatment of common cardiovascular problems. The rationale and mechanisms of these interventions will be described. Many of these approaches have proven to be extremely safe, effective, and cost effective, both by themselves and also when integrated with conventional interventions in this frequently high-risk area of medicine.

OBJECTIVE OF THIS CHAPTER

In this chapter, the most current use of naturopathic medicine for cardiovascular conditions will be described, in an attempt to inform and guide clinical practice of integrative cardiology where rigorous evidence may not yet always exist or where the existing evidence is not well accepted. The focus here will be on the naturopathic management of common cardiovascular problems. Other chapters in the book will address some areas that are typically included in naturopathic protocols, such as smoking cessation, exercise, stress management, emotions, spirituality, and quality control. These subjects will not be covered here; the focus will be a comprehensive overview of nutrition, dietary supplements, and herbal medicines. The intention is to describe the scientific evidence for the naturopathic approach to cardiovascular diseases. The reader is referred to the references for more specific information on dosages, mechanisms, and details on statistical significance of the clinical trials cited. It is hoped that the reader will appreciate the value of naturopathic medicine as a distinct discipline and see the desirability of collaborative care for patients with cardiac diseases.

Naturopathic medicine is a system of primary health care-an art, science, philosophy, and practice of diagnosis, treatment, and prevention of illness.

Naturopathic medicine is distinguished by the principles that underlie and determine its practice. These principles are based upon the objective observation of the nature of health and disease, and are continually reexamined in the light of scientific advances. Methods used are consistent with these principles and are chosen upon the basis of patient individuality. Naturopathic physicians are primary health-care practitioners, whose diverse techniques include modern and traditional, scientific and empirical methods that complement mainstream medical practice by contributing to the patient's best interests, satisfying a demand not met by conventional healthcare, and diversifying the approach to healing.

Naturopathic medicine encompasses a wide range of practices. Nutrition, vitamins, minerals, and other dietary supplements, including herbal and homeopathic medicines, physical therapies, lifestyle and psychological counseling are considered to be the mainframe of naturopathic healthcare. In some jurisdictions, prescription drugs, parenteral medicines, injection therapies, acupuncture, minor surgery, and natural childbirth are also included in the scope of practice.

The principles of naturopathic medicine are as follows:

The Healing Power of Nature (Vis Medicatrix Naturae): Naturopathic medicine recognizes an inherent self-healing process in the person that is ordered and intelligent. Naturopathic physicians act to identify and remove obstacles to healing and recovery, and to facilitate and augment this inherent self-healing process.

Identify and Treat the Causes (Tolle Causam): The naturopathic physician seeks to identify and remove the underlying causes of illness, rather than to merely eliminate or suppress symptoms.

First Do No Harm (Primum Non Nocere): To avoid harming the patient, a naturopathic physician utilizes methods and medicinal substances that minimize the risk of harmful side effects, using the least force necessary to diagnose and treat, and acknowledge, respect, and work with the individual's self-healing process.

Doctor as Teacher (Docere): Naturopathic physicians educate their patients and encourage self-responsibility for health. They also recognize and employ the therapeutic potential of the doctor-patient relationship.

Treat the Whole Person: Naturopathic physicians treat each patient by taking into account individual physical, mental, emotional, genetic, environmental, social, and other factors. Since total health also includes spiritual health, naturopathic physicians encourage individuals to pursue their personal spiritual development.

Prevention: Naturopathic physicians emphasize the prevention of disease-assessing risk factors, heredity and susceptibility to disease, and making appropriate interventions in partnership with their patients to prevent illness. Naturopathic medicine is committed to the creation of a healthy world in which humanity may thrive.

The education of a naturopathic physician is as rigorous and demanding as it is at conventional medical schools. A licensed naturopathic physician (ND) has graduated from a 4-year graduate level naturopathic medical school and is educated in all of the same basic sciences as an MD but also studies naturopathic approaches to therapy with a strong emphasis on disease prevention and optimizing wellness. In addition to a standard medical curriculum, the naturopathic physician is required to complete 4 years of training in clinical nutrition, acupuncture, homeopathic medicine, botanical medicine, psychology, and counseling. A naturopathic physician must pass national professional board exams in order to be licensed by a state or jurisdiction as a primary care general practice physician. Residency programs are highly competitive and are typically hospital and/or clinic based. Additional information on naturopathic medical schools can be found at http://www.aanmc.org/. Licensed naturopathic doctors in the United States, Canada can be found at www.naturopathic.org and www.naturopathicassoc.ca.

Nutrition and supplements

Nutrition is a major contributor to cardiovascular health and is a major determinant of body weight, blood pressure (BP), blood glucose, lipids, endothelial function, inflammation, coagulation, and cardiac rhythm. Primary and secondary prevention of cardiovascular disease usually calls for dietary modifications and nutritional supplementation. The merits of various heart-healthy dietary regimes can be debated, but in clinical practice the bottom line is patient compliance and adherence to dietary recommendations. Most conventional physicians recognize their "nutritional deficiency" in their medical education and training. In contrast, naturopathic physicians are trained as experts in nutrition, dietary supplements, and helping patients make therapeutic lifestyle changes. This book's chapter on diet will contain most of the evidence and recommendations generally provided by naturopathic physicians and therefore will not be duplicated here. However, condition-specific dietary recommendations will be briefly enumerated.

Herbal and homeopathic medicine

Naturopathic physicians are experts in herbal medicine as well, and employ specific herbs and formulas in the treatment of cardiovascular disease. The majority of conventionally trained physicians have comparatively little knowledge about herbal medicines, and their primary concern with herbs regards potential interactions with cardiovascular medications. These concerns are justified in some cases; the reader is referred to web-based databanks as this information is continually being updated (herbalgram.com; www.naturaldatabase.com).

There are sparse published studies on the homeopathic treatment of heart disease, and only a couple will be referenced in this chapter. Homeopathy, due to the individualizing of prescriptions, does not lend itself well to randomized trials.

Chelation therapy

Chelation therapy is utilized only by a minority of naturopathic physicians. Most "chelation doctors" are conventionally trained. Chelation therapy has been summarily dismissed by mainstream medicine, although it offers a promising alternative to bypass surgery, angioplasty, and coronary stenting. This chapter will discuss the evidence for this controversial treatment.

Conclusion

Some of the perspectives and recommendations in this chapter will differ from those found in mainstream publications, including the ACCF Complementary Medicine Expert Consensus Document.[1] A problem in many trials and reviews of dietary supplements is that conventional researchers, reviewers, and editors do not always recognize the crucial subtleties of product quality. For a supplement to be subjected to a fair trial, it must be well characterized in purity, potency, and be delivered in the appropriate form. For example, there are many studies on vitamin E and cardiovascular risk which, when subjected to meta-analysis, present a conflicting and confusing picture of whether it is protective or harmful. In naturopathic practice, vitamin E is generally prescribed in the form of natural dl tocopherol, mixed tocopherols, or gamma tocopherol. Rarely is synthetic vitamin E used, although it has been the subject of many of the vitamin E studies. What constitutes product quality for herbal preparations can be even more problematic. Equating quality with strength is a common error. Quality in plant preparations must recognize a balanced combination of complexities that requires intelligent consideration for each plant and its associated substances, including an examination of solvents, simplified fractions, isolated phytochemicals, and standardization.

HYPERLIPIDEMIA

Reconsidering cholesterol

Statins effectively lower total cholesterol, triglycerides, and low-density lipoprotein (LDL) cholesterol. Statins are known to reduce coronary artery disease (CAD)-associated morbidity and mortality in patients with hypercholesterolemia and even in the setting of normocholesterolemia. Additional benefits of statins include atherosclerotic plaque stabilization and regression and reduction of C-reactive protein (CRP). An understanding of why naturopathic and integrative physicians may recommend alternatives to statins must begin with an appreciation for the vital function played by cholesterol in human metabolism. Cholesterol is the precursor to all the glucocorticoids, mineralo-corticoids, and sex hormones. Thus, low cholesterol-whether due to an innate error of metabolism or induced by cholesterol-lowering diets and drugs-can be expected to disrupt the production of adrenal hormones and contribute to blood sugar problems, edema, mineral deficiencies, chronic inflammation, difficulty in healing, allergies, asthma, reduced libido, infertility, and various reproductive problems.

Unfortunately, statins themselves are not without adverse effects. Bedsides the usual common suspects, sleep disturbance may occur with the lipophilic statins (simvastatin, atorvastatin). The most serious, although infrequent, adverse events encountered with statins are hepatotoxicity and myositis. All 5-hydroxy-3-methylglutaryl coenzyme A (HMG-CoA) reductase inhibitors can induce a coenzyme Q10 (CoQ10) deficiency, thought to be responsible for myalgia and fatigue, with the possibility of contributing to heart failure. Myopathy usually occurs in combination with other pharmacological agents, and the risk of muscle damage is higher if the patient is hypothyroid or has hepatic or renal impairment. Finally, there is evidence that simvastatin, at clinical blood concentrations, is immunosuppressive.[2]

Naturopathic physicians recommend dietary and lifestyle changes (exercise, stress reduction) to prevent and treat hyperlipidemia in patients. For established hyperlipidemic patients, who do not comply or respond to this conservative approach, an evidence-based therapeutic algorithm is suggested.

Diet

Saturated and trans fatty acids directly damage endothelial function as well as increase and oxidize serum LDL cholesterol. High-density lipoprotein (HDL) cholesterol is reduced by trans fatty acids. Omega-3 fatty acids reduce triglycerides, stabilize membranes, inhibit platelet aggregation, and are anti-inflammatory. Soluble fibers such as psyllium, guar gum, pectin, and oat bran reduce LDL-C, and there is data from numerous studies demonstrating a reduced risk for myocardial infarctions (MIs) and death from coronary heart disease (CHD) in those who consume higher amounts of dietary fiber. Walnuts and almonds also reduce LDL-C, although the improvement in serum lipids associated with the consumption of nuts does not explain the magnitude of the CHD risk reduction of approximately 40–50% found in large epidemiologic studies.[3] Nuts, especially walnuts and almonds, contain not only omega-3 fatty acids but other cardioprotective nutrients such as vitamin E, arginine, magnesium, folate, plant sterols, and soluble fiber.[4] Although plant stanol/sterol lowers LDL-C and total cholesterol, no trials have studied their effects on cardiovascular risk.[1] Naturopathic physicians do not generally recommend plant stanol/sterol esters in the form of margerine or other butter substitutes.

Soy-based foods have cholesterol-lowering, estrogenic, and antioxidant properties. They promote increased vascular reactivity, improve arterial compliance, and are antithrombotic. Studies have shown that making multiple dietary changes simultaneously is more effective than simply changing one aspect of the diet. In a study of hyperlipidemic patients, a diet high in plant sterols, soy-protein foods, almonds, and fibers from oats, barley, psyllium, okra, and eggplant was nearly as effective as 20 mg/day of lovastatin in reducing LDL-C and highly sensitive C-reactive protein (hsCRP).[5]

One of the dietary factors thought to play a large role in the significant lower mortality from CAD associated with the Mediterranean Diet is olive oil. Polyphenols from extra virgin olive oil are thought to be responsible for inhibiting the oxidation of LDL. And lastly, the best documented benefit of moderate alcohol intake is an increase in HDL.[6] Based on a single randomized trial, adherence to the DASH (Dietary Approaches to Stop Hypertension) diet and taking multi-vitamins was found to raise HDL levels by 21–33%. Based on meta-analyses, adherence to a low-carbohydrate diet was found to raise HDL by 10% and consumption of soy protein with isoflavones was found to raise HDL by 3%.[6a]

When dietary, exercise, and stress management recommendations are insufficient in treating hyperlipidemia, naturopathic physicians resort to an evidence-based approach which begins with those natural medicines that are validated by randomized controlled trials, systematic reviews, laboratory research, and the effects of interventions in the clinical practice setting. Currently, many naturopathic physicians treat hyperlipidemia that is unresponsive to therapeutic lifestyle changes with red yeast rice.

Red yeast rice—a "kinder, gentler" statin?

Red yeast rice (RYR) is a fermented product of rice on which red yeast (Monascus purpureus) has been grown, and has been used in China for centuries as a medicinal food to promote "blood circulation." In Chinese cuisine it is used to make rice wine and to make "Peking Duck" red. RYR contains lovastatin and has been shown in clinical trials to favorably impact lipid profiles of hypercholesterolemic patients.[2]

RYR's HMG-CoA reductase activity comes from a family of compounds called monacolins. Monacolin K is lovastatin, comprising 0.2% of the total product. RYR contains eight other monacolins, all of which have HMG-CoA reductase-lowering ability. Other active ingredients in RYR include sterols, isoflavones, and monounsaturated fatty acids. A daily dosage of 2.4 g of RYR contains 4.8 mg lovastatin, making it extremely unlikely that the effects achieved with RYR are solely due to the lovastatin content, which is generally dosed at 20–40 mg daily. The other monacolins, sterols, and isoflavones probably contribute significantly and synergistically to achieve the lipid profile improvements seen with RYR.

RYR reliably lowers total cholesterol, LDL, and triglycerides and raises HDL in approximately the same amounts as found in the first human study carried out with 1.2 g/day RYR for 8 weeks in hypercholesterolemic adults, which reduced total cholesterol by 23%, LDL by 31%, and triglycerides by 34%. Serum HDL levels increased by 20%.

Toxicity evaluation of RYR in animals and humans has shown no toxicity. Side effects have been limited to headaches and gastrointestinal (GI) discomfort. The same contraindications as for lovastatin are prudent. Because HMG-CoA reductase inhibitors reduce production of CoQ10, supplementation with tocotrienol CoQ10 is advised. When comparing the value of a drug to a natural alternative, the safety factors and cost must be considered. Often, the ramifications of a nutrient, in contrast to a drug, are not side effects but side benefits.

Niacin

Combined use of niacin with a statin is an attractive option, since these types of medication have the best records in clinical trials for reduction in cardiovascular events and improvement in progression/regression of coronary lesions, and even low doses of niacin potentiates the lipid-lowering effects of statins. As with fibrate-statin combinations, safety concerns exist with combining statins and niacin.[7] According to a retrospective analysis of all FDA reports of statin-induced rhabdomyolysis, only 4 of 871 cases were attributed to combination therapy with niacin. Prospective trials in more than 400 patients have not encountered myopathy or significant hepatotoxicity. This experience includes 165 patients who took a statin in combination with Niaspan, an extended-release niacin. However, substantial transaminase elevations occurred with the use of sustained-release niacin (Nicobid) given twice daily. The niacin-statin treatment regimens gave augmented LDL-C reduction along with favorable changes in high-density lipoprotein cholesterol (HDL-C), lipoprotein(a), and triglycerides. This combination therapy can therefore be used safely as long as (1) careful attention is given to niacin formulation and dosing, (2) liver functions are monitored, and (3) patients are educated to recognize symptoms of myopathy.

A 68% reduction in carotid artery intimal medial thickening was achieved when adding extended-release niacin to statin therapy in patients with coronary heart disease on a statin with an LDL-C<130 mg/dL and an HDL-C<45 mg/dL. No change in this measure was seen in a statin-only group.)[8] A 60% reduction of coronary events was also found with niacin plus statins compared to statins alone. HDL was increased a significant 21% in the niacin plus statin patients (from 39 to 47 mg/dL). Triglycerides were significantly improved with niacin plus statin versus statin-alone (134 mg/dL and 164 mg/dL, respectively). A post hoc analysis comparing patients with diabetes/metabolic syndrome or no diabetes, showed progression in both placebo groups, lowest progression of intimal medial thickness in the niacin plus statin group, and a significantly lower progression in patients without diabetes/metabolic syndrome taking niacin. A single-tablet combination of extended release niacin and lovastatin has shown efficacy greater than either drug alone and without an increased safety risk over the manual combination of its individual components.[9]

A long-term, open-label study of 814 dyslipidemic patients with or without CHD reported a 47% reduction in LDL, 41% reduction in triglycerides, and 30% increase in HDL after 16 weeks of therapy with monthly titration from lovastatin 10 mg/day-niacin ER 500 mg/day to lovastatin 40 mg/day-niacin 2000 mg/day, with the effect persisting during 1 year of follow-up. Levels of HDL continued to increase during the study to 41% by study end. The side effects of niacin, which may occur at the dosages often required for therapeutic efficacy, ranging from flushing and pruritus to hepatoxicity and impaired glucose tolerance, often prove troubling for both patient and practitioner. The need for a safer approach to niacin supplementation has resulted in the investigation of niacin esters. Inositol hexaniacinate, in numerous trials, has been found to be virtually free of the side effects associated with conventional niacin therapy. Niacin in even modest amounts will potentiate the effects of statins, and CoQ10 in small doses will prevent the deficiency of this nutrient which is induced by statins. This author uses a compounded preparation of RYR (300 mg), niacin (25 mg), and CoQ10 (5 mg), two capsules twice daily, in the treatment of hyperlipidemic patients, with reliable, consistent results, at a cost of approximately $30 per month, compared to $37 or more per month for 20-mg generic lovastatin.

Phytosterols

Inhibition of absorption of intestinal cholesterol rather than inhibition of cholesterol synthesis via statins may provide an excellent alternative route in both lowering cholesterol and reducing risk of CVD. A wealth of evidence shows that the supplementation of plant sterols will decrease absorption of cholesterol by 30–66% leading to reductions in both total and LDL-C of between 5–20%, irrespective of initial cholesterol concentration.[10] The FDA recommends that the daily requirement of phytosterols to achieve benefits is 1.6 g phytosterol esters divided over two meals per day. Phytosterols have been found to provide an additional 10–20% reduction in LDL when combined with a statin.[11] The combination of fish oils and phytosterols also provides comprehensive preventative protection for CVD. Regular consumption of phytosterols has been observed to be accompanied by decreases in absorption of fat-soluble vitamins.[12] However, a closer examination of adverse effects of phytosterols indicates that the extent to which fat-soluble vitamins may be decreased is minimal and likely to have no clinical implications.[13]

Policosanol

Sugarcane may seem an unlikely source for natural lipid-lowering substances, but a mixture of alcohols isolated and purified from sugarcane, known as policosanol, has demonstrated considerable efficacy in benefiting cardiovascular biomarkers in over 50 Cuban studies, representing tens of thousands of people. In addition to sugarcane (Saccharum officinarum), policosanol occurs in other plants and beeswax, and its main component is octacosanol. Studies are underway to determine the optimal synergetic proportions of polyaliphatic cosanols. Policosanol appears to cause decreased synthesis and increased degradation of HMG-CoA reductase, unlike statins, which competitively inhibit the enzyme. Policosanol has also demonstrated a dose-dependent ability (typically 5–10 mg twice daily) to reduce oxidized LDL and decrease platelet aggregation in humans. It has also improved various other measures of cardiovascular function. A meta-analysis of randomized controlled trials (from a total of 4596 patients from 52 eligible studies) concluded that plant sterols and stanols and policosanol were well tolerated and safe.[14] Policosanol was more effective than plant sterols and stanols for LDL-level reduction and more favorably altered the lipid profile, approaching antilipemic drug efficacy. In a randomized, double-blind, placebo-controlled trial involving 40 subjects with mild hypercholesterolemia, supplementation with a policosanol supplement (20 mgld) was not found to be any more effective than a placebo in altering lipid levels, C-reactive protein, or nuclear magnetic resonance-determined lipoprotein profile among subjects over the course of 8 weeks events.[14a]

Guggul

The mukul myrrh tree (Commiphora mukul), a native of India, secretes the substance guggul (also known as guggulu or guggulipid) when its bark is injured. Guggul has been used in Ayurvedic medicine for thousands of years to treat arthritis and obesity. Guggul extracts were first used in Asia to help manage cholesterol levels and are becoming increasingly popular in the United States. It is believed that guggul can reduce total cholesterol, LDL cholesterol, and triglycerides.[15]

Studies of the efficacy of guggul for hypercholesterolemia have produced conflicting results. Information currently available indicates that guggul may be effective for lowering total cholesterol and triglycerides in patients on a non-Western diet. The one study involving a typical American diet did not show any benefits; in fact, patients taking guggul had slight increases in LDL cholesterol.[16] The effectiveness of guggul may therefore depend on dietary practices. Although most adverse effects have not been serious, the one reported case of rhabdomyolysis raises concern, especially if guggul is used in conjunction with other lipid-lowering therapies. Also, since lipid control may require ongoing management, the long-term effects of guggul should be assessed.

Omega-3 fatty acids

A systematic review of 97 randomized clinical trials (more than 275,000 people) has revealed that omega-3 fatty acids are more effective than statins in reducing both heart disease-related mortality and all-cause mortality.[17] The only interventions that produced statistically significant reductions in both total and cardiac mortality were statins (13% and 22%) and omega-3 fatty acids (23% and 32%). The heterogeneity of the patient populations and the interventions studied makes definitive extrapolations for the general population difficult to draw. Some trials enrolled patients who had survived a MI; other patients had angina or were status-post angioplasty. One study was a primary prevention trial in high-risk patients without established heart disease. Omega-3 fatty acids produced an average reduction in serum cholesterol levels of only 2%, compared to a 20% reduction for statins. A marked triglyceride-lowering effect was seen with omega-3 fatty acids, but a variable, and not particularly strong effect was observed on LDL-C. Omega-3 fatty acids exert a number of other cardioprotective effects such as antiarrhythmic activity, inhibiting platelet aggregation, reducing plasma viscosity, and fibrinogen. Omega-3 fatty acids do not appear to reduce hsCRP levels in healthy people, despite their anti-inflammatory activity, so its benefit on heart disease may be due to these other activities, and may be most effective for people who do not have elevated LDL-C and hsCRP.[18]

Krill oil

Krill is a zooplankton crustacean (Euphausia superba) rich in omega-3 fatty acids that also contains vitamins A and E, astaxanthin, and a novel flavonoid. A multi-center, 3-month, prospective, randomized study followed by a 3-month controlled follow-up was performed on 120 patients treated with 1 and 1.5 g krill oil daily in patients able to maintain a healthy diet and with blood cholesterol levels between 194 and 348 mg/dL. A sample size of 30 patients per group was randomly assigned to one of four groups. Group A received krill oil at a body mass index (BMI)-dependent daily dosage of 2–3 g daily. Patients in Group B were given 1–1.5 g krill oil daily, and Group C was given fish oil at a dose of 3 g daily. Group D was given a placebo containing microcrystalline cellulose. Krill oil 1–3 g/day was found to be effective for the reduction of glucose, total cholesterol, triglycerides, LDL, while increasing HDL compared to both fish oil and placebo.[19]

Garlic

Garlic shows modest, short-term effects on lipids. Naturopathic physicians do not generally rely on garlic supplements as a major intervention for hyperlipidemia, but instead advocate including it as a component of a heart healthy, anti-inflammatory diet, along with other foods such as onions, ginger, and turmeric.

The data described above supports the concept that statins are not the "only game in town" for the management of hyperlipidemia. For many people, a well-designed program of diet, lifestyle changes, and nutritional supplements might be as successful as, or more successful than statins for cardiac disease prevention. A successful naturopathic intervention is likely to improve not only cardiovascular disease risk, but many other aspects of overall health, as well.

BEYOND LIPIDS–PREDICTIVE MEDICINE AND PRIMARY PREVENTION

Half of all heart attacks and strokes in the United States occur in people with normal cholesterol levels, and 20% of all events occur in people with no major risk factors. It has been repeatedly verified that hsCRP levels, when added to the traditional ways of measuring risk, enhances detection of the high-risk patient and affords the opportunity to lower risk through diet, supplements, exercise, smoking cessation, and other early interventions, improving our ability to not only predict but to prevent thrombotic occlusion. This has been termed "predictive medicine," that is, early disease diagnosis, which addresses the underlying causes and prevention of acute coronary syndromes.

C-reactive protein

CRP is found in high levels in inflammatory fluids and in both the intimal layer of the atherosclerotic aortic artery and the foam cells within the lesions of atherosclerotic plaque. CRP has been found in the fatty streak of the aorta and is the key in many of the inflammatory sequences that promote the progression of atherosclerosis. CRP stimulates monocytes to release tissue factor, a protein that is central to the initiation of coagulation reactions, complement activation, and the neutralizing of platelet-activation factor. Together, these reactions promote a thrombotic response.

Measurement of hsCRP adds prognostic information at all levels of LDL, at all levels of the Framingham Risk Score, and at all levels of the metabolic syndrome. It is crucial to measure hsCRP to assess the dual-goal therapy of not only reduction of oxidized LDL-C but of hsCRP levels as well.[20] (See Figs. 16–1 and 16–2.)

However, not all patients who get an LDL reduction from statins also get an hsCRP reduction; in fact, there is almost no relationship between the change in LDL and hsCRP. The best way to lower hsCRP is by diet, exercise, and smoking cessation. Foods with an anti-inflammatory effect include garlic, ginger, tumeric, olive oil, flaxseed oil, nuts, seeds, avocado, and cold-water fish. Pro-inflammatory foods should be avoided: fatty meats, whole milk products, margerine, vegetable shortening, fried foods, hydrogenated oils, sugar, and caffeine. In addition, the following supplements may be helpful: bromelain and other proteolytic enzymes, fish oil, L-arginine, vitamins B_6, C, E, folic acid, and RYR. Prospective studies show clearly that higher CRP levels are associated with higher coronary heart disease (CHD) incidence and mortality, but the cardiology community has largely de-emphasized this association in recent years. To some extent, this may reflect a commercial rather than a scientific imperative: there may be an attempt by some to discourage use of other risk markers in favor of lipid markers and the subsequent prescription of statin drugs.

On the other hand, the unwillingness of many cardiologists to embrace CRP as a fully-fledged risk factor may be due to an uncertainty as to whether CRP is a passive marker of risk, an active participant in the disease process, or both. Is a high CRP level an actual driver of heart disease or merely a hapless passenger on the road to MI? Is there a causal connection or merely an association?

Like many other things in medicine, our confusion about CRP may reflect our desire for simple "yes or no" answers, and "one size fits all" solutions. In truth, CRP elevation may mean different things in different people.

A patient's specific CRP genotype may influence CRP synthesis, which in turn, could mediate the onset of subclinical and clinical CV events. Alternatively, CRP may increase the propensity toward acute ischemic events through indirect

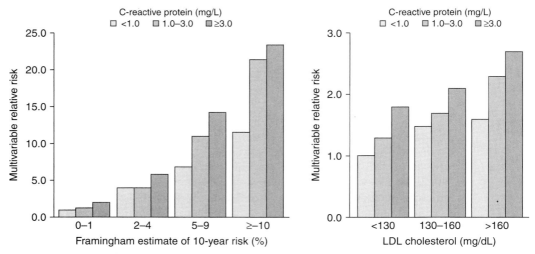

FIGURE 16-1 *Multivariable-adjusted relative risks of cardiovascular disease according to levels of C-reactive protein and the estimated 10-year risk-based on the Framingham Risk Score as Currently Defined by the National Cholesterol Education Program and according to levels of C-reactive protein and categories of LDL cholesterol. To convert values for LDL cholesterol to millimoles per liter, multiply by 0.02586. (With permission from Ridker PM, Hennekens CH, Buring JE, et al. C-reactive protein and other markers of inflammation in the prediction of cardio-vascular disease in women. NEJM. 2000 March 23;342:836.)*

effects, such as causing a procoagulant phenotype through induction of tissue factor and expression of plasminogen activator inhibitor (PAI)-1 by vascular endothelial cells or monocytes.

Attempts to add CRP to traditional CV risk modeling protocols, with the ultimate objective of improving targeted therapy, have led to widely divergent conclusions.[20a]

The burning question is whether CRP truly has a causal role in heart disease. Principles of Mendelian randomization have been applied to try and tease out an answer. We know there are polymorphisms in the CRP gene that influence CRP levels. These genetic variations, however, are not related to any of the factors that confound observational studies, such as smoking, obesity, or socioeconomic status.

Groups defined on the basis of CRP genotype have long-term differences in CRP levels. If CRP is causally related to CHD, the genotypic variations should be reflected as variations in CHD risk. New data obtained from studies in elders suggest that certain CRP gene variants are, in fact, linked with increased incidence of cardiovascular events.[20b] The data also suggest that CRP polymorphisms may reflect lifetime exposure to CRP more accurately than CRP serum concentrations measured at a single point in time. This implies that when it comes to the negative impact of CRP, lifetime exposure matters more than isolated, short-term elevations.

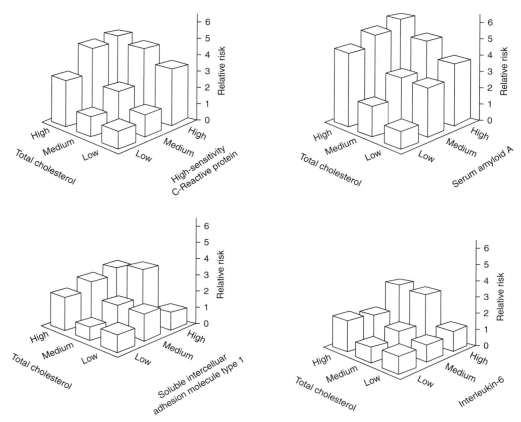

FIGURE 16-2 *Relative risk of cardiovascular events among apparently healthy postmenopausal women. According to base-line plasma levels of total cholesterol and markers of inflammation, each marker of inflammation improved risk-prediction models based on lipid testing alone, an effect that was strongest for hsCRP and serum amyloid A. (With permission from Pai JK, Pischon T, Ma J, et al. Inflammatory markers and the risk of CHD in men and women. NEJM. 2004 Dec 16; 351:2599.)*

Randomized, controlled trials of CRP-lowering should provide a more definitive answer to the question of whether CRP causes CHD. Until these studies are completed, however, the CRP debate will likely continue, yet the evidence still weighs in favor of comprehensive cardiometabolic risk assessment that includes both hsCRP and homocysteine.[23a]

Beyond homocysteine

Hyperhomocysteinemia has been recognized as an independent risk factor for cardiovascular disease. The mechanism by which it impairs vascular function may involve oxidative-endothelial injury and dysfunction, vascular smooth muscle cell growth and collagen synthesis, lipid peroxidation and platelet activation, and hypercoagulability.[21] Optimizing the methionine-homocysteine pathways with twice daily doses of betaine (3 g), vitamins B_6 (60 mg) and B_{12} (500 mg), and folic acid (1 g) offers the possibility for primary and secondary prevention and treatment.[22]

Beyond their effect on homocysteine, high-dose folic acid and 5-methyltetrahydrofolate (5–30 mg/d) have recently been shown to enhance nitric oxide (NO) bioavailability and restore endothelial function and demonstrate important potential for the prevention of atherosclerosis and inflammatory disorders of the vascular endothelium.[23]

FIBRINOGEN

Fibrinogen has been identified as an associative risk element by the American Heart Association.[24] Fibrinogen is a plasma glycoprotein which is synthesized by the liver and is involved in the final steps of coagulation in response to vascular or tissue injury. Aside from its role in thrombosis, fibrinogen has a number of actions that add to its participation in atherosclerosis and CAD including: regulation of cell adhesion and proliferation; vasoconstriction at sites of vascular injury; stimulation of platelet aggregation; influence on blood viscosity. Clinically, it is important to consider both genetic and environmental influence on fibrinogen levels. These include gender (males have higher values), tobacco use, use of drugs (i.e., some statins, hormone replacement therapy, and oral contraceptives), excess weight, sedentary lifestyle, stress, inflammatory processes, and diabetes.[25] Factors that decrease fibrinogen include smoking cessation, weight loss, exercise, alcohol, fibrates, and niacin. To lower fibrinogen below 300 mg/dl, the following supplements will be helpful: inositol hexanicotinate, vitamin C, bromelain, fish oil, curcumin, nattokinase, and lactobacillus plantarum.

LIPOPROTEIN-PLA2

Lipoprotein-associated Phospholipase A2 or Lp-PLA2, when elevated, and hsCRP values have been shown in several studies to be independently predictive of CVD risk and, when elevated together, equal very high risk.[26] Lp-PLA2 is an enzyme which circulates primarily in association with LDL and is believed to have a causal role in atherosclerosis. Once small dense LDL within the intima becomes oxidized, Lp-PLA2 cleaves it to generate two pro-inflammatory mediators. As elevated Lp-PLA2 levels are indicative of an activated or progressing atherosclerotic process, Lp-PLA2 testing is additive and complementary to hsCRP testing (which instead reflects acute phase inflammatory response). An elevated Lp-PLA2 value has been demonstrated as a predictor of future events and is a warning signal that the inflammatory process of atherosclerosis is active. It may thus be used to increase aggressiveness of therapy targeting known risk factors. Elevated levels of Lp-PLA2 levels have been shown to be significantly reduced by both statin and fenofibrate therapies.

Vitamin D and vascular function—beyond-way beyond-rickets

Because the intakes required to prevent many of the long latency diseases (such as cardiovascular disease, metabolic syndrome, and diabetes) are higher than those required to prevent the respective index diseases (scurvy, beri-beri, rickets, etc.), recommendations based solely on preventing the index diseases are no longer biologically defensible.[27] The recommended adequate intakes for vitamin D are inadequate, and, in the absence of exposure to sunlight, a minimum of 1000 IU/day vitamin D_3 is required to maintain a healthy concentration of 25-hydroxy-vitamin D_3 in the blood.[28]

Metabolic syndrome

Finally, it would be remiss to not recognize the metabolic syndrome and its relevance to cardiovascular disease, given the increased attention it has received in the last few years. Metabolic syndrome consists of multiple, interrelated risk factors of metabolic origin that appear to directly promote the development of atherosclerotic cardiovascular disease and are strongly associated with Type II diabetes. Metabolic syndrome is a complex disorder of multifactorial etiology. The most important risk factors are abdominal obesity and insulin resistance. Other metabolic risk factors are atherogenic dyslipidemia, high BP, high plasma glucose levels, a prothrombotic state, and a proinflammatory state. Other conditions that may promote the metabolic syndrome include sedentary lifestyle, aging, hormonal imbalance, and genetic or ethnic predisposition.

Fat as an endocrine organ

Adipose tissue has recently emerged as an active endocrine organ that secretes a variety of metabolically important substances, collectively called adipocytokines or adipokines.[29] Study of the effects of the adipokines leptin, adiponectin, and resistin on the vasculature has shown their potential role in the pathogenesis of vascular disease. Leptin is associated with arterial wall thickness, decreased vessel distensibility, and elevated hsCRP levels. Leptin possesses procoagulant and antifibrinolytic properties, and it promotes thrombus and atheroma formation, probably through the leptin receptors by promoting vascular inflammation, proliferation, and calcification, and by increasing oxidative stress. Adiponectin inhibits the expression of the intracellular adhesion molecule ICAM-1, vascular c. adhesion molecule (VCAM-1), and P selectin. Therefore, it interferes with monocyte adherence to endothelial cells and their subsequent migration to the subendothelial space, one of the initial events in the development of atherosclerosis. Adiponectin also inhibits the transformation of macrophages to foam cells in vitro and decreases their phagocytic activity. Resistin was named for its ability to promote insulin resistance. Resistin increases the expression of the adhesion molecules VCAM-1 and ICAM-1, up-regulates the monocyte chemoattractant chemokine-1, and promotes endothelial cell activation via endothelin (ET-1) release. From this perspective of the metabolically acitve adipocyte, the association with obesity and cardiovascular disease becomes even clearer.

Primary prevention

Before addressing specific naturopathic treatments for various cardiac conditions, it is important not to overlook the obvious: primary prevention. The adage "prevention is the best medicine," is unquestionably true of heart disease. Since traditional risk factors account for only half of the cases of CAD, a more proactive preventive course would be to make the necessary changes which will impact those risk factors, along with addressing dietary nutrients and their biochemical pathways, which have been shown to have a significant impact on CAD, and which may account for some of the traditional risk factors and part of the other half of CAD incidence. These nutrients and pathways include B vitamins, vitamins C, D, and E, beta carotene, lipoic acid, betaine, CoQ10, glutathione, polyphenols/flavonoids, methionine metabolism, cholesterol metabolism and excretion, and the amino acids L-arginine, L-carnitine, glycine, lysine, and taurine. Ensuring efficient functioning of these interconnected pathways can have a significant positive impact on the multifactorial process of CAD. Hyperlipidemia, hypertension, and family history of premature CAD may not be a problem unto themselves, but an end-result of nutrient deficiencies caused by inadequate dietary intake or genetic predisposition toward decreased utilization and/or decreased enzyme activity.

Metabolic cardiology is the term for a paradigm of heart disease prevention and treatment that employs a regimen to protect the senescent heart against stress, combining metabolic therapy (CoQ10, alpha lipoic acid, magnesium orotate, and omega 3 polyunsaturated fatty acids) with physical exercise and mental stress reduction. The preliminary results of this program have been promising. The aging heart has a diminished capacity to recover from stress that is not readily predictable by cardiac content of intact mitochondrial DNA.[30]

CORONARY ARTERY DISEASE

Diet

The prevalence of CAD is considerably less in Mediterranean and Pacific Rim countries than in the United States at equivalent cholesterol levels. Common to these cultures is a diet high in fruits, vegetables, legumes, whole grains, nuts, fish, and mono- and polyunsaturated oils. Dairy products and meat are consumed in low-to-moderate amounts. Alcohol is consumed in moderation. The Lyon Diet Heart Study tested the effectiveness of a Mediterranean diet (modified by substituting alpha-linolenic acid-enriched canola oil margerine for olive oil), on cardiovascular risk after a first MI.[31] After an average follow-up of 46 months, subjects on the diet had 72% fewer cardiovascular events and 60% lower all-cause mortality. These findings were reproduced with an Indo-Mediterranean diet, reducing cardiovascular events by 45% and sudden cardiac death by 66%.[32]

Fish and omega-3 fatty acids from fish affect CHD outcomes by decreasing triglycerides, ventricular arrhythmias, fibrinogen, platelet aggregation, inflammation, BP, and cell proliferation. Omega-3 fatty acids also improve arterial compliance, endothelial function, heart rate variability, and mood (depression).

Most of the prospective, controlled intervention trials with either cold water fish or omega-3 fatty acid capsules have demonstrated reduced cardiovascular events. Because of genetic polymorphisms, it may be that only certain patients may benefit from omega-3 fatty acids to prevent post-angioplasty restenosis.[33]

Nuts are strongly cardioprotective as well. In a prospective study of 86,016 women without previously diagnosed CHD, eating 5 oz of nuts per week was associated with a relative risk (RR) of 0.66 of coronary events adjusted for risk factors and independent of fiber, fruit, and vegetable supplements. Prospective data from the Physicians' Health Study demonstrated consumption of nuts two or more times a week significantly reduced the risk of sudden cardiac death (RR) of 0.53 and a RR of 0.70 for total CHD deaths compared with men who rarely or never consumed nuts.[3] The association between nut consumption and sudden cardiac death became stronger after adjustment for lifestyle, cardiac risk factors, and diet.

Olive oil, when phenol rich as in extra virgin olive oil, has been shown to be cardioprotective in epidemiological studies and in mildly dyslipidemic patients is associated with favorable changes in circulating markers of cardiovascular risk.[34]

Tea drinking appears to be protective against CHD in a number of epidemiologic studies. An inverse association was found between tea drinking and advanced aortic atherosclerosis, stronger for fatal events than for nonfatal events.[35] Results are inconclusive for clinical and case control studies. A prospective cohort study of 1,900 patients hospitalized with an acute MI followed for 3.8 years found a significantly reduced hazard ratio for subsequent total and cardiovascular mortality of 0.56 for heavy tea drinkers (more than 14 cups per week) compared to non-tea drinkers.[36] A clinical study has shown that consumption of black tea improves brachial artery flow-mediated dilation in patients with CAD and further research has shown that the benefits of black tea consumption on endothelial function may not be attributable to tea catechins or a systemic antioxidant or anti-inflammatory effect. Chronic dietary flavonoid status appears to relate to endothelial function, possibly suggesting that other flavonoids or polyphenolic components of tea favorably influence vascular health and risk for cardiovascular disease.[37] Despite the favorable epidemiology and mechanistic investigations, no studies to date have prospectively documented a reduction in cardiovascular risk with tea drinking.

Alcohol intake, in moderation, has shown in epidemiologic studies that the incidence of MI, angina pectoris, and coronary-related deaths are inversely related. Many mechanisms for this effect have been suggested; the best documented one being an increase in HDL cholesterol by alcohol. Studies have shown that moderate drinkers are less likely to suffer ischemic stroke, peripheral vascular disease, and death following an acute MI. [36] Moderate consumption of alcohol-containing beverages does not appear to result in significant morbidity; however, heavy alcohol consumption can result in cardiomyopathy, hypertension, hemorrhagic stroke, cardiac arrhythmia, and sudden death. Alcohol ingestion poses such a number of health hazards with irresponsible consumption that the American Heart Association (AHA) recommends that physicians and patients discuss the adverse and potentially beneficial aspects of moderate drinking.[38] The mechanisms underlying the effects of alcohol on cardiovascular disease have been limited to lipid metabolism and the hemostatic system; those related to wine consumption have also been extended to specific anti-inflammatory, antioxidant, and NO-related vaso-relaxant properties of its polyphenolic constituents.[39]

Antioxidants are potentially useful in preventing both atherosclerosis and its complications by retarding LDL oxidation and by inhibiting the proliferation of smooth muscle cells, platelet adhesion and aggregation, the expression and function of adhesion molecules, and the synthesis of leukotrienes. Antioxidants may improve endothelial function, reduce ischemia, and stabilize atherosclerotic plaques to prevent plaque rupture. Despite lipoprotein oxidation's biologically plausible role in atherogenesis, several studies have reported inconsistent effects of antioxidants on clinical coronary end points.[40]

VITAMIN E

There is an ongoing controversy about the effect of supplemental tocopherol and its ability to reduce risk of cardiovascular events in randomized trials. The meta-analysis published in late 2004 concluded that vitamin E in dosage greater than 400 IU/day may increase all-cause mortality and should be avoided.[41] The article set off a maelstrom of lurid headlines and backlash. What's the truth about this meta-analysis? Statisticians criticized the study as being too far-reaching in its conclusions and unpersuasive that vitamin E might be unsafe. Others criticized the study for what was overlooked. The authors did not investigate at all dozens of observational studies involving millions of people that show vitamin E supplementation can be beneficial and completely safe. Moreover, the studies that allegedly showed evidence of the harmful effects of vitamin E considered sick populations already at high risk of death: patients with advanced heart disease, cancer, Alzheimer's disease, and renal failure. Even the authors of the paper themselves admit: "High dosage trials (greater than 400 IU/day) were often small and were performed in patients with chronic diseases. The generalization of the findings to healthy adults is uncertain." Additionally, these studies mostly looked at the effects of synthetic vitamin E, when most naturopathic and integrative physicians prescribe natural mixed tocopherols, which supply gamma tocopherol and tocotrienols, and recommend vitamin E not as an isolated nutrient, as in most of the studies included in the meta-analysis, but as a component of a balanced program of antioxidant supplementation.[42]

The Nurses Health Study of approximately 90,000 nurses published over 10 years ago suggested that the incidence of heart disease was 30–40% lower among nurses with the highest intake of vitamin E from diet and supplements. The apparent benefit was mainly associated with intake of vitamin E from dietary supplements. High vitamin E intake from food was not associated with significant cardiac risk reduction.

The Institute of Medicine (IOM) position on vitamin E flies in the face of the meta-analysis warning against high doses of vitamin E. IOM states on its web site (ods.od.nih.gov/factsheets/vitamine.asp), "The general health risk of too much vitamin E is low." The IOM has set an upper tolerable level for vitamin E at 1000 mg or 1500 IU/day. This upper limit represents the maximum intake for a nutrient that is likely to pose no risk of adverse health effects in most healthy people in the general population. Clearly, before any action is taken to discourage the use of vitamin E, further studies are needed to prove any lack of safety.

Some of the discrepancies in trial outcomes may result from the doses of vitamin E used in the trials. Human studies have shown a direct dose-response effect up to 1200 IU daily for anti-inflammatory effects and inhibition of CRP. Supplementation with 1200 IU alpha-tocopherol was able to reduce elevated CRP by 33% in nondiabetic controls after 3 months, and a similar trial found a 48% reduction in CRP with 800 IU in patients with Type II diabetes after 4 weeks.[43] A placebo-controlled, double-blind study of 104 carotid endarterectomy patients determined the effects of short-term alpha-tocopherol supplementation (500 IU/day) on lipid oxidation in plasma and advanced atherosclerotic lesions.[44] The vitamin E group showed significant increase in plasma alpha-tocopherol concentrations, a 40% increase (compared with placebo patients) in circulating LDL-associated alpha-tocopherol), and their LDL was less susceptible to ex vivo oxidation than that of the placebo group. Alpha-tocopherol concentrations in lesions correlated significantly with those in plasma, suggesting that plasma alpha-tocopherol levels can influence lesion levels. There was a significant inverse correlation in lesions between cholesterol-standardized levels of alpha-tocopherol and 7-hydroxycholesterol, a free radical oxidation product of cholesterol. These results may explain why studies using less than 500 IU alpha-tocopherol per day failed to demonstrate benefit of antioxidant therapy. Better understanding of the pharmacodynamics of oral antioxidants is required to guide future clinical trials. It is also apparent that using alpha-tocopherol alone is inadequate for complete protection from LDL oxidation. Tocopherol is recycled by ascorbate and, although ascorbate is not lipophilic and is unable to enter the LDL particle, it has the ability to prevent LDL oxidation in human cell lines.

VITAMIN C

A meta-analysis of nine studies evaluating dietary intake of vitamin E, carotenoids, and vitamin C, with a 10-year follow-up to check for coronary disease, found that antioxidant vitamins were only weakly related to reduced incidents of coronary heart disease, but subjects who took more than 700 mg of vitamin C daily in supplement form reduced their risk by 25% compared to those who took no supplements.[45]

L-ARGININE

In 1998, Furchgott, Ignaro, and Murad were awarded the Nobel Prize in Medicine for their discovery of "nitric oxide as a signaling molecule in the cardiovascular system." Since then, NO has been the focus of intense research (more than 27,000 references in Pub Med are found for "arginine" and "nitric oxide"). L-arginine is converted by endothelial nitric oxide synthase (eNOS) into NO. Vitamin C and folic acid are essential cofactors for eNOS. Folate in large doses (5–30 g/day) can significantly push this conversion. Another form of arginine, asymmetric dimethylarginine (ADMA) has been found to inhibit eNOS. ADMA competes with arginine for binding with eNOS, causing down-regulation of this enzyme. Elevated ADMA occurs in many clinical conditions including hyperlipidemia, hyperhomocysteinemia, CAD, angina pectoris, congestive heart failure (CHF), peripheral vascular disease, hypertension, diabetes mellitus, chronic renal failure, preeclampsia, and erectile dysfunction (ED).[46] By inhibiting the production of NO, ADMA can stimulate atherosclerosis and impair vascular flow. L-arginine has been shown to significantly mitigate these effects, independent of ADMA status. However, using plasma ADMA as a marker for vascular risk may give physicians a means to predict which patients are most likely to benefit from L-arginine supplementation. Ordinary L-arginine, while shown to be helpful, is rapidly absorbed and metabolized; its half-life in humans is less than 1 hour. Therefore it does not have a sustained effect unless it is taken in frequently and continuously. A controlled-release form of L-arginine has been developed, which allows a twice daily dose to maintain an effective concentration. This is available in the United States and Canada as "Perfusia-SR" and is available at perfusia-sr.com or from Thorne Research at www.thorne.com. (Cost of a month's supply is $32.95 plus shipping.)

NO can only be produced by the vascular endothelial cells when they contain adequate amounts of L-arginine, since L-arginine is the only substrate for the creation of NO. NO in turn is responsible for a number of critical vascular functions, including smooth muscle relaxation and subsequent vasodilation, inhibition of platelet aggregation, monocyte adhesiveness, and smooth muscle proliferation. NO is also vital to maintaining normal BP, myocardial function, inflammatory response, apoptosis, and antioxidant function. Other effects of arginine are seen in endocrine and immune functions. It stimulates the release of catecholamines, insulin, glucagons, prolactin, growth hormone, increases natural killer-cell activity and decreases pro-inflammatory cytokines.

Myocardial PET scans have shown significant improvement in myocardial perfusion following supplementation with sustained-release L-arginine (preliminary results from a study by K. Loance Gould, MD, University of Texas Medical School, Houston, TX). Sustained-release L-arginine has demonstrated synergistic endothelium-dependent vasodilatory effects when taken with simvastatin. The vascular benefits of HMG-CoA reductase inhibitors are in part due to their ability to up-regulate eNOS gene expression.

ED affects an estimated 54% of men aged 65–70, and is considered an indicator of vascular compromise. Existing research on L-arginine and ED appears promising and suggests that at least some men will experience improved sexual function. Insofar as most of the studies conducted to date have used a nonsustained release form of L-arginine, it is expected that once a clinical trial is completed with the controlled-release formulation, the effects of arginine on vascular function will be more fully appreciated. No significant adverse effects have been noted with arginine supplementation.

EDTA chelation therapy—alternative, adjunctive, or integrative?

Bypass surgery, angioplasty, and stenting are expensive, invasive, risky procedures with poor cost-effectiveness and are limited to being palliative since they fail to treat the underlying atherosclerotic occlusive process. Re-occlusion of the treated vessels and the progression of occlusive disease in untreated vessels are common. EDTA chelation therapy appears to achieve revitalization of the myocardium, and is a viable alternative or adjunct to revascularization, halting atherosclerotic progression, restoring cardiac functionality, extending survival, and improving quality of life, especially when integrated together with nutrients, lifestyle-dietary revision, exercise, and medications as necessary. Chelation therapy has not been subjected to vast numbers of clinical trials, and has been stubbornly regarded as still less than proven by mainstream medicine.[47,48] A $30 million NIH-funded clinical trial (TACT) is currently underway to assess its safety and efficacy in 4000 post-MI patients at over 100 research sites. In launching this study, the safety of intravenous (IV) EDTA was accepted as firmly established.[49] Two meta-analyses suggest chelation therapy benefits 87–88% of patients.[50]

EDTA chelation therapy employs IV administration of ethylene diamine tetraacetic acid along with nutrients and stabilizers, and is most effective when used as part of a comprehensive, individualized treatment program. Chelation has negligible risk, the materials are affordable, and the procedure is available from over 8000 physicians in the United States. The peer-reviewed protocol approved by the American Board of Chelation Therapy and the International Board of Chelation Therapy involves IV infusion of an osmotically standardized EDTA solution over 1.5–3 hours. The solution contains magnesium, potassium, B vitamins, vitamin C, sodium bicarbonate, procaine, and heparin. Frequency of treatment is generally once or twice weekly; for symptomatic patients a series of 30 or more treatments may be necessary. The therapy benefits all forms of atherosclerotic occlusive disease. No distinct mechanism has been established for the benefits of EDTA, although many are postulated. Contraindications are limited to the rare patient intolerant to EDTA, acute lead encephalopathy, and patients on renal dialysis. Renal damage, only occurring in those with preexisting renal insufficiency, is estimated to occur in less than 1 in 30,000 patients.[51]

Thrombosis prevention

Since the leading cause of death in the Western world results from the formation of an abnormal blood clot inside a blood vessel, it is paramount for healthy persons to take steps to optimize the prevention of thrombosis. Platelet aggregators include adenosine diphosphate (ADP), thromboxane and serotonin (5-HT). Fibrin, formed from fibrinogen in a complex coagulation cascade, binds platelets together to form a clot. Platelet aggregation inhibitors and vasodilators oppose the action of aggregators and fibrin and include NO, prostacyclin (also known as prostaglandin I2), tissue plasminogen activator, and anticoagulants such as antithrombin III (activated by heparin) and proteins C and S. In the healthy body, a balance is created between the opposing factors of the complex clotting system: coagulants versus anticoagulants; vasodilators versus vasoconstrictors; and platelet aggregators versus platelet aggregator inhibitors. The beauty of nutritional supplements is that they support the natural homeostatic and hemostatic mechanisms to maintain balance.

Platelet adherence to endothelia plaque is part of the atherosclerosis cascade. Platelet-derived growth factor increases thrombus formation. Although anticoagulants such as Coumadin and heparin are the conventional treatment of choice for thrombosis prevention, thrombi from hypercoagulability are considered to be uncommon. There are many risk factors for hypercoagulable states, including MI, prolonged bed rest, cardiac failure, heart valve replacement, hyperlipidemia, atrial fibrillation, cardiomyopathy, oral contraceptives, and thrombocytosis. The underlying causes of thrombosis, besides hypercoagulability, are endothelial injury, circulatory stasis, and alterations in arterial blood flow. Because so many factors can contribute to coagulation and therefore should be considered for prevention, it is difficult for conventional drug therapy to control them all, and it can exert control on only some crucial steps in the coagulation cascade.

Bleeding is the primary adverse effect of Coumadin therapy, and is related to dosage, length of therapy, underlying clinical state, and the use of other drugs that can affect coagulation or interfere with Coumadin metabolism. There is an extremely long list of contraindications and drug interactions, including acetominophen, lovastatin, thyroid hormones, estrogens, and oral contraceptives. Use with aspirin and NSAIDS increase the risk of bleeding. Aspirin, vitamin E, fish oil, garlic, ginkgo, and numerous other phytomedicines inhibit platelet adhesion and aggregation and are classified as antiplatelet agents. There is much debate and confusion about the interactions between dietary supplements and prescription antithrombotic medications regarding clot formation.[52] There has been apprehension that certain supplements put patients at risk for bleeding problems by adding to the overall effects of Coumadin. As a result, some physicians advise patients on Coumadin to avoid any supplement that could possibly cause increased bleeding. This ultra-cautious approach deprives patients of beneficial supplements and prevents the use of antiplatelet agents that act on hemostatic mechanisms, separate from those of Coumadin, to reduce more effectively the risk of thrombosis. There are studies that confirm the importance of lowering the risk of thrombosis by such a two-pronged approach using an agent with antiplatelet activity in addition to Coumadin.[53] Just as the INR is used to monitor Coumadin therapy, bleeding times can be used to titrate the proper dose of antiplatelet agents. Contrary to earlier reports, a 2003 study showed that CoQ10 does not effect Coumadin's anticoagulation mechanisms.[54] Perhaps of greater concern is the finding that polymorphisms in the cytochrome P450 CYP2C9 resulting in impaired hydroxylation of S-warfarin have been associated with warfarin dose requirement and 3.68 risk of bleeding complications.

Several studies have shown that homocysteine increases blood coagulation by inhibiting tissue fibrinogen activators. The result is increased levels of fibrinogen and fibrin.[55] As noted earlier in this chapter, in order to reduce blood homocysteine levels, adequate amounts of betaine, folic acid, vitamin B_{12}, and vitamin B$_6$ are usually required. Ideal levels of homocysteine are under 7 μmol/L of blood.

Foods with proven antiplatelet actions include green tea, fish, tumeric, garlic, onions, tomatoes, grapes, grapefruit, melons, and strawberries. The extracts of some of these foods are even more therapeutic. Discussion of omega-3 fatty acids and Nattokinase will be found later in this chapter in the section on arrhythmias.

The amino acid N-acetyl-L-cysteine (NAC) inhibits platelet aggregation by several mechanisms, including increasing the antiplatelet aggregating effects of L-arginine.[56] NAC also affects platelet-derived growth factor, a key player in fibrosis. Ginseng has demonstrated an inhibitory effect on platelet aggregation.[57] Ginseng may inhibit activation of platelets through multiple components and multiple pathways, which is different from that of aspirin (derived only through inhibition on arachidonic acid metabolism which then suppresses platelet aggregation). Low-dose aspirin is widely recommended to help prevent abnormal platelet aggregation, thus reducing heart attack and stroke risk. One tablet daily is recommended for its anticlotting and anti-inflammatory effects. Some people may require more than 81 mg of aspirin daily, which can be determined by their bleeding time.

The effects of exercise on fibrinogen levels have been extensively studied. Several studies demonstrate that regular exercise lowers fibrinogen levels and reduces the risk of thrombosis.

HYPERTENSION

High BP is an even stronger predictor of cardiovascular risk than high cholesterol and Type II diabetes. Scientific studies directly correlate high BP with decreased longevity. The purpose of this section is to provide a protocol that can be followed that will prevent the development of hypertension, and thus, the development of hypertensive vascular disease, as well as adjuvant therapy to ongoing, conventional medical treatment. This requires an initial focus on understanding the mechanisms behind the development of hypertension; a symptom of many underlying disease processes that frequently precedes and further aggravates the progression of a number of common cardiovascular-related diseases.

At the organ level, excess dietary sodium triggers a well-characterized, coordinated sequence of physiological events that typically causes some degree of hypertension, particularly in those genetically predisposed to the effects of salt, or who, as a result of aging or other nutritional and environmental factors are otherwise sensitized to sodium intake. The amount of salt in the typical American diet greatly exceeds what is obtained from a wholesome diet, and this level of sodium chloride intake is pharmacological, with profound but insidious effects. Blood isotonicity is very carefully regulated by many interconnected systems. Retention of excess sodium chloride and fluid is pathological. This retained salt water expands the volume of the plasma compartment, increases demands on the heart to pump more volume (increased cardiac output), and thus, raises BP.

At the tissue level, there is strong evidence that regulatory processes within vascular smooth muscle and vascular endothelial cells are dysfunctional and/or compromised by the affects of hypertension, declining testosterone levels, aging, and other nutritional and hormonal imbalances.

Since an exact cause of hypertension is not clearly understood in approximately 90–95% of those affected, this has led to the term "essential hypertension," or idiopathic hypertension. Staying mindful of the concept of hypertension as a symptom, rather than a disease in and of itself, helps to focus attention on the underlying processes that result in elevated BP, and how one can intervene in these processes in such as way as to reverse the pathophysiology. Thus, instead of telling patients that the "cause of your high BP is unknown," we can educate them about what they can do to address the imbalances that result in hypertension. Evidence is particularly strong for linkage of the angiotensinogen gene.[58] This gene is presumed to code for a collection of proteins that regulate the renin-angiotensin-aldosterone axis. Many environmental factors determine the expression of this gene and the degree of hypertension that results in particular individuals. The manipulation of these factors through salt restriction, other dietary change, decreased alcohol intake, and stress, can reduce or eliminate hypertension.

A subgroup of people, approximately 20%, have essential hypertension with low plasma renin activity (PRA). This group, and those with normal renin levels, are salt sensitive and should restrict it. Another 25–30% of people with essential hypertension have a reduced adrenal (aldosterone) response to sodium, and are termed "nonmodulators." They are salt sensitive because of a genetic defect in renal excretion of sodium, and are not sensitive to dietary intake of salt. A final subgroup possesses high renin levels probably related to overactivity of the adrenergic system. Secondary hypertension is caused by renal, adrenal, and other endocrine dysfunctions, including insulin resistance.

Commonly, physicians and patients believe that by eliminating the hypertension, that is, by merely reducing BP, the increased risk and mortality associated with underlying cardiovascular disease will be reversed. Unfortunately, controlling only one aspect of hypertensive disease, the elevated BP, reduces only part of the cardiovascular risk associated with hypertension.

What we call "hypertension" is a powerful indicator of disease in other body systems, such as left ventricular hypertrophy associated with congestive heart failure, that may exist prior to and progress independently of the hypertension. Any and all associated conditions must be considered to successfully treat hypertension. It must also be remembered that people are different. The same elevation of BP that leads to the diagnosis of "essential" hypertension may result from many different "primary" causes. Hypertension is just one shared clinical manifestation. The implication is that when asking, "Is this drug or integrated therapy good, or preferred for hypertension?" the answer is, "It depends." For example, the salt-sensitive hypertensive patient sometimes responds to dietary salt restriction and to certain drug classes differently from an individual who is not salt sensitive. Therefore, it is worthwhile to consider the associated underlying cardiovascular disease when considering the treatment protocols present in the various chapters of this text.

High normal BP is not benign—prehypertension

The risk of cardiovascular complications begins at a relatively high normal BP and is also associated with such disorders as the metabolic syndrome. The Framingham database has demonstrated that beginning with systolic BP as low as 117 mm Hg, there is a progressive increase in risk of cardiovascular events including death, MI, stroke, and congestive heart failure. Between a systolic BP of 120 mm Hg and 139 mm Hg, there is a 2.5-fold greater risk for women and a 1.6-fold greater risk for men.[59] Among the higher-risk individuals are subjects with metabolic syndrome, whose criteria for definition includes slightly elevated BP of >/= 135/85 mm Hg. Metabolic syndrome increases coronary heart disease and stroke risk two- to threefold, and cardiovascular disease mortality by four- to fivefold. Lifestyle change is critical as a therapeutic approach because of its numerous benefits. For example, for every 10 kg of weight lost, there is a 5–20 mm Hg reduction in systolic BP; dietary sodium reduction can lower systolic BP by 2–8 mm Hg in those who are salt sensitive; regular physical activity lowers systolic BP by at least 4–9 mm Hg; and moderation of alcohol consumption lowers systolic BP by 2–4 mm Hg. Dietary change (see in the diet section) smoking cessation, and stress management also contribute significantly to lowering BP. One of the new concepts in JNC7 was the inclusion of the BP classification of prehypertension, which encompasses individuals with systolic BP between 120 and 139 mm Hg and/or diastolic BP between 80 and 89 mm Hg.[59] For this group, lifestyle modification is indicated without active pharmacotherapy unless there is a compelling indication for an individual drug class. For example ACE inhibitors and angiotensin receptor blockers consistently decrease the rate of onset of Type II diabetes.

Hypertension as an antecedent to heart failure

Aggressive treatment strategies for heart failure must begin with prevention, and hypertension represents a major contributing factor. Some have estimated that as many as 90% of persons with heart failure have an antecedent history of hypertension. JNC 7 reported the following benefits of lowering BP: a 50% average reduction in the incidence of heart failure; a 35–40% average reduction in the incidence of stroke; and a 20–25% average reduction in the incidence of MI. Central to the pathobiology of heart failure is neurohumoral activation, which involves both the renin-angiotensin-aldosterone system and the sympathetic nervous system. High levels of angiotensin acting through its specific AT1 receptor results in sodium and water retention, cell growth, vasoconstriction, and further activation of the sympathetic nervous system. Both angiotensin II and norepinephrine have deleterious effects on the heart, which include hypertrophy, apoptosis, ischemia, arrhythmias, remodeling, and fibrosis, which directly contribute to excess morbidity and mortality that accompany heart failure. There are a number of deleterious effects of the renin-angiotensin-aldosterone system that have emerged from in vitro studies and animal observations and which support a direct role in the pathobiology of CV diseases, including heart failure. Deleterious effects directly attributable to aldosterone include myocardial fibrosis, catecholamine potentiation, ventricular arrhythmias, endothelial dysfunction, and potassium and magnesium loss.[60]

Diet

Besides maintaining optimal body weight, a healthy diet containing a high proportion of plant foods can have a major impact on BP. Studies have shown that the DASH (Dietary Approaches to Stop Hypertension) diet, which emphasizes poultry, fish, fruits, vegetables, whole grains, low-fat dairy products, and nuts, and which is low in sodium and provides a large supply of potassium, magnesium, and fiber, can reduce BP as much as some prescription drugs.[61] Tobacco and stimulant drugs should be avoided, as these substances boost BP and can injure the sensitive endothelium that lines the blood vessels. Caffeinated beverages are a controversial topic among hypertension specialists. Caffeine appears to raise the BP of some people but not others. Caffeine certainly does not appear to help control BP and thus probably should be avoided.

Supplements

The list of supplements that can help lower BP is lengthy, and includes CoQ10, omega-3 fatty acids, fiber, garlic, lipoic acid, magnesium, potassium, L-arginine, N-acetylcysteine, taurine, vitamins B_6 and C, hawthorn, mistletoe, and rauwolfia among others. Some of these substances are more useful than others; some are backed by considerable scientific study, while others are not.[62]

Unfortunately, the medical treatment of hypertension is fraught with difficulty. Antihypertensives are notorious for their many adverse effects, including depression and sexual dysfunction. Because of these side effects, it has been estimated that half of those who take antihypertensive medications eventually quit taking them, usually within 3 months of starting treatment. Patients with hypertension will seek care from naturopathic physicians to help them reduce or discontinue prescription medications, and for recommendations on dietary supplements that may help them achieve this goal.

Magnesium is probably the best example in a well-established body of research indicating that specific nutrients are highly effective in treating and-even more importantly-preventing high BP. Because magnesium is not plentiful in foods, supplementation may be effective in both preventing and controlling high BP. Many physicians are unaware that diuretics flush magnesium as well as potassium from the body. Large epidemiological studies suggest a relationship between magnesium and BP. However, the fact that foods high in magnesium (fruits, vegetables, nuts, whole grains) are frequently high in potassium and dietary fiber has made it difficult to evaluate independent effects of magnesium on BP in these epidemiologic studies. Magnesium is a major factor in relaxing the smooth muscles within the blood vessels, thereby reducing peripheral vascular resistance and BP. In addition, magnesium reduces nerve and muscle excitability and stabilizes cardiac conductivity. Because of magnesium's primary role in BP regulation, for decades scientists have called magnesium a "physiologic calcium channel blocker" because magnesium directly offsets the constriction of blood vessels caused by calcium. Calcium channel blockers have been developed to do what magnesium does. In 2000, doctors in the United States wrote more than 95 million prescriptions for calcium antagonists. These drugs are not only costly, but they can also cause side effects such as dizziness, palpitations, fatigue, and peripheral edema.

Numerous independent clinical studies have shown that patients with hypertension of diverse etiologies exhibit hypomagnesemia in serum or tissues, or both. Numerous other randomized controlled trials have found that oral magnesium supplementation can produce dose-dependent significant reductions in BP. These and other studies create a compelling body of evidence for the use of magnesium in preventing and treating hypertension. In some studies, magnesium failed to reduce BP significantly, though these studies typically were too brief in duration for the magnesium to reach maximum effect, or they used inadequate amounts or poorly absorbed types of magnesium.[63]

In other studies, oral magnesium supplementation has further lowered BP in people already receiving beta-blockers or diuretics. Although these reports are highly suggestive, other clinical trials have demonstrated no BP effects of magnesium supplementation. As emphasized earlier, these controversies may not be resolved no matter how many progressively larger or more expensive clinical trials are performed, as long as hypertensive subjects are considered as a homogeneous group, which they are not, neither pathophysiologically in general, or with respect to their magnesium metabolism in particular.

As early as 1983, it was observed that despite a uniform intracellular magnesium deficit, hypertensive subjects exhibit a range of extracellular magnesium values, within the normal range, that seem to be closely related to the activity of pressor hormone systems such as the renin-angiotensin system. Patients with normal to high plasma renin activity have lower serum magnesium values that predict a hypotensive response to magnesium supplementation. These are the patients who respond best to beta blockers, converting enzyme inhibitors, or angiotensin-II blockers-drugs that block the secretion, activation, or action of the renin-angiotensin system. Interestingly, these drugs may also increase serum magnesium levels. Other hypertensive patients who have low PRA and/or salt sensitivity may exhibit no response or even a mild pressor response to magnesium. These patients may respond better to calcium supplements. Grouping all subjects together according to only BP levels as if they were the same obscures the dramatic magnesium responses in those with high PRA; the net result for the entire group might appear modest or nil.

Hence, progress in this area will require a priori identification of subgroups of patients on the basis of PRA, dietary salt sensitivity, reproducible and sensitive measures of extracellular magnesium, and other criteria useful in identifying subjects for whom oral magnesium supplementation will be particularly effective. As previously articulated, hypertension is a heterogenous phenomenon, not a uniform epidemiologically defined condition.[64] For now, all patients should at least increase their magnesium intake to achieve current

RDA standards (magnesium deficiency is the second-most common mineral deficiency in the United States population, after iron). Similar to current recommendations for dietary salt restriction in hypertension, magnesium supplementation beyond these levels should only be used on a trial basis for 1–6 months and continued only if a clear-cut response is observed. Magnesium deficiency is rarely recognized because there is no simple, widely available test for magnesium deficiency. Mainstream medical laboratories measure the total serum (blood) magnesium. This measurement is not very helpful; even if one is severely magnesium deficient, the body will maintain a normal blood level of magnesium by drawing magnesium from cells and bone. Developing a reliable test that can accurately reflect magnesium levels in the tissues has been a challenge because less than 1% of the body's total magnesium is contained in the blood, whereas about 55% resides in bone, 26% in muscle, and 18% in other tissues. Yet such measurement is possible. Specialty laboratories can perform magnesium analyses on ionized blood, red blood cells, hair, and cells swabbed from the inner side of the cheek.[65]

Oral magnesium is usually well tolerated in people with normal kidney function. The dose-limiting factor is diarrhea. Symptoms of magnesium toxicity are rare and include weakness, slowed heart rate, reduced tendon reflexes, and somnolence. Magnesium does interfere with the absorption of digoxin.

CoQ10 is the predominant form of ubiquinone in humans, and has been called "cholesterol's reclusive cousin." Studies have clearly shown the potential benefit of CoQ10 in the treatment of hypertension.[66] Clinical trials of patients on medication for essential hypertension given CoQ10 in a dosage dependant on its blood level have shown that patients have been able to gradually decrease antihypertensive drug therapy during the first 1–6 months. In a review of eight studies, the mean decrease in systolic BP was 16 mm Hg and in diastolic BP, 10 mm Hg. More than half of these patients were able to completely discontinue between one and three antihypertensive drugs after starting CoQ10.[67] Reduction in BP may not be from any direct antihypertensive effect of CoQ10, but possibly by mitigating underlying physiological states resulting in hypertension.[68]

Omega-3 fatty acids have been the subject of a meta-regression analysis. These 36 trials of fish oil, of which 22 had a double-blind design, found that the intake of a median dose of 3.7 g/day of fish oil provided statistically significant reductions of both systolic and diastolic pressures. Effects were greater in populations over age 45 and in hypertensive individuals.[69] Several publications have cautioned about the long-term safety of fish oil in doses sufficient to lower BP due to potential prolongation of bleeding time, a possible decline in renal function due to decreased production of the renal vasodilator prostaglandin E2, eructations, and the sensation of a fishy taste. Bleeding time can be monitored, and the possible decline in renal function is merely a theoretical concern. Stabilized forms of fish oil are available that do not cause eructations or leave a fishy taste.

Omega-3 fatty acids may be particularly effective in hypertensive heart transplant recipients. In a double-blind placebo-controlled randomized study of

45 clinically stable patients studied 1–12 years after heart transplantation, patients given 3.4 g/day of omega-3 fatty acids for 1 year had no change in BP or vascular resistance, and renal function was maintained. By comparison, those on placebo had increases in 24-hour ambulatory BP, systemic vascular resistance (14 percent), and serum creatinine concentration.[70]

L-*Arginine*, as noted earlier in this chapter, improves not only endothelial function but has a hypotensive effect as well. This is currently a dynamic area of research, with many studies published and underway.[71]

Herbs

Small pilot clinical trials, animal studies, and in vitro work has been conducted on a variety of herbal preparations that have traditionally been used in the treatment of hypertension, including Crataegus oxycantha and monogyna (Hawthorn), Terminalia arjuna, Olea africana and europa (Olive Leaf), Viscum album (European Mistletoe), Achillea wilhelmsii (Yarrow), Nigella sativa (Black Cumin Seeds), Coleus forskohlii, Rauwolfia serpentina (Indian Snakeroot), and Allium sativum (Garlic).[72]

Rauwolfia is arguably the herb that naturopathic physicians have traditionally employed more than others to cause significant reduction in BP. It contains reserpine and must be used cautiously. Rauwolfia can interact with MAO inhibitors, exacerbate cholelithiasis, gastric ulcer, ulcerative colitis, and cause drowsiness, dizziness, arrhythmia, bradycardia, and parkinsonism. Excessive doses can cause depression. Maximum daily dose is 600 mg daily corresponding to 6 mg total alkaloids.

The hawthorn berry is considered an adaptogenic in regard to normalizing BP. Hawthorn derives much of its hypotensive and weight management properties through its diuretic action. Also, its ACE inhibiting factors interrupt the renin-angiotensin sequence, resulting in lower BP and improved cardiac output.[73]

Olive leaf extract has been shown in both laboratory and clinical settings to have beta-adrenergic antagonistic, hypotensive, and vasodilating properties.[74]

In animals, Taraxacum leaf has been shown to have diuretic activity, stimulating the loss of excess water and promoting weight loss. Taraxacum leaf was shown to have diuretic activity in rats and mice comparable to furosemide (Lasix). It produced a 30% loss of body weight in mice and rats in a 30-day period, with much of the weight loss attributed to the loss of excess amounts of extracellular water. Unlike furosemide, which causes potassium loss, Taraxacum is a rich source of potassium, capable of replacing the potassium lost through diuresis.

Proanthocyanidins (PCO) are antioxidants and ACE inhibitors found in pine bark and grape seed. Grape seed extracts are available that contain from 92–95% PCO content; pine bark extracts vary from 80–85%. An extract of French maritime pine park (Pycnogenol) has demonstrated a statistically significant ability to allow hypertensive patients to reduce prescribed dosages of the common calcium channel blocker nifedipine by 40% in a randomized controlled trial. Those taking Pycnogenol had significantly higher levels of 6-ketoprostagland in ketoprostag F1, a vasodilator, and lower concentrations of endothelin-1, a potent vasoconstrictor.[75]

Red wine polyphenols have been demonstrated to partially prevent cardio-vascular remodeling and vascular dysfunction in induced hypertensive rats via the increase of NO-synthase activity and prevention of oxidative stress.[76]

Homeopathy

In a randomized double-blind crossover study, the effects of antihypertensive pharmacotherapy were compared with those of homeopathic treatment in 10 patients with essential hypertension. The BP lowering effect under pharmacotherapy was superior to that with homeopathy, where it was negligible and statistically not significant. However, there was no difference in improvement of subjective complaints of the patients with the two treatments. The crossover design was less suitable than a design with parallel treatment groups because of the long duration of such a study and the observed carry-over effect.[77]

CONGESTIVE HEART FAILURE

Diet

The dietary recommendations given for hypertension earlier in this chapter are appropriate for most people with congestive heart failure, especially if the congestive heart failure is due to long-term hypertension.

Alcohol drinking, when heavy, is associated with increased risk of non-CAD-heart failure and the apparent protection by alcohol drinking against CAD-heart failure risk provides confirmation of a protective effect of alcohol against CAD.[78]

CoQ10

CoQ10 is known to be highly concentrated in heart muscle cells due to the high energy requirements of this cell type. Congestive heart failure (from a wide variety of causes) has been strongly correlated with significantly low blood and tissue levels of CoQ10. Assessment of CoQ10 status is generally based on plasma measurements, but these are influenced by a number of physiological factors and may not represent cellular concentrations. Platelets, lymphocytes, and fibroblasts may provide suitable alternatives for CoQ10 measurement. The severity of heart failure correlates with the severity of CoQ10 deficiency. This CoQ10 deficiency may well be a primary etiologic factor in some types of heart muscle dysfunction, while in others it may be a secondary phenomenon. Whether primary, secondary, or both, this deficiency of CoQ10 appears to be a major treatable factor in the otherwise inexorable progression of heart failure.

Pioneering trials of CoQ10 in heart failure involved primarily patients with idiopathic dilated cardiomyopathy. CoQ10 was added to standard treatments for heart failure such as diuretics, digoxin, and ACE inhibitors. Several trials involved the comparison between supplemental CoQ10 and placebo on heart function as measured by echocardiography. Ejection fraction showed a gradual and sustained improvement in tempo with a gradual and sustained improvement in patients' symptoms of fatigue, dyspnea, chest pain, and palpitations. The degree of improvement was occasionally dramatic with some patients developing a normal heart size and function on CoQ10 alone. Most of these dramatic cases were patients who began CoQ10 shortly after the onset of congestive heart failure. Patients with more established disease frequently showed clear improvement but not a return to normal heart size and function.

In nine randomized trials of CoQ10 in heart failure published up to 2003, there were non-significant trends toward increased ejection fraction and reduced mortality.[67] The majority of the clinical studies of the treatment of heart disease with CoQ10 have shown significantly improved heart muscle function while producing no adverse effects or harmful drug interactions. Concerns about the design of these studies have limited their acceptance. The limited data from well-designed trials indicates some benefit with CoQ10 in ejection fraction and end diastolic volume. Diastolic relaxation is more highly energy demanding than systole and thus more highly dependent on CoQ10.

Administration of CoQ10 to heart transplant candidates led to a significant improvement in functional status, clinical symptoms, and quality of life.[79] However, there were no objective changes in echocardiographic measurements or atrial natriuretic factor and tumor necrosis factor blood levels. CoQ10 may serve as an optional addition to the pharmacologic armamentarium of patients with end-stage heart failure. The apparent discrepancy between significant clinical improvement and unchanged cardiac status requires further investigation.

Even brief exposure to atorvastatin causes a marked decrease in plasma CoQ10 concentration. If for no other reason, because of this it is prudent to add CoQ10 in patients with heart failure who are on statins.[80]

Crataegus oxycantha (hawthorn)

The berries and flowers of Crataegus oxycantha have been used traditionally as cardiac tonics and diuretics in a variety of functional heart disorders. Crataegus extracts exert a wide range of positive actions on heart function. The primary cardiovascular protective activity of Crataegus is generally attributed to its oligomeric proanthocyanadins (OPCs) highly concentrated in the leaves, berries, and flowers. Laboratory studies have suggested that these procyanidins stimulate a pseudo laminar shear stress response in endothelial cells, which helps restore endothelial function and underlies the benefit from treatment with hawthorn extract in heart failure.[81] Due to the flavonoid content, extracts of Crataegus exert considerable antioxidant and collagen-stabilizing effects, enhancing integrity of the blood vessels. Extracts of Crataegus reduce plasma lipids by enhancing cholesterol degradation to bile acids, promoting bile flow, suppressing cholesterol biosynthesis, and inhibiting LDL oxidation.[82]

Because of these actions, it can be safely and effectively utilized for cardiac conditions for which digitalis is not indicated. It may also have a potentiating effect on digitalis, necessitating a reduction in the dosage of digitalis. Crataegus provides subjective and objective benefits in individuals with congestive heart failure stage NYHA-II. Patients report improvement in subjective symptoms, such as reduced performance, shortness of breath, and ankle edema, improved BP, heart rate, and the change in heart rate in response to exercise. Crataegus exerts mild BP-lowering activity, which appears to be a result of a number of diverse pharmacological effects. It dilates coronary vessels, inhibits angiotensin-converting enzyme, acts as an inotropic agent, and possesses mild diuretic activity.

A meta-analysis was performed of eight randomized, double-blind, placebo-controlled clinical trials ($n = 632$) of the use of hawthorn extract alone to treat patients with chronic heart failure (NYHA classes I-III).[83] For the physiologic outcome of maximal workload, treatment with hawthorn extract was more beneficial than placebo. The pressure-heart rate product also showed a beneficial decrease with hawthorn treatment. Symptoms such as dyspnea and fatigue improved significantly with hawthorn treatment as compared with placebo. Reported adverse events were infrequent, mild, and transient; they included nausea, dizziness, and cardiac and gastrointestinal complaints. The authors concluded that there is a significant benefit from hawthorn extract as an adjunctive treatment for chronic heart failure. In a study involving 217 general practitioners, 952 patients with heart failure (NYHA II) were enrolled, 588 patients receiving Crataegus special extract WS 1442 (Crataegutt novo 450) either as an add-on therapy or as a monotherapy (Crataegus cohort) and 364 patients receiving therapy without hawthorn (comparative cohort).[84] After 2 years, the three cardinal symptoms of heart failure-fatigue, stress dyspnea, and palpitations were significantly less marked in the Crataegus cohort than in the comparative cohort. Patients in the Crataegus cohort received markedly fewer drugs than the patients in the comparative cohort (ACE-inhibitors, cardiac glycosides, diuretics, and beta-blockers).

Another placebo-controlled, randomized, parallel group, multicenter trial showed the efficacy and safety of Crataegus (Crataegisan) in patients with cardiac failure NYHA class II.[85] A total of 143 patients were treated with Crataegus or placebo for 8 weeks. The primary variable for the evaluation of efficacy was the change in exercise tolerance determined with bicycle exercise testing. Secondary variables included the blood pressure-heart rate product (BHP). Subjective cardiac symptoms at rest and at higher levels of exertion were assessed by the patient. The difference between the treatment groups was significantly in favor of Crataegus. The medication was well tolerated and had a high level of patient acceptability.

The combination homeopathic Crataegus preparation Cralonin was tested for noninferiority to standard treatment for mild cardiac insufficiency in a multicenter nonrandomized cohort study in patients with NYHA class II heart failure. Cralonin contains Crataegus tincture plus Kali carbonicum D3 and Spigelia anthelmia D2. Patients received Cralonin ($n = 110$) or ACE inhibitor/diuretics ($n = 102$) for 8 weeks. Cralonin was found to be comparable to usual ACE inhibitor/diuretics treatment for mild cardiac insufficiency on all parameters except BP reduction.[86]

Traditionally, several herbal preparations have been used in the naturo-pathic treatment of heart failure. Isolation of cardiac glycosides from digitalis, convallaria, strophanthus, and squill and determination of their chemical structures initiated biochemical and pharmacological studies. The scientific advances led to an understanding of cardiac muscle contractility and the Na-K pump as the cellular receptor for the inotropic action of digitalis. Examination of putative endogenous ligands to the receptor revealed some endogenous cardiac glycosides of similar or identical structures as those found in digitalis, strophanthus, and squill. Increased concentrations of these glycosides are found in patients with heart failure. Further investigations are needed to determine whether the secretion of glycosides might be a physiologic response to a diminished cardiac output.[87]

Exercise

Researchers analyzed data from nine trials involving 801 people with heart failure and showed a better chance of survival in those taking part in supervised exercise programs. Of the people in the trials, 395 received exercise training for at least 8 weeks and 406 in the control group received usual care. All the people were monitored for at least 3 months. There were 88 (22%) deaths in the exercise group, after an average of 618 days and 105 (26%) deaths in the control group, after an average of 421 days.[88] The benefits were seen without regard to the underlying cause of heart failure and extended equally to all age groups and among men and women. Admissions to hospitals were lower in the exercise group as well. The exercise groups also stayed out of the hospital longer. Average times to hospital admission were 426 days for the exercise group versus 371 days in the control group. Currently, exercise is not widely prescribed for people with chronic heart failure due to lack of evidence of its long-term effectiveness. The NIH is currently conducting a large multicenter trial that hopefully will provide more definitive information.

ARRYTHMIAS

Atrial fibrillation is the most common cardiac arrhythmia in Europe and North America, and recently it was described as an epidemic. Treatment and management of this arrhythmia consists of using drugs, external electrical cardioversion, and in extreme cases, internal electrical pacing. Despite treatment, this arrhythmia continues to impact on morbidity and mortality. The possible benefits from dietary interventions and supplements in relation to the primary and secondary prevention of atrial fibrillation have largely been overlooked. In such patients, anticoagulation with warfarin is currently recommended. Warfarin therapy carries significant risks (especially bleeding), inconveniences (the cost of prothrombin time monitoring, the need for rigid dietary stability, the concerns of drug and herbal interactions), and other concerns (the issue of generic formulation substitution).

Whether or not a patient is taking warfarin, bleeding times should also be utilized to assess platelet aggregation. They need to be targeted to approximately 6–8 minutes (reference range of 2–10 minutes). Additionally, fibrinogen levels need to be targeted to an optimal 250 mg/dL of whole blood with a reference range of 215–519 mg/dL. When these optimal numbers are achieved, chronic coagulation risk management has been optimized in all physiological parameters. Most patients on warfarin have bleeding times at 3–5 rather than 6–8 minutes and also have fibrinogen levels well over 250 mg/dL. Smoking raises fibrinogen and some smokers have levels in the 600s. Warfarin has been shown to inhibit fibrinolysis in some studies, making it more difficult to achieve the target level of 250 mg/dL for fibrinogen.

It is both fundamental to naturopathic medicine and a basic treatment guideline to first use essential nutrients to affect coagulation markers before selecting specialty products. An essential nutrient is defined as one our body cannot biosynthesize that is essential for a range of biochemical and physiological processes. From a hierarchal perspective, the main class of "essential" nutrients that have a significant impact on inhibiting platelet aggregation and stimulating some fibrinolysis are essential fatty acids (EFAs).

Fish oil

Fish oil, as a source of omega-3 fatty acids or a blend of fish, flax, and borage oils as a source of blended omega-3 and omega-6 fatty acids, is where we begin our protocol in clinical practice, with a minimum dose of 2 g tid with meals for 100 lb. individuals increasing by 3 g daily for every 100 lb. This starting dose is assessed with monthly bleeding times and fibrinogen levels. If our targets are not reached, we increase the dose up to a maximum of 6 g tid. This dose is maintained on an ongoing basis. If dose elevations have not resulted in targeted goals, we lower the dose back to 2 g tid and move on to adding Nattokinase to the protocol. In addition to the aforementioned effects of omega-3 fatty acids, they also have antiarrhythmic activity.[89] In a double-blind trial, people with ventricular premature complexes were supplemented for 16 weeks with either 15 ml (1 tbsp)/day of fish oil or a similar amount of safflower oil as placebo. Patients taking the fish oil had a significantly reduced frequency of abnormal heartbeats compared with those receiving placebo, and 44% of those receiving fish oil experienced at least a 70% reduction in the frequency of abnormal beats.[90]

Nattokinase

Nattokinase is an extract of the fermented soybean product known as natto. It inactivates plasminogen activator inhibitor Type I and potentiates fibrinolytic activity.[91] There is a broad range of quality in the fibrinolytic activity measured in fibrinolytic units (FU) among Nattokinase products. Some contain vitamin K naturally occurring in Natto and others do not. Using a product higher in FU and lower in vitamin K is best in order to allow for increasing the dose of Nattokinase without vitamin K levels being raised. The softgel in an oil base is absorbed better and more effective in reaching target levels than the dry capsule.

The protocol begins with 1 softgel bid on an empty stomach an hour away from meals for a 100 lb. individual, increased based on body weight up to 2, 3, or 4 bid until target levels are reached after 30 days of medication.

If the patient is taking other supplements that have an effect on coagulation, their dose needs to be consistent in combination with the warfarin they are taking and/or with the EFAs and Nattokinase. Such products include vitamins C, E, and K, bromelain, garlic, ginkgo, ginger, and Panax ginseng. Drug-nutrient interactions may occur; they are not true contraindications, and are easily managed with consistent dosing and proper monitoring of INR, bleeding times, and fibrinogen level.[92]

Magnesium and potassium

A double-blind trial investigating the effect of oral magnesium supplementation on arrhythmic episodes in people with congestive heart failure found that those people taking 3.2 g/day of magnesium chloride (equivalent to 384 mg/day of elemental magnesium) had between 23% and 52% fewer occurrences of specific types of arrhythmia during the 6-week study, compared with those taking placebo. Lower serum concentrations of magnesium have been found to be associated with a higher incidence of arrhythmia in a large population study. A study of patients hospitalized with new onset atrial fibrillation found to have potassium and/or magnesium deficiency showed a statistically significant restoration of sinus rhythm after magnesium administration compared to controls.[93] Two meta-analyses of randomized controlled trials found that intravenous magnesium is associated with a significant reduction in the incidence of atrial fibrillation after coronary artery bypass surgery.[94,95] In addition, another meta-analysis found that administration of prophylactic magnesium reduced ventricular arrhythmias after cardiac surgery by 48%.[96]

Patients taking hydrochlorothiazide for high BP had a significant reduction in arrhythmias when supplemented with 1 g twice per day of potassium hydrochloride (supplying 1040 mg/day of elemental potassium). Those results were not improved by adding 500 mg twice per day of magnesium hydroxide (supplying 500 mg/day of elemental magnesium) to the potassium. Low serum concentrations of potassium were found to be associated with a higher incidence of arrhythmia in a large population study.

Herbs

An animal study showed that an extract of Crataegus significantly reduced the number of experimentally induced arrhythmias. An active constituent in Corydalis, dl-tetrahydropalmatine (dl-THP), exerted an antiarrhythmic action on the heart in a preliminary human trial. Other herbs that have demonstrated antiarrhythmic effects, but need further research, include Adonis vernalis, Allium cepa/sativa (garlic and onion), Amni visnaga, Atropa belladonna, Berberine alkaloids, Capsella bursa pastoris, Cinnamomum camphoraa, Convallaria majalis, Digitalis purpurea, Drimia maritime (Squill), Ginkgo biloba, Leonurus cardiaca, Olea europaea (Olive leaf), Rauwolfia serpentina, and Strophanthus kombe. Acetyl-L-carnitine is used in Europe to treat cardiac arrhythmia.

VALVULAR HEART DISEASE

Because of the anatomical nature of valvular disease, prevention may be the best approach to this disorder. For example, there is evidence that the deposition of apolipoprotein A, B, and E (protein variations of LDL cholesterol) on the aortic valve creates a binding site for calcium. Aortic valve stenosis is often described as a calcification process. Fibrinogen may also contribute to this process by depositing on aortic valves, further adding to deposit buildup by binding with calcium deposits already present on valves. Studies also implicate a chronic inflammatory process that promotes calcium infiltration into the aortic valve.

Preventing or curbing the progression of aortic-valve disease may involve lowering homocysteine, fibrinogen, and apolipoproteins A, B, and E in the blood. Supplementing with magnesium and vitamin K_1 may be especially effective in preventing aortic valve calcification. Nutrients that safely inhibit many chronic inflammatory reactions include fish oil, curcumin, and ginger. (See the sections earlier in this chapter for suggestions on lowering homocysteine, CRP, fibrinogen, and apolipoprotein levels.)

Mitral valve prolapse

Magnesium deficiency may be part of the mechanism of the mitral valve prolapse (MVP) syndrome.[97] However, determinations of magnesium concentration in blood serum and hemolysates of red blood cells in this disease revealed divergent results. Patients with the mitral valve prolapse syndrome ($n = 49$) and 30 healthy individuals were matched by age and gender. The concentration of magnesium was measured in blood plasma and lysates of lymphocytes isolated from venous blood. The magnesium concentration in plasma was similar in both the patients and the healthy controls. By contrast, the magnesium concentration in lysates of lymphocytes was significantly lower in the patients with mitral valve prolapse syndrome than in the controls.[98]

Herbs

The bark powder of *T. arjuna* has been found to have antianginal, decongestive, and hypolipidemic effects. A study to evaluate the role of *T. arjuna* in ischemic mitral regurgitation (IMR) following acute MI was conducted in 40 patients randomly divided into 2 groups of 20 each. They were given placebo or 500 mg of *T. arjuna* in addition to anti-ischemic treatment. After 1 and 3 months of follow up, patients receiving adjuvant *T. arjuna* showed significant decrease in IMR, improvement in atrial filling phase and considerable reduction in anginal frequency.[99] Much research is needed to gain an insight into the multitude of bioactivities reported in the traditional literature for other preparations of herbal medicines (such as Convallaria) which have been used for vavular heart disorders, as well as the use of L-carnitine, which has been found to be deficient in patients with MVP and has resolved the symptoms associated with MVP in case reports.

Prophylaxis of endocarditis

It has long been known that bacteremias caused by medical or dental procedures may cause endocarditis in patients with specific types of congenital or acquired heart disease. In the 1940s, it was thought that the administration of antibiotics before such procedures would prevent endocarditis. However, the beneficial effect of this preventive measure on the incidence of endocarditis did not live up to its expectations. It became clear that prophylaxis was not 100% efficacious in humans, although it did prevent endocarditis in animals. A controlled study into the protective effect of prophylaxis in humans has never been carried out. Such a trial would require a very large number of patients because of the rarity of the disease after a single bacteremic episode in a patient at risk. Also, such an approach is considered unethical. In the last decade it has become obvious from case-control studies that endocarditis prophylaxis is not a very effective preventive measure but that it reduces an already small risk even further. In MVP without regurgitation, prophylaxis is not worthwhile.[100]

CONCLUSION

Blanket naturopathic recommendations for patients with cardiac conditions cannot be made. One must always individualize the treatment approach to the patient, that is, statin drugs and anti-hypertensives may be contraindicated in some patients, or produce unacceptable side effects, or not work. For these patients, natural medicines such as RYR, L-arginine, and magnesium may be appropriate, although facile attempts to incorporate these options integratively should not be done without close medical monitoring. There are other recommendations here that have wide applicability in integrative cardiology, for example an anti-inflammatory diet and folic acid. This chapter adds information about the effectiveness of naturopathic interventions on heart disease and indicates that most have few adverse effects, and many positive side benefits. Overall, however, further studies are needed with larger numbers of patients and for longer periods before some of these recommendations can be more widely implemented. The ultimate goal should be to create an effective integrative approach to the prevention and treatment of cardiovascular disease that is patient-centered, comprehensive, cost-effective, and involves shared decision-making and communication between various caregivers.

REFERENCES

1. Vogel JHK, Bolling SF, Costello RB, et al. Integrating complementary medicine into cardiovascular medicine: a report of the American College of Cardiology Foundation Task Force on Clinical Expert Consensus Documents (Writing Committee to Develop an Expert Consensus Document on Complementary and Integrative Medicine). J Am Coll Cardiol. 2005;46:184–221. [PMID: 15992662.]

2. Patrick L, Uzick M. Cardiovascular disease: CRP and the inflammatory disease paradigm: HMG-CoA reductase inhibitors, alpha-tocopherol, red yeast rice, and olive oil polyphenols. A review of the literature. Alt Med Rev. 2001;6(3):248–71. [PMID: 11410071.]

3. Albert CM, Gaziano JM, Willett WC, et al. Nut consumption and decreased risk of sudden cardiac death in the Physicians' Health Study. Arch Int Med. 2002;162:1382–7. [PMID: 12076237.]

4. Ros E, Nunez I, Perez-Heras A, et al. A walnut diet improves endothelial function in hypercholesterolemic subjects: a randomized crossover trial. Circulation. 2004;109(13):1,609–11,61. [PMID: 15037535.]

5. Jenkins DJA, Kendall CWC, Marchie A, et al. Effects of a dietary portfolio of cholesterol-lowering foods vs. lovastatin on serum lipids and C-reactive protein. JAMA. 2003;290:502–10. [PMID: 12876093.]

6. Mukamal KJ, Maclure M, Muller JE, Sherwood JB, Mittleman MA. Prior alcohol consumption and mortality following acute myocardial infarction. JAMA. 2001;285:1965–70. [PMID: 11308432.]

6a. Crawford P, Paden SL, Park MK, Clinical inquiries: What is the dietary treatment for low HDL cholesterol? J Fam Pract, 2006;55(12):1076–8.

7. Shek A, Ferrill MJ. Statin-fibrate combination therapy. Ann Pharmacother. 2001;35:908–17. [PMID: 11485144; PMID: 15537681.]

8. Taylor AJ, Sullenberger LE, Lee HJ, et al. Arterial biology for the investigation of the treatment effects of reducing cholesterol (ARBITER) 2. A double-blind, placebo-controlled study of extended-release niacin on atherosclerosis progression in secondary prevention patients treated with statins. Circulation. 2004;110. [PMID: 15537681.]

9. Worz CR, Bottorff M. Treating dyslipidemic patients with lipid-modifying and combination therapies. Pharmacotherapy. 2003 May;23(5):625–37. [PMID:12741437.]

10. St-Onge MP, Jones PJ. Phytosterols and human lipid metabolism: efficacy, safety and novel foods. Lipids. 2003;38:4. [PMID: 12848281.]

11. Simons LA. Additive effect of plant sterol-ester margarine and cerivastatin in lowering low density lipoprotein cholesterol in primary hypercholesterolemia. Am J Cardiol. 2002;90:737.

12. Maki Kc, et al. Lipid responses to plant-sterol-enriched reduced-fat spreads incorporated into a National Cholesterol Education Program Step I diet. Am J Clin Nutr. 2001;74:33.

13. Santosa S, et al. Plant sterols: evidence to support a health claim. Int J Nat Med. Summer 2005 (online journal).

14. Chen JT, Wesley R, Shamburek RD, Pucino F, et al. Meta-analysis of natural therapies for hyperlipidemia: plant sterols and stanols versus policosanol. Pharmacotherapy. 2005 Feb;25(2):171–83. [PMID: 15767233.]

14a. Dulin MF, Hatcher LF, et al. Policosanol is ineffective in the treatment of hypercholesterolemia: a randomized controlled trial, Am J Clin Nutr, 2006;84(6):1543–8.

15. Shields KM, Moranville MP. Guggul for hypercholesterolemia. Am J Health Syst Pharm. 2005 May 15;62(10):1012–4. [PMID: 15901582.]

16. Szapary PO, Wolfe ML, Bloedon LT, et al. Guggulipid for the treatment of hypercholesterolemia: a randomized controlled trial. JAMA. 2003 Aug 13;290(6):765–72. [PMID: 12915429.]

17. Studer M, Briel M, Leimenstoll B, et al. Effect of different antilipidemic agents and diets on mortality: a systematic review. Arch Intern Med. 2005;165:725–30. [PMID: 15824290.]

18. Geelen A, Brouwer IA, Schouten EG, et al. Intake of n-3 fatty acids from fish does not lower serum concentrations of C-reactive protein in healthy subjects. Eur J Clin Nutr. 2004;58:1440–2. [PMID: 15100717.]

19. Bunea R, El Farrah K, Deutsch L. Evaluation of the effects of neptune krill oil on the clinical course of hyperlipidemia. Altern Med Rev. 2004;9(4):420–8.[PMID: 15656713.]

20. Ridker PM, Cannon CP, Morrow D, et al. Pravastatin or atorvastatin evaluation and infection therapy-thrombolysis in myocardial infarction 22 (PROVE IT-TIMI 22) investigators. C-reactive protein levels and outcomes after statin therapy. N Engl J Med. 2005 Jan 6;352(1):20–8. [PMID: 15635109.]

20a. Cook NR, et al. Ann Intern Med. 2006;145:21–9; Lloyd-Jones DM, et al. Ann Intern Med 2006;145:35–42.

20b. Lange LA, et al. JAMA. 2006;296:2703–2711.

21. Hackam DG, Anand SS. Emerging risk factors for atherosclerotic vascular disease: a critical review of the evidence. JAMA. 2003;290:932–40. [PMID: 12928471.]

22. Liem A, Reynierse-Buitenwerf GH, Zwinderman AH, et al. Secondary prevention with folic acid: effects on clinical outcomes. J Am Coll Cardiol. 2003;41:2105–13. [PMID: 12821232.]

23. Spijkerman AM, Smulders YM, Kostense PJ, et al. S-adenosylmethionine and 5-methyltetrahydrofolate are associated with endothelial function after controlling for confounding by homocysteine: the Hoorn Study. Arterioscler Thromb Vasc Biol. 2005 Apr;25(4):778–84. [PMID: 15692102.]

23a. van Oijen MG, Vlemmix F, et al. Hyperhomocysteinaemia and vitamin B12 deficiency: the long-term effects in cardiovascular disease. Cardiology, 2007;107(1):57–62.

24. Danesh J, Lewington S, Thompson SG, et al. Plasma fibrinogen level and the risk of major cardiovascular diseases and nonvascular mortality: an individual participant meta-analysis. JAMA. 2005;294(14):1799–809. [PMID: 16219884.

25. Vischetti M, Zito F, Donati MB, et al. Analysis of gene-environment interaction in coronary heart disease: fibrinogen polymorphisms as an example. Ital Heart J. 2002 Jan;3:18–23. [PMID: 11899584.]

26. Khuseyinova N, Imhof A, Rothenbacher D, et al. Association between Lp-PLA2 and coronary artery disease: focus on its relationship with lipoproteins and markers of inflammation and hemostasis. Atherosclerosis. 2005 Sep;182(1):181–8. [PMID:16115490.]

27. Heaney RP. Long-latency deficiency disease: insights from calcium and vitamin D. Am J Clin Nutr. 2003 Nov;78(5):912–9. [PMID: 14594776.]

28. Holick MF. Vitamin D: importance in the prevention of cancers, type 1 diabetes, heart disease, and osteoporosis. Am J Clin Nutr. 2004 Mar;79(3):362–71. [PMID: 14985208.]

29. Kougias P, Chai H, Lin PH, et al. Effects of adipocyte-derived cytokines on endothelial functions: implication of vascular disease. J Surg Res. 2005 Jun 1; 126(1):121–9. [PMID: 15916985.]

30. Rosenfeldt F, Miller F, Nagley P, et al. Response of the senescent heart to stress: clinical therapeutic strategies and quest for mitochondrial predictors of biological age. Ann NY Acad Sci. 2004 Jun;1019:78–84. [PMID: 15246998.]

31. Kris-Etherton P, Eckel RH, Howard BV, et al. AHA science advisory: Lyon Diet Heart Study. Benefits of a Mediterranean-style, National Cholesterol Education Program/American Heart Association Step I dietary pattern on cardiovascular disease. Circulation. 2001;103:1823–5. [PMID: 11282918.]

32. Singh RB, Dubnov G, Niaz MA, et al. Effect of an Indo-Mediterranean diet on progression of coronary artery disease in high-risk patients (Indo-Mediterranean Diet Heart Study): a randomised single-blind trial. Lancet. 2002;360:1455–61. [PMID: 12433513.]

33. de Lorgeril M, Salen P. Dietary prevention of post-angioplasty restenosis. From illusion and disillusion to pragmatism. Nutr Metab Cardiovasc Dis. 2003 Dec; 13(6):345–8. [PMID: 14979680.]

34. Visioli F, Caruso D, Grande S, et al. Virgin Olive Oil Study (VOLOS): vasoprotective potential of extra virgin olive oil in mildly dyslipidemic patients. Eur J Nutr. 2005 Mar;44(2):121–7. [PMID: 15309433.]

35. Geleijnse JM, Launer LJ, Van der Kuip DA, et al. Inverse association of tea and flavonoid intakes with incident myocardial infarction: the Rotterdam Study. Am J Clin Nutr. 2002;75:880–6. [PMID: 11976162.]

36. Mukamal KJ, Maclure M, Muller JE, et al. Tea consumption and mortality after acute myocardial infarction. Circulation. 2002 May 28;105(21):2476–81. [PMID: 12034652.]

37. Widlansky ME, Duffy SJ, Hamburg NM, et al. Effects of black tea consumption on plasma catechins and markers of oxidative stress and inflammation in patients with coronary artery disease. Free Radic Biol Med. 2005 Feb 15;38(4):499–506. [PMID: 15649652.]

38. Goldberg IJ, Mosca L, Piano MR, et al. AHA Science Advisory: wine and your heart: a science advisory for healthcare professionals from the Nutrition Committee, Council on Epidemiology and Prevention, and Council on Cardiovascular Nursing of the American Heart Association. Circulation. 2001;103:472–5. [PMID:11157703.]

39. de Gaetano G, Di Castelnuovo A, Donati MB, et al. The mediterranean lecture: wine and thrombosis-from epidemiology to physiology and back. Pathophysiol Haemost Thromb. 2003 Sep-2004 Dec;33(5–6):466–71. [PMID: 15692262.]

40. Gotto AM. Antioxidants, statins, and atherosclerosis. J Am Coll Cardiol. 2003 Apr 2; 41(7):1205–10. [PMID: 12679223.]

41. Miller ER, Pastor-Barriuso R, Dalal D, et al. Meta-analysis: high-dosage vitamin E supplementation may increase all-cause mortality. Ann Intern Med, 2004;142:37–46. [PMID: 15537682.]

42. Houston M. Meta-analysis, metaphysics and mythology-scientific and clinical perspective on the controversies regarding vitamin E for the prevention and treatment of disease in humans. J Am Nutraceu Assn. 2005;8:4–7. [Online at: www.ana-jana.org]

43. Singh U, Jialal I. Anti-inflammatory effects of alpha-tocopherol. Ann NY Acad Sci. 2004 Dec;1031:195–203. [PMID: 1575314.]

44. Carpenter KL, Kirkpatrick PJ, Weissberg P, et al. Oral alpha-tocopherol supplementation inhibits lipid oxidation in established human atherosclerotic lesions. Free Radic Res. 2003;37:1235–44. [PMID: 14703736.]

45. Knekt P, Ritz J, Pereira MA, et al. Antioxidant vitamins and coronary heart disease risk: a pooled analysis of 9 cohorts. Am J Clin Nutr. 2004;80(6):1508–20. [PMID: 15585762.]

46. Boger RH, Ron ES. L-arginine improves vascular function by overcoming the deleterious effects of ADMA, novel cardiovascular risk factor. Alt Med Rev. 2005;10(1):14–2. [PMID: 15771559.]

47. Anderson TJ, Hubacek J, Wyse DG, et al. Effect of chelation therapy on endothelial function in patients with coronary artery disease: PATCH substudy. J Am Coll Cardiol. 2003;41:420–5. [PMID: 12575969.]

48. Villarruz MV, Dans A, Tan F. Chelation therapy for atherosclerotic cardiovascular disease. Cochrane Database Syst Rev. 2002;4:CD002785. [PMID: 12519577.]

49. Wong SS, Nahin RL. National center for complementary and alternative medicine perspectives for complementary and alternataive medicine research in cardiovascular diseases. Cardiol Rev. 2003;11:94–8. [PMID: 12620133.].

50. Chappell LT, Stahl JP, Evans R. EDTA chelation treatment for vascular disease: a meta-analysis using unpublished data. J Advancement Med. 1994;7:131–42).

51. Hininger I, Waters R, Osman M, et al. Acute prooxidant effects of vitamin C in EDTA chelation therapy and long-term antioxidant benefits of therapy. Free Radic Biol Med. 2005;38:156–507. [PMID: 15917185.]

52. Heck AM, DeWitt BA, Lukes AL. Potential interactions between alternative therapies and warfarin. Am J Health Syst Pharm. 2000 Jul 1;57(13):1221–7. [PMID: 10902065.]

53. Hurlen M, Abdelnoor M, Smith P, et al. Warfarin, aspirin, or both after myocardial infarction. N Engl J Med. 2002 Sep 26;347(13):969–74. [PMID: 12324552.]

54. Engelsen J, Nielsen JD, Hansen KF. Effect of CoQ10 and Ginkgo biloba on warfarin dosage in patients on long-term warfarin treatment. A randomized, double blind, placebo-controlled cross-over trial. Ugeskr Laeger. 2003 Apr 28;165(18):1868–71. [PMID: 12772396.]

55. Durand P, Prost M, Loreau N, et al. Impaired homocysteine metabolism and atherothrombotic disease. Lab Invest. 2001 May;81(5):645–72. [PMID: 11351038.]

56. Anfossi G, Russo I, Massucco P, et al. N-acetyl-L-cysteine exerts direct anti-aggregating effect on human platelets. Eur J Clin Invest. 2001 May;31(5):452–61. [PMID: 11380598.]

57. Wang J, Xu J, Zhong JB. Effect of radix notoginseng saponins on platelet activating molecule expression and aggregation in patients with blood hyperviscosity syndrome. Zhongguo Zhong Xi Yi Jie He Za Zhi. 2004;24:312–16. [PMID: 15143716.]

58. Kosachunhanun N, Hunt RC, Hopkins PN, et al. Genetic determinants of nonmodulating hypertension. Hypertension. 2003;42(5):901–908. [PMID: 14530292.]

59. Chobanian AV, Bakris GL, Black HR, et al. Seventh report of the Joint National Committee on prevention, detection, evaluation, and treatment of high blood pressure (JNC7). Hypertension. 2003;42:1206–52. [PMID: 14656957.]

60. Pitt B. Effect of aldosterone blockade in patients with systolic left ventricular dysfunction: implications of the RALES and EPHESUS studies. Mol Cell Endocrinol. 2004;217:53–8. [PMID: 15134801.]

61. Svetkey LP, Simons-Morton DG, Proschan MA, et al. Effect of the dietary approaches to stop hypertension diet and reduced sodium intake on blood pressure control. J Clin Hypertens. 2004 Jul;6(7):373–81. [PMID: 15249792.]

62. Wilburn AJ, King DS, Glisson J, et al. The natural treatment of hypertension. J Clin Hypertens. 2004 May;6(5):242–8. [PMID: 15133406.]

63. Gums JG. Magnesium in cardiovascular and other disorders. Am J Health Syst Pharm. 2004 Aug 1;61(15):1569–76. [PMID: 15372830.]

64. Townsend MS, Fulgoni VL,III, Stern JS, et al. Low mineral intake is associated with high systolic blood pressure in the Third and Fourth National Health and Nutrition Examination Surveys: could we all be right? Am J Hypertens. 2005 Feb; 18(2 Pt 1):261–9. [PMID: 15752955.]

65. Rosanoff A. Magnesium and hypertension. Clin Calcium. 2005 Feb;15(2):255–60. [PMID: 15692166.]

66. Burke BE, Neuenschwander R, Olson RD. Randomized, double-blind, placebo-controlled trial of CoQ10 in isolated systolic hypertension. South Med J. 2001 Nov; 94(11):1112–7. [PMID: 1178068.]

67. Rosenfeldt F, Hilton D, Pepe S, et al. Systematic review of effect of coenzyme Q10 in physical exercise, hypertension and heart failure. Biofactors. 2003;18(1–4):91–100. [PMID: 1469592.]

68. Hodgson JM, Watts GF. Can coenzyme Q10 improve vascular function and blood pressure? Potential for effective therapeutic reduction in vascular oxidative stress. Biofactors. 2003;18(1–4):129–36. [PMID: 14695928.]

69. Geleijnse JM, Giltay EJ, Grobbee DE, et al. Blood pressure response to fish oil supplementation: metaregression analysis of randomized trials. J Hypertens. 2002 Aug; 20(8):1493–9. [PMID: 12172309.]

70. Holm T, Andreassen AK, Aukrust P, et al. Omega-3 fatty acids improve blood pressure control and preserve renal function in hypertensive heart transplant recipients. Eur Heart J. 2001 Mar;22(5):428–36. [PMID: 11207085.]

71. Perticone F, Sciacqua A, Maio R, et al. Asymmetric dimethylarginine, L-arginine, and endothelial dysfunction in essential hypertension. J Am Coll Cardiol. 2005 Aug 2; 46(3):518–23.[PMID: 16053968.]

72. Khosh F, Khosh M. Natural approach to hypertension. Alt Med Rev. 2001;6(6): 590–8. [PMID: 11804549.]

73. Lacaille-Dubois<CHECK FOR AU INITIALS>, Franck U, Wagner H. Search for potential angiotensin converting enzyme (ACE)-inhibitors from plants. Phytomedicine. 2001 Jan;8(1):47–52.) [PMID: 1129223.]

74. Somova L, Shode FO, Mipando M. Cardiotonic and antidysrhythmic effects of oleanolic and ursolic acids, methyl maslinate and uvaol. Phytomedicine. 2004 Feb; 11(2–3):121–9. [PMID: 1507016.]

75. Liu X, Wei J, Tan F, et al. Pycnogenol, French maritime pine bark extract, improves endothelial function of hypertensive patients. Life Sci. 2004;74:855–62. [PMID: 14659974.]

76. Pechanova O, Bernatova II, Babal P, et al. Red wine polyphenols prevent cardiovascular alterations in L- NAME-induced hypertension. J Hypertens 2004;22: 1551–9.[PMID: 15257179.]

77. Hitzenberger G, Korn A, Dorcsi M. Controlled randomized double-blind study for the comparison of the treatment of patients with essential hypertension with homeopathic and with pharmacologically effective drugs. Wien Klin Wochenschr. 1982 Dec 24; 94(24):665–70. [PMID: 6763404.]

78. Klatsky AL, Chartier D, Udaltsova N, et al. Alcohol drinking and risk of hospitalization for heart failure with and without associated coronary artery disease. Am J Cardiol. 2005 Aug 1;96(3):346–51. [PMID: 160544.]

79. Berman M, Erman A, Ben-Gal T, et al. Coenzyme Q10 in patients with end-stage heart failure awaiting cardiac transplantation: a randomized, placebo-controlled study. Clin Cardiol. 2004 May;27(5):295–9. [PMID: 15188947.]

80. Rundek T, Naini A, Sacco R, et al. Atorvastatin decreases the coenzyme Q10 level in the blood of patients at risk for cardiovascular disease and stroke. Arch Neurol. 2004;61:889–92.[PMID: 15210526.]

81. Corder R, Warburton RC, Khan NQ, et al. The procyanidin-induced pseudo laminar shear stress response: a new concept for the reversal of endothelial dysfunction. Clin Sci (Lond). 2004 Nov;107(5):513–7. [PMID: 15324299.]

82. Quettier-Deleu C, Voiselle G, Fruchart JC. Hawthorn extracts inhibit LDL oxidation. Pharmazie. 2003 Aug;58(8):577–81. [PMID: 12967038.]

83. Pittler MH, Schmidt K, Ernst E. Hawthorn extract for treating chronic heart failure: meta-analysis of randomized trials. Am J Med. 2003 Jun 1;114(8):665–74. [PMID: 12798455.]

84. Habs M. Prospective, comparative cohort studies and their contribution to the benefit assessments of therapeutic options: heart failure treatment with and without

Hawthorn special extract WS 1442. Forsch Komplementarmed Klass Naturheilkd. 2004 Aug;11 Suppl 1:36–9. [PMID: 15353901.]

85. Degenring FH, Suter A, Weber M, et al. A randomised double blind placebo controlled clinical trial of a standardised extract of fresh Crataegus berries (Crataegisan) in the treatment of patients with congestive heart failure NYHA II. Phytomedicine. 2003;10(5):363–9. [PMID: 12833999.]

86. Schroder D, Weiser M, Klein P. Efficacy of a homeopathic Crataegus preparation compared with usual therapy for mild (NYHA II) cardiac insufficiency: results of an observational cohort study. Eur J Heart Fail. 2003 Jun;5(3):319–26. [PMID: 12798830.]

87. Norn S, Kruse PR. Cardiac glycosides: from ancient history through Withering's foxglove to endogeneous cardiac glycosides. Dan Medicinhist Arbog. 2004;119–32. [PMID: 15685783.]

88. Piepoli MF. Exercise training-meta-analysis of trials in patients with chronic heart failure. BMJ. 2004;328:189. [PMID: 14729656.]

89. Singer P, Wirth M. Can n-3 PUFA reduce cardiac arrhythmias? Results of a clinical trial. Prostaglandins Leukot Essent Fatty Acids. 2004;71:153–9. [PMID: 15253884.]

90. Harrison RA, Elton PJ. Is there a role for long-chain omega3 or oil-rich fish in the treatment of atrial fibrillation? Med Hypotheses. 2005;64(1):59–63.[PMID: 15533612.]

91. Suzuki Y, Kondo K, Matsumoto Y, et al. Dietary supplementation of fermented soybean, natto, suppresses intimal thickening and modulates the lysis of mural thrombi after endothelial injury in rat femoral artery. Life Sci. 2003 Jul 25;73(10):1289–98. [PMID: 12850244.]

92. Milner M. Naturopathic management of coagulation in chronic atrial fibrillation. Naturopathic Doctors News and Review. Sept 2005;23.

93. Cybulski J, Budaj A, Danielewicz H, et al. A new-onset atrial fibrillation: the incidence of potassium and magnesium deficiency. The efficacy of intravenous potassium/magnesium supplementation in cardioversion to sinus rhythm. Kardiol Pol. 2004 Jun;60(6):578–81 [PMID: 15334158.]

94. Alghamdi AA, Al-Radi OO, Latter DA. Intravenous magnesium for prevention of atrial fibrillation after coronary artery bypass surgery: a systematic review and meta-analysis. J Card Surg. 2005 May-Jun;20(3):293–9. [PMID: 15854101.]

95. Miller S, Crystal E, Garfinkle M, et al. Effects of magnesium on atrial fibrillation after cardiac surgery: a meta-analysis. Heart. 2005 May;91(5):618–23. [PMID: 15831645.]

96. Shiga T, Wajima Z, Inoue T, et al. Magnesium prophylaxis for arrhythmias after cardiac surgery: a meta-analysis of randomized controlled trials. Am J Med. 2004 Sep 1;117(5):325–33. [PMID: 15336582.]

97. Bobkowski W, Nowak A, Durlach J. The importance of magnesium status in the pathophysiology of mitral valve prolapse. Magnes Res. 2005 Mar;18(1):35–52. [PMID: 15945614.]

98. Kitlinski M, Stepniewski M, Nessler J, et al. Is magnesium deficit in lymphocytes a part of the mitral valve prolapse syndrome? Magnes Res. 2004 Mar;17(1):39–45. [PMID: 15083568.]

99. Dwivedi S, Aggarwal A, Agarwal MP, et al. Role of Terminalia arjuna in ischaemic mitral regurgitation. Int J Cardiol. 2005 Apr 28;100(3):507–8. [PMID: 15837100.]

100. van der Meer JT. Prophylaxis of endocarditis. Neth J Med. 2002 Dec;60(11):423–7. [PMID: 12685488.]

17

HOMEOPATHY

Maryann Ivons

INTRODUCTION

In the late 1800s, a German physician, Dr Samuel Hahnemann, frustrated by the medical practices of his day that had a tendency to kill more often than it cured, described a new system of medicine. After extensive experimentation with smaller and smaller doses of medicinal substances already in use, Dr Hahnemann found that continuing to decrease the size of the dosage increased the therapeutic results while eliminating the side effects normally attributed to the substance used.

Dr Hahnemann and the practitioners of his day did not have the knowledge of physiology, biochemistry, anatomy, and the other medical sciences we take for granted today. However, being a man of science himself, he strove to explain the observations he had made in his long experimentation with the medications at his disposal. He developed a philosophic model called the "Law of Similiars"— Like Cures Like. He postulated that substances that would have an adverse effect on an organism, if used in very small doses would cure those same symptoms.

We have no idea if this is technically true, we still don't understand how Homeopathy works. There has been no good basic research into the mechanism of action of homeopathic medicine, but for the doctors who use it and the patients who benefit from it, the positive effects of this medical modality are undeniable.

It is important to remember that just because we don't understand how something works, that does not mean that it does not exist. DNA, for example, has always been a double helix and the basis of organic life on this planet. It did not come into existence when Watson and Crick identified it and described its action. Much in the same way, homeopathy has always worked. Just because we don't understand the mechanism of action does not mean that we should dismiss it. It is important not to get fixated on a 200-year-old explanation that has no basis in the science we understand today.

Homeopathy is not an easy discipline. What can be therapeutic, can also do harm if not used correctly. Professionals who do not understand the modality well and do not have experience in its use should not practice homeopathy. Homeopathic practitioners spend years studying materia medica, learning to use the repertory, taking cases, and seeing patients. It is very important to have this experience to effectively and safely practice this type of medicine.

HOMEOPATHIC PHILOSOPHY

Theory of disease: vital force

Samuel Hahnemann believed that all disease was caused by an imbalance of the vital force. This was a very different concept from the practitioners of his time. The vital force is that part of an organism that makes it alive, rather than dead. He believed that very person's vital force is unique. Disease occurs when the vital force of an organism becomes imbalanced. The imbalance can occur from causes arising within the organism itself, or from external forces impinging on the organism. These external influences are termed exciting causes. He felt that the response of the vital force to imbalances had to do with both the innate vitality of the patient and the strength of the exciting cause.

Vitality of the patient depends on many things; the genetic make up of the person, nutrition, and environment—all the things we recognize today that affect the health of any individual. As all medical practitioners know, some people are more susceptible to disease than others. They may also have areas of weakness in their body inherited from their parents and grandparents. These predispositions can, in some ways, predict the types of the diseases that may appear in a patient as well as how they will respond to stressors in their environment.

External causes of imbalance of the vital force include infectious agents, environmental problems, and lifestyle choices. Poverty, malnutrition, bad habits, such as smoking, poor diet, or excessive stress, all impinge on an organism in various and unique ways. Not all people are affected by outside stresses in the same way. I'm sure we all have patients who eat perfectly, have excellent habits, get plenty of rest, and still seem to be unwell. There are others who smoke and drink but live to be a hundred, and never have any problems at all.

Disease states

Hahnemann described three disease states, acute, chronic, and pseudo-chronic. The acute state is described as short-lived and self-limiting. Either the patient will fully recover or they will die. The acute state is initiated by an exciting cause. Most familiar to us would be some type of an organism such as typhoid or viral influenza. But, also, these states can be initiated by traumas such as a motor vehicle accident.

In an attempt to cope with these insults, the organism manifests a set of symptoms that are designed to clear the body of the problem and reestablish balance. For instance, in a viral upper respiratory infection, the organism produces a lot of mucus and a cough in order to rid the body of the elements of the virus. In general, left untreated, these diseases will resolve over time. If the vital force is too weak to deal with the acute disease, the organism will descend into a chronic disease state.

In allopathic medicine, chronic disease describes a long-standing case where illness has a recurrent pattern, such as heart disease or asthma. To a homeopath, chronic disease is the failed attempt of the vital force to deal with some acute problem in the past or an imbalance that arises from some innate problem generated from within the organism. The symptoms elicited by the organism are not strong enough to resolve these problems and so the disease lingers on and on. These symptoms are also not strong enough to actually damage the organism unto death, nor can they restore the balance of the vital force.

The constellation of symptoms that describe this chronic state of a patient are referred to as the "constitutional state" of the patient. Hahnemann described the chronic state arising from internal factors as a miasm. The concept of miasm is extremely interesting, but very hard to explain and is one of the most misunderstood concepts in all of homeopathy.

Hahnemann saw the miasma as the foundation of all disease. It can be described as a predisposition to disease with which one is born. To read more about miasma and the philosophy of disease in homeopathy, refer to the *Organon of Medicine*, by Samuel Hahnemann.

Pseudo-chronic disease refers to a disruption in the vital force that is initiated by an outside influence that, unlike the acute disease, lingers. It is fostered by what is termed a "maintaining cause." For instance, an otherwise healthy person who starts to live with a smoker may develop symptoms of sinusitis. They fall into that state due to the chronic upper respiratory irritation. The pseudo-chronic state only needs the maintaining cause to be removed for balance to be restored to the organism.

In order to understand how homeopaths view disease, it is important to understand how they view the organism. We picture an individual as composed of three planes of being: mental, emotional, and physical. The physical plane also has a hierarchy of layers—from the deep layers involving the immune and endocrine systems to the most superficial layer of the skin. When the disease process starts to occur, the organism will generate symptoms on the level or plane that it considers the least harmful to the organism in order to reinstate balance. Thus, the most benign symptoms appear first on the most superficial levels.

If the symptoms on that level are suppressed or ignored, the organism will attempt to express symptoms at deeper levels. If the imbalance continues to be ignored or suppressed, more and increasingly serious symptoms will appear on progressively deeper layers.

From a homeopathic perspective, a classic example of this process can be seen in children who have eczema. When the eczema is suppressed by treatment with steroids, the child may develop asthma. We feel that original diagnosis of eczema was actually the expression of the miasmatic state of that child. It's usually accompanied by a constellation of other symptoms that are specific to that vital force. If the eczema is treated homeopathically, it disappears and the asthma never results.

Herring's law of cure

Just as the organism gets sick in specific ways, it also gets well in specific ways. Dr Constantine Herring, a nineteenth century physician, described what he termed the "Law of Cure." After many years of observing patients, he noticed that improvement of symptoms that lead to cure followed a specific pattern. This pattern has become a road map for evaluation of homeopathic treatment, although it can also be applied to allopathic treatment.

To reflect the return of balance in the vital force, symptoms need to disappear from the deepest level to the outmost level, from the top of the organism to the bottom, and from the most recent symptoms to the oldest symptoms, that is the reverse order of their appearance. When assessing symptoms, there are a number of possible outcomes that can appear:

> *Aggravation:* The symptoms that the patient came in will get worse. This is a good sign for homeopaths, because the remedy is working on the problem. Aggravations are transient and the organism ends up better in general after the aggravations disappear. Cure is the end of this process.

> *Palliation:* The presenting symptom gets well, but all the other symptoms stay the same. For example, if a person comes in complaining of headaches and depression, then the headaches disappear, but the depression remains and nothing else changes.

> *Suppression:* This happens in the same way homeopathically as it does with allopathic therapies. The presenting symptom disappears and a deeper symptom appears. If we use the example above, the headache would improve and the emotional symptoms would worsen. This is exactly opposite of Herring's law and very detrimental to the patient.

> *Proving:* This is an outcome particular to homeopathy. Proving happens when a patient is given an incorrect medication and develops symptoms that they have never had before. However, the new symptoms that the patient complains of are particular to the remedy they were given. We will discuss this process later in the chapter.

Homeopathic medications

Materials become homeopathic medications by a process called potentization. Potentization involves the serial dilution and secussed, or shaking, of the material to be potentized. Homeopaths refer to these potentized medications as "remedies." For a more detailed explanation, refer to my book, *Homeopathy for Nurses*.

In order to determine the properties of a medication that is potentized, a procedure called *proving* is followed. Proving is the way that homeopathic medications are evaluated and the therapeutic properties of that medication discovered. Provings are done on healthy people. These people are given a repeated small dose of the remedy until symptoms appear, then the person doing the proving chronicles those symptoms. Each proving is done by a group of people, the more people that are involved with each proving the more complete the information. The symptoms of each prover are gathered together, collated and evaluated to articulate the "picture" of that particular remedy.

According to the theory of homeopathic medicine, there is one single remedy, the similimum, that will cover the symptoms expressed by an individual at any time and that single remedy should be given in the minimum dose required to cover the symptoms and to affect a change in the organism.

THE MEDICINES

Unlike allopathic medicine, there are no homeopathic medications specifically for a disease. That is to say, there are no remedies for asthma or cardiac disease or arrhythmias per se. Remedies reflect a complex of symptoms that describe a state of a particular patient's vital force. It is true, however, that some remedies may have specific tissue affinities, which are reflected in the provings and also in clinical practice. The biggest mistake, and therefore the failure of homeopathic remedies to affect a good outcome, is usually reflected in the failure of the practitioner to prescribe the medications properly. Practitioners who prescribe homeopathic medicines in an allopathic way are bound to fail most of the time. Occasionally they hit on the right remedy, but usually for the wrong reasons.

In order to prescribe a homeopathic remedy effectively and safely, a good case must be taken and the symptoms that the patient relates must be matched to the medication that the patient is given.

Even though I stress that there is no such thing as "acute homeopathy," there are homeopathic medication that are effective for acute medical conditions. Medical emergencies such as cardiac arrhythmia or anaphylactic shock can be treated effectively with homeopathic medications. This is certainly not to suggest that one should use homeopathic medications instead of allopathic medications in these very serious situations. It's just to explain that there are remedies that cover these medical emergencies.

Homeopathic tools: materia medica

A materia medica is a book that lists homeopathic medications, both proven and unproven. They usually consist of a general description of the medication, followed by symptoms related to various parts of the body that describe the attributes of that medication. Materia medicas have been with us for a very long time and they can reflect general use or can be disease specific. Many modern materia medicas which include new provings are now available, but the old standards, particularly, *Homeopathic Materia Medica and Repertory* by W. Bourke, MD, are still widely in use. I will include a list of various materia medicas at the end of the chapter.

Repertories

Like materia medica, repertories are indispensable tools for practitioners of homeopathy. Repertories are a list of symptoms organized by body parts, generalities, and other categories that have symptoms under them organized in a very specific way. Under those symptoms are lists of remedies that can be cross-referenced in materia medica. The classic repertory is the *Repertory of Homeopathic Materia Medica*, by JP Kent. All modern repertories are based on this repertory. All new repertories have been modernized and expanded but any new additions made follow the basic pattern set down by Kent 150 years ago.

The language of the repertory will be unfamiliar to most practitioners. The process of case taking and repertorization is time consuming and a little frustrating at first. The practitioner must take the symptoms of the patient, and then translate them to the language of the repertory. The symptoms listed in the repertories are referred to as "rubrics." Under each rubric is listed a group of remedies. When you have found all the rubrics that you are going to use you must cross-reference the remedies under them to find those common to all or most of the rubrics. When you have gotten the list of the common remedies, you read the materia medica of each to find the appropriate medication for that case. For further discussion and in depth look at how to use a repertory, I would refer you to *A Tutorial and Workbook for Homeopathic Repertory* by Karen B Allen.

As you can imagine, this process is time consuming. However, repertorization is uniquely suited to the computer. There are a number of programs available to do the legwork. The two most popular are MacRepertory and Radar. There is a materia medica program available with each. These materia medica programs contain whole libraries of books and journals from more than 200 years of homeopathic writing.

Potentized

Materials that are potentized can be drawn from any source, plant, animal, or mineral. Potentized medications that are proven and have an extensive history in clinical practice are called polycrests. These medications have a long medical track record and have been used for at least 200 years.

The first potentized substance that Dr Hahnemann used was Cinchona officinalis, quinine. Over the years, it has been helpful treating a number of different conditions including anemia, gastritis, and influenza. Each potentized substance has its own unique set of properties and treats a range of symptoms specific to the realm of that medication.

Therapeutics

Given the nature of homeopathic treatment, it might be misleading to divide this section into disease categories. But for the purpose of this book, we will use them, because it will be more familiar to most of the practitioners using this text. I shall describe how homeopathic treatment can be helpful in the treatment of each of these diagnoses.

HYPERTENSION

Hypertension is a ubiquitous problem in this country and is quite difficult to treat successfully, due to the multifactorial nature of the problem. If hypertension had one physiologic cause, it would be relatively easy to find a medication that addressed that cause and to treat the hypertension. Unfortunately, that is not the case. As any physician knows, hypertension is a potential symptom of many conditions, some of them physiologic, but many of them emotional. Most commonly we find a combination of both. Because cardiology tends to look at the physical causes of disease, hypertension is addressed as a purely physical problem. Patients are given medications that target vascular physiology, like calcium channel blockers or beta-blockers. If they do not respond to one class of medication then another is available. Unfortunately, many of these medications have side effects that patients may find so distressing that they quit the medication. This can lead to very dangerous consequences. These medications are unable to effectively treat this problem in the long run. It is generally frustrating and ineffective to treat a problem if you do not know what caused it.

Hypertension is a symptom that can be the result of noncompliant blood vessels as in arterial sclerotic disease. It can be a manifestation of pathologies in the kidneys. It can also arise if the blood vessels spasm for some reason. The vast majority of cases of hypertension in the United States are due, at least in part, to the stresses that a person encounters in their lives. Those compounded with poor eating habits and lack of exercise produce the cocktail problems we treat as hypertension. Medications alone do not address the complete picture. Homeopathic treatment looks at the whole person. It can balance patients so that they will be more able to handle the stressors in their lives and make the changes that can lead to a healthier lifestyle. If hypertension remains, it is more effectively treated with conventional medications.

CARDIAC ARRHYTHMIAS

Homeopathy is also an effective adjunct therapy for cardiac arrhythmias. It may be indicated either acutely or as a constitutionally. Constitutional homeopathy can help a patient who has a history of arrhythmia, particularly if the arrhythmia is triggered by stressful events in a patient's life. I have found homeopathy is particularly useful in acute episodes of pharmacogenomics of arrhythmia therapy (PAT) or atrial fibrillation.

MYOCARDIAL INFARCT

Chest pain can be effectively treated by a first responder who understands homeopathy. If the patient receives the remedy that reflects their symptoms, the chances of survival are very much increased. I want to emphasize that this is not a substitute for emergency medical intervention.

While there are no remedies specifically for chest pain, as we have stated before, here are a few of the homeopathic medications that have an affinity for the cardiovascular system: aconitum, arnica, aurum, argentum nitricum, cactus grandiflora, convallaria, crategus, and digitalis. An excellent resource is *Desktop Companion to Physical Pathology* by Dr Roger Morrison, MD. This book will give you a very good idea of the remedy pictures of multiple homeopathic medications that treat not only arrhythmias, but also chest pain and other heart conditions.

ARTERIAL SCLEROTIC HEART DISEASE

Arterial sclerotic heart disease is another multifactorial problem. Genetic predisposition, life style choices, and possibly environmental factors all contribute to the development of this condition.

Constitutional homeopathy, once again, is the best strategy to start with. It balances the whole system and can help the patient realize the necessity of making the lifestyle changes that will ultimately lead to better health.

There is no direct correlation with the use of homeopathic medications and the lowering of cholesterol levels. However, it is reasonable to postulate that a person in a constitutional state of balance may metabolize cholesterol and triglycerides more efficiently. Hyperlipidemia, like hypertension, is a disease that the allopathic community addresses as a single entity. The standard of practice is to treat the numbers regardless of why they are elevated.

While homeopathy can be helpful in many of these cases, the mechanism of action is unclear. It is probable that the homeopathic medication treats both the physical and the emotional state of the patient.

CARDIOVASCULAR SURGERY

Although I have stressed that homeopathy is not well suited for "one size fits all," prescribing, there appears to be an exception to this rule when dealing with surgeries. I have developed a protocol that seems to decrease the postsurgical complications in patients either with anesthesia or bleeding. Postsurgical homeopathics can also decrease the amount of pain medication patients require and speed wound healing and recovery.

I use this protocol for any surgery that my patients have scheduled. The homeopathic surgical protocol that I use is as follows:

- The day before surgery, Arnica 6c and Phosphorus 6c are alternated every 3 hours while awake.
- The day of surgery, the patient gets up in the morning and takes Arnica 6c as soon as they get out of bed. Phosphorus 6c is taken as close as possible to entering surgery.
- After surgery, the patient takes Arnica 30c as soon as possible and may repeat it up to every 3 hours, as needed, after that for pain control. It is important to discuss this protocol with the anesthesiologist before the patient initiates it.

Like all other modalities, homeopathy works best when it is part of a comprehensive therapeutic regime, but if homeopathy is to be a successful therapeutic tool, it must be prescribed by practitioners who know how to use it. I would encourage physicians to attend introductory seminars or case conferences to learn more about this fascinating, sometimes frustrating, yet amazingly powerful medical modality.

BIBLIOGRAPHY

Allen KB. A tutorial and workbook for the homeopathic repertory. Redmond (WA): Homeopathic Tutorials; 1994.

Boericke W. Homeopathic materia medica and repertory. London, England: B. Jain Publishers; 1998.

Hahnemann S. The organon of medicine, first inaugural English translation of the Sixth Edition, Blaine (WA): Cooper Publishing; 1962.

Ivons M. Homeopathy for nurses. Orlando (FL): Bandido Books; 2004.

Kent JT. Repertory of the homeopathic materia medica. 6th edition. New Delhi, India: World Homeopathic Links; 1989.

Morrison, R. Desktop companion to physical pathology. Nevada City (CA): Hahnemann Clinic Publishing; 1998.

Resources

Homeopathic Academy of Naturopathic Physicians
1412 W. Washington St.
Boise, ID. 83702
208-336-3309
208-367-9242 (FAX)
www.bmathiew@spro.net

National Center for Homeopathy
801 N. Fairfax St., Suite 306
Alexandria, VA. 22314
703-548-7790
703-548-7792 (FAX)
www.homeopathic.org

Directory of Homeopathic Organization:
www.extendedyears.com/lib/4010.html

4

MECHANISTIC AND PHYSIOLOGICAL LINKS BETWEEN CAM AND THE CARDIOVASCULAR SYSTEM

18

PSYCHOLOGICAL RISK FACTORS AND PATHOPHYSIOLOGICAL PATHWAYS INVOLVED IN CORONARY ARTERY DISEASE: RELEVANCE TO COMPLEMENTARY MEDICINE INTERVENTIONS

Willem J. Kop and Jennifer L. Francis

INTRODUCTION

Cardiovascular disease (CVD) is the leading cause of mortality in industrialized countries. In the United States, over 900,000 deaths (37.3% of all deaths) were attributable to cardiovascular disease in 2003. The American Heart Association reports that over 70 million Americans have one or more forms of cardiovascular disease. The most common cardiovascular disorder is hypertension (65 million people), and the most prevalent diseases are coronary artery disease (CAD) (13 million) and cerebrovascular events (5.5 million). Based on the Framingham Heart Study, the lifetime risk of CAD in 50-year-old disease-free individuals is approximately 50%. Thus, cardiovascular disease is a major public health problem.

Major improvements have been accomplished in risk reduction and survival of acute coronary syndromes. Because cardiovascular disease is a multifactorial disorder with various genetic and environmental risk factors, it is likely that a multidisciplinary approach will be needed to optimize cardiovascular health and prevent incident and recurrent cardiac events. Pharmacological interventions and revascularization procedures have been extremely successful in reducing cardiovascular morbidity and mortality. However, patients with cardiovascular disease often use complementary (alternative) medicine strategies to potentially further optimize health and reduce risk of adverse health outcomes. Complementary therapies are defined here as practices that are not currently considered an integral part of conventional medical practice and are used instead of or in combination with conventional medical treatment. Although some overlap exists, this chapter makes a distinction between complementary therapies (such as acupuncture and herbal medicine), psychological interventions (e.g., relaxation, cognitive behavioral therapy), and health behavior modification (e.g., exercise, dietary interventions, and smoking cessation). It is estimated that approximately 40% of patients with general medical conditions use complementary medicine techniques. This trend may partly reflect the increasing appreciation of the "whole person" in health and disease, and the lack of confidence in traditional medicine by the general public. Complementary therapies encompass a diverse range of health care approaches. These approaches include meditation, biofeedback, acupuncture, chiropractic interventions, herbal medicine, and massage. The National Institutes of Health and the National Center for Alternative and Complementary Medicine have issued a joint report on the use of complementary medicine in cardiovascular health care.[1] The pathophysiological processes described in the following sections may prove useful for the identification of potentially overlapping mechanisms by which psychological and complementary therapies are beneficial in reducing cardiovascular risk. In addition, such information can promote the development of novel integrative interventions.

Evidence suggests that both chronic and acute psychological factors increase the risk of CAD.[2-5] These psychological risk factors can be categorized as: chronic personality traits (e.g., hostility), episodic factors (e.g., depression and exhaustion), and acute psychological triggers (e.g., anger). An increasing number of studies suggests that the immune system plays an important role in the relationship between these psychological risk factors and future coronary syndromes.[6-9] It is important to differentiate between CAD as gradual disease process and its clinical manifestations as acute coronary syndromes (i.e., myocardial infarction [MI] and sudden cardiac death). A brief description of the pathophysiology of CAD will be reviewed first, followed by psychological CAD risk factors and their purported biobehavioral mechanisms relevant to CAD. This chapter concludes with possible clinical implications and directions for future research in complementary medicine.

BRIEF OVERVIEW OF THE PATHOPHYSIOLOGY OF CAD

The development of acute coronary syndromes is based on plaque, blood, and myocardial vulnerability markers.[10] These vulnerability markers are part of the atherosclerotic disease process and are influenced by the immune system, lipid metabolism, and a wide range of other pro-atherogenic factors. Clinical manifestations of CAD may be symptomatic (i.e., angina pectoris and its equivalents) without permanent structural myocardial damage. In addition, clinical manifestations of CAD may present as life-threatening acute coronary syndromes such as myocardial infarction and sudden cardiac death.[10-13] Acute coronary syndromes commonly occur in the presence of underlying coronary atherosclerosis.

Gradual atherosclerotic plaque development can be viewed as a "response to injury" because atherosclerosis causes damage to the coronary vessel wall.[14,15] Several pathophysiological classifications of coronary vascular injury have been formulated based on the extent of damage to the arterial wall.[10,11;16-18] The severity of coronary disease will be used here to clarify effects of psychosocial factors on CAD progression and its clinical manifestations as acute coronary syndromes.

Initial stages of coronary atherosclerosis are characterized by fatty streaks, which are associated with functional alterations of the endothelium (the lining cells of the vessel wall) without substantial reductions in the vessel diameter. Hypercholesterolemia, circulating vasoactive amines, chemical irritants such as tobacco smoke, and inflammatory processes promote endothelial dysfunction.[16,17] These early lesions also involve accumulation of lipids, macrophages, and T-lymphocytes in the arterial vessel wall.[15,19] Fatty streaks are never associated with cardiac symptoms and may either disappear or develop into atheromata (i.e., atherosclerotic lesions).[19] Platelets, endothelial cells, and macrophages may secrete several growth factors that initiate proliferation and migration of smooth muscle cells to other layers of the vessel wall. Endothelial dysfunction and smooth muscle cell proliferation may result in lesions of the more inward (intimal) layers of the coronary vascular wall. These coronary lesions display fibrin deposits and/or lipid-laden phagocytes (i.e., foam cells). Endothelial activation can be caused by low-density lipoprotein (LDL) cholesterol modification by oxidation resulting in the release of phospholipids. Platelets first respond to activated endothelium and may further increase endothelial activation by their glycoproteins (Ib and IIb/IIIa). Subsequently, a capsule-like fibrous layer of smooth muscle cells is formed, which covers the lipid lesion and predominantly collagen-based matrix. The atherosclerotic lesion is also infiltrated by T-cells, macrophages, and mast cells, particularly at sites where the plaque grows. These activated immune cells produce inflammatory cytokines which can be detected in the systemic circulation.

Atherosclerotic plaques at the advanced stage of CAD are characterized by severe damage to all layers of the vessel wall, including the elastic lamina. Because of the thin layer of lipid-laden lesions, plaque rupture can easily occur, causing blood-clot formation and development of severe vascular lesions, even when obstructive luminal narrowing has not yet developed. When collagen is exposed to circulating blood, platelet adhesion and aggregation, as well as coagulation and fibrinolytic processes, are involved in the formation and stabilization of the blood clot. Evidence indicates that advanced coronary lesions progress to total occlusion three times as often as less severe lesions.[20,21] In most instances, however, these advanced lesions do not significantly impair coronary blood flow (<75% luminal stenosis). The nature and speed of the progression from moderate to severe lesions are mediated by immunological processes and are associated with major clinical consequences, including unstable anginal complaints and acute coronary syndromes.

Chest pain and shortness of breath are indicative of CAD and are referred to as anginal symptoms. These symptoms occur when CAD has progressed to become flow-limiting (i.e., >50% stenosis of luminal diameter). When increased cardiac demand occurs (e.g., in response to exercise or acute mental arousal) in the setting of reduced coronary supply, myocardial ischemia may ensue, which may lead to symptoms of chest pain and other angina equivalents.

Acute coronary syndromes are often the first clinical manifestations of CAD and occur in vulnerable individuals with advanced lesions.[16,22] Acute coronary syndromes commonly occur in the setting of relatively stable but nonobstructive (<75% stenosis) atherosclerotic plaques as a result of plaque rupture or endothelial erosion. Myocardial infarction develops as a consequence of acute sustained cardiac ischemia.[16,22] Sudden cardiac death is often preceded by acute myocardial ischemia[23] and, therefore, may be triggered by the same pathophysiological factors as those involved in myocardial ischemia. In addition to rupture of relatively stable coronary lesions, sudden progression of a nonobstructive lesion to a large and occlusive thrombus may result in acute coronary occlusion and subsequent myocardial infarction.[18] It is estimated that plaque rupture and thrombus formation account for approximately 50% of acute coronary syndromes.[15]

In summary, the atherosclerotic process is characterized by gradual progression from fatty streaks, associated with minor endothelial injury, via intimal damage (atheromata) to thrombus formation. Initial CAD stages involve arterial engulfment of lipids, macrophages, and T-cells, platelet adhesion and aggregation, as well as smooth muscle cell proliferation. At progressed CAD stages, thrombosis and impaired fibrinolysis contribute to the development of severe coronary lesions. Prolonged coronary disease often results in gradual vessel narrowing, which may be accompanied by anginal complaints. When CAD has progressed gradually over a long period of time, acute coronary syndromes may not occur as a consequence of the protective effects of well-developed collateral coronary blood supply. In contrast, the disruption of relatively small atherosclerotic plaques plays a crucial role in the pathogenesis of acute myocardial infarction. Thus, it is important to differentiate between the stage of anatomical CAD progression and its clinical manifestation as an acute coronary syndrome.

PSYCHOLOGICAL RISK FACTORS FOR CAD

The role of psychological factors in the progression of CAD and acute coronary syndromes has been documented in a large body of studies.[2,3,5] The nature and magnitude of the associations between psychological factors with the onset of acute coronary syndromes are influenced by the severity of underlying CAD (Fig. 18-1). Thus, consistent with the pathophysiology of CAD, it is important to differentiate between chronic and acute psychological factors in the progression of CAD.[4,24] Chronic psychological risk factors may promote the onset of initial stages of atherosclerosis by sympathetic nervous system-mediated pathophysiological pathways (e.g., lipid deposition and inflammatory processes) and/or as a result of their association with known CAD risk factors (e.g.,

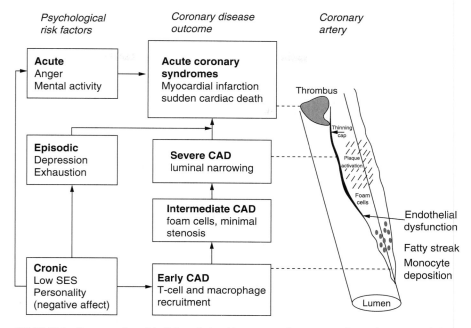

FIGURE 18-1 *Conceptual model of the relationships among chronic, episodic, and acute psychologi-*
cal risk factors for coronary syndromes. Acute psychological factors can trigger ischemia and
plaque instability in vulnerable patients, which can lead to acute coronary syndromes (myocardial
ischemia and sudden cardiac death). Episodic psychological factors have physiological correlates
that are involved in the progression of severe coronary disease to acute coronary syndromes.
Chronic psychological factors promote the onset of early atherosclerosis, especially in the setting of
genetic vulnerability, adverse health behaviors, and other environmental risk factors. In addition,
chronic psychological factors are related to increased frequency and elevated responsiveness to acute
psychological factors and promote the risk of developing episodic factors. (Modified from Kop, 2003)

hypertension, smoking, lipids, and obesity). At advanced stages of CAD, acute
psychological risk factors may trigger acute coronary syndromes, including
myocardial infarction or malignant arrhythmias.

Prior investigations have shown that psychological risk factors for coronary
disease can be classified into three broad categories, based on their duration and
temporal proximity to coronary syndromes:[2] (1) chronic factors, such as negative personality traits (e.g., hostility) and low socioeconomic status; (2) episodic
factors with a duration of several weeks up to 2 years, among which are depression and exhaustion; and (3) acute factors, including mental stress and outbursts
of anger. Accumulating evidence indicates that the stage of coronary disease is a
major determinant of the mechanisms involved in coronary disease progression
and acute coronary syndromes. It is also known that the duration of psychological distress influences the nature of the accompanying immune system parameters.[25–27] In the following sections, evidence for the adverse cardiovascular risk
associated with each of these three categories of psychological factors will be

reviewed, followed by the potential pathophysiological and immune system mediators. Other pathophysiological processes may also mediate the risk associated with psychological factors, including blood coagulation, platelet aggregation, endothelial dysfunction, and vasoconstriction,[4] but those fall beyond the scope of this chapter.

Chronic psychological risk factors

Hostility and the Type A behavior pattern have been extensively investigated as CAD risk factors. In the late 1950s, Friedman and Rosenman demonstrated that the Type A behavior pattern (i.e., an antagonistic personality, combined with competitiveness, and a sense of time pressure) was associated with incident myocardial infarction as well as cardiovascular risk factors.[28–30] Later studies have indicated that hostility is the toxic component of Type A behavior. Hostility is a relatively stable personality trait characterized by cynical mistrust, aggressive responding, and an overall antagonistic attitude.[31,32] Most studies report an association between hostility/Type A behavior and severity of underlying coronary disease[33,34] as well as first myocardial infarction.[31,35,36] The potential importance of hostility for early onset CAD is supported by the stronger association between hostility and MI in younger (<55 years of age) than older men.[33–35] In contrast, evidence for the predictive value of hostility/Type A behavior for recurrent coronary events is less consistent.[37,38]

The physiological pathways involved in the relationship between chronic psychological factors and CAD involve increased sympathetic nervous system activity and exaggerated reactivity to acute challenges. Direct adverse effects of elevated sympathetic activity on early CAD include elevated blood pressure and damage of vasculature as a result of arterial lipid deposition. In addition to the consequences of sympathetic hyperactivity, chronic psychological risk factors affect CAD progression indirectly by their association with persistent cardiovascular risk factors such as hypertension, circulating lipids, and blood clotting factors.[30,39]

An additional potential mechanism accounting for chronic psychological risk factors involves elevated responsiveness to acute environmental challenges (e.g., mental distress) of catecholamines and hemodynamic measures; referred to as "hyperreactivity." Hyperreactivity plays an important role at the advanced CAD stages (see below), but may also promote early CAD processes. Increased catecholamine reactivity may specifically affect increased cardiac demand, as well as coronary constriction[22] and increased tendency for clot formation.[40] These acute challenge-induced (patho)physiological changes may increase the risk of ischemia and subsequent acute coronary syndromes in vulnerable patients.

Recent investigations have examined relationships between psychological traits and immune system functioning. Since the early 1940s, it has been well-documented that macrophages and lipids interact at the early stages of CAD.[41] Atherosclerosis may initially be promoted by immunosuppressive effects of persistent psychological distress, whereas at later CAD stages, reduced immunocompetence will become ineffective because of the inherent silencing effects of the atherosclerotic process.[8] One potential mechanism would be that hostility promotes early CAD progression by adversely affecting the normal phagocytic function of macrophages.[42] Gidron et al. have demonstrated that hostility is positively correlated with the percentage of monocytes among patients with acute coronary syndromes.[43] Some evidence also supports associations between hostility and hyperlipidemia and elevated levels of oxidized lipids. Other evidence indicates that plasma IL-6 is independently associated with anger and hostility in otherwise healthy individuals.[44]

In addition to hostility, other psychological traits such as trait anxiety as well as sociological factors—particularly low socioeconomic status—may act as additional sources of persistent exposure to psychological distress. Low socioeconomic status is associated with adverse cardiovascular health outcome,[45] which is mediated, in part, by increased cardiovascular risk factors and adverse health behaviors,[46,47] including measures of chronic low-grade inflammation.[48]

In summary, chronic psychological traits are associated with persistent alterations in biological parameters that are known to be associated with gradual CAD progression. The elevated risk factors associated with chronic psychological risk factors (e.g., hyperlipidemia) may also interact with inflammatory or infectious processes, thereby indirectly promoting CAD progression. In addition to these indirect effects, some evidence suggests elevated immune responses to acute challenging conditions in hostile individuals. It is well documented that sympathetic nervous system tone and reactivity are elevated among hostile individuals. Clinical investigations examining chronic psychological factors are limited by their essentially observational study designs. Thus, both hostility and low socioeconomic status can be construed as chronic risk indicators that promote atherosclerosis and affect cardiovascular risk. These chronic factors may also increase the chance of other more proximate psychological risk factors such as episodes of exhaustion and frequent occurrences of acute psychological arousal. The direct consequences of increased sympathetic nervous system activity for the psychoneuroimmunological components of gradual CAD progression require further investigation.

Episodic psychological risk factors

Episodic psychological risk factors are transient and recurring, with a duration ranging from several weeks to 2 years.[2,49] Episodic risk factors are associated with a two- to threefold elevated risk for adverse coronary events. Depression is considered to be the core episodic risk factor in behavioral cardiology. A wide range of studies indicate that depression is predictive of first and recurrent myocardial infarction and sudden cardiac death.[50–53] It is still debated whether depression reflects one single underlying pathologic process, or whether a group of distinct disorders with overlapping characteristics is involved in adverse CAD risk.[54]

Independent of the research on depression and CAD, clinical and experimental studies have shown that extreme fatigue is among the most common premonitory symptoms of acute coronary syndromes.[55–57] This state has been referred to as "exhaustion" (i.e., lack of energy, increased irritability, and demoralization) and is also an episodic risk factor. The original label was "vital exhaustion" with the term "vital" referring to the far-reaching consequences of this condition on daily life functioning (similar to vital depression). The predictive value of exhaustion for adverse cardiovascular events has been demonstrated in prospective studies examining healthy and CAD populations.[58–60] The extent to which exhaustion reflects the same construct as depression is not fully understood, but some evidence suggests that depression and exhaustion are not entirely overlapping conditions[52,61] and have different biological concomitants.[24,54,62]

Depression is characteristically associated with increased activation of the corticotropin-releasing hormone (CRH) system and hence elevated cortisol levels, particularly when patients primarily present with melancholia. Both central norepinephrine as well as hypothalamic CRH are the main effectors of the general adaptation response.[63] In addition to neuroendocrine correlates, episodic risk factors are related to hemostatic cardiovascular risk factors including impaired fibrinolysis,[62,64,65] increased platelet adhesion and aggregation,[66] as well as sympathetic overactivity and decreased parasympathetic activity.[67] Research has also demonstrated that episodic factors are related to a range of blood clotting factors, including fibrinogen, factor VII, and PAI-1.[68] Studies have also found moderately elevated hemodynamic responsiveness among individuals with episodic risk factors,[69] but this has not been consistently documented in CAD patients.[51,70] It is not known whether the variability in reactivity finding reflects a blunted hyperresponsiveness in a subgroup of individuals exposed to prolonged psychological challenges, as a result of increased allostatic load.[71,72] In general, episodic risk factors are characterized by an overall imbalance of normal homeostatic function.

Evidence indicates that atypical forms of depression (i.e., hyperphagia and hypersomnia and mood reactivity), are characterized by inactivation of the CRH system and reduced norepinephrine levels.[54] Weight gain and hypersomnia often occur in exhausted individuals and in other conditions where fatigue is a primary symptom. Therefore, evidence suggests that typical melancholic depression is associated with different neurohormonal concomitants than those observed in exhaustion and atypical forms of depression. The clinical nature of depression (i.e., melancholic depression versus exhaustion) may influence the association between depressive symptoms and immune system parameters. Episodic risk factors may elevate the risk of acute coronary syndromes in the setting of advanced CAD by their association with thrombotic factors and plaque rupture.

Depression and exhaustion are associated with decreased parasympathetic nervous system activity in CAD patients, which may contribute to elevations in pro-inflammatory cytokines. Immune system correlates of depression have been reviewed in detail elsewhere.[73–78] Depression is associated with increased numbers of peripheral leukocytes (particularly neutrophils and monocytes), decreased lymphocytes, elevated cytokine production, lower natural killer (NK) cell activity, and a decreased proliferative response of lymphocytes to mitogenic stimulation.[25,75,77] The psychoneuroimmunology literature generally categorizes the immunosuppressive correlates of depression along with the long-term immunological consequences of distressing behavioral or emotional states (e.g., bereavement, separation, and daily hassles).[25] Our group,[79] as well as others,[80–84] has consistently found elevated CRP levels among individuals with depressive symptoms. These associations may be mediated, in part, by being overweight and other adverse health behaviors.[85] Patients with depression and/or exhaustion also have increased levels of antibody to several herpes viruses, including CMV. Elevated pathogen burden has been documented by Appels and colleagues (2000) in patients undergoing coronary angioplasty[86] and by Miller et al. (2005) in postmyocardial infarction patients.[87]

In summary, some of the correlates of depression and exhaustion (e.g., increased levels of leukocytes, cytokines, and antibodies to viruses) are also associated with elevated risk for acute coronary syndromes. These markers of a proinflammatory state in depression may promote CAD progression by enhancing macrophage and lipid deposition processes at early stages of atherosclerosis. More importantly, low-grade inflammation may alter the stability of atherosclerotic plaques and increase the risk of plaque rupture leading to acute coronary syndromes. The latter mechanism is of particular importance because the duration of episodic risk factors may not be long enough to initiate and sustain an atherosclerotic process. This notion is further supported by the finding that although depression may have long-term predictive values for adverse CAD outcomes, no consistent associations have been found between episodic risk factors and CAD severity. In addition, the predictive value of episodic risk factors decreases when the follow-up exceeds 2 years. These factors indicate that plaque activation, rather than gradual CAD progression, may be primarily involved in the adverse risk associated with episodic psychological risk factors. Because of the recurring nature of episodic risk factors, longitudinal studies are needed to further our understanding of the time trajectory of psychological and immunological factors in patients at risk for acute coronary syndromes.

Acute psychological risk factors

Outbursts of acute anger as well as natural disasters can trigger acute coronary syndromes.[88–91] Cardiac ischemia is the primary cause of most acute coronary syndromes. Laboratory and field studies have confirmed that mental activities and emotions can provoke myocardial ischemia[4] and life-threatening arrhythmias[92] in vulnerable patients. Ischemic responses occur in 30–70% of stable CAD patients in response to tasks such as public speech, anger recall, mental arithmetic with harassment, and the Stroop color word test.[4]

Acute mental arousal is associated with a shift toward increased sympathetic nervous system activity and decreased parasympathetic (vagal) activity, accompanied by elevated circulating catecholamines and increased cardiac demand (i.e., elevated blood pressure, heart rate, and cardiac contractility). These ischemic responses to acute psychological risk factors result from increased cardiac demand and decreased coronary supply.[4] Markers of decreased coronary supply include: impaired dilation of the coronary vessels,[93,94] decreases in plasma volume,[95] and increased platelet activity and blood clotting tendency.[96,97] The resulting imbalance between increased cardiac demand and decreased coronary blood supply may result in myocardial ischemia. Hemodynamic responses to acute mental and physical challenges can lead to plaque rupture, and increased platelet aggregation may promote acute coronary thrombus formation.

Acute immune system responses may also play a role in CAD progression. The effects of acute mental arousal on the immune system are complex,[98] and both increased and decreased numbers of lymphocytes and NK cells have been reported. Most studies show increases in B-cells and CD8+ T-cells and decreases in CD4+ T-cells in response to acute-challenge tasks. Cytokines increase with psychological challenge (e.g., undergoing coronary angioplasty)[99], suggesting at least a partial activation of the immune system.[100] Acute phase proteins (CRP and fibrinogen),[97,101,102] as well as adhesion molecules,[103] increase during mental challenge tasks. The effects of acute laboratory challenge tasks on immune parameters are also mediated in part by the increased hemoconcentration following laboratory tasks.[104] It has been demonstrated that the acute immune system response may be exaggerated among individuals with cardiovascular risk factors, such as hypertension. Patients with hypertension display larger numbers of circulating white blood cells compared with normotensives.[105] Hypertensive patients also show a greater increase in the number of circulating CD3+CD8+, CD8+CD62L T-cells, as well as increased expression of the endothelial CD11a ligand, ICAM-1, suggesting that patients with hypertension exhibit increased leukocyte adhesion.[105]

In summary, acute psychological challenges induce a partial activation of the immune system. These immune system changes may trigger acute coronary syndromes by activation and subsequent rupture of vulnerable atherosclerotic plaques.[106] Moreover, immune activation may directly interact with several blood-clotting factors and indirectly promote thrombus formation and coronary vasoconstriction by interfering with normal endothelial function. Acute immune system activation may further result in reduced perfusion of coronary arteries distal to the culprit lesion and decrease perfusion of the microcirculation.[107] The immune activation component of the acute response to challenges, therefore, may be more important than the immunosuppressive component in the pathophysiology of acute coronary syndromes.

EFFECTS OF PSYCHOLOGICAL INTERVENTIONS ON CARDIOVASCULAR DISEASE OUTCOMES

Cardiovascular behavioral medicine interventions have primarily targeted coronary disease patients and individuals with elevated cardiovascular risk factors. These psychological interventions can be grouped into three broad categories: (a) interventions targeting chronic psychological risk factors such as hostility; (b) interventions aimed at improving episodic risk factors such as depression and exhaustion; and (c) interventions addressing health behaviors (e.g., smoking cessation, weight reduction, exercise). The latter category has multiple complementary medicine-based intervention options, which are beyond the scope of this chapter. Interventions for chronic psychological factors commonly address lifestyle factors and coping strategies for handling acute stressors. In vulnerable patients, the effects of chronic psychological risk factors are primarily mediated by elevated acute stress responses. Therefore, the efficacy of intervention programs on acute and chronic psychological risk factors will be considered simultaneously. Ornish and colleagues have successfully applied a combination of stress management (meditation and group support) and lifestyle changes (exercise, low-fat vegetarian diet) in reducing recurrent cardiac events and reversing progressive coronary disease.[108,109] The Recurrent Coronary Prevention Project is one of the most convincing investigations in this area.[110] The trial randomized 862 post-myocardial infarction patients to group therapy sessions consisting of relaxation, self-monitoring of Type A behaviors and stress, and cognitive-behavioral techniques ($N = 592$) or usual care ($N = 270$). The intervention resulted in significant reduction of recurrent events (12.9% vs. 21.2%)[111] and reduced mortality in patients with less severe coronary disease at study entry.[110] It has further been demonstrated that this project not only decreased global Type A behavior but also hostility, depression, and anxiety.[112] A more recent study by Blumenthal et al. revealed that stress management reduced recurrent cardiac events and ischemia in patients with stable coronary disease,[113] which has recently been replicated.[114] Denollet and colleagues have demonstrated that a multifactorial rehabilitation program using both group and individual sessions for 3 months resulted in significant clinical benefits including reduced negative affect and resulted in a significant reduction in 9-year all-cause mortality (OR 0.2; 95% CI 0.1–0.7; $p = 0.016$).[115] The nonrandom assignment to the control group in some of these studies may have introduced a potential bias toward positive results.

These positive results have not been consistently replicated, however. Jones and West (1996) conducted a randomized multicenter intervention trial in 2,328 consecutive and unselected post-myocardial infarction patients and their spouses using psychotherapy and counseling, relaxation training, and stress management in groups of outpatients over 7 weeks.[116] The intervention was not successful in reducing anxiety or depression, and there was no reduction in secondary cardiac events or 1-year mortality. Lisspers and colleagues conducted a lifestyle intervention program in coronary angioplasty patients which resulted in decreased Type A behavior and chest pain, but the intervention did not decrease other psychological measures (e.g., trait anger, depression, anxiety), nor did it reduce recurrent cardiac events within 1 year (23% in both groups).[117] Failure of these interventions may have resulted from their ineffectiveness in reducing psychological risk factors relevant to CAD progression.

Interventions targeting episodic psychological risk factors have addressed depression and exhaustion in patients with CAD. One of the landmark studies in this area was conducted by Frasure-Smith and Prince (1985) in post-myocardial infarction patients. Nurses provided emotional and instrumental support when patients reported increased distress levels. The active intervention program had a significant reduction in mortality compared to a randomized control group.[118] A more recent replication study was not successful in reducing recurrent cardiac events.[119] The recent Enhancing Recovery in Coronary Heart Disease

(ENRICHD) trial enrolled 2,481 post-myocardial infarction patients at eight medical centers in the United States.[120] The 6-month active treatment consisted of individual and group cognitive behavioral therapy sessions targeted at modifying thought patterns and behaviors contributing to depressive symptoms, and the comparison group received usual care. Patients with persistently high levels of depression were also referred for additional psychiatric evaluation and prescribed antidepressant medication. Reductions in depression were stronger in the treatment group (8.6 scale units reduction in Beck Depression Inventory (BDI)) versus the control group (5.9 units reduction in BDI; $p < 0.001$). After 3 years, mortality and reinfarction rate in the active treatment group was 24.4% versus 24.2% in the control condition.[120] Thus, psychological interventions can significantly reduce (not eliminate) episodic risk factors, but most have not been successful in reducing subsequent cardiac events.

Similar results are found for exhaustion. In a randomized psychological intervention trial of 710 angioplasty patients, exhaustion remained present in patients with a previous history of CAD. Furthermore, clinical event rates were similar in the active treatment arm (22%) and standard of care control condition (20%; RR = 1.09; 95% CI = 0.79–1.5).[121] This result is similar to the aforementioned observations in angioplasty patients by Lisspers et al.[117]

A series of pharmacological interventions aimed at reducing depression in patients with CAD have been conducted. The strongest trial at this point is the double blind, randomized placebo-controlled, multinational Sertraline Antidepressant Heart Attack Randomized Trial (SADHART) in 369 patients with myocardial infarction or unstable angina.[122] The active treatment group significantly improved on a clinical rating scale compared with the placebo condition, but no differences were found on the Hamilton Depression Rating Scale (8.4 + 0.4 vs. 7.8 + 0.4 units reduction; $p = 0.14$). The recurrent cardiac event rate during treatment tended to be lower (14.5%) in the treatment than the placebo group (22.4%; RR = 0.77; 95% CI = 0.51–1.16; nonsignificant).

In summary, the initial psychological intervention studies demonstrated beneficial effects on both psychological risk factors as well as recurrent cardiac events. In contrast, more recent studies have failed to support these positive results. A few excellent reviews and meta-analyses have been published on the efficacy of psychological interventions in reducing recurrent cardiac events.[123–125] On an average, psychological and educational interventions reduce cardiac mortality by 34% and recurrent myocardial infarction by 29%.[123] These effects are at least as strong as those obtained by traditional medical interventions such as β-adrenergic medication.

CONCLUSIONS AND FUTURE DIRECTIONS

Chronic and acute psychological factors increase the risk of CAD and its clinical manifestations as acute coronary syndromes. The increased risks for cardiovascular disease outcomes are mediated by plausible biobehavioral mechanisms, including immune system-related processes and psychological intervention studies demonstrate that efforts aimed at reducing chronic and episodic psychological risk factors are important but complicated endeavors. Residual depression and other indicators of psychological distress are common in patients with cardiovascular disease. Approximately 50% of depressed cardiac patients continue to have depressive symptoms after psychological or pharmacological intervention. In addition to residual depression, another factor contributing to null findings in controlled trials is the high spontaneous recovery rate. It is well established that subthreshold depression is a strong predictor of adverse cardiovascular outcomes. Thus, it is not surprising that the suboptimal reduction in episodic risk factors is not paralleled by a subsequent reduction in recurrent cardiac events. Complementary medicine techniques may prove beneficial in further reducing distress levels and other subthreshold psychological risk factors. The success of complementary techniques in cardiovascular disease has been reviewed previously by the joint committee of the National Heart Lung and Blood Institute and the National Center for Complementary and Alternative Medicine.[1] Additional research is needed to investigate potential synergism between psychosocial and complementary medicine techniques in optimizing treatment for patients at risk of adverse cardiovascular health outcomes. Increasing evidence suggests that it is important to match psychological interventions to patient characteristics and needs. One reason why some interventions have been unsuccessful in improving psychological risk factors is that patients were not preselected for their need for psychological interventions. A triage system based on the type of psychological risk factor (acute, episodic, and chronic) may improve treatment allocation and outcome. Acute stress disorders occasionally occur in the setting of myocardial infarction, including acute emotional reactions to the onset of a life-threatening disease. Other issues may involve major life events such as divorce, decease of a loved one, and job loss. These acutely distressing factors are relatively rare but should be the primary targets of psychological interventions before other approaches are considered. Episodic risk factors (depression and exhaustion) are crucially important in patients at risk for recurrent cardiac events. Interventions targeted at these episodic risk factors generally improve patients' quality of life but may also promote cardiovascular health outcomes. The current literature suggests that these factors are unlikely to fully remit by psychological or pharmacological interventions, and a combined approach with complementary medicine techniques may prove more successful in eradicating these risk factors. Chronic psychological risk factors, such as hostility, can be successfully altered when focusing on acutely challenging situations. Successful treatment components include stress-coping strategies, anger management, and conflict reduction.[126]

Understanding of biobehavioral pathways may improve the development and monitoring of successful intervention strategies. Immune system parameters may be of particular importance in the integration of psychological and complementary medicine techniques as treatment options for cardiovascular disease. Inflammation causes central nervous system responses as well as psychological states similar to depression and exhaustion.[100,127] The immune system (e.g., inter-leukin-1 and tumor necrosis factor-α) can indeed activate the HPA axis.[100,128] This negative feedback loop may account for the immunosuppressive state in episodic risk factors. Evidence of immunological influences on the central nervous system is supported by observations that cytokines mediate nonspecific responses to infection such as malaise, fatigue, fever, slow wave sleep, apathy, and irritability. Fatigue and malaise are also common side effects of the parenteral administration of certain cytokines. More research is needed to establish the clinical importance of the bidirectional relationship between immune system parameters and brain function, particularly in vulnerable populations with depressive symptoms.[129] In summary, the relationship between episodic risk factors and immune system parameters is bidirectional, such that central nervous system correlates of depressive symptoms result in immune system changes, and vice versa.

Complementary medicine techniques may be of particular importance if psychological risk factors coincide with adverse health behaviors. Psychological risk factors do not exist in a vacuum and often coincide with adverse health behaviors such as smoking, poor diet, nonadherence to medication regimen, and sedentary life style. In addition, immune system parameters and other biological cardiovascular risk factors are also related to traditional CAD risk factors (e.g., hypertension, smoking, dyslipidemia, obesity). Smoking cessation and weight reduction should be primary foci of intervention for patients with these risk factors. Addressing self-efficacy and promoting behavior change are major components of such interventions. Exercise has well-established positive effects on mood and plays an important role in cardiac rehabilitation. It is important to note that lifestyle changes per se do not necessarily improve psychological risk factors.[117] Furthermore, active lifestyle intervention may decrease rather than improve patient satisfaction with medical care.[130]

Psychological interventions are most effective in reducing recurrent cardiac events if they have initial beneficial effects on more proximal medical (e.g., blood pressure, exercise tolerance) and psychological (e.g., depression) measures that are risk factors for these cardiac events.[123] A combination of pharmacological, complementary medicine, and psychological intervention will be needed to optimally reduce psychological risk factors in patients at high risk of recurrent cardiac events.

ACKNOWLEDGMENTS

Preparation of this manuscript supported by grants from the NIH (HL066149; HL069751). The opinions and assertions expressed herein are those of the authors and are not to be construed as reflecting the views of the USUHS or the US Department of Defense.

REFERENCES

1. Lin MC, Nahin R, Gershwin ME, Longhurst JC, Wu KK. State of complementary and alternative medicine in cardiovascular, lung, and blood research: executive summary of a workshop. Circulation. 2001;103(16):2038–41.
2. Kop WJ. Chronic and acute psychological risk factors for clinical manifestations of coronary artery disease. Psychosom Med. 1999;61(4):476–87.
3. Rozanski A, Blumenthal JA, Kaplan J. Impact of psychological factors on the pathogenesis of cardiovascular disease and implications for therapy. Circulation. 1999; 99(16):2192–217.
4. Krantz DS, Kop WJ, Santiago HT, Gottdiener JS. Mental stress as a trigger of myocardial ischemia and infarction. Cardiology Clinics. 1996;14(2):271–287.
5. Suls J, Bunde J. Anger, anxiety, and depression as risk factors for cardiovascular disease: the problems and implications of overlapping affective dispositions. Psychol Bull. 2005;131(2):260–300.
6. Kop WJ. The predictive value of vital exhaustion in the clinical course after coronary angioplasty. Maastricht:Datawyse. 1994.
7. Kop WJ. The integration of cardiovascular behavioral medicine and psychoneuroimmunology: new developments based on converging research fields. Brain Behav Immun. 2003;17(4):233–7.
8. Fricchione GL, Bilfinger TV, Hartman A, Liu Y, Stefano GB. Neuroimmunologic implications in coronary artery disease. Adv Neuroimmunol. 1996;6(2):131–42.
9. Kop WJ, Cohen N. Psychological risk factors and immune system involvement in cardiovascular disease. In: Ader R, Felten DL, Cohen N, editors. Psychoneuroimmunology. San Diego (CA): Academic Press; 2001:525–44.
10. Naghavi M, Libby P, Falk E, et al. From vulnerable plaque to vulnerable patient: a call for new definitions and risk assessment strategies: Part I. Circulation 2003; 108(14):1664–72.
11. Naghavi M, Libby P, Falk E et al. From vulnerable plaque to vulnerable patient: a call for new definitions and risk assessment strategies: Part II. Circulation. 2003; 108(15):1772–8.
12. Braunwald E. Heart disease. Philadelphia, London, Toronto, Montreal, Sydney, Tokyo, WB Saunders; 1988.
13. Alonzo AA, Simon AB, Feinleib M. Prodromata of myocardial infarction and sudden death. Circulation. 1975;52:1056–62.
14. Ross R. The pathogenesis of atherosclerosis: an update. N Eng J Med. 1986;314: 488–500.
15. Ross R. Atherosclerosis—an inflammatory disease. N Engl J Med. 1999;340(2):115–26.
16. Fuster V, Badimon L, Badimon JJ, Chesebro JH. The pathogenesis of coronary artery disease and the acute coronary syndromes (1). N Engl J Med. 1992;326:242–50.
17. Fuster V, Badimon L, Badimon JJ, Chesebro JH. The pathogenesis of coronary artery disease and the acute coronary syndromes (2). N Engl J Med. 1992;326(5):310–18.
18. Falk E, Shah PK, Fuster V. Coronary plaque disruption. Circulation. 1995;92(3): 657–71.
19. Hansson GK. Inflammation, atherosclerosis, and coronary artery disease. N Engl J Med. 2005;352(16):1685–95.
20. Ambrose JA, Tannenbaum MA, Alexopoulos D, et al. Angiographic progression of coronary artery disease and the development of myocardial infarction. J Am Coll Cardiol. 1988;12(1):56–62.

21. Giroud D, Li JM, Urban P, Meier B, Rutishauer W. Relation of the site of acute myocardial infarction to the most severe coronary arterial stenosis at prior angiography. Am J Cardiol. 1992;69(8):729–732.
22. Muller JE, Abela GS, Nesto RW, Tofler GH. Triggers, acute risk factors and vulnerable plaques: the lexicon of a new frontier. J Am Coll Cardiol. 1994;23(3):809–13.
23. Davies MJ, Thomas A. Thrombosis and acute coronary-artery lesions in sudden cardiac ischemic death. N Engl J Med. 1984;310(18):1137–40.
24. Kop WJ. Acute and chronic psychological risk factors for coronary syndromes: moderating effects of coronary artery disease severity. J Psychosom Res. 1997;43(2):167–81.
25. Segerstrom SC, Miller GE. Psychological stress and the human immune system: a meta-analytic study of 30 years of inquiry. Psychol Bull. 2004;130(4):601–30.
26. Herbert TB, Cohen S. Stress and immunity in humans: a meta-analytic review. Psychosom Med. 1993;55(4):364–79.
27. Benschop RJ, Rodriguez-Feuerhahn M, Schedlowski M. Catecholamine-induced leukocytosis: early observations, current research, and future directions. Brain Behav Immun. 1996;10(2):77–91.
28. Friedman M, Rosenman R. Association of specific overt behavior pattern with blood and cardiovascular findings: blood cholesterol level, blood clotting time, incidence of arcis senilis and clinical coronary artery disease. JAMA. 1959;169:1286–96.
29. Welin L, Tibblin G, Svardsudd K, et al. Prospective study of social influences on mortality. The study of men born in 1913 and 1923. Lancet. 1985;915–18.
30. Suarez EC, Williams RB, Kuhn CM, Zimmerman EH, Schanberg SM. Biobehavioral basis of coronary-prone behavior in middle-age men. Part II: Serum cholesterol, the Type A behavior pattern, and hostility as interactive modulators of physiological reactivity. Psychosom Med. 1991;53(5):528–37.
31. Barefoot JC, Dahlstrom WG, Williams RB. Hostility, CHD incidence, and total mortality: a 25-year follow-up study of 255 physicians. Psychosom Med. 1983;45(1): 59–63.
32. Engebretson TO, Matthews KA. Dimensions of hostility in men, women, and boys: relationships to personality and cardiovascular responses to stress. Psychosom Med. 1992;54(3):311–23.
33. Williams RB, Barefoot JC, Haney TL, et al. Type A behavior and angiographically documented coronary atherosclerosis in a sample of 2,289 patients. Psychosom Med. 1988 Mar–Apr;50(2):139–52.
34. Siegman AW, Dembroski TM, Ringel N. Components of hostility and the severity of coronary artery disease. Psychosom Med. 1987;49(2):127–35.
35. Meesters CM, Smulders J. Hostility and myocardial infarction in men. J Psychosom Res. 1994;38(7):727–34.
36. Shekelle RB, Gale M, Ostfeld AM, Paul O. Hostility, risk of coronary heart disease, and mortality. Psychosom Med. 1983;45(2):109–14.
37. Shekelle RB, Gale M, Norusis M. Type A score (Jenkins Activity Survey) and risk of recurrent coronary heart disease in the aspirin myocardial infarction study. Am J Cardiol. 1985;56(4):221–5.
38. Ragland DR. Type A behavior and outcome of coronary disease. N Engl J Med. 1989;319(22):1480–1.
39. Williams RB, Suarez EC, Kuhn CM, Zimmerman EA, Schanberg SM. Biobehavioral basis of coronary-prone behavior in middle-aged men. Part I: Evidence for chronic SNS activation in Type As. Psychosom Med. 1991;53(5):517–27.
40. Markovitz JH, Matthews KA. Platelets and coronary heart disease: potential psychophysiologic mechanisms. Psychosom Med. 1991;53:643–68.

41. Leary T. The genesis of atherosclerosis. Arch Pathol. 1941;32(4):507–55.
42. Adams DO. Molecular biology of macrophage activation: a pathway whereby psychosocial factors can potentially affect health. Psychosom Med. 1994;56(4):316–27.
43. Gidron Y, Armon T, Gilutz H, Huleihel M. Psychological factors correlate meaningfully with percent-monocytes among acute coronary syndrome patients. Brain Behav Immun. 2003;17(4):310–15.
44. Suarez EC. Plasma interleukin-6 is associated with psychological coronary risk factors: moderation by use of multivitamin supplements. Brain Behav Immun. 2003; 17(4):296–303.
45. Marmot MG, Shipley MJ, Rose G. Inequalities in death—specific explanations of a general pattern? Lancet. 1984; May 5;1(8384):1003–6.
46. Winkleby MA, Jatulis DE, Frank E, Fortmann SP. Socioeconomic status and health: how education, income, and occupation contribute to risk factors for cardiovascular disease. Am J Public Health. 1992; 82(6):816–20.
47. Kraus JF, Borhani NO, Franti CE. Socioeconomic status, ethnicity, and risk of coronary heart disease. Am J Epidemiol. 1980;111(4):407–14.
48. Owen N, Poulton T, Hay FC, Mohamed-Ali V, Steptoe A. Socioeconomic status, C-reactive protein, immune factors, and responses to acute mental stress. Brain Behav Immun. 2003;17(4):286–95.
49. Appels A, Kop WJ, Meesters CM, Markusse R, Golombeck B, Falger PR. Vital exhaustion and the acute coronary syndromes. In: Maes S, Leventhal H, Johnston M, editors. International review of health psychology. New York: John Wiley & Sons; 1994:65–95.
50. Wulsin LR, Singal BM. Do depressive symptoms increase the risk for the onset of coronary disease? A systematic quantitative review. Psychosom Med. 2003;65(2): 201–10.
51. Carney RM, Freedland KE, Rich MW, Jaffe AS. Depression as a risk factor for cardiac events in established coronary heart disease: a review of possible mechanisms. Ann Behav Med. 1995;17(2):142–9.
52. Appels A. Depression and coronary heart disease: observations and questions. J Psychosom Res. 1997;43(5):443–52.
53. Lesperance F, Frasure-Smith N. Depression in patients with cardiac disease: a practical review. J Psychosom Res. 2000;48(4–5):379–91.
54. Gold PW, Goodwin FK, Chrousos GP. Clinical and biochemical manifestations of depression. Relation to the neurobiology of stress (1). N Engl J Med. 1988;319(6): 348–53.
55. Appels A, Otten F. Exhaustion as precursor of cardiac death. Br J Clin Psychol. 1992;31:351–6.
56. Kuller L, Cooper M, Perper J. Epidemiology of sudden death. Arch Intern Med. 1972;129:714–9.
57. McSweeney JC, Cody M, O'Sullivan P, Elberson K, Moser DK, Garvin BJ. Women's early warning symptoms of acute myocardial infarction. Circulation. 2003;108(21):2619–23.
58. Prescott E, Holst C, Gronbaek M, Schnohr P, Jensen G, Barefoot J. Vital exhaustion as a risk factor for ischaemic heart disease and all-cause mortality in a community sample. A prospective study of 4084 men and 5479 women in the Copenhagen City Heart Study. Int J Epidemiol. 2003;32(6):990–7.
59. Appels A, Mulder P. Excess fatigue as a precursor of myocardial infarction. Eur Heart J. 1988;9:758–64.

60. Kop WJ, Appels AP, Mendes de Leon CF, de Swart HB, Bar FW. Vital exhaustion predicts new cardiac events after successful coronary angioplasty. Psychosom Med. 1994;56:281–7.
61. Kopp MS, Falger PR, Appels A, Szedmak S. Depressive symptomatology and vital exhaustion are differentially related to behavioral risk factors for coronary artery disease. Psychosom Med. 1998;60(6):752–8.
62. Raikkonen K, Lassila R, Keltikangas-Jarvinen L, Hautanen A. Association of chronic stress with plasminogen activator inhibitor-1 in healthy middle-aged men. Arterioscler Thromb Vasc Biol. 1996;16(3):363–7.
63. Selye H. The stress of life. New York, McGraw Hill; 1977.
64. Pietraszek MH, Takada Y, Nishimoto M, Ohara K, Takada A. Fibrinolytic activity in depression and neurosis. Thromb Res. 1991;63:661–6.
65. Kop WJ, Hamulyak K, Pernot K, Appels A. Relationship between blood coagulation and fibrinolysis to vital exhaustion. Psychosom Med. 1998;60:352–8.
66. Bruce EC, Musselman DL. Depression, alterations in platelet function, and ischemic heart disease. Psychosom Med. 2005;67 Suppl 1:S34–6.
67. Carney RM, Freedland KE, Veith RC. Depression, the autonomic nervous system, and coronary heart disease. Psychosom Med. 2005;67 Suppl 1:S29–33.
68. von KR, Mills PJ, Fainman C, Dimsdale JE. Effects of psychological stress and psychiatric disorders on blood coagulation and fibrinolysis: a biobehavioral pathway to coronary artery disease? Psychosom Med. 2001;63(4):531–44.
69. Kibler JL, Ma M. Depressive symptoms and cardiovascular reactivity to laboratory behavioral stress. Int J Behav Med. 2004;11(2):81–7.
70. Kop WJ, Appels A, Howell RH, et al. Relationship between vital exhaustion and stress-induced myocardial ischemia. Ann Behav Med. 1997;19:159. (Ref type: Abstract.)
71. McEwen BS. Protective and damaging effects of stress mediators. N Engl J Med. 1998;338(3):171–9.
72. Seeman TE, Singer BH, Rowe JW, Horwitz RI, McEwen BS. Price of adaptation—allostatic load and its health consequences. Macarthur studies of successful aging. Arch Intern Med. 1997;157(19):2259–68.
73. Kop WJ, Gottdiener JS. The role of immune system parameters in the relationship between depression and coronary artery disease. Psychosomat Med. 2005;67 Suppl 1: 537–41.
74. Stein M, Miller AH, Trestman RL. Depression, the immune system, and health and illness. findings in search of meaning. Arch Gen Psychiat. 1991;48(2):171–7.
75. Weisse CS. Depression and immunocompetence: a review of the literature. Psychol Bull. 1992;111(3):475–89.
76. Maes M. Evidence for an immune response in major depression: a review and hypothesis. Prog Neuropsychopharmacol Biol Psychiat. 1995;19(1):11–38.
77. Herbert TB, Cohen S. Depression and immunity: a meta-analytic review. Psychol Bull. 1993;113(3):472–86.
78. Zorrilla EP, Luborsky L, McKay JR, et al. The relationship of depression and stressors to immunological assays: a meta-analytic review. Brain Behav Immun. 2001;15(3):199–226.
79. Kop WJ, Gottdiener JS, Tangen CM, et al. Inflammation and coagulation factors in persons >65 years of age with symptoms of depression but without evidence of myocardial ischemia. Am J Cardiol. 2002;89(4):419–24.
80. Ladwig KH, Marten-Mittag B, Lowel H, Doring A, Koenig W. Influence of depressive mood on the association of CRP and obesity in 3205 middle aged healthy men. Brain Behav Immun. 2003;17(4):268–75.

81. Empana JP, Sykes DH, Luc G, et al. Contributions of depressive mood and circulating inflammatory markers to coronary heart disease in healthy European men: the Prospective Epidemiological Study of Myocardial Infarction (PRIME). Circulation. 2005;111(18):2299–305.

82. Miller GE, Stetler CA, Carney RM, Freedland KE, Banks WA. Clinical depression and inflammatory risk markers for coronary heart disease. Am J Cardiol. 2002;90(12):1279–83.

83. Lesperance F, Frasure-Smith N, Theroux P, Irwin M. The association between major depression and levels of soluble intercellular adhesion molecule 1, interleukin-6, and C-reactive protein in patients with recent acute coronary syndromes. Am J Psychiat. 2004;161(2):271–7.

84. Panagiotakos DB, Pitsavos C, Chrysohoou C, et al. Inflammation, coagulation, and depressive symptomatology in cardiovascular disease-free people; the ATTICA study. Eur Heart J. 2004;25(6):492–9.

85. Douglas KM, Taylor AJ, O'Malley PG. Relationship between depression and C-reactive protein in a screening population. Psychosom Med. 2004;66(5):679–83.

86. Appels A, Bar FW, Bar J, Bruggeman C, de Baets M. Inflammation, depressive symptomtology, and coronary artery disease. Psychosom Med. 2000;62(5):601–5.

87. Miller GE, Freedland KE, Duntley S, Carney RM. Relation of depressive symptoms to C-reactive protein and pathogen burden (cytomegalovirus, herpes simplex virus, Epstein-Barr virus) in patients with earlier acute coronary syndromes. Am J Cardiol. 2005;95(3):317–21.

88. Mittleman MA, Maclure M, Sherwood JB, et al. Triggering of acute myocardial infarction onset by episodes of anger. Determinants of Myocardial Infarction Onset Study Investigators. Circulation. 1995;92(7):1720–25.

89. Dobson AJ, Alexander HM, Malcolm JA, Steele PL, Miles TA. Heart attacks and the Newcastle earthquake. Med J Aust. 1991;155(11–2):757–61.

90. Trichopoulos D, Katsouyanni K, Zavitsanos X, Tzonou A, Dalla-Vorgia P. Psychological stress and fatal heart attack: the Athens (1981) earthquake natural experiment. Lancet. 1983;1(8322):441–3.

91. Meisel SR, Kutz I, Dayan KI, et al. Effect of Iraqi missile war on incidence of acute myocardial infarction and sudden death in Israeli civilians. Lancet. 1991;338(8768):660–1.

92. Verrier RL. Mechanisms of behaviorally induced arrhythmias. Circulation. 1987;76:I48–56.

93. Yeung AC, Vekshtein VI, Krantz DS, et al. The effect of atherosclerosis on the vasomotor response of coronary arteries to mental stress. N Engl J Med. 1991;325(22):1551–6.

94. Kop WJ, Krantz DS, Howell RH, et al. Effects of mental stress on coronary epicardial vasomotion and flow velocity in coronary artery disease: Relationship with hemodynamic stress responses. J Am Coll Cardiol. 2001;37(5):1359–66.

95. Patterson SM, Gottdiener JS, Hecht G, Vargot S, Krantz DS. Effects of acute mental stress on serum lipids: mediating effects of plasma volume. Psychosom Med. 1993;55(6):525–32.

96. Patterson SM, Krantz DS, Gottdiener JS, Hecht G, Vargot S, Goldstein DS. Prothrombotic effects of environmental stress: changes in platelet function, hematocrit, and total plasma protein. Psychosom Med. 1995;57(6):592–9.

97. Jern C, Eriksson E, Tengborn L, Risberg B, Wadenvik H, Jern S. Changes of plasma coagulation and fibrinolysis in response to mental stress. Thromb Haemost. 1989;62:761–1.

98. Ader R, Cohen N, Felten D. Psychoneuroimmunology: interactions between the nervous system and the immune system. Lancet. 1995;345(8942):99–103.

99. Schulte HM, Bamberger CM, Elsen H, Herrmann G, Bamberger AM, Barth J. Systemic interleukin-1 alpha and interleukin-2 secretion in response to acute stress and to corticotropin-releasing hormone in humans. Eur J Clin Invest. 1994;24(11):773–7.

100. Dantzer R, Kelley KW. Stress and immunity: an integrated view of relationships between the brain and the immune system. Life Sci. 1989;44(26):1995–2008.

101. Kop WJ, Zhu J, Doyle MP, et al. Mental stress and exercise effects on immune system and blood coagulation parameters in patients with coronary artery disease following coronary angioplasty (abstract). Ann Behav Med. 2004; S069.

102. Dugue B, Leppanen EA, Teppo AM, Fyhrquist F, Grasbeck R. Effects of psychological stress on plasma interleukins-1 beta and 6, c-reactive protein, tumour necrosis factor alpha, anti-diuretic hormone and serum cortisol. Scand J Clin Lab Invest. 1993;53(6):555–61.

103. Mills PJ, Dimsdale JE. The effects of acute psychologic stress on cellular adhesion molecules. J Psychosom Res. 1996;41(1):49–53.

104. Marsland AL, Herbert TB, Muldoon MF, et al. Lymphocyte subset redistribution during acute laboratory stress in young adults: mediating effects of hemoconcentration. Health Psychol. 1997;16(4):341–8.

105. Mills PJ, Farag NH, Hong S, Kennedy BP, Berry CC, Ziegler MG. Immune cell CD62L and CD11a expression in response to a psychological stressor in human hypertension. Brain Behav Immun. 2003;17(4):260–7.

106. Libby P, Egan D, Skarlatos S. Roles of infectious agents in atherosclerosis and restenosis: an assessment of the evidence and need for future research. Circulation. 1997;96(11):4095–103.

107. Entman ML, Ballantyne CM. Inflammation in acute coronary syndromes. Circulation. 1993;88(2):800–3.

108. Gould KL, Ornish D, Scherwitz L, et al. Changes in myocardial perfusion abnormalities by positron emission tomography after long-term, intense risk factor modification. JAMA. 1995;274(11):894–901.

109. Ornish D, Scherwitz LW, Billings JH, et al. Intensive lifestyle changes for reversal of coronary heart disease. JAMA. 1998;280(23):2001–7.

110. Powell LH, Thoresen CE. Effects of type A behavioral counseling and severity of prior acute myocardial infarction on survival. Am J Cardiol. 1988;62(17):1159–63.

111. Friedman M, Thoresen CE, Gill JJ, et al. Alteration of Type A behavior and its effect on cardiac recurrences in post myocardial infarction patients: summary results of the recurrent coronary prevention project. Am Heart J. 1986;112(4):653–665.

112. Mendes de Leon CF, Powell LH, Kaplan BH. Change in coronary-prone behaviors in the recurrent coronary prevention project. Psychosom Med. 1991;53(4):407–19.

113. Blumenthal JA, Jiang W, Babyak MA, et al. Stress management and exercise training in cardiac patients with myocardial ischemia. Effects on prognosis and evaluation of mechanisms. Arch Intern Med. 1997;157(19):2213–23.

114. Blumenthal JA, Sherwood A, Babyak MA, et al. Effects of exercise and stress management training on markers of cardiovascular risk in patients with ischemic heart disease: a randomized controlled trial. JAMA. 2005;293(13):1626–34.

115. Denollet J, Brutsaert DL. Reducing emotional distress improves prognosis in coronary heart disease: 9-year mortality in a clinical trial of rehabilitation. Circulation. 2001;104(17):2018–23.

116. Jones DA, West RR. Psychological rehabilitation after myocardial infarction: multicentre randomised controlled trial. BMJ. 1996;313(7071):1517–21.

117. Lisspers J, Sundin O, Hofman-Bang C, et al. Behavioral effects of a comprehensive, multifactorial program for lifestyle change after percutaneous transluminal coronary angioplasty: a prospective, randomized controlled study. J Psychosom Res. 1999;46(2):143–54.

118. Frasure-Smith N, Prince R. The ischemic heart disease life stress monitoring program: impact on mortality. Psychosom Med. 1985;47(5):431–5.

119. Frasure-Smith N, Lesperance F, Prince RH, et al. Randomised trial of home-based psychosocial nursing intervention for patients recovering from myocardial infarction. Lancet. 1997;350(9076):473–9.

120. Berkman LF, Blumenthal J, Burg M, et al. Effects of treating depression and low perceived social support on clinical events after myocardial infarction: the Enhancing Recovery in Coronary Heart Disease Patients (ENRICHD) Randomized Trial. JAMA. 2003;289(23):3106–16.

121. Appels A, Bar F, van der PG, et al. Effects of treating exhaustion in angioplasty patients on new coronary events: results of the randomized exhaustion intervention trial (EXIT). Psychosom Med. 2005;67(2):217–3.

122. Glassman AH, O'Connor CM, Califf RM, et al. Sertraline treatment of major depression in patients with acute MI or unstable angina. JAMA. 2002;288(6):701–9.

123. Dusseldorp E, van ET, Maes S, Meulman J, Kraaij V. A meta-analysis of psychoeducational programs for coronary heart disease patients. Health Psychol. 1999;18(5):506–19.

124. Linden W. Psychological treatments in cardiac rehabilitation: review of rationales and outcomes. J Psychosom Res. 2000;48(4–5):443–54.

125. Sebregts EH, Falger PR, Bar FW. Risk factor modification through nonpharmacological interventions in patients with coronary heart disease. J Psychosom Res. 2000;48(4–5):425–41.

126. Smith TW, Ruiz JM. Psychosocial influences on the development and course of coronary heart disease: current status and implications for research and practice. J Consult Clin Psychol. 2002;70(3):548–68.

127. Goodkin K, Appels A. Behavioral-neuroendocrine-immunologic interactions in myocardial infarction. Med Hypotheses. 1997;48(3):209–14.

128. Sapolsky R, Rivier C, Yamamoto G, Plotsky P, Vale W. Interleukin-1 stimulates the secretion of hypothalamic corticotropin-releasing factor. Science. 1987;238(4826):522–4.

129. Tracey KJ. The inflammatory reflex. Nature. 2002;420(6917):853–9.

130. Meland E, Laerum E, Maeland JG. Life style intervention in general practice: effects on psychological well-being and patient satisfaction. Qual Life Res. 1996;5(3):348–54.

131. Kop WJ, Appels A, Mendes de Leon CF, Bar FW. The relationship between severity of coronary artery disease and vital exhaustion. J Psychosom Res. 1996;40:397–05.

19

INTEGRATIVE CARDIOLOGY: MECHANISMS OF CARDIOVASCULAR ACTION OF ACUPUNCTURE

John C. Longhurst and Stephanie C. Tjen-A-Looi

INTRODUCTION

Acupuncture is one of the few areas of integrative medicine for which the mechanism of cardiovascular action has been explored.[1,2] Over the last two decades, studies in both China and the United States have used a number of experimental preparations that lend themselves to acupuncture and careful measurement of cardiovascular function. This chapter describes investigations carried out in the United States that have explored the peripheral and central neurobiological mechanisms of acupuncture's influence on cardiovascular function, particularly blood pressure. These studies have been sponsored by the National Institutes of Health, National Heart, Lung and Blood Institute. The experimental paradigm used in these studies has been to investigate the influence of acupuncture in a feline model of demand-induced myocardial ischemia or short-term reflex hypertensive responses to visceral organ stimulation, including activation of chemosensitive sensory endings in the gallbladder with bradykinin (BK) or distension of the stomach with a balloon. These conditions simulate sensory nerve stimulation during inflammation and food ingestion, both of which are known to evoke profound sympathoexcitatory reflex cardiovascular responses.[3–6] The influence of acupuncture on the hemodynamic response to exercise also has been studied,[7] since exercise is well known to raise blood pressure.[8–13] The rationale for superimposing acupuncture on cardiovascular excitatory reflexes is that, for the most part, acupuncture has little or no influence on baseline blood pressures of normotensive humans or animals.[7] Conversely, elevated blood pressure in genetically hypertensive rats can be lowered by acupuncture for up to 10–12 hours.[14]

ACUPUNCTURE IN MYOCARDIAL DEMAND-INDUCED ISCHEMIA, RELATIONSHIP TO THE OPIOID SYSTEM

In a chloralose-anesthetized feline preparation (Fig. 19-1), we either partially occluded the left anterior descending coronary artery or fully ligated a diagonal branch of this artery, such that, under baseline conditions there was sufficient flow through the epicardial vessel and innate collaterals to meet myocardial oxygen requirements (partial occlusion group) or enough flow to limit infarction to <1% of the left ventricle (complete occlusion group).[15] When chemosensitive sensory nerve endings in the gallbladder were stimulated with BK applied to the serosal surface, a sympathoexcitatory reflex was induced, which included an increase in blood pressure of 30–50 mm Hg. During this reflex stimulation, there was an increase in myocardial oxygen demand, noted as an increase in the double product. Using sonomicrometer crystals to measure regional wall thickening, we found that during the increase in myocardial oxygen demand there was a reduction in local myocardial function in the area just distal to the partially occluded coronary vessel, signifying regional demand-induced myocardial ischemia. Compared to a sham control without nerve stimulation, 30 minutes of low-frequency (5 Hz) low-intensity (0.5 mA, 0.5 ms duration) bilateral stimulation of the median nerves at a level that was sufficient to produce moderate paw twitches significantly reduced the reflex increase in blood pressure and virtually eliminated the regional ischemic wall dysfunction. Evaluation of the afferent fibers activated by the median nerve stimulation showed that approximately two-thirds were low-threshold myelinated fibers (Group III), while one-third were high-threshold unmyelinated fibers (Group IV). We chose the median nerve since it is positioned directly beneath the Jianshi-Neiguan acupoints along the pericardial meridian (P 5–P 6), which are stimulated in the treatment of patients with cardiovascular disease. In this first experiment, we opted to directly stimulate the median nerve rather than to try acupuncture to verify that the principal neural pathway under the pericardial meridian was stimulated. Measurement of coronary blood flow, using a Doppler flow transducer over the partially ligated coronary artery demonstrated no improvement of flow during or following median nerve stimulation. We concluded that stimulation of the median nerve, to simulate acupuncture at the Neiguan-Jianshi acupoints, through a mechanism that involves activation of both Group III and Group IV somatic afferent nerve fibers, reverses myocardial ischemic dysfunction in a model of demand-induced ischemia. Furthermore, we concluded that this beneficial effect of acupuncture was mediated by a decrease in myocardial oxygen demand, caused by the reduction of the increase in the reflex-induced blood pressure elevation, rather than an improvement in blood supply to the heart. Interestingly, the improvement in ischemic dysfunction began 15 minutes after starting median nerve stimulation and lasted for at least an hour after terminating neural stimulation, indicating that this response far outlasted the period of stimulation, reminiscent of early studies indicating that acupuncture has a prolonged action.[14]

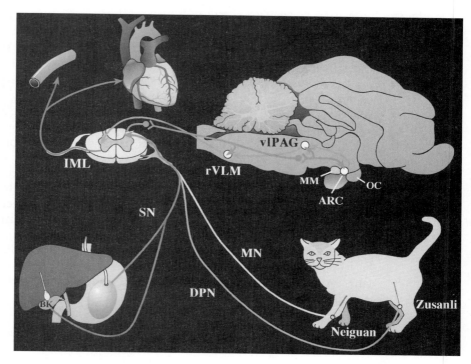

FIGURE 19-1   *Experimental evaluation of peripheral and central neural mechanisms of action of acupuncture on the cardiovascular system of anesthetized cats. Because acupuncture has been shown to be most effective in lowering elevated blood pressure (BP), we repetitively stimulated either chemosensitive afferent nerve fibers in the gallbladder with bradykinin (BK) or mechanosensitive gastric afferent endings by balloon distension to reflexly increase BP for 1–2 minutes repetitively (10–15 episodes) over a 1–2 hour period. Acupuncture needles were inserted at Neiguan (P 5) and Zusanli (ST 35), acupoints along pericardial and stomach meridians were stimulated either mechanically or electrically with low-frequency (2–4 Hz) low-intensity (1–3 mA) for 30 minutes. Acupuncture lowered the reflex increases by 40–50% beginning 10–15 minutes after initial application for a period that frequently exceeded 1 hour after termination of acupuncture stimulation (total time of inhibition, 1–2 hours). In a series of protocols, we have investigated the afferent pathways involved in transmission of the acupuncture sensory neural signals in the median and deep peroneal nerves (MN, DPN), and central neural processing in the rostral ventral lateral medulla (rVLM), hypothalamic arcuate nucleus (ARC) near the optic chiasm (OC) and mammillary bodies (MM), and the midbrain ventral lateral periaqueductal gray (vlPAG). See text for explanation of results of these studies. The brain stem rVLM is a particularly important site for signal processing and acupuncture influence, since it provides premotor bulbospinal projections to the IML thoracic spinal cord, where preganglionic sympathetic neurons exit to innervate the heart and blood vessels. Our studies have shown that neurons in the rVLM receive input from visceral organs like the gallbladder and the stomach, as well as somatic afferents from acupoints like Neiguan and Zusanli. During acupuncture modulatory neurotransmitters, including opioid peptides like endorphins and enkephalins and nonopioid peptides like nociceptin, released through a long-loop pathway that involves the ARC and the vlPAG, inhibit activity in premotor sympathetic neurons in the rVLM to ultimately reduce sympathetic outflow and elevated BP.*

In a subsequent study employing the same animal model of partial coronary occlusion, we again determined that low-frequency (4 Hz), low-intensity (2–5 mA, 0.5 ms) electroacupuncture (EA) at the Jianshi-Neiguan (P 5–P 6) acupoints bilaterally reduced the demand-related regional wall dysfunction following stimulation of the gallbladder with BK.[16] We chose EA since this form of acupuncture can be controlled precisely with respect to frequency, intensity, and duration of stimulation. In this and all subsequent studies we have employed EA using one needle at each of two closely located acupoints, one needle acting as a cathode and one as an anode, so that there is minimal current spread throughout the body. In this study, we also observed that the nonspecific opioid antagonist naloxone administered either intravenously or through microinjection of a small volume (100 nL) bilaterally into the nucleus paragigantocellularis lateralis of the rostral ventral lateral medulla (rVLM) reversed the acupuncture response immediately after termination of the 30-minute period of stimulation, indicating that the acupuncture-cardiovascular response is mediated through the opioid system and that the rVLM serves as one important site for central integration of the acupuncture-cardiovascular response. The rVLM is a source of bulbospinal sympathetic premotor fibers and hence serves as an important brain stem region in cardiovascular control.[17,18]

ACUPUNCTURE REGULATION OF REFLEX BLOOD PRESSURE ELEVATION DURING GASTRIC DISTENSION AND EXERCISE

In addition to our studies on the influence of acupuncture in myocardial ischemia caused by reflex increases in blood pressure during chemical stimulation of the gallbladder, we have investigated the ability of acupuncture to regulate reflex elevations in blood pressure in both a rodent (rat) model during activation of mechanosensitive receptors by gastric distension and in humans during exercise.[19,7]

Inflation of a balloon in the rat stomach to degrees of distension achieved during food ingestion (20 mm Hg),[20,21] reflexly increases blood pressure by 20–30 mm Hg. We found that 30 minutes of low-frequency (2 Hz), low-intensity (1–2 mA) EA performed bilaterally at the pericardial meridian over the median nerve (Jianshi-Neiguan acupoints, P 5–P 6) as well as at the stomach meridian located over the deep peroneal nerve (Zusanli-Shangquxu acupoints, ST 36–ST 37) but not over the gallbladder meridian, located over the superficial peroneal nerve (Guangming-Xuanzhong control acupoints, GB 37–GB 39), reduced the reflex increase in blood pressure by approximately 45%. The responses began within 10 minutes of instituting EA and lasted longer following termination of EA at Jianshi-Neiguan (40 minutes) compared to Zusanli-Shangquxu (10 minutes). A new finding in this study was the observation of point-specific responses to EA. In this respect, we found that stimulation of acupoints over the median nerves caused longer suppression of the reflex blood pressure elevations than stimulating acupoints over the deep peroneal nerves. Furthermore, there was no influence on the reflex cardiovascular response during stimulation of acupoints over superficial somatic nerves. The reduction in cardiovascular reflex blood pressure responses following EA at Jianshi-Neiguan occurred over a range of gastric transmural distension pressures from 5 to 41 mm Hg elicited by graded distension of the stomach with a balloon from 5 to 21 mL. Finally, we observed that naloxone administered either intravenously or microinjected unilaterally into the rVLM rapidly reversed the EA-related inhibition of the blood pressure reflex, thus confirming our studies of opioid-related EA mechanisms in cats during gallbladder stimulation.

The effect of 30 minutes of low-frequency (2 Hz), low-intensity (1–2 mA) EA at several sets of acupoints, including: (1) Jianshi-Neiguan (P 5–P 6) found along the pericardial meridian over the median nerves, (2) Hegu-Lique (LI 4–L 7) along the large intestine and lung meridians overlying the median and ulnar nerves, and (3) Guangming-Zuanzhong (GB 37–GB 39) located along the gallbladder meridian over the superficial peroneal nerve, on the hemodynamic response to exercise was evaluated in healthy adult subjects of both sexes.[7] Subjects completed one of two exercise protocols involving electronically braked bicycle ergometry. One protocol involved a ramp increase in workload, increasing 10 watts each minute to exhaustion. The second protocol was a constant load that was individualized for each subject to allow them to exercise to exhaustion in 8–12 minutes. During the second protocol, we assessed the subjects' breath to breath maximal oxygen consumption and anaerobic (lactate) threshold by measuring their gas exchange. EA at any of the three sets of acupoints did not alter resting blood pressure. We found that in 70% of subjects, EA at either the Jianshi-Neiguan or Hegu-Lique acupoints, but not at the Guangming-Xuanzhong acupoints, reduced exercise-induced increases in systolic and mean arterial blood pressures but not diastolic blood pressure or heart rate. EA reduced the blood pressure responses during both exercise protocols. Additionally, the calculated rate-pressure product, an index of myocardial oxygen demand was reduced by EA.[22] The observation was that EA suppresses blood pressure elevations and the increased maximal double product achieved during exercise confirms our experimental observations in feline and rodent models during visceral stimulation and suggests that acupuncture might have a beneficial effect on patients with coronary artery disease, who experience angina during exercise stress. Furthermore, the absence of effect during stimulation of the Guangming-Xuanzhong acupoints confirms our earlier experimental animal data and suggests that this acupoint can be used as a good negative control point in studies of the cardiovascular effects of acupuncture, to assess the magnitude of placebo-related responses during acupuncture.[23] The observation that acupuncture works in 70% of subjects is consistent with responses in our experimental preparations and has been verified by others.[24,25]

AFFERENT PATHWAYS MEDIATING THE CARDIOVASCULAR INFLUENCE OF ACUPUNCTURE

Acupuncturists typically ask patients to tell them about the sensation experienced during acupuncture, specifically to determine if the patient senses deqi. Deqi, is described as a sensation of heaviness, fullness, or numbness, rather than overt pain.[26] Deqi represents a radiating paresthesia and demonstates that neural pathways underlying the acupoint have to be stimulated for acupuncture to be most effective. However, if the patient experiences pain, the practitioner typically will reduce the degree of stimulation. The absence of pain suggests that Group III, but perhaps not Group IV, sensory fibers generally are stimulated during acupuncture. Although our initial study of acupuncture using single-unit sensory nerve recordings showed that both Group III (finely myelinated) and Group IV (unmyelinated) afferents are activated by the stimulation parameters used with acupuncture.[15] most early studies employing measurements of multiunit compound action potentials[27] concluded that the finely myelinated afferents were responsible for transmitting the afferent stimulation by acupuncture to the CNS. The problem with using multiunit recordings to assess activation of nerve pathways is that very small, unmyelinated fibers that generate relatively smaller action potentials may not be recorded.

To evaluate the importance of Group IV fibers more fully, we employed a model involving administration of capsaicin to neonatal rats. Capsaicin, a pungent ingredient extracted from hot peppers, is a neurotoxin, which, if administered early in life, causes the loss of most unmyelinated sensory nerve fibers.[28] In adult animals (~90 days of age), we assessed the impact of capsaicin treatment on the EA response. First, we observed that neonatal capsaicin eliminated many (75%) of the Group IV afferents but very few of the Group III afferents using single-unit recordings of the proximal median nerve. These data were confirmed by noting a significant reduction in substance P-containing neurons in the T_1–T_5 dorsal root ganglia, the location for cell bodies of primary afferent nerves supplying the forelimb. Substance P is a marker of small diameter nerve fibers, particularly Group IV afferents.[28] The capsaicin-treated group showed virtually no effect of 30 minutes of low-frequency (2 Hz), low-intensity (1–2 mA, 0.5 ms) EA at Jianshi-Neiguan (P 5–P 6) acupoints bilaterally during repeated gastric distension. Conversely, a control group treated with the vehicle for capsaicin responded to EA with a reduction in the distension-induced blood pressure response of approximately 40%, similar to our previous study. These data demonstrate the importance of unmyelinated somatic sensory afferent fibers in the median nerve in the EA-related inhibition of blood pressure during gastric distension. The study does not eliminate a role for finely myelinated sensory nerve fibers during EA. Thus, although acupuncture at Jianshi-Neiguan acupoints ordinarily is not associated with the perception of pain, this study shows that the cardiovascular response to EA is dependent upon activation of unmyelinated Group IV afferents in the median nerve.[29]

POINT SPECIFICITY

Point specificity is defined as differential physiological or clinical responses to stimulation of specific acupoints, with some acupoints causing a profound response and others causing a small or no response at all.[19] Although our initial study suggested that electrical stimulation of some acupoints during EA cause longer reductions in the reflex blood pressure responses to distension of the stomach, while others cause no cardiovascular response (and hence can serve as control points). There was no comprehensive study of the cardiovascular influence during separate stimulation of a large number of acupoints, nor have there been any studies of the central neural regions that receive and integrate somatic input and thus confer point-specific cardiovascular responses. As such, in the feline model of gallbladder stimulation with BK, we evaluated the cardiovascular response during low-frequency (2–4 Hz), low-intensity (4 mA, 0.5 ms) stimulation of acupoints located at Neiguan-Jianshi (P 5–P 6) along the pericardial meridian over the median nerve, Shousanli-Quchi (LI 10–LI 11) on the large intestine meridian over the deep radial nerve, Hegu-Lique (LI 4–L 7) on the large intestine and lung meridians over branches of the median and superficial radial nerves, Zusanli-Shangjiuxu (ST 36–ST 37) along the stomach meridian over the deep peroneal nerve, Pianli-Wenlui (LI 6–LI 7) on the large intestine meridian over the superficial radial nerve, and Youngquan-Zhiyin (K 1–BL 67) along the kidney and bladder meridians over terminal branches of the tibial nerve.[30] In one protocol, we evaluated the influence of stimulating each individual set of acupoints on the reflex cardiovascular response.

In a second protocol the responses of a group of rVLM cardiovascular neurons was measured using micropipettes for extracellular recordings during stimulation of each set of points. To carefully identify rVLM cells that functioned as sympathoexcitatory sympathetic premotor neurons, capable of altering sympathetic outflow to the heart and vascular system, we used a combination of baroreceptor stimulation or inactivation, frequency domain coherence analysis, time domain pulse-triggered averaging, and antidromic stimulation from the intermediolateral (IML) region of the spinal cord to determine if these cells represented cardiovascular sympathoexcitatory and sympathetic premotor neurons. We found that stimulation at Jianshi-Neiguan or Shousanli-Quchi each caused similar large reductions in the reflex blood pressure response, averaging 40% that lasted for 70 and 60 minutes, respectively. Hegu-Lique and Zusanli-Shangjiuxu led to more modest decreases, averaging 20–30%, and lasting for ~30 minutes. Pianli-Wenlui and Youngquan-Zhiyin did not influence the gallbladder-blood pressure reflex. Concordant changes in rVLM neuronal evoked response were observed during short-term stimulation of each of these sets of acupoints. Prolonged stimulation for 30 minutes during EA reduced activity of these rVLM neurons in a graded fashion that paralleled the point-specific effects of EA on the blood pressure responses. Thus, point specificity exists in EA with some acupoints exerting a strong cardiovascular influence, others a more moderate effect, and still others causing no response. The rVLM, an important area that receives input from many cardiovascular afferent systems, including barore-ceptors and chemoreceptors, and regulates sympathetic outflow, was identified as a brain stem nucleus that processes input from somatic sensory nerves acti-vated during acupuncture. During short-term stimulation of acupoints, neu-ronal activity in the rVLM increases but following prolonged somatic afferent stimulation, as occurs during the clinical application of acupuncture, neuronal activity in the rVLM is suppressed, most likely through a mechanism that relies, in part, on the production of opioid neurotransmitter modulators.

MODALITY OF STIMULATION, INFLUENCE OF MANUAL AND EA, AND STIMULATION FREQUENCY

We recently evaluated afferent mechanisms that are effective in initiating the optimal cardiovascular responses during acupuncture.[31] While manual acupunc-ture (MA) has been practiced for almost 3000 years, EA has been introduced more recently as a potent alternative because it can be standardized and is thus quite reproducible.[32] While there are differences in the influence of these two modes of acupuncture stimulation, a careful comparison between these two modalities has not been performed. We therefore carefully matched MA and EA using low-frequency stimulation (~2 Hz) applied for 120 seconds every 10 minutes over a 30-minute period and found virtually identical effects on the cardiovas-cular reflex response to gastric distension in rats. The only difference in response was a slightly more prolonged effect of EA as compared to MA, lasting for 30 and 20 minutes, respectively, after termination of stimulation. The shorter response to EA in this experiment, compared to our previous studies of EA noted above, likely derived from the intermittent rather than a continuous form of stimulation. We also found that both forms of stimulation caused nearly identical responses of afferent single units recorded in the median nerve. It is not surprising, therefore, that the inhibitory influence of MA and EA on the gastric distension blood pressure reflex was nearly identical.

Scientific reports have suggested that both low- (2–6 Hz) and high- (100 Hz) frequency EA or transcutaneous electrical stimulation (TENS) can modulate sympathetic vasomotor changes and pain.[33,34] Thus, we also evaluated the influ-ence of frequency of EA stimulation.[31] We found that low-frequency EA (2 Hz) caused large reductions in the reflex cardiovascular response to gastric disten-sion, while higher frequencies (50 and 100 Hz) did not alter the gastric reflex. In concert with our previous study,[15] the effectiveness of low-frequency EA was demonstrated to rely on sensory neural responses, since we observed only a modest response at 10 Hz and no afferent response at 20 Hz. Thus, high fre-quencies of acupuncture appear to block the ability of somatic afferents to con-duct information to the CNS. This conclusion was confirmed in a very recent study[35] in which sympathoexcitatory sympathetic premotor neurons in the rVLM were found to respond similarly to MA and EA, specifically low-frequency, not high-frequency EA. This study raises considerable question about the ability of high-frequency EA to provide afferent input to the CNS to regulate sympathetic outflow. Differences between this and previous studies from other laboratories may be that, in other species and/or in other situations, such as in studies of pain, high frequency EA may provide sufficient input to the spinal cord to allow sufficient segmental influence of afferent neural transmission to influence spinal centers involved in pain modulation. Alternatively, high-frequency acupuncture may modulate cellular activity in higher neural centers more concerned with processing pain as compared to the cardiovascular centers (rVLM), which we have studied. A final difference may be related to the species studied. Perhaps, in contrast to the cat, afferent systems in rats respond differently to higher levels of stimulation. However, afferent nerves in mammalian species respond similarly to electrical stimulation suggesting that a species difference is unlikely. The absence of significant response of the somatic nerves to frequencies of 20 Hz suggests that the clinical or physiological responses to high-frequency stimulation (>20 Hz) could be a placebo effect. The response to high-frequency TENS cannot be directly compared with acupuncture, since the neural response to external stimulation may be quite different than the response to a needle placed in or immediately adjacent to a neural pathway. TENS uses much higher currents and likely involves stimulation of much larger areas than that occurring during EA, which involves discrete stimulation of a single major somatic neural pathway. As such, it is quite possible that afferent information during TENS may be very different from needle acupuncture. In summary, in contrast to low-frequency acupuncture, high-frequency EA is not an effective inhibitory cardiovascular stimulus. Although the literature suggests that high-frequency EA or TENS may regulate pain, it is uncertain if there is sufficient input to the CNS to evoke responses over and above placebo. It is also difficult to extrapolate from studies utilizing TENS since this form of stimulation likely is quite different than EA.

WHAT CONSTITUTES A GOOD CONTROL FOR ACUPUNCTURE, THE ISSUE OF PLACEBO

Many trials of acupuncture, including both basic and clinical studies are limited by inadequacy of the control procedure used to evaluate for a nonspecific or placebo response. Mayer[23] suggested that the strongest control for acupuncture involves stimulation with an acupuncture needle either at an inactive acupuncture point along a meridian or in the same segment outside a meridian, but that simply tapping the skin with a needle to simulate acupuncture constitutes a weak control. We question the adequacy of stimulation outside a meridian as a control since a large bundle of afferent fibers would not be stimulated sufficiently to cause the sensation of deqi, thus allowing the patient and certainly the acupuncturist to discern differences between active and control stimulation. Using a tablet placebo and comparing acupuncture to ususal therapy without any surrogate form of acupuncture stimulation are still weaker and really are unacceptable controls. It is important to control for placebo responses since acupuncture, like most medial therapies, can be associated with clinical responses simply by virtue of a nonspecific interaction between the therapist and the patient.[1,36] Our studies of point specificity[31,30,19,7] indicate that inactive acupoints along meridians can be readily identified as control points in studies of acupuncture's influence on the cardiovascular system.

This type of control has a particular advantage in humans because major neural pathways are stimulated to induce a feeling of deqi, which makes it difficult for patients and potentially even the acupuncturist to distinguish between active acupuncture stimulation and the control acupoint. Hence there is a possibility of double blinding, if the patient and the acupuncturist are not informed about the clinical endpoint. In our recent study of the effects of MA and EA.[3] we observed that insertion of a needle in active acupoints, for example, Jianshi-Neiguan (P 5–P 6), without any subsequent mechanical or electrical stimulation, caused only very brief afferent fiber excitation and, as such, did not stimulate median nerve afferent fibers for a sufficiently long period to inhibit the cardiovascular excitatory response to gastric distension. Thus, simple insertion of a needle at an active acupuncture point may be one of the best controls to use in acupuncture studies. This observation, however, brings into question the practice of some acupuncturists of needle insertion without stimulation, as a presumed active intervention that causes an acupuncture response beyond placebo. Our data suggest that stimulation of an inactive acupoint along a known meridian or needle insertion without any form of mechanical or electrical insertion constitute the best controls to compare with active acupuncture stimulation. All studies of acupuncture should be judged by the controls they include for comparison.

CENTRAL NEURAL MECHANISMS IN ACUPUNCTURE

The rVLM serves as an important brain stem region involved in processing somatic afferent information during acupuncture stimulation. For example, we have demonstrated in both feline and rodent experimental models that microinjection of small quantities of naloxone (100 nL, 10 nM) either unilaterally or bilaterally into the rVLM reverses the reflex blood-lowering effect of EA at Jianshi-Neiguan (P 5–P 6).19,16. To more thoroughly evaluate opioid receptor subtype(s) involved in this response, we examined the response to blockade of μ-δ- and κ-opioid receptors by unilaterally microinjecting (100 nL) specific receptor antagonists or agonists into the rVLM as a surrogate for EA, using the model of BK-gallbladder stimulation to evoke reflex increases in blood pressure in association with EA (2 Hz, 1–2 mA) at Jianshi-Neiguan acupoints.[3,7] Like nonspecific antagonism with naloxone, blockade of either μ- or δ-opioid receptors eliminated the blood pressure-lowering effect of EA, while substitution of μ or δ receptor agonists for EA caused an acupuncture-like reduction of the reflex blood pressure response. In contrast, blockade of κ-opioid receptors caused only modest inhibition of the EA-blood pressure response and the κ receptor agonist did not alter the reflex. These studies suggest that endorphins and endomorphin, the principal endogenous ligands for μ-opioid receptors and enkephalins, the ligand for δ-opioid receptors, function as the principal rVLM opioid peptides that modulate the reflex increase in blood pressure during low-frequency EA at the Jianshi-Neiguan acupoints. In contrast, dynorphin does not appear to serve an important role in EA modulation of rVLM processing of visceral afferent-induced reflex increases in blood pressure.

There are many neurotransmitters and neuromodulators in brain stem nuclei concerned with cardiovascular regulation. Recently we investigated the role of nociceptin, [38] or Orphanin FQ, a recently identified opioid-like peptide that is distributed in neurons throughout the CNS, including the rVLM.[39–42] In fact, nociceptin has been found to inhibit neuronal activity in the rVLM,[43] although there also is evidence to indicate that nociceptin can exert excitatory actions.[44] To study the action of this opioid-like peptide, we employed microinjection of the native molecule, as an alternative to EA, as well as local blockade with a newly synthesized antagonist directed against its primary receptor, opioid receptor-like (ORL)-1. We found that, like EA, nociceptin (100 nL, 10 nM) administered unilaterally into the rVLM inhibited the reflex blood pressure response to gastric distension. In contrast, inhibition of activity of the ORL-1 receptor promptly reversed the inhibitory influence of 20 minutes of low-frequency, low-intensity (2 Hz, 1–2 mA, 0.5 ms) EA at Jianshi-Neiguan (P 5–P 6). The influence of nociceptin was found to be entirely distinct from the opioid system since it persisted even after naloxone had been administered. Thus, nociceptin serves as an additional modulatory neurotransmitter in the rVLM in the influence of EA in cardiovascular blood pressure regulation, through a mechanism that is separate from the opioid system.

EA has a prolonged duration of action that has been observed in both human and experimental animal studies. The long-term influence of EA is clinically relevant since although each episode of acupuncture lasts for only a few minutes (15–45 minutes), clearly a sustained effect on cardiovascular function potentially would allow practitioners to treat patients once or twice a week to achieve a satisfactory clinical response. The rVLM appears to be a center that likely promotes this prolonged response, since it processes input from multiple afferent inputs including those from both somatic and visceral systems activated during EA, as well as during excitatory reflexes associated with gallbladder or gastric stimulation. We have completed an electrophysiological-pharmacological study examining the activity of sympathoexcitatory neurons in this region of the medulla.[45] We identified a population of premotor sympathoexcitatory neurons that could be driven antidromically from the IML columns of the thoracic (T_2-T_4) spinal cord (which provides sympathetic outflow to the heart) and by baroreceptor stimulation, which received convergent input from the Jianshi-Neiguan acupoints (somatic afferents) and gallbladder (splanchnic nerve visceral afferents). Thus, this group of neurons incorporated all the characteristics of cells that are capable of modulating sympathetic outflow to the heart and vascular system. Furthermore, these neurons received information from somatic afferents that are activated during acupuncture and from the visceral afferents that convey sensory neural input from the gallbladder and stomach. We found very interesting responses during the extracellular recordings of evoked rVLM neuronal activity resulting from stimulation of the splanchnic and median nerves. For example, a group of sympathoexcitatory premotor neurons in this region displayed increased activity during stimulation of the two afferent pathways. Simultaneous stimulation of the median and splanchnic nerves caused neural occlusion, noted as a smaller response compared to the individual responses to stimulation of either afferent pathway alone. The phenomenon of neural occlusion was short-lived, lasting only as long the period of combined stimulation occurred and hence could not account for prolonged response attributed to acupuncture. In fact, when we stimulated the median nerve afferent pathway for a period of 30 minutes to simulate EA, we observed prolonged suppression of the evoked response to splanchnic nerve stimulation. Prolonged inhibition that lasted for 50 or more minutes after the termination of acupuncture occurred in a subgroup comprising a little more than half of the sympathoexcitatory premotor rVLM neurons. We speculate that this long-term suppression of neuronal responsiveness is dependent upon activation of long loop pathways, located perhaps in the hypothalamus and midbrain that participate in the EA-cardiovascular response, a working hypothesis that we are now exploring.

Iontophoresis of naloxone reversed this prolonged acupuncture-related inhibitory response, analogous to blockade of the acupuncture-induced cardiovascular reflex inhibition by intravenous and regional rVLM microinjection of naloxone.[45] This study therefore demonstrates that EA profoundly and for a prolonged time period inhibits the activity of a special population of neurons in the rVLM that regulate sympathetic outflow to the cardiovascular system. Additional studies will be required to determine the mechanisms underlying the prolonged influence of EA. Possible candidates include long-term synaptic inhibition and changes in the gene regulation of expression of inhibitory neurotransmitters such as opioid peptides, nociceptin, and γ-amino butyric acid (GABA).

HYPOTHALAMIC AND MIDBRAIN REGIONS INVOLVED IN CARDIOVASCULAR MODULATION BY EA

We have employed immunohistochemical techniques combined with fluorescence light and confocal laser microscopy to identify other regions in the brain that participate in the long loop EA-cardiovascular response. Using c-Fos, an early immediate gene expressed in neurons activated during relatively brief afferent stimulation,[46] as occurs during EA, we observed increased expression in both the ventral medulla as well as in the ventrolateral periaqueductal gray (vlPAG) following 30 minutes of low-frequency, low-intensity EA (2 Hz, 1–4 mA, 0.5 ms pulses) at the Jianshi-Neiguan (P 5–P 6) acupoints.[47] The PAG, and particularly the vlPAG, may process information during acupuncture that ultimately regulates the cardiovascular system.[48] In fact, this midbrain region contains opioid receptors[49] and projects to neurons concerned with pain and cardiovascular regulation in the rVLM.[50–52] Using separate antibodies to identify cytoplasm of cells containing β-endorphin, enkephalin (both met- and leu-enkephalin), and Fos-labeled nuclei (responsive to stimulation of Jianshi-Neiguan acupoints), we observed that activated nuclei in neurons were co-localized with cytoplasmic enkephalin in the rVLM and rarely in the vlPAG. There was no co-localization of Fos with β-endorphin in either the rVLM or the vlPAG. However, in both brain stem regions we observed, using confocal laser microscopy to provide high resolution, many Fos-labeled neurons situated in close proximity (0.2–15 μm) to axons or dendrites containing β-endorphin or enkephalin. Thus, both the rVLM and the vlPAG appear to be parts of a long loop pathway that processes sensory somatic information input during acupuncture at Jianshi-Neiguan acupoints overlying the median nerve. Through a mechanism that involves both β-endorphin and enkephalin interaction with classical excitatory neurotransmitters (possibly glutamate), these brain stem regions modulate visceral reflex input to limit the increase in blood pressure associated with visceral organ chemical or mechanical stimulation. In this respect, new evidence from studies employing microdialysis in the rVLM of cats to recover small quantities of extracellular fluid suggests that low-frequency EA (2 Hz) at Jianshi-Neiguan acupoints reduces the increase in glutamate associated with brief stimulation of the splanchnic nerve.[53,54]

Recent electrophysiological studies indicate the presence of a long-loop pathway that is activated during EA. This pathway involves the arcuate nucleus in the ventral hypothalamus, the vlPAG in the midbrain, possibly the midline medullary nuclei, including the nucleus raphe obscurus, possibly the nucleus raphe magnus, and nucleus raphe pallidus and ultimately the rVLM. We have shown that the arcuate nucleus, like the rVLM and the vlPAG, is a potentially important center that receives excitatory visceral and somatic information, for example during splanchnic (afferent pathway from the gallbladder and stomach) and median nerve stimulation (afferent pathway from Jianshi-Neiguan acupoints).[55] The arcuate nucleus is a major site of synthesis of opioid peptides[56,57] and provides an excitatory projection to the vlPAG. The vlPAG, as noted above, also receives both somatic and visceral excitatory input and projects to the rVLM, where it causes inhibition of activity of cardiovascular excitatory premotor sympathetic neurons.[58] Thus, inhibition of neuronal activity in either the arcuate nucleus or the vlPAG with microinjection of kainic acid interrupts the modulatory influence of EA on the reflex increase in blood pressure during gallbladder stimulation, while stimulation of these regions with D, L-homocysteic acid can lead to an EA-like inhibition of sympathoexcitatory reflex increase in blood pressure. These initial studies suggest that the long-loop pathway activated during EA, which inhibits sympathetic outflow to the heart and vascular system and thus reduces blood pressure, includes the arcuate nucleus, the vlPAG, and the rVLM, located in the hypothalamus, midbrain, and medulla, respectively. This pathway appears to be activated only after prolonged (>10–15 minutes) somatic nerve stimulation during acupuncture. The inhibitory connection between the vlPAG and the rVLM is critical for the EA-related modulation of sympathetic outflow and reflex increases in blood pressure.

CONCLUSIONS

In the last 10 years, we have gained many new perspectives on the peripheral and central neural mechanisms that underlie acupuncture's influence on the cardiovascular system. We know that it is capable of limiting increases in blood pressure and myocardial ischemia that result from increased demand for oxygen. Acupuncture needles stimulate major neural pathways beneath points located along meridians, which serve as road maps directing practitioners where they should stimulate. Stimulation during either manual or EA activates both finely myelinated and unmyelinated somatosensory pathways that provide information to several locations in the brain, including the arcuate nucleus in the ventral hypothalamus, the ventrolateral periaqueductal gray in the midbrain, and most importantly the rVLM, which regulates sympathetic outflow from the thoracic spinal cord. We know that low-frequency, low-intensity EA is more effective than high-frequency EA but is very similar to MA when the two forms of stimulation are matched for frequency and duration. We also have learned that, with respect to its action on the cardiovascular system, acupuncture is very effective at certain acupoints on the arm and leg that overlie deep neural pathways and is less effective at acupoints located over very superficial somatic nerves.

However, there are several aspects of acupuncture that we still do not fully understand. The first is why it has such a long mechanism of action. One part of the answer is the apparent long-loop pathway through the hypothalamus and midbrain that it activates. However, it seems clear that the long-term effect is related to chronic alterations in the brain, perhaps with neurotransmitter synthesis or altered baseline discharge activity of the medullary neurons that regulate sympathetic outflow. Second, we do not fully understand all of the interactions between the various regions of the brain and the neurotransmitter systems involved. Clearly opioids and opioid-like neurotransmitters are involved. But how about other inhibitory neurotransmitters, like GABA? Also, what is the importance of EA-mediated activation in some regions (arcuate nucleus and rVLM) during short-term stimulation and inhibition in other regions (vlPAG-rVLM) during more prolonged stimulation as occurs normally during acupuncture. And, are the neurotransmitters-neuromodulators acting pre- or postsynaptically to influence neuronal responsiveness and activity. Third, are other regions of the brain involved and does acupuncture influence the cardiovascular system through other mechanisms, for example, the parasympathetic nervous system or the humoral system, such as the renin-angiotensin system? Thus, while much work has been done, much more remains to allow a complete understanding of how acupuncture can influence cardiovascular function. We believe that a better understanding, particularly a mechanistic understanding, in addition to rigorous randomized, well-controlled clinical trials will aid substantially in increasing acceptance of this promising integrative medical modality by the western medical and scientific communities.

REFERENCES

1. Longhurst JC. Acupuncture's beneficial effects on the cardiovascular system. Prevent Cardiol. 1998;1(4):21–33.
2. Lin MC, Nahin R, Gershwin ME, Longhurst JC, Wu KK. State of complementary & alternative medicine in cardiovascular, lung and blood. Circulation. 2001;103:2038–41. [PMID: 11319191.]
3. Ordway GA, Longhurst JC. Cardiovascular reflexes arising form the gallbladder of the cat: effects of capsaicin, bradykinin and distension. Circ Res. 1983;52:26–35. [PMID: 6129075.]
4. Longhurst JC, Spilker HL, Ordway GA. Cardiovascular reflexes elicited by passive gastric distension in anesthetized cats. Am J Physiol. 1981;240:H539–45. [PMID: 7223905.]
5. Longhurst JC, Ibarra J. Reflex regional vascular responses during passive gastric distension in cats. Am J Physiol. 1984;247:R257–65. [PMID: 6147100.]
6. Longhurst JC. Reflex effects from abdominal visceral afferents. In: Zucker IH, Gillmore JP, editors. Reflex control of the circulation. Caldwell (NJ): Telford Press; 1991. p. 551–77.
7. Li P, Ayannusi O, Reed C, Longhurst J. Inhibitory effect of electroacupuncture (EA) on the pressor response induced by exercise stress. J Autonom Clin Res. 2004;14:182–8.
8. Stebbins CL, Longhurst JC. Potentiation of the exercise pressor reflex by muscle ischemia. J Appl Physiol. 1989;66:1046–53. [PMID: 2496081.]
9. Stebbins CL, Reimus W, Longhurst JC. Effect of muscle ischemia on the exercise pressor reflex. Clin Res. 1987;35(3):576A.
10. Stebbins CL, Brown B, Levin D, Longhurst JC. Reflex effect of skeletal muscle mechanoreceptor stimulation on the cardiovascular system. J Appl Physiol. 1988;65:1539–47. [PMID: 3182517.]
11. Longhurst JC, Mitchell JH. Reflex control of the circulation by afferents from skeletal muscle. In: Guyton AC, Cowley JAW, editors. Cardiovascular physiology III: international review of physiology.Baltimore (MD): University Park Press; 1979. pp. 125–48.
12. Daniels JW, Stebbins CL, Longhurst JC. Comparision of hemodynamic response to static and dynamic contractions at equivalent tension-time indexes. FASEB J. 1999;13:A449.
13. Longhurst JC. Neural regulation of the cardiovascular system. In: Squire LR, Bloom FE, McConnel SK, Roberts JL, Spitzer NC, Zigmond MJ, editors. Fundamental neuroscience. 2nd edition. San Diego (CA): Academic Press; 2003. pp. 935–66.
14. Yao T, Andersson S, Thoren P. Long-lasting cardiovascular depression induced by acupuncture-like stimulation of the sciatic nerve in unanaesthetized spontaneously hypertensive rats. Brain Res. 1982;240:77–85.
15. Li P, Pitsillides KF, Rendig SV, Pan H-L, Longhurst JC. Reversal of reflex-induced myocardial ischemia by median nerve stimulation: a feline model of electroacupuncture. Circulation. 1998;97:1186–94. [PMID: 9537345.]

16. Chao DM, Shen LL, Tjen-A-Looi S, Pitsillides KF, Li P, Longhurst JC. Naloxone reverses inhibitory effect of electroacupuncture on sympathetic cardiovascular reflex responses. Am J Physiol. 1999 June;276(Heart Circulation Physiology 45): H2127–34. [PMID: 10362696.]

17. Bauer RM, Iwamoto GA, Waldrop TG. Ventrolateral medullary neurons modulate pressor reflex to muscular contraction. Am J Physiol. 1989;257(26):R1154–61. [PMID: 2589541.]

18. Stornetta RL, Morrison S, Ruggiero DA, Reis D. Neurons of rostral ventral lateral medulla mediate somatic pressor reflex. Am J Physiol Regulatory Integrative Comp Physiol. 1989;256:R448–62. [PMID: 2464948.]

19. Li P, Rowshan K, Crisostomo M, Tjen-A-Looi S, Longhurst J. Effect of electroacupuncture on pressor reflux during gastric distention. Am J Physiol. 2002;283: R1335–45. [PMID: 12388466.]

20. Davison JS, Grundy D. Modulation of single vagal efferent fibre discharge by gastrointestinal afferents in the rat. J Physiol (Lond). 1978;284(69):82. [PMID:731576.]

21. Deutsch J. The stomach in food satiation and the regulation of appetite. Prog Neurobiol. 1978;10,135–153. [PMID: 715223.]

22. Kitamura K, Jorgensen CR, Gobel FL, Taylor HL, Wang Y. Hemodynamic correlates of myocardial oxygen consumption during upright exercise. J Appl Physiol. 1972;32:516–22. [PMID:5026501.]

23. Mayer DJ. Acupuncture: an evidence-based review of the clinical literature. Ann Rev Med. 2000;51:49–63. [PMID: 10774452.]

24. Morey SS. NIH issues consensus statement on acupuncture. Am Fam Physician. 1998 May 15;57(10):2545–6.

25. Stux G, Pomeranz B. Basics of acupuncture. Berlin: Springer-Verlag; 1998.

26. Andersson S. The functional background in acupuncture effects. Scand J Rehab Med, Suppl. 1993;29:31–60. [PMID:8122076.]

27. Xiao YF, Li P. Effect of deep peroneal nerve stimulation on renal nerve discharge under different levels of blood pressure in rabbits. Acta Physiol Sin. 1983;35:432–9.

28. Nagy JI, Iversen L, Goedert M, Chapman D, Hunt SP. Dose-dependent effects of capsaicin on primary sensory neurons in the neonatal rat. J Neurosci. 1983;3:399–406. [PMID: 6185658.]

29. Tjen-A-Looi S, Fu L-W, Zhou W (Syuu Y), Longhurst JC. Role of unmyelinated fibers in electroacupuncture cardiovascular responses. Auton Neurosci Basic Clin. 2005;118:43–50. [PMID: 15881777.]

30. Tjen-A-Looi S, Li P, Longhurst J. Medullary substrate and differential cardiovascular response during stimulation of specific acupoints. Am J Physiol Regulatory Integrative Comp Physiol. 2004;287:R852–62. [PMID: 15217791.]

31. Zhou W, Fu L-W, Tjen-A-Looi S, Li P, Longhurst J. Afferent mechanisms underlying stimulation modality-related modulation of acupuncture-related cardiovascular responses. J Appl Physiol. 2005;98(3):872–80. [PMID:15531558.]

32. Ernst E, White A. Acupuncture: a scientific appraisal. Butterworth Heinemann;1999.

33. Ernst M, Lee MH. Sympathetic vasomotor changes induced by manual and electrical acupuncture of the Hoku point visualized by thermography. Pain. 1985;21(1):25–33. [PMID: 3982836.]

34. Han JS, Chen XH, Sun SL, Xu XJ, Yuan Y, Yan SC, et al. Effect of low- and high-frequency TENS on Met-enkephalin-Arg-Phe and dynorphin A immunoreactivity in human lumbar CSF. Pain. 1991;47(3):295–8. [PMID: 1686080.]

35. Zhou W (Syuu Y), Tjen-A-Looi S, Longhurst JC. Brain stem mechanisms underlying acupuncture modality-related modulation of cardiovascular responses in rats. J Appl Physiol. 2005. [PMID: 15817715.]

36. Longhurst J. The ancient art of acupuncture meets modern cardiology. Cerebrum Dana Forum Brain Sci. 2001;3(4):48–59.

37. Li P, Tjen-A-Looi S, Longhurst JC. Rostral ventrolateral medullary opioid receptor subtypes in the inhibitory effect of electroacupuncture on reflex autonomic response in cats. Autonom Neurosci Basic Clin. 2001;89:38–47. [PMID: 11474645.]

38. Crisostomo M, Li P, Tjen-A-looi SC, Longhurst JC. Nociceptin in rVLM mediates electroacupuncture inhibition of cardiovascular reflex excitatory response in rats. J Appl Physic. 2005;98(6):2056–63. [PMID: 15649868.]

39. Anton B, Fein J, To T, Li X, Silberstein L, Evans CJ. Immunohistochemical localization of ORL-1 in the central nervous system of the rat. J Comp Neurol.1996;368:229–51. [PMID:8725304.]

40. Houtani T, Nishi M, Takeshima H, Nukada T, Sugimoto T. Structure and regional distribututunion of nociceptin/orphan FQ precursor. Biochem Biophys Res Commun. 1996;219:714–9. [PMID: 8645247.]

41. Neal CJ, Mansour A, Reinscheid R, Nothacker H-P, Civelli O, Akil H, Watson SJ. Opioid receptor-like (ORL1) receptor distribution in the rat central nervous system: comparison of ORL1 receptor mRNA expression with 125I-[14Tyr]-orphanin FQ binding. J Comparative Neurol. 1999;412:563–605. [PMID: 10464356.]

42. Schulz M, Schreff M, Nuss D, Gramsch C, Hollt V. Nociceptin/orphanin FQ and opioid peptides show overlapping distribution but not co-localization in pain modulatory brain regions. Neuro Report. 1996;7:3021–5. [PMID: 9116232.]

43. Chu XP, Xu NS, Li P, Wang JQ. The nociceptin receptor mediated inhibition of the rat rostral ventrolateral medulla neurons in vitro. Eur J Pharmacol. 1999;364:49–53. [PMID: 9920184.]

44. Arndt M, Wu D, Soong Y, Szeto H. Nociceptin/orphanin FQ increases blood pressure and heart rate via sympathetic activation in sheep. Peptides. 1999;20:465–70. [PMID: 10458516.]

45. Tjen-A-Looi S, Li P, Longhurst JC. Prolonged inhibition of rostral ventral lateral medullary premotor sympathetic neuron by electroacupuncture in cats. Autonom Neurosci Basic Clin. 2003;106 (2):119–31. [PMID: 12878081.]

46. Guo Z, Lai H, Longhurst J. Medullary pathways involved in cardiac sympathoexcitatory reflexes in the cat. Brain Res. 2002;925:55–66. [PMID: 11755900.]

47. Guo Z-L, Moazzami A, Longhurst J. Electroacupuncture induces c-Fos expression in the rostral ventrolateral medulla and periaqueductal gray in cats: relation to opioid containing neurons. Brain Res. 2004;1030:103–15. [PMID: 15567342.]

48. Lee JH, Beitz AJ. The distribution of brain-stem and spinal cord nuclei associated with different frequencies of electroacupuncture analgesia. Pain. 1993;52:11–28. [PMID: 8446432.]

49. Wang H, Wessendorf MW. Mu and delta-opiod receptor mRNAs are expressed in periaqueductal gray neurons projecting to the rostral ventromedial medulla. Neuroscience. 2002;109(3):619–34. [PMID: 11823071.]

50. Lovick TA. Projections from the diencephalon and mesencephalon to nucleus paragigantocellularis lateralis in the cat. Neuroscience. 1985;14(3):853–61. [PMID: 3990961.]

51. Punnen S, Willette R, Krieger AJ, Sapru HN. Cardiovascular response to injections of enkephalin in the pressor area of the ventrolateral medullla. Neuropharmacology. 1984;23:939–46. [PMID: 6090967.]

52. VanBockstaele EJ, Aston-Jones G, Pieribone VA, Ennis M, Shipley MT. Subregions of the periaqueductal gray topographically innervate the rostral ventral medulla in the rat. J Comp Neurol. 1991, 309:305–27. [PMID: 1717516.]

53. Zhou W, Fu L, Tjen-A-Looi S, Guo Z, Longhurst J. Glutamate's role in a visceral sympathoexcitatory reflex in rostral ventrolateral medulla of cats. Am J Physiol Heart Circ Physiol. (In press).

54. Fu L-W, Syuu YZW, Guo Z-L, Longhurst JC. Acupuncture modulates release of glutamate in the rVLM during stimulation of visceral afferents. J Neurosci. 2004.

55. Li P, Tjen-A-Looi S, Longhurst J. Excitatory projections from arcuate nucleus to ventrolateral periaqueductal gray in electroacupuncture inhibition of cardiovascular reflexes. Am J Physiol. In press.

56. Cuello AC. Central distribution of opioid peptides. In: Hughes J, editor. British Medical Bulletin. Churchill Livingstone; 1983. p. 11–6.

57. Bach FW, Yaksh TL. Release into ventriculo-cisternal perfusate of beta-endorphin and met-enkephlin-immunoreactivity: effects of electrical stimulation in the arcuate nucleus and periaqueductal gray of the rat. Brain Res. 1995;690:169–76. [PMID: 8535833.]

58. Tjen-A-Looi S, Li P, Longhurst J. Midbrain vlPAG inhibits rVLM cardiovascular sympathoexcitatory. Am J Physiol. In press.

CHAPTER

20

THE EMOTIONAL BASIS OF CORONARY HEART DISEASE

Robert A. Vogel

INTRODUCTION

The emotional contribution to organic illness is accepted by both traditional and alternative medicine. Compared with traditional medicine, alternative medicine focuses more directly on the link between emotions and organic disease, and more often utilizes supportive, relaxing, and focusing interventions. Coronary heart disease is a good example of an organic disease with a strong emotional basis. Emotions, traditional risk factors, and coronary heart disease are complexly interrelated. A better understanding of how emotions affect the management of coronary artery disease is useful because emotional distress:

- Commonly masquerades as cardiac symptoms
- Accentuates improper lifestyle and risk factor burden
- Constitutes an independent risk factor for coronary heart disease
- May trigger acute cardiovascular events
- Frequently follows cardiovascular events
- Serves as a barrier to accepted treatment
- Constitutes an important therapeutic opportunity

Although diet and physical activity are well recognized for their direct and indirect contributions to coronary heart disease, emotional causes and consequences remain largely ignored by many practitioners. Cardiologists do not often discuss emotional problems with their patients due to limited familiarity with effective treatments and recommendations. As a result, the emotional origins and consequences of coronary heart disease often go unrecognized and untreated. This chapter considers the epidemiological evidence linking emotions and coronary heart disease, probable pathophysiological mechanisms, and evolving treatment options. The goal of this chapter is to enable cardiologists and other physicians dealing with coronary disease to become more proactive with the emotional issues of their patients, and to seek the assistance of mental health professionals when needed. A detailed review of this topic was recently published.[1]

EVIDENCE LINKING EMOTIONS AND CORONARY HEART DISEASE

There is strong evidence linking both negative and positive emotions and chronic stressors to coronary heart disease. Atherogenic emotions include depression, anxiety, hostility, anger, and pessimism. Protective emotional factors include optimism and emotional vigor and flexibility. Lack of social support, lower socioeconomic status, and work and family stress greatly magnify the impact of emotional distress on coronary heart disease. It is also important to recognize that negative emotions both contribute to and result from heart disease.

Depression

Both depressed mood and clinical depression have been linked to increased coronary heart disease events, such as myocardial infarction and poorer outcome after coronary events and interventions. Even mild depressive symptoms appear to have measurable consequences.[2] A comparison of the coronary heart disease risk associated with traditional and emotional risk factors was carried out as part of the Framingham Heart Study.[3] In this study, depressed mood increased the risk of a coronary heart disease event by about 50%, whereas clinical depression increased it almost threefold. The magnitude of increased risk associated with the spectrum of depression was at least as great as for diabetes, hypertension, smoking, and dyslipidemia. A highly significant correlation between negative emotions, predominately depression and anxiety, and the incidence of coronary heart disease was also found prospectively in older men without heart disease or diabetes participating in the Normative Aging Study, even after adjusting for other risk variables.[4]

Both short- and long-term mortality after myocardial infarction are also strongly predicted by depressive symptoms. Six-month mortality of men and women experiencing myocardial infarction was more than four times greater in depressed individuals (Mental Health Diagnostic Interview Schedule) than in nondepressed individuals.[5] There is a continuous graded relationship between severity of depression and mortality following myocardial infarction. Five-year mortality after myocardial infarction was approximately four times greater in subjects with a Beck Depression Inventory ≥19 compared with those with a depression index <5.[5] Those subjects with intermediate depression indexes had intermediate mortality rates. Depressive symptoms were the strongest predictors of short-term decline in health status in subjects with heart failure.[6] In contrast, when anxiety and depression were individually considered in men experiencing myocardial infarction, only anxiety independently predicted postmyocardial infarction cardiac events and increased health-care consumption.[7] The association between depression and morbidity was no longer statistically significant after anxiety was considered.

Anxiety

Anxiety may be associated with the progression of atherosclerosis and coronary heart disease events. Of the several forms of anxiety, phobic disorders have been the most strongly associated with sudden cardiac death.[1] Men without known heart disease but with sustained anxiety (Spielberger Inventory) had twice the progression of carotid intima-media thickness over 4 years compared with those without anxiety.[8] During the 20 years of follow-up of the Normative Aging Study, men with the highest level of anxiety had 2.4 times greater risk of experiencing a first coronary heart disease event than those with the lowest level of anxiety.[9] Worry about social conditions had the strongest association with heart disease risk. The risk of fatal coronary events was increased 3.2 times and the risk of sudden death was increased 5.7 times.[10] The impact of anxiety and depression are not limited to major morbidity and mortality after myocardial infarction. These negative emotions adversely affect daily functioning, ability to return to work, and the presence of continued cardiac symptoms, such as angina.[11]

Other studies suggest an absent or even inverse relationship between anxiety and coronary heart disease. A history of anxiety disorder was associated with a decreased likelihood of coronary artery disease in women undergoing coronary arteriography in the WISE study.[12] No correlation between anxiety and coronary calcification was found in an Army study, but somatic complaints were associated with decreased calcification.[13] These findings underscore the contribution of anxiety to somatic symptoms, which often take the form of chest pain, palpitations, difficulty breathing, and other cardiac symptoms. More than three-quarter of patients with panic disorders present in primary care situations with somatic complaints only.[14,15] The inverse relationship between anxiety and the presence of coronary disease in these latter studies may be explained by the increased medical attention sought by anxious patients.

Hostility

Hostility and anger proneness are also strongly associated with coronary heart disease. The prospective Atherosclerosis in Communities (ARIC) study found that high-trait anger increased the risk of coronary heart disease myocardial infarction (coronary heart disease death) by 2.7 times compared with low anger after multivariate adjustment.[16] Intermediate grades of anger had lesser risk and lower but significant risk was observed for revascularization. In the 16-year follow-up of the Multiple Risk Factor Intervention Trial (MRFIT), men with high hostility (Interpersonal Hostility Assessment Technique) were 1.6 times more likely to be victim of cardiovascular disease than men with low hostility and were more than 5 times more likely to die if they experienced a nonfatal event during the study.[17]

Social connectedness and support

Emotional traits, such as anger proneness interact with social functioning. Social support can be generally divided into two broad categories, social networks which describe the size, structure, and frequency of interpersonal contact and functional support which includes the type and amount of resources provided by the social networks and perceived support which focus on the subjective satisfaction that would be available if needed.[1] Low structural support is associated with increased coronary disease mortality for individuals living alone, lacking confidence, and suffering from social isolation. In a 2-year study of 223 subjects with coronary artery disease, the association of high cynical hostility (State-Trait-Anger-Expression-Inventory, Cook-Medley Cynical Hostility Scale) and low social support greatly increased angiographic progression (30-fold).[18] As expected, the interplay between negative emotions and low social support also contributes to the development of carotid atherosclerotic disease.

A combination of high hostility and low social support was reported to be associated with carotid artery plaques, especially in individuals with high family predisposition.[19] Anger appears to increase the likelihood of coronary disease development, as well. In 18- to 30-year-old subjects, the odds of having any coronary artery calcification was 2.6 times greater in those with high-trait hostility compared with low hostility and were 9.6 times more likely to have a calcium score greater than 20.[20]

Optimism/pessimism

Common wisdom touts the medical benefit of "thinking positively" and being optimistic. Individuals who foresee a pleasant future, especially those who believe that they can control their own future, appear to derive several health benefits. Emotional vitality comprising energy, enthusiasm, optimism, coping flexibility, and senses of purpose and self-worth are key components of mental health.[1] In a sense, depression and anxiety are the opposites of emotional vitality.

Although not studied as extensively as depression, anxiety, and hostility, optimism appears to retard the development of coronary heart disease. A 10-year follow-up of men in the Normative Aging Study revealed that highly optimistic subjects (Optimism-Pessimism Scale of the Minnesota Multiphasic Personality Inventory) had 56% less nonfatal myocardial infarction and coronary heart disease death than did highly pessimistic men.[21] Graded levels of risk correlated with varying levels of optimism. Outcomes after a coronary event also appear to be better in optimistic individuals. In a study of 309 consecutive patients undergoing coronary bypass surgery, optimistic persons were significantly less likely to be rehospitalized for subsequent problems, including sternal wound infections, angina, myocardial infarction, and revascularization procedures compared with pessimistic patients.[22] The approximate 50% fewer complications were independent of traditional sociodemographic and medical factors, as well as measures of self-esteem, depression, and neuroticism. Striving, time-conscious personality Type A has been variably associated with increased coronary heart disease risk, but these individuals experience better survival after myocardial infarction, perhaps due to better adherence to medical care.[23] Personality Type D individuals characterized by negative emotions, especially in social interactions, had a fourfold increase in coronary events after percutaneous coronary intervention with a drug-eluting stent in a recent trial.[24]

Chronic stressors

As with emotional distress, psychosocial stressors contribute to the development of coronary heart disease. Chronic stress initiates both physical (e.g., obesity, hypertension) and emotional atherogenic factors. For example, individuals experiencing high job strain have higher rates of depression compared to those without job strain.[25] Chronic stress has clearly identified physical consequences. Hypothalamic-pituitary-adrenal dysfunction accompanies chronic stress and increased dysfunction occurs especially at lower socioeconomic levels.[1] Lower socioeconomic level is associated with increases in coronary heart disease, which can only be attributed in part to associated increases in traditional risk factors.[26] The direct influence of chronic stress on atherosclerosis has been well documented in experimental studies. Watanabe rabbits either caged separately to mimic social isolation and those caged repetitively with different other animals develop more atherosclerosis.[27]

The most studied chronic stressor is job stress, but debate exists on its definition and measurement. Two models of job-related stress have been predominately employed. The job strain model is a matrix approach that places individuals with high job demands and hazards and low job latitude or choice at the highest level of stress. The effort/reward imbalance model is also a matrix approach, which places those with the highest effort and least financial and emotional reward at the highest level of stress. Work-related busyness is often confused with true stress. In fact, many successful, achieving busy professionals encounter far less true job stress than do lower level workers performing routine, often repetitive tasks. The creativity, control over their tasks, extensive financial return, and social regard usually more than offsets the high demands and long work hours of busy professionals.

In a 14-year Swedish study, workers with low work control experienced 1.8 times more cardiovascular mortality compared with workers with more control.[28] Workers with both low control and low support had 2.6 times more mortality. A longer duration of work stress had more adverse effect. Similar results were reported from a 26-year Finnish study that found that the combination of high work demands and low job control was associated with a 2.2-fold increase in cardiovascular mortality.[29] Although these results were independent of traditional coronary risk factors, effort-reward imbalance predicted increased serum cholesterol and body mass index. In the Kuopio Ischemic Heart Disease Risk Factor Study, men with high job demands and low economic reward had greater 4-year progression of carotid artery intima-media thickness.[30] Increased job strain is also associated with greater somatic complaints. As a consequence, increased job stress does not appear to predict the presence or severity of coronary stenoses in individuals undergoing coronary arteriography.[31]

Family stress

Marital quality, caregiver strain, and child rearing are also associated with coronary heart disease. Following myocardial infarction, women reporting marital stress experienced a higher frequency of recurrent cardiac events during 5 years of follow-up compared to women with less marital stress.[32] The atherogenic potential of marital stress is further supported by a recent study that found a higher prevalence of subclinical atherosclerosis and accelerated disease progression among women reporting marital dissatisfaction.[33] The cardiac impact of marital stress extends beyond coronary artery disease. Four-year mortality rates for men and women with congestive heart failure reporting marital dissatisfaction were approximately twice that of those reporting better marital quality.[34] In this study, marital quality was at least as predictive of survival as was New York Heart Association functional assessment. This finding underscores the need for physicians to delve into the emotional issues of their patients with cardiac disease.

Caregiver strain is another important chronic stressor. In the Nurses' Health Study, caregiving for an ill spouse was associated with nearly twofold risk of experiencing a coronary heart disease event over a 4-year follow-up period.[35] This study did not stratify caregiver strain according to the emotional appraisal of the subject's experience. Other research suggests that highly meaningful, altruistic experience can be of psychological benefit.[1] When caregivers were divided into those with and without a sense of emotional strain, the Caregivers Health Effects study reported increase death rate only among those reporting increased strain.[36]

Child-rearing is another source of both emotional reward and distress. Several studies indicate that rearing large families is associated with excess coronary heart disease. In the British Women's Heart and Health study, minimum coronary heart disease risk was associated with raising two children.[37] For each additional child raised, coronary heart disease risk increased about 30% for both parents. Increasing family size correlated with increased obesity, diabetes, serum triglycerides, and decreased high-density lipoprotein cholesterol.

PATHOPHYSIOLOGY

Atherosclerotic coronary artery disease is a chronic inflammatory, proliferative, thrombotic disease initiated by risk factors. The subintimal deposition of lipids and endothelial dysfunction are early manifestations. Acute emotional distress is associated with tachycardia, hypertension, and increased cardiac output due to increased sympathetic activity, as well as endothelial dysfunction, platelet activation, and inflammation.[1] Chronic depression is also associated with increased sympathetic activity manifest by higher levels of circulating norepinephrine. The increased sympathetic tone results in higher fasting heart rates, diminished heart rate variability, baroreflex dysfunction, and increased QT variability. For example, diminished heart rate variability is associated with autonomic dysfunction and is a strong, independent predictor of sudden death in patients with coronary heart disease.[38] In a large study of patients experiencing acute myocardial infarction, depression was associated with four indexes of diminished heart rate variability, which were independent of other risk factors. These autonomic disturbances likely explain the high mortality rate observed in depressed patients after myocardial infarction.

Acute and chronic emotional distress affects the hypothalamic-pituitary-adrenal axis, resulting in hypercortisolemia, decreased diurnal variation in serum cortisol, and decreased sex hormones.[1] The increased cortisol results in central obesity, insulin resistance, hypertriglyceridemia, and diminished high-density lipoprotein cholesterol. The combination of chronic stress and high glucocorticoids stimulates a preferential desire to ingest sweet and fatty foods,[39] leading to more obesity. A desire for these "comfort foods" results from the effect of glucocorticoids on dopaminergic transmission in the midbrain associated with motivation and reward, specifically dealing with food preferences.[1] Increases in cortisol also contribute to baroreflex impairment observed in stressful circumstances.[40]

The increase in sympathetic activity associated with acute emotional distress directly induces coronary vasoconstriction and ischemia. Laboratory-induced mental stress triggers signs of ischemia in 40–70% of stable coronary heart disease patients, who have treadmill-induced ischemia.[41] Signs of ischemia include chest pain, ST-segment depression, wall motion abnormalities, and decreased ejection fraction. Spontaneous emotions produce the same signs of ischemia. Ambulatory ST-segment monitoring over 48 hours was compared with self-reported positive and negative emotions in 132 subjects with coronary heart disease and evidence of ischemia.[42] Feelings of severe tension, frustration, and sadness were associated with a threefold increase in ST-segment depression in the hour after the reported emotion. Lesser levels of negative emotions were associated with little increase in ischemia. In contrast, physical activity resulted in an approximate doubling of likelihood of ischemia. An intense feeling of happiness was associated with a small, but statistically insignificant decrease in ischemia.

Endothelial function, inflammation, and platelet activation

Beyond the traditional risk factors of lipids, blood pressure, and diabetes, emotional distress affects the pathophysiological processes of endothelial dysfunction, inflammation, and platelet activation, which are both chronically atherogenic and initiate acute cardiovascular events. Several studies have documented a decrease in endothelium-dependent vasodilation resulting from acute emotional distress. Brachial artery flow-mediated dilation, a noninvasive measurement of nitric oxide availability, has been the most often utilized technique for studying acute and chronic changes in endothelial function. In a study of 23 healthy subjects, a 3-minute mental stress task decreased flow-mediated dilation by about 50% within 10 minutes and lasting at least 45 minutes.[43] The pre-administration of an endothelin-A receptor blocker prevented the impairment. The administration of norepinephrine did not produce a similar decrease in flow-mediated dilation, suggesting that the emotional stress was not directly related to increased sympathetic tone. An experimental distressing confrontation rapidly decreased flow mediated dilation, which remained impaired for about 4 hours.[44] Alterations of endothelial function are also associated with chronic emotional symptomatology. Flow-mediated dilation is significantly reduced in subjects with depressive symptomatology, as measured by a Beck Depression Index score ≥10.[45] The use of antidepressive medication in this study was associated with an improvement in flow-mediated dilation.

A second association of emotional distress is an increase in circulating markers of inflammation, which along with endothelial dysfunction contributes to both the chronic development of atherosclerosis and to acute plaque rupture. The prospective epidemiological study of myocardial infarction of healthy, middle-aged men found that depressive mood (Welsh depression subscale) was associated with both the incidence of coronary events and increased inflammatory markers including C-reactive protein, interleukin-6, and intercellular adhesion molecule-1.[46] Correction for traditional risk factors did not diminish these associations. Although all of the inflammatory markers are associated with an increased coronary disease risk, the correlation of depressive mood remained after correcting for the inflammatory markers, suggesting additional etiological pathways. Similar increases in intercellular adhesion molecule-1, E-selectin, and monocyte chemoattractant protein were found in 31 young subjects with major depressive syndromes compared with 29 healthy controls.[47] More than 50% reductions in flow-mediated dilation were also observed. There were no significant differences between the groups in traditional risk factors. In contrast, increases in C-reactive protein and interleukin-6 were found in a study of 50 depressed individuals compared with the same number of healthy controls, which was partly explained by increases in body mass index, but not cigarette smoking or subclinical infection.[48]

Alterations of platelet function have also been observed in depressed individuals. In the Sertraline Antidepressant Heart Attack Randomized Trial (SAD-HART), platelet factor-4, β-thromboglobulin, platelet/endothelial cell adhesion molecule, and thromboxane were decreased by selective serotonin reuptake inhibition.[49]

Effect-associated aspects of daily living

Several positive and negative Effect-associated aspects of every day living may have pronounced effects on endothelial function and inflammation. These observations identify potential pathways by which supportive alternative therapies may affect vascular health. Whereas more than 14,000 studies have investigated depressive factors, fewer than 500 studies have been devoted toward positive daily interactions. Pet ownership is an emotionally supportive factor and has been widely recommended for stress reduction. Physical contact with pets acutely lowers heart rate and blood pressure and chronic ownership is associated with persistent reductions in these parameters.[50] This study also demonstrated that pet owners experienced lesser increases in blood pressure and pulse with mental arithmetic and cold pressor testing. In a complementary study, the support afforded by pet ownership reduced mental stress-associated hypertension more than did antihypertensive medication.[51]

Considering the extensive time commonly devoted to watching media, our research group has studied the effect of video viewing on vascular function. We found that healthy young volunteers experienced significant decreases in flow-mediated dilation after watching a troubling video.[52] The same individuals experienced significant increases in flow-mediated dilation following watching a humorous video. Neither change could be explained by hemodynamic factors, suggesting a direct effect on endothelial function. As noted above, vasoconstrictive factors such as endothelin-A appear to be responsible for the affect of negative emotions on endothelial dysfunction. Alternately, the mechanisms by which positive emotions and interactions, such as laughter and pets, improve vascular function are not yet clear. Numerous other aspects of daily functioning, such as sleep deprivation, have also been shown to increase markers of inflammation.[53] These data suggest that both emotional and situational life issues affect the same atherogenic pathways as do traditional risk factors.

IDENTIFYING EMOTIONAL DISTRESS

Since emotional issues often precipitate somatic complaints and play both direct and indirect roles in atherogenesis, cardiologists and other physicians treating heart disease need to be sensitive to their patients' emotional problems. Some symptoms, such as palpitations and shortness of breath can be of either cardiac origin or denote emotional distress. Asking patients about emotional and psychosocial issues conveys the message that these factors are relevant and important.[1] Screening, whether by structured questionnaire or by informal discussion should be directed to emotional factors, such as depression, chronic stressors, such as work or family strain, and somatic complaints, such as fatigue and sleep deprivation. Suggested areas of inquiries include:[1]

- Mood
- Energy level
- Sleep patterns
- Pressure at work and home
- Relaxation activities
- Social support
- Financial difficulties
- Personal concerns

As noted above, both acute stress and adverse daily occurrences contribute to the endothelial dysfunction and inflammation that underlie coronary heart disease.

Acute coronary events, such as myocardial infarction, represent truly life-changing events. Depressive disorders frequently follow coronary events and are associated with poor prognosis and impaired patient compliance with proven therapies. During the post-event period, inquiry about emotional and psychosocial problems may be perceived as threatening, and may elicit denial, defensiveness, and resentment.[1] Openly addressing these issues and placing them in the context of standard therapy can help address patients concerns and fears.

BEHAVIORAL INTERVENTIONS

Lifestyle interventions

Behavioral interventions can be divided into lifestyle management and psychopharmacological interventions. Although usually thought of as a physical cardiac intervention, structured exercise training has important emotional benefit, especially after a coronary event or intervention. Supervised exercise is useful in setting safe limits for physical activity and reassuring patients that they can resume daily activities. Beyond these benefits, physical activity is an excellent antidepressant, with an efficacy equivalent to pharmacological intervention. In a 16-week study comparing the effect of exercise, sertraline, and both in older subjects with major depression, exercise and drug therapy had equal efficacy, both of which were equivalent to the combination.[54] Follow-up of these subjects at 6 months revealed persistence of the antidepressant effects of continued exercise.[55] As with other lifestyle management therapies, referral of patients to organized, monitored exercise programs insures the best compliance and efficacy.

Relaxation training and stress management techniques include muscle relaxation, guided imagery, diaphragmatic breathing, biofeedback, problem solving, and appropriate goal setting. Recommendations for vacations, hobbies, yoga, music, pets, and pleasurable activities may have similar effectiveness.[1] Poor social or structural support should be addressed with concrete suggestions involving support groups and social worker assistance. Work and/or home stress should be addressed with formal or informal counseling.

Psychosocial interventions

Psychosocial interventions, such as stress reduction counseling, are often employed in comprehensive cardiac rehabilitation programs. A meta-analysis of 23 studies demonstrated that the addition of psychosocial interventions to post-infarction cardiac rehabilitation reduced cardiac mortality and recurrent infarctions over 2 years of follow-up.[56] The efficacy of psychosocial interventions appears to affect outcomes in a complex fashion. When stress reduction accompanies counseling, the risk for subsequent mortality and reinfarction are reduced, whereas higher morbidity and mortality occur when stress is not reduced.[57] The failure to respond to psychosocial intervention may identify individuals at high risk for subsequent events.

Stand-alone psychosocial intervention programs have been employed in coronary heart disease with mixed results. Using group therapy directed toward decreasing type A behavior and negative effect, the Recurrent Coronary Prevention Project Study observed a reduction in coronary heart disease mortality and nonfatal myocardial infarction.[58] The Ischemic Heart Disease trial reduced coronary events using a home-based stress-reduction program.[59] Two other large trials did not reduce coronary events, but neither program successfully reduced psychosocial stress.[1] One trial did observe significantly less coronary mortality at 1 year in a subgroup that experienced a reduction in psychological stress. The largest stand-alone trial, the Enhanced Recovery in Coronary Heart Disease Patient (ENRICHD) study, evaluated the effect of individual cognitive and group therapy and use of selective serotonin reuptake inhibitors on post-infarction subjects with depression and/or perceived low social support.[60] No difference in the primary endpoint of all-cause mortality and nonfatal infarction was observed between the treatment and control groups. This lack of effect was attributed to only a modest difference in psychosocial functioning between the treatment groups, perhaps due to more aggressive therapy in the routine medical care arm, which employed cardiac rehabilitation.

Pharmacological intervention

Considerably less data are available on the efficacy of pharmacological therapy in coronary heart disease. The Sertraline Antidepressant heart Attack Randomized Trial (SADHART) demonstrated that a selective serotonin reuptake inhibitor could be safely used for the treatment of clinical depression in patients with coronary heart disease.[61] A trend toward reduced coronary events was observed in this trial, although it was not powered to evaluate efficacy on events. A large observational study supports the safety of selective serotonin reuptake inhibitors in coronary heart disease, but tricyclic antidepressants were associated with a twofold increase in myocardial infarction.[62] A recent case-control study suggests that the safety of selective serotonin reuptake inhibitors is primarily dependent on their receptor affinity.[63]

SUMMARY

Considerable evidence suggests that emotional factors play large role in the genesis and expression of coronary heart disease. Physicians often neglect coronary heart disease-associated emotional distress. Negative affect, chronic stress, perceived social support, and personality disorders significantly increase coronary risk. They also interfere with compliance with lifestyle and pharmacological therapies. Alternately, positive emotions are associated with reduced coronary risk. Some of the atherogenic effect of emotions can be attributed to their association with traditional risk factors. A major portion of this impact, however, results from direct effects on vascular biology, including endothelial dysfunction and inflammation. In addition to their effect on coronary heart disease, emotional disorders commonly present as cardiac somatic complaints, which need to be distinguished from organic disease. Cardiac rehabilitation employing psychosocial counseling can improve negative affect, and when successful reduce subsequent coronary events. The selective serotonin reuptake inhibitors are the preferred treatment for significant depressive disorders in coronary heart disease patients. The close association of emotional functioning and coronary heart disease probably explains a significant portion of the efficacy of some alternative medical treatments.

REFERENCES

1. Rozanski A, Blumenthal JA, Davidson KW, Saab PG, Kubzansky L. The epidemiology, pathophysiology, and management of psychosocial risk factors in cardiac practice. J Am Coll Cardiol. 2005;45:637–51.
2. Lesperance F, Frasure-Smith N, Bourassa MG. Five-year risk of cardiac mortality in relation to initial severity and one-year changes in depression symptoms after myocardial infarction. Circulation. 2002;105:1049–53.
3. Suadicani P, Hein HO, Gyntelberg F. Are social inequalities as associated with the risk of ischaemic heart disease a result of psychosocial working conditions? Atherosclerosis. 1993;101:165–75
4. Todaro JF, Shen B-J, Niaura R, Spiro A, Ward KD. Effect of negative emotions on frequency of coronary heart disease (The Normative Aging Study). Am J Cardiol. 2003;92:901–6.
5. Frasure-Smith N, Lesperance F, Talajic M. Depression following myocardial infarction. Impact on 6-month survival. JAMA. 1993;270:1819–25.
6. Rumsfeld JS, Havranek EH, Masoudi FA, et al. Depressive symptoms are the strongest predictors of short-term declines in health status in patients with heart failure. J Am Coll Cardiol. 2003;42:1811–7.
7. Strik JJMH, Denoller J, Louisberg R, Honig A. Comparing symptoms of depression and anxiety as predictors of cardiac events and increased health care consumption after myocardial infarction. J Am Coll Cardiol. 2003;42:1801–7.
8. Paterniti S, Zureik M, Ducimetiere P, Touboul P-J, Feve J-M, Alperovitch A. Sustained anxiety and 4-year progression of carotid atherosclerosis. Arterioscler Thromb Vasc Biol. 2001;21:136–41.
9. Kubzansky LD, Kawachi I, Spiro A, Weiss ST, Vokonas PS, Sparrow D. Is worrying bad for your heart? A prospective study of work and coronary heart disease in the Normative Aging Study. Circulation. 1997;95:818–24.
10. Kawachi I, Sparrow D, Vokonas PS, Weiss ST. Symptoms of anxiety and risk of coronary heart disease. The Normative Aging Study. Circulation. 1004;90:2225–9.
11. Sullivan MD, LaCroix AZ, Spertus JA, Hecht J. Five-year study of the effects of anxiety and depression in patients with coronary artery disease. Am J Cardiol. 2000;86:1135–7.
12. Rutledge T, Reis S, Olson M, et al. History of anxiety disorders is associated with a decreased likelihood of angiographic coronary artery disease in women with chest pain: the WISE study. J Am Coll Cardiol. 2001;37:780–5.
13. O'Malley PG, Jones DL, Feuerstein IM, Taylor AJ. Lack of correlation between psychological factors and subclinical coronary artery disease. N Engl J Med. 2000;343:1298–304.

14. Fleet RP, Dupuis G, Marchand A, et al. Panic disorder in coronary artery disease patients with noncardiac chest pain. J Psychosom Res. 1998;44:81–90.

15. Kirmayer LJ, Robbins JM, Dworkin M, Yaffe MJ. Somatization and the recognition of depression and anxiety in primary care. Am J Psychiatry. 1993;150:734–41.

16. Williams JE, Paton CC, Siegler IC, Eigenbrodt ML, Nieto FJ, Tyroler HA. Anger proneness predicts coronary heart disease risk. Prospective analysis from the Atherosclerosis Risk in Communities (ARIC) Study. Circulation. 2000;101:2034–9.

17. Matthews KA, Gump BB, Harris KF, Haney TL, Barefoot JC. Hostile behaviors predict cardiovascular mortality in the Multiple Risk Factor Intervention Trial. Circulation. 2004;109:66–70.

18. Angerer P, Siebert U, Kothny W, Muhlbauer D, Mudra H, von Shacky C. Impact of social support, cynical hostility and anger expression on progression of coronary atherosclerosis. J Am Coll Cardiol. 2000;36:1781–8.

19. Know SS, Adelman A, Ellison RC, et al. Hostility, social support, and carotid artery atherosclerosis in the National Heart, Lung, and Blood Institute Family Heart Study. Am J Cardiol. 2000;86:1086–9.

20. Iribarren C, Sidney S, Bild DE. et al. Association of hostility with coronary artery calcification in young adults. JAMA. 2000;283:2546–51.

21. Kubzansky LD, Sparrow D, Vokonas P, Kawachi I. Is the glass half empty or half full? A prospective study of optimism and coronary heart disease in the Normative Aging Study. Psychosom Med. 2001;63:910–6.

22. Scheier MF, Metthews KA, Owens JF, et al. Optimism and rehospitalization after coronary artery bypass graft surgery. Arch Intern Med. 1999;159:829–35.

23. Ragland DR, Brand RJ. Type A behavior and mortality from coronary heart disease. N Engl J Med. 1988;318:65–9.

24. Pedersen SS, Lemos PA, van Vooren PR, et al. Type D personality predicts death or myocardial infarction after bare metal stent or sirolimus-eluting stent implantation. J Am Coll Cardiol. 2004;44:997–1001.

25. Mausner-Dorsch H, Eaton WW. Psychosocial work environment and depression: epidemiologic assessment of the demand-control model. Am J Public Health. 2000;90:1765–70.

26. Ruberman W, Weinblatt E, Goldberg JD, Chaudhary B. Psychosocial influences on mortality after myocardial infarction. N Engl J Med. 1984;311:552–9.

27. McCabe PM, Gonzales JA, Zaias J, et al. Social environment influences the progression of atherosclerosis in the Wantanabe heritable hyperlipidemic rabbit. Circulation. 2002;105:354.

28. Johnson JV, Stewart W, Hall EM, Fredlund P, Theorell T. Long-term psychosocial work environment and cardiovascular mortality among Swedish men. Am J Public Health. 1996;86:324–31.

29. Kivimaki M, Luukkonen R, Ruhimaki H, Vahtera J, Kirjonen J. Work stress and risk of cardiovascular mortality: prospective cohort study of industrial employees. BMJ. 2002;325:857–60.

30. Lynch J, Krause N, Kaplan GA, Salonen R, Salonen JT. Workplace demands, economic reward, and progression of carotid atherosclerosis. Circulation. 1997;96:302–7.

31. Hlatky MA, Lam L, Lee KL, et al. Job strain and the prevalence and outcome of coronary artery disease. Circulation. 1995;92:327–33.

32. Orth-Gomer K, Wamala SP, Horsten M, Schenck-Gustafson K, Schneiderman N, Mittleman MA. Marital stress worsens prognosis in women with coronary heart disease: the Stockholm Female Coronary Risk Study. JAMA. 2000;284:3008–14.

33. Gallo LC, Troxel WM, Kuller LH, et al. Marital status, marital quality, and athero-sclerotic burden in postmenopausal women. Psychosom Med. 2003;65:952–62.

34. Coyne JC, Rohrbaugh MJ, Shoham V, Sonnega JS, Nicklas JM, Cranford JA. Prognostic importance of marital quality for survival of congestive heart failure. Am J Cardiol. 2001;88:526–9.

35. Lee S, Colditz GA, Berkman LF, Kawachi I. Caregiving and risk of coronary heart disease in U.S. women: a prospective study. Am J Prev Med. 2003;24:113–9.

36. Schultz R, Beach SR. Caregiving as a risk factor for mortality: the Caregiver Health Effects Study. JAMA. 1999;282:2215–9.

37. Lawlor DA, Emberson JR, Ebrahim S, et al. Is the association between parity and coronary heart disease due to biological effects of pregnancy or adverse lifestyle risk factors associated with child-rearing? Findings from the British Women's Heart and Health Study and the British Regional Heart Study. Circulation. 2003;107:1260–4.

38. Carney RM, Blumenthal JA, Stein PK, et al. Depression, heart rate variability, and acute myocardial infarction. Circulation. 2001;104:2024–8.

39. Dallman MF, La Fluer S, Pecoraro NC, Gomez F, Houshyar H, Akana SF. Minireview: glucocorticoids—food intake, abdominal obesity, and wealthy nations in 2004. Endocrinology. 2004;145:2633–8.

40. Broadley AJM, Korszun A, Abdelaal E, et al. Inhibition of cortisol production with metyrapone prevents mental stress-induced endothelial dysfunction and baroreflex impairment. J Am Coll Cardiol. 2005;46:344–50.

41. Sheps DS, McMahon RP, Becker L, et al. Mental stress-induced ischemia and all-cause mortality in patients with coronary artery disease. Results from the Psychophysiological Investigations in Myocardial Infarction Study. Circulation. 2002;105:1780–4.

42. Gullette ECD, Blumenthal JA, Babyak M, et al. Effects of mental stress on myocar-dial ischemia during daily life. JAMA. 1997;277:1621–6.

43. Spieker LE, Hurlimann D, Ruschitzka F, et al. Mental stress induces prolonged endothelial dysfunction via endothelin-A receptors. Circulation. 2002;105:2817–20.

44. Ghiadoni L, Donald AE, Cropley M, et al. Mental stress induces transient endothe-lial dysfunction in humans. Circulation. 2000;102:2473–78.

45. Sherwood A, Hinderliter AL, Watkins LI, Waugh RA, Blumenthal JA. Impaired endothelial function in coronary heart disease patients with depressive symptoma-tology. J Am Coll Cardiol. 2005;46:656–9.

46. Empana JP, Sykes DH, Luc G, et al. Contributions of depressive mood and circulat-ing inflammatory markers to coronary heart disease in healthy European men. The Prospective Epidemiological Study of Myocardial Infarction (PRIME). Circulation. 2005;111:2299–305.

47. Rajagopalan S, Brook R, Rubenfire M, Pitt E, Young E, Pitt B. Abnormal brachial artery flow-mediated vasodilation in young adults with major depression. Am J Cardiol. 2001;88:196.

48. Miller GE, Stetler CA, Carney RM, Freedland KR, Banks WA. Clinical depression and inflammatory risk markers for coronary heart disease. Am J Cardiol. 2002;90:1279–83.

49. Serebruany VL, Glassman AH, Malinin AI, et al. Platelet/endothelial biomarkers in depressed patients treated with the selective serotonin reuptake inhibitor sertraline after acute coronary events. The Sertraline Antidepressant Heart Attack Randomized Trial (SADHART) platelet substudy. Circulation. 2003;108:939–44.

50. Allen K, Blascovich J, Mendes WB. Cardiovascular reactivity and the presence of pets, friends, and spouses: the truth about dogs and cats. Psychosom Med. 2002;64:727–39.

51. Allen K, Shykoff BE, Izzo JL. Pet ownership, but not ACE inhibitor therapy, blunts home blood pressure responses to mental stress. Hypertension. 2001;38:815–20.
52. Miller M, Mangano C, Park Y, Goel R, Plotnick G, Vogel R. Impact of cinematic viewing on endothelial function. Heart. (in press).
53. Meier-Ewert HK, Ridker PM, Rifai N, et al. Effect of sleep loss on C-reactive protein, an inflammatory marker of cardiovascular risk. J Am Coll Cardiol. 2004;43:678–83.
54. Blumenthal JA, Babyak MA, Moore KA, et al. Effects of exercise on older patients with major depression. Arch Intern Med. 1999;159:2349–56.
55. Babyak M, Blumenthal JA, Herman S, et al. Exercise treatment for major depression: maintenance of therapeutic effect at 10 months. Psychosom Med. 2000;62:633–8.
56. Linden W, Stoussel C, Maurice J. Psychosocial interventions for patients with coronary artery disease: a meta-analysis. Arch Intern Med. 1997;156:745–52.
57. Dusseldorp E, van Elderen T, Maes S, Meulman J, Kraaij V. A meta-analysis of psychoeducational programs for coronary heart disease patients. Health Psychol. 1999;18:506–19.
58. Friedman M, Thoresen CE, Gill J, et al. Alteration of type A behavior and its effect on cardiac recurrences in postmyocardial infarction patients: summary results of the Recurrent Coronary Prevention Project. Am Heart J. 1986;112:653–65.
59. Frasure-Smith N, Prince R. The Ischemic Heart Disease Life Stress Monitoring Program: impact on mortality. Psychosom Med. 1985;47:431–45.
60. The ENRICHD Investigators. Effects of treating depression and low perceived social support on clinical events after myocardial infarction: the Enhanced Recovery in Coronary Heart Disease Patients (ENRICHD) randomized trial. JAMA. 2003; 289:3106–16.
61. Glassman AH, O'Connor CK, Califf RM, et al. Sertraline treatment of major depression in patients with acute MI or unstable angina. JAMA. 2002;288:701–9.
62. Cohen HW, Gibson G, Alderman MH, et al. Excess risk of myocardial infarction in patients treated with antidepressant medications: association with use of tricyclic agents. Am J Med. 2000;108:2–8.
63. Sauer WH, Berlin JA, Kimmel SE. Selective serotonin reuptake inhibitors and myocardial infarction. Circulation. 2001;104:1894–8.

21

NONTRADITIONAL APPROACHES TO LIPOPROTEIN METABOLISM MANIPULATION

H. Robert Superko

INTRODUCTION

With the relative success of the pharmacologically induced cholesterol-lowering trials, interest has increased in possible nontraditional methods of lipoprotein manipulation. The agents discussed in this chapter include alcohol, artihcoke, cinnamon, polycosinol, red rice yeast, and vitamin E.

In March 2003, the FDA unveiled new rules designed to ensure that dietary supplements are produced in clean plants, are genuine, and remain uncontaminated. In addition to quality and cleanliness, they set standards for inspections and record-keeping. The FDA has the power to remove products from the market if they are adulterated or contain subpotent or superpotent levels of the wrong ingredients, or contaminants. Methods of enforcing of these rules are unclear.

A large number of patients utilize dietary supplements. A report from the Kaiser Permanente Medical Care program in Northern California reported that 84% of women aged 65–84 years used dietary supplements in the past year. About 82% used a vitamin/mineral supplement, 59% a supplement other than vitamins, 32% a nonmineral supplements including herbs.[1]

ALCOHOL

Oral alcohol consumption has been employed for thousands of years as a medicinal product. Only recently has it been suggested that it may have beneficial effects in regard to coronary heart disease (CHD) risk. Large risk association studies have reported a statistically significant relationship between the amount of alcohol consumed and reduced CHD risk.[2] Reputedly beneficial metabolic effects of alcohol consumption include increased high-density lipoprotein cholesterol (HDL-C), improved thrombolysis, and reduced platelet adhesion.

In deciding whether to use such associations to make medical recommendations to patients, at least four issues must be addressed. *First*, association studies only suggest a physiological relationship and no matter how many variables are used in the multivariant regression equation, a successful prospective randomized trial is commonly required prior to adoption as a clinical tool. The only National Institutes of Health-funded randomized prospective trial of alcohol consumption demonstrated that a rise in HDL-C did occur with daily alcohol consumption. However, it was also reported that the increase was in the HDL3 subfraction and not in the reputedly more beneficial HDL2 subfraction.[3] *Second*, alcohol consumption is well established to be associated with adverse health outcomes such as alcoholism, hepatic disease, and hypertension.[4-6] *Third*, alcohol consumption impairs fine motor skills and judgement that may result in harm. *Fourth*, the reputed beneficial cardiovascular effects of alcohol consumption may be linked to specific polymorphisms such as genetic variation in alcohol dehydrogenase-1C, and thus not be applicable to the entire population.[7] In France, the WHO reports that the leading cause of death are external causes, including automobile accidents and suicide, often linked to alcohol consumption.[8]

Thus, no matter how popular the notion that alcohol consumption may be beneficial to cardiovascular health, we urge caution in recommending this to patients.

ARTICHOKE

Medicinal properties of artichoke (*Cynara scolymus*) have been described since ancient times and generally promoted as an artichoke leaf extract (ALE). Beneficial properties have been historically attributed to its choleretic activity and antidyspeptic action, although some inhibition of cholesterol biosynthesis and low-density lipoprotein (LDL) oxidation may occur. In rats, ALE has been reported to increase total bile acid concentration.[9]

Two randomized trials have reported some blood cholesterol reduction with ALE.[10] After 42 days of treatment, total blood cholesterol reduction from 299 mg/dL to 244 mg/dL (-18%) was reported, which was significantly different from the placebo group.

Artichoke may have cardiovascular benefits other than blood lipid effects. In human hyperlipidemic subjects administered artichoke juice, brachial flow-mediated vasodilation was increased and markers of vascular cell adhesion decreased including VCAM-1 and ICAM-1.[11]

CINNAMON

It has been suggested that cinnamon extract (*Cinnamomi cassiae*) may have antidiabetic attributes that may have beneficial effects on lipoproteins. However, clinical data is sparse. In a diabetic animal model, cinnamon extract was reported to decrease blood sugar in a dose dependent manner and this was associated with higher HDL-C levels along with reduced triglycerides and total cholesterol.[12] One study in human volunteers revealed some benefit in humans as well. About 60 subjects with Type II diabetes were randomized to placebo or 1, 3, or 6 g cinnamon per day for 40 days. In this investigation no change in HDL-C was noted but triglycerides were reduced 23–30% and LDL-C 7–27%.[13]

POLICOSANOL

Policosanol is a mixture of alcohols isolated from sugarcane (*Saccharum officinarum* L.) that has been researched primarily in Cuba. It is reported to consist of 66% octacosanol, 12% triacontanol, and 7% hexacosanol, with other minor components.[14] Several potentially beneficial effects are attributed to policosanol, including improved blood lipids, reduced LDL oxidation potential, decreased platelet aggregation, and decreased smooth muscle proliferation. It is believed to reduce LDL-C by decreasing 3-hydroxy-3-methyl-glutaryl-CoA (HMG-CoA) synthesis and increasing its degradation.

Studies in patients with elevated blood cholesterol levels have reported LDL-C reductions of approximately 20%. Change in HDL-C does not appear to be consistent with some investigations revealing an increase and others a decrease. The majority of older studies did not incorporate a randomized placebo-controlled design, making it difficult to interpret the data. Recently a German multicenter, randomized, placebo-controlled, parallel-group trial of the effect of 12 weeks of policosanol (10, 20, 40, 80 mg/day) compared to placebo was reported in 143 subjects.[15] Subjects had LDL-C values at baseline of approximately 187 mg/dL, HDL-C of approximately 51 mg/dL, and triglycerides of approximately 175 mg/dL. There was no significant reduction in LDL-C and no dose response that could be demonstrated. Side effect incidence has been difficult to determine since only postmarketing studies were available for analysis. The recent well-designed study by Berthold and colleagues confirms a low incidence of side effects in this 12-week study. This lack of lipid effect had been previously reported in a smaller investigation of 58 subjects who were randomized to either wheat germ policosanol (20 mg) mixed in chocolate pellets or placebo mixed in chocolate pellets for 4 weeks.[16]

RED YEAST RICE

Red yeast rice extract has been used since at least the Tang dynasty (AD 800) in China for the treatment of heart disease patients.[17] Relatively recently it was determined that HMG-CoA reductase inhibition action can be linked to naturally occurring substances called monacolins. Monacolin K is also named mevinolin or lovastatin.[18] The active agent is *Monascus purpureus*, which is derived from fermented rice and contains greater than nine different monacolins in addition to β-sitosterol, campesterol, stigmasterol, sapogenin, isoflavones, and monounsaturated fatty acids.[19]

Blood lipid and pathological effects of one product, cholestin, have been tested in animal models. In cholesterol-fed rabbits, cholestin treatment (0.4 or 1.35 g/kg/day) significantly reduced LDL-C and Apo B, and increased HDL-C.[20] Examination of arterial segments revealed a significant reduction in sudanophilic area from 81% in the control group to 17–30% in the cholestin-treated groups. A similar rabbit model of atherosclerosis was used to investigate the combined effect of red yeast rice and policosanol on lipids and atherosclerosis.[21] Red yeast rice significantly reduced lipid infiltration into the aortic wall but the combination of red yeast rice and policosanol was most effective in preventing atherosclerosis build in this cholesterol-fed rabbit model of atherosclerosis.

There are many red yeast rice products and lovastatin generally comprises approximately 0.2% of the total product. Daily doses of 2.4 g of red yeast rice is roughly equivalent to 4.8 mg lovastatin. Many of the clinical trials employing the FDA-approved lovastatin product utilized 20–40 mg/day lovastatin.

Quality control for monacolin content and potential toxic byproducts is a concern. Citrinin is a toxic fermentation product of red yeast rice and creates a potential health hazard when ingested. Nine commercial products have been tested for monacolin and citrinin content. The monacolin content varied between 9% and 0.6% wet weight and only one of nine preparations had a full complement of 10 monacolin compounds. The toxic citrinin product was found in 78% of the preparations.[19] Anaphylaxis due to *M. purpureus*-fermented rice has been reported and the FDA has the right to regulate this product.[22,23]

Public interest in red yeast rice or Colestin is generated due to the effect on LDL-C reduction and the belief that a "natural" product has superior benefits in regard to efficacy and safety, when compared to pharmaceutical products. Relatively small studies that utilized control or placebo groups demonstrate an approximate 20–30% reduction in LDL-C, 15–35% reduction in triglycerides, and 0–20% increase in HDL-C.[24] In a small randomized, placebo-controlled trial of cholestin in HIV-related dyslipidemia, a 32% reduction in LDL-C with no change in triglycerides or HDL-C was reported.[25]

Xuezhikang is an extract of cholestin that has been approved by the FDA. The effect on cholesterol, lipoprotein(a) (Lp[a]) and highly sensitive C-reactive protein (hsCRP) has been reported. A nonrandomized study reported the effect of two doses of xuezhikang on blood lipids and hsCRP. Administration of 1200 or 2400 mg/day xuezhikang resulted in respectively a 23% and 32% reduction in LDL-C, a 13% and 23% reduction in triglycerides, and no change in HDL-C. HsCRP was reduced 22% and 25% with 1200 or 2400 mg/day xuezhikang. About 60 CHD patients were randomized to 300 mg bid cholestin or placebo for 6 weeks. In this relatively short-term study, Xuezhikang was reported to significantly ($p < 0.05$) reduce fasting and post-fat meal load triglycerides and Lp(a).[26] Fasting LDL-C was reduced 30%, triglycerides 25%, and Lp(a) 23% ($p < 0.05$). HDL-C increased 16% ($p < 0.05$). These changes were accompanied by a significant reduction in hsCRP.

VITAMIN E

The role of oxidation in the atherogenic process has been well elucidated.[27,28] Less clear is the possible potential benefit of antioxidant therapy. Vitamin E has been established to provide antioxidant protection in vitro.[29] Studies in humans have associated increased lipoprotein oxidation potential with increased CHD risk.[30]

Susceptibility of lipoproteins to oxidation is in-part due to inherited lipoprotein issues that result in a particle more, or less, susceptible to oxidative damage. LDL subclass pattern B subjects have a threefold increased CAD risk, independent of other risk factors and lipoproteins.[31] It has been shown to have a significantly increased rate of oxidation in LDL subclass fraction 1, which includes triglyceride-rich remnant particles. Lipoproteins from LDL pattern B subjects have significantly less antioxidant content (such as vitamin E) compared to pattern A subjects, particularly in the IDL region.[32]

The result of the Cambridge Heart Antioxidant Study (CHAOS) raised optimism that antioxidation therapy may provide cardiovascular benefit. In 2002 CHD patients undergoing angiography, a significant reduction in nonfatal myocardial infraction (MI) was reported after 17 months of treatment with 400–800 IU/day α-tocopherol.[33] A slightly higher, but not statistically significant, incident of fatal MI and total CVD death was noted in the vitamin E compared to placebo group, but this was offset by a significant 66% reduction in nonfatal MI ($p = 0.0001$). The initial optimism has been cooled by the reports of the HOPE and HDL Atherosclerosis Treatment Study (HATS) trials. The HOPE trial utilized a large cohort randomized to vitamin E and no beneficial cardiovascular benefit could be attributed to the vitamin E therapy.[34] The HATS tested the hypothesis that treatment with a statin plus nicotinic acid, with or without an antioxidant cocktail that included vitamin E, vitamin C, β-carotene, and selenium, would reduce cardiovascular events and arteriographic progression.[35] HATS successfully demonstrated a significant reduction in both clinical events and arteriographic coronary artery change in the group randomized to statin plus nicotinic acid. However, the addition of the antioxidant cocktail blunted the ability of nicotinic acid to increase HDLC and significantly blunted the reduction in clinical events and arteriographic benefit. This pivotol study suggests that such a cocktail might be detrimental by decreasing benefit associated with a statin plus nicotinic acid combination treatment in CHD patients with low HDL-C and heralds the end of a long romance with antioxidant supplements.[36]

REFERENCES

1. Gordon NP, Schaffer DM. Use of dietary supplements by female seniors in a large Northern California health plan. BMC Geriatr. 2005;5:4.
2. Gaziano JM, Gaziano TA, Glynn RJ, Sesso HD, Ajani UA, Stampfer MJ, et al. Light-to-moderate alcohol consumption and mortality in the Physicians' Health Study enrollment cohort. J Am Coll Cardiol. 2000 Jan;35(1):96–105.

3. Haskell WL, Camargo C, Jr, Williams PT, Vranizan KM, Krauss RM, Lindgren FT, et al. The effect of cessation and resumption of moderate alcohol intake on serum high-density-lipoprotein subfractions. A controlled study. N Engl J Med. 1984 Mar 29;310(13):805–10.

4. Adachi M, Brenner DA. Clinical syndromes of alcoholic liver disease. Dig Dis. 2005;23(3–4):255–63.

5. Bathgate AJ. UK Liver Transplant Units. Recommendations for alcohol-related liver disease. Lancet. 2006 Jun 24;367(9528):2045–6.

6. Puddey IB, Beilin LJ. Alcohol is bad for blood pressure. Clin Exp Pharmacol Physiol. 2006 Sep;33(9):847–52.

7. Younis J, Cooper JA, Miller GJ, Humphries SE, Talmud PJ. Genetic variation in alcohol dehydrogenase 1C and the beneficial effect of alcohol intake on coronary heart disease risk in the Second Northwick Park Heart Study. Atherosclerosis. 2005 Jun;180(2):225–32. Epub 2005 Jan 15.

8. http://www.euro.who.int/eprise/main/WHO/Progs/CHHFRA/burden/20050

9. Saenz Rodriguez T, Garcia Gimenez D, de la Puerta Vazquez R. Choleretic activity and biliary elimination of lipids and bile acids induced by an artichoke leaf extract in rats. Phytomedicine. 2002 Dec;9(8):687–93.

10. Pittler MH, Thompson CO, Ernst E. Artichoke leaf extract for treating hypercholesterolaemia. Cochrane Database Syst Rev. 2002;(3):CD003335.

11. Lupattelli G, Marchesi S, Lombardini R, Roscini AR, Trinca F, Gemelli F, et al. Artichoke juice improves endothelial function in hyperlipemia. Life Sci. 2004 Dec 31; 76(7):775–82.

12. Kim SH, Hyun SH, Choung SY. Anti-diabetic effect of cinnamon extract on blood glucose in db/db mice. J Ethnopharmacol. 2005 Oct 3; [Epub ahead of print.]

13. Khan A, Safdar M, Ali Khan MM, Khattak KN, Anderson RA. Cinnamon improves glucose and lipids of people with type 2 diabetes. Diabetes Care. 2003 Dec; 26(12):3215–8.

14. Arruzazabala ML, Noa M, Menendez R, et al. Protective effect of policosanol on atherosclerotic lesions in rabbits with exogenous hypercholesterolemia. Braz J Med Biol Res. 2000;33:835–40.

15. Berthold HK, Unverdorben S, Degenhardt R, Bulitta M, Gouni-Berthold I. Effect of policosanol on lipid levels among patients with hypercholesterolemia or combined hyperlipidemia. JAMA. 295:2262–9.

16. Lin Y, Rudrum M, van der Wielen RP, Trautwein EA, McNeill G, Sierksma A, Meijer GW. Wheat germ policosanol failed to lower plasma cholestrol in subjects with normal to mildly elevated cholesterol concentrations. Metabolism. 2004 Oct; 53(10):1309–14.

17. Patrick L et al. www.thorne.com/altmedrev

18. Huang HN, Hua YY, Bao GR, Xie LH. The quantification of monacolin K in some red yeast rice from Fujian province and the comparison of the other product. Chem Pharm Bull (Tokyo). 2006 May;54(5):687–9.

19. David Heber, Audra Lembertas, Qing-Yi Lu, Susan Bowerman, VavLiang W. Go. An analysis of Nine Proprietary Chinese Red Yeast Rice Dietary Supplements: Implications of Variability in Chemical Profile and Contents. The Journal of Alternative and Complementary Medicine. 2001 Apr;7(2):133–9.

20. Wei W, Li C, Want Y, Su H, Zhu J, Kritchevsky D. Hypolipdemia and anti-atherogenic effects of long-term Cholestin in cholesterol red rabbits. J Nutr Biochem. 2003; 14:314–8.

21. Setnikar I, Senin P, Rovati LC. Antiatherosclerotic efficacy of policosanol, red yeast rice extract and astaxanthin in the rabbit. Arzneimittelforschung. 2005;55:312–7.
22. Wigger-Alberti W Bauer A, Hipler UC, Elsner P. Anaphylaxis due to Monascus purpureus-fermented rice (red yeast rice). Allergy. 1999;1330–1.
23. Ruth SoRelle. Sentinel Emergency Departments Report Safety Net Frayed by Uninsured and Managed care. Circulation. 2000;102;e9012.
24. Wang et al. A multi-center clinical trial of the serum lipid-lowering effect of Monascus purpureus (red yeast) rice preparation from TCM. Cur Ther Res. 1997; 58:964–78.
25. Keithley et al. A pilot study of the safety and efficacy of cholestin in treating. HIV-related dyslipidemia. Nutrition. 2002;18:201–4.
26. Lie L, Zhao SP, Cheng YC, Li YL. Xuezhikang decreases serum lipoprotein(a) and c-reactive protein concentrations in patients with coronary heart disease. Clin Chem. 2003;49:1347–52.
27. Steinberg D. Beyond cholesterol. Modifications of low-density lipoprotein that increase its atherogenicity. NEJM. 1989;320:915–21.
28. Steinberg D. Antioxidant vitamins and coronary heart disease. NEJM. 1993;328:1487–9.
29. Laranjinha J, Cadenas E. Redox cycles of caffeic acid, alpha-tocopherol, and ascorbate: implications for protection of low-density lipoproteins against oxidation. IUBMB Life. 1999 Jul;48(1):57–65.
30. Chait A, Brazg RL, Tribble DL, Krauss RM. Susceptibility of small, dense, low-density lipoproteins to oxidative modification in subjects with the atherogenic lipoprotein phenotype, pattern B. Am J Med. 1993;94:350–6.
31. Superko HR, Chronos NA. Hypercholesterolemia and dyslipidemia. Issues for clinicians. Curr Treatment Options in CV Med. 2004;5:35–50.
32. Tribble DL, van den Berg JJM, Motchnik PA, Ames BN, Lewis DM, Chait A, et al. Oxidative susceptibility of low density lipoprotein subfractions is related to their Ubiquinol-10 and alpha-tocopherol content. Proc Natl Acad Sci USA. 1994;91:1183–7.
33. Stephens NG, Parsons A, Schofield PM, Kelly F, Cheeseman K, Mitchinson MJ. Randomised controlled trial of vitamin E in patients with coronary disease: Cambridge Heart Antioxidant Study (CHAOS). Lancet. 1996;347:781–6.
34. Heart Outcomes Prevention Evaluation Study Investigators. NEJM. 2000;342: 154–60.
35. Brown GB, Zhao XQ, Chait A, Fisher LD, Cheung MC, Morse JS, et al. Simvastatin and niacin, antioxidant vitamins, or the combination for the prevention of coronary disease. NEJM. 2001;345:1583–92.
36. Brown BG, Cheung MC, Lee AC, Zhao XQ, Chait A. Antioxidant vitamins and lipid therapy: end of a long romance? Arterioscler Thromb Vasc Biol. 2002 Oct 1;22(10): 1535–46.

PART

5

SPECIAL CONSIDERATION AREAS

22

HERBS FOR MENOPAUSE AND CARDIOVASCULAR DISEASE

Sara L. Warber

INTRODUCTION

Prior to 2002, hormone replacement therapy (HRT) was promoted as the standard of care for women during menopause. HRT was effective in reducing symptoms of hot flashes and night sweats, but perhaps more importantly HRT was thought to reduce cardiovascular risks as well as risk of osteoporosis. In 2002, the Women's Health Initiative randomized controlled cardiovascular disease prevention trial (RCT) of estrogen plus progestin versus placebo in healthy postmenopausal women was stopped prematurely.[1] The study showed increased risk of coronary heart disease, invasive breast cancer, stroke, and pulmonary embolism. On balance, these risks outweighed the benefits of reductions in colorectal cancer, endometrial cancer, and hip fractures. Overnight, women and their physicians needed to rethink and explore new territory in order to consistently promote both menopausal and cardiovascular health. For many women, who were already using or interested in alternative medicine, this became an opportunity to experiment with many herbs and supplements to meet their needs. For physicians, it has meant delving into a new knowledge base, deciphering risks versus benefits, and embracing a pluralistic approach to both menopause and cardiovascular health.

This chapter provides some guidance in the use of herbs for both of these problems. It covers approaches to the patient encounter, resources for the busy clinician, brief reviews of major herbs for menopausal symptoms and cardiovascular health, and a suggested holistic plan. Engaging in the discussion with women about these topics may be time consuming, but brings potential rewards in enhanced health for women in the menopausal years.

STRATEGY AND RESOURCES

In order to effectively counsel women in their quest for relief of menopausal symptoms and pursuit of cardiovascular health, it is important to have a consistent strategy. The first principle is to establish a mutually respectful trusting relationship. Women are sensitive to issues of respect and many will have done extensive research prior to engaging in a discussion with their physician. Seek out their knowledge and use it as a starting place for the conversation.

Always ask about supplement use, even if you think that it is unlikely. For all new patients, I recommend that they bring all supplement containers to the first appointment and the clinic staff documents these for the chart. Experience has taught me that women often change the supplements based on advice from family and friends or what is readily available. I emphasize choosing a limited number of supplements and using brands that have been tested by independent third party investigators such as consumerlab.com or NSF.

Invariably, I need to learn about new herbs or refresh my knowledge of familiar ones. For quick, on-the-fly updates, I use naturaldatabase.com or eFacts.com. Each database summarizes the available literature in easy to use formats. Naturaldatabase.com is useful because you can look up actual brand names of products and follow links to learn about various ingredients. eFacts.com has a useful drug–herb interaction checker. For more in-depth information, I use CAM on PubMed sponsored by the National Center for Complementary and Alternative Medicine at the National Institutes of Health. It is limited to searching articles classified under the complementary medicine Mesh heading thus leading to efficient searching for clinical purposes. Having these databases readily available on your computer and using them frequently will go a long way toward improving your confidence in making recommendations. The remainder of this chapter will summarize the evidence to date on herbs for menopausal symptoms and herbs for cardiovascular health. Keep in mind, however, that this is one of the fastest growing fields in medicine and new insights are published frequently!

HERBS FOR MENOPAUSE

Soy

Controversy exists about the benefit of soy for reduction of hot flashes and protection from heart disease or osteoporosis. Soy foods contain phytoestrogens. There are three classes of phytoestrogens: isoflavones found primarily in soy products, lignans found in most fiber-rich foods, and coumestans found in many plants. Adding to the controversy about whether to recommend soy is the concern related to possible negative effects of phytoestrogens on endometrial hyperplasia and breast cancer. It is important to differentiate between studies done with soy protein versus those done with soy isoflavones versus those with soy whole foods in the diet.

Four studies on the effect of supplementation with soy isoflavones on menopausal symptoms have been reported. A randomized controlled trial (RCT) was done using 100 mg of soy isoflavone supplementation daily versus a purified soy protein and glucose placebo. About 80 women studied for 4 months showed a significant decrease, for the isoflavone group, in vasomotor complaints, insomnia, and depression. Two other investigators conducted placebo-controlled trials and found that both groups, isoflavone (80–90 mg/day) and placebo, had significant reductions in hot flushes after 3 or 6 months.[2]

An uncontrolled trial documented reductions in hot flashes over 4 months in 80% of the participants with just 35 mg/day of soy isoflavone.[3] Two 3-month studies of soy protein and soy flour showed similar mixed results. Soy protein was more effective than placebo in reducing hot flashes by 45% versus 30% ($p < 0.01$),[4] while soy flour and the placebo, wheat flour, both significantly reduced hot flashes and other menopausal symptoms in another study.[5] These data point out the high rate of placebo effect in menopause trials, which makes it difficult to sort out the difference in effects of soy isoflavones and soy protein. It does appear that higher doses (100 mg of soy isoflavones or 60 g of soy protein) may be beneficial in reducing menopausal symptoms and hot flashes.

Because of its estrogen-like effects, soy isoflavones, soy protein, and dietary soy also have been examined for their effects on bone loss, cognition, and the cardiovascular system. An RCT of isoflavones and an epidemiological study of dietary soy both showed that modest increases in bone mineral content were associated with higher soy intake.[6] Two other studies do not document improvements in bone mineral density.[7,8] Another RCT showed improved cognition with 110 mg of soy isoflavones daily.[9] It has been shown that 25–30 g of soy protein per day is sufficient to decrease serum cholesterol levels in those with initially high serum levels. However, studies using isolated isoflavone supplements have not shown any effect on lipids.[10,11] In a case-control study involving 947 women, higher isoflavone and lignan intake lowered endometrial cancer risk.[12] It is reasonable to recommend whole food soy products in the diet for their probable benefit accompanied by low risk. Women with or at risk for breast cancer should limit soy intake because the benefit to risk ratio is not as favorable based on preliminary animal studies.[13]

Flaxseed

Flaxseed is particularly high in lignan and phytoestrogens and of flaxseed daily intake of 40 g has been shown to be as effective as oral estrogen-progesterone therapy to control mild menopausal symptoms. It did not improve lipid profiles in women with hypercholesterolemia, but did lower serum insulin and glucose levels.[14] In another RCT using the same dose of 40 g ground seed daily for 3 months, post-menopausal women experienced a decrease in total cholesterol by 6%, Apo A-1 by 6%, and Apo B by 7.5%. There was no stimulation of bone metabolism.[15] Subsequently a year-long RCT comparing flaxseed to wheat germ placebo showed that flaxseed produced clinically minor reduction in total cholesterol, no change in bone mineral density, and a reduction in menopausal symptoms equivalent to placebo.[16] Current investigations focus on flaxseed as a source of the omega-3 fatty acid, α-linolenic acid, a precursor for eicosapentaenoic acid (EPA).[17] Thus flaxseed may be a reasonable substitute for fish oil supplementation.

Black cohosh (Cimicifuga racemosa)

Black cohosh has been used for both menstrual and menopausal conditions in Europe for over 50 years. Four older randomized trials of black cohosh, with a total of 345 menopausal women, lasting 3–6 months, support its efficacy in reducing menopausal somatic complaints.[18–21] In one of the larger and more recent studies, leutenizing hormone (LH), follicle-stimulating hormone (FSH), prolactin, estradiol, and vaginal cell proliferation were not different between two doses of black cohosh and placebo; supporting its safety.[19] A 5th trial showed that black cohosh decreased LH but not FSH.[22] A new large RCT ($n = 304$) confirms utility of 40 mg of isopropanolic extract of black cohosh for menopausal symptoms.[23] And, in a large observational study, 2016 Hungarian women, treated for 3 months experienced significant reductions in total symptom scores, hot flashes, sweating, insomnia, and anxiety ($p < .001$ in each case).[24]

Two studies have examined the effect of black cohosh in breast cancer survivors, many of whom suffered hot flashes as a side effect of taking tamoxifen. One study showed that both placebo and black cohosh improved symptoms.[25] Another larger trial using standardized black cohosh in the form of CR BNO 1055 (Menoem/Klimadynon) showed a significant reduction in percentage of women with severe hot flashes in the black cohosh group (24.4%) compared to control (73.9%, $p < 0.01$).[26] There were no serious adverse events and only 11 minor adverse events in the latter study. In women without breast cancer, CR BNO 1055 is as effective as conjugated estrogens in reducing menopausal symptoms, but with no effect on endometrial thickening.[27]

The most studied product, Remifemin, is currently standardized to 1 mg of triterpines per 20 mg tablet. The recommended dose is 20 mg two times per day. No drug interactions have been identified. The most common side effect is GI disturbance. A study in rats revealed no toxicity at 90 times the typical human dose. No mutagenicity or teratogenicity has been identified, but use during pregnancy can cause premature birth.[28,29] Multiple studies have attempted to determine whether black cohosh acts through estrogen receptors or via other mechanisms.[30] Black cohosh did not have estrogenic activity in a highly sensitive recombinant estrogen receptor system[31] and did not stimulate growth of human breast cancer cells, but instead inhibited their growth.[32]

Red clover (Trifolium pretense)

Red clover contains isoflavones similar to soy products. One large ($n = 252$)[33] and four small ($n = 30–51$) RCTs[34–37] have been conducted with mixed results on hot flashes. Two of the small trials showed reductions in number of hot flashes in the isoflavone groups.[35, 37] The other two small trials revealed no difference when compared to placebo. The large multicenter trial demonstrated a statistically significant 41% reduction in the number of hot flashes in the group taking a higher dose (82 mg isoflavones), compared to the lower dose group (34%) or placebo (36%).[33] Others have shown that red clover isoflavones increase arterial compliance,[38] increase HDL,[39] decrease trigycerides,[40,41] increase bone density,[39] improve cognitive function,[42] and did not increase breast density.[43] Two forms of bioassay support estrogen receptor activity[31] and promotion of proliferation of estrogen-sensitive breast cancer cells.[32] Thus, red clover should be avoided by women with breast cancer or a family history of breast cancer. For other women, taking a higher dose (82 mg isoflavones) may be effective in reducing hot flashes.

Dong quai (Angelica sinensis)

Dong quai is commonly recommended as part of a mixture of other herbs.[44] Indications include menopausal symptoms, irregular menses, vaginal dryness, dysmenorrhea, and palpitations. A single RCT examined the 6-month administration of 4.5 g powdered root or placebo, and found decreased hot flashes in both dong quai and placebo groups.[45] The lack of estrogenic effects in a trial on vaginal cytology, endometrial thickness, and serum estrogens is corroborated by a recent study that assayed estrogen activity using a highly sensitive human estrogen receptor and yeast recombinant system.[31] Dong quai contains psoralen that can cause photodermatitis and safrole which is carcinogenic, as well as several coumarins. Dong quai should not be used by women on anticoagulants or with heavy menstrual flow or with fibroids because of increased risk of bleeding.

Evening primrose oil (Oenothera biennis)

Evening primrose oil (EPO) is often used for premenstrual symptoms as well as menopausal symptoms. A single RCT compared 500 mg EPO plus 10 mg natural vitamin E to placebo in 56 women over 6 month's time.[46] EPO was no more effective than placebo for hot flashes except in decreasing the maximum number of night flushes. Side effects of nausea were relieved by taking the supplement with food. This appears to be a benign supplement, which may benefit some women.

Chaste tree berries (Vitex agnus castus)

Chaste tree berries are popular for PMS, menstrual irregularities, secondary amenorrhea, and are recommended for menopausal symptoms as well. Studies in the 1940s and 1950s established progestin-like effects, supporting the use for premenstrual symptoms. Others have demonstrated prolactin-inhibiting effects based on dopaminergic actions.[47] Two small studies of essential oils from the leaf or berry have shown effectiveness for self-reported menopausal symptoms.[48,49] Side effects in trials of chaste tree berry include GI symptoms, headache, rash, itching, and increased menstrual flow. No estrogen activity was found in a high-sensitivity recombinant estrogen receptor system.[31] Therefore, the mechanism of action is more likely based on the progestin-like effects. This herb deserves further study.

Wild yam (Dioscorea villosa)

Wild yam creams have been touted for their effects on menopausal symptoms. Wild yam contains diosgenin that can be converted into progesterone in the laboratory and was once a source of semisynthetic hormones. The human body cannot make this conversion, so it is unknown whether wild yam acts as a progestin in vivo. A single RCT of a one teaspoon mixture of 100 g wild yam, 2 g flax oil, 100 mg geranium oil, and 10 mg α-tocopherol applied twice per day versus placebo showed no difference in flushing, mood, breast symptoms, libido, or energy levels. There was also no difference in lipids, estradiol, FSH, or LH in the 3-month trial.[50] Almost half of the participants dropped out because of unrelieved symptoms further suggesting that yam cream may not be useful for menopausal symptoms.

HERBS FOR CARDIOVASCULAR DISEASE

Artichoke leaf (Cynara scolymus)

Animal studies have shown that artichoke leaf inhibits cholesterol synthesis and LDL oxidation. In humans, 1800 mg dry powder per day artichoke leaf results in a 10% improvement in total cholesterol, 17% improvement in LDL cholesterol compared to placebo.[51] A recent study showed that brachial flow-mediated vasodilation, vascular cell adhesion molecule-1, intercellular adhesion molecule-1, and E-selectin, markers of endothelial function, are all improved by 20 mL/day of frozen artichoke juice; however, reductions in lipid markers were not different from those in the control group.[52] Interestingly, other recent studies have focused on the efficacy of artichoke leaf for dyspepsia.[53,54] Artichokes are part of the Compositae, that is, the ragweed family, and allergy is common, usually producing dermatitis, so it is important to ask about this type of allergy before suggesting artichoke leaf. Obstruction of bile ducts or gallstones are contraindications to using artichoke leaf.

Bilberry fruit (Vaccinium myrtillus)

In Italy, bilberry fruit is used for varicose veins, venous insufficiency, and atherosclerosis. In vitro and animal studies indicate that bilberry fruit inhibits edema formation, platelet aggregation, and thrombus formation. In humans, there are preliminary studies that show positive effects on the peripheral vasculature.[55] Bilberries combined with lingonberries and black currants increase serum concentrations of quercetin by 32–51%.[56] Quercetin, a flavonoid, has been shown to affect platelet intracellular signaling and reduce platelet aggregation in humans.[57]

No adverse effects have been reported. The dose is 4–8 g of dried fruit taken with water several times per day or 80–160 mg dry extract (25% anthocyano-sides) taken three times per day.[55]

Turmeric (Curcuma longa)

The dietary spice turmeric contains an important polyphenol, curcumin that possesses both anti-inflammatory and anticancer properties following oral or topical administration. Curcumin is also a potent antioxidant with effects on cyclooxygenases and glutathione S-transferases.[58] In vitro studies show that curcumin inhibits platelet aggregation.[59] In rabbits and in humans it also decreases lipid peroxidation and lipid levels, thus possibly protecting against both atherogenesis and thrombotic sequelae.[60,61] The human dose is 1.5–3 g root powder per day. Some patients may experience contact dermatitis.

Fenugreek seed (Trigonella foenum-graecum)

Fenugreek seed has hypoglycemic effects when studied in rats and dogs. Glycoxidation is thought to be one of the mechanisms contributing to oxidized LDL and atherogenesis. An early study in human diabetics reports decreased cholesterol when taking 6 g/day crushed fenugreek seeds.[62] In another study, a hydroalcoholic extract (1 g/day) of fenugreek seeds significantly decreased serum triglycerides and increased HDL cholesterol as compared to placebo ($p < 0.05$). The fenugreek seed extract also improved glycemic control and decreased insulin resistance in the mild Type-II diabetic subjects.[63]

Garlic (Allium sativa)

The German Commission E approves the use of garlic for elevated blood lipids and prevention of age-related vascular changes.[62] Herbalists also use garlic for hypertension. The intact garlic bulb contains alliin. When garlic bulbs are crushed alliin is converted to allicin, the pharmacologically active moiety, and the one to which products are standardized. Garlic affects CAD by modestly reducing serum cholesterol, blood pressure, and thrombus formation.

In numerous animal studies, garlic prevents the formation of atherosclerotic plaques and reverses existing lesions. Two meta-analyses have shown that overall garlic lowered cholesterol by about 9–12%.[64,65] In one study, trigycerides were also significantly decreased and HDL cholesterol was unchanged.[65] Another meta-analysis of eight trials supports the use of garlic as an antihypertensive.[66] All trials used the same preparation (Kwai®) given over at least 4 weeks. Systolic blood pressure was lowered by 11.1 mm Hg (95% CI 5.0–17.2) and diastolic blood pressure was lowered by 6.5 mm Hg (95% CI 3.4–9.6). A double blind RCT of garlic that followed 152 subjects for 4 years showed that garlic reduced development of atherosclerosis, thus supporting the role of garlic in overall cardiovascular care.[67] In a recent pilot study of Aged Garlic Extract (AGE), used over 1 year's time, the AGE group had a significantly smaller increase in calcium score measured by electron beam tomography (7.5 +/− 9.4%) versus the placebo group who had an average increase of 22.2 +/− 18.5% ($p = 0.046$). There were no significant differences in individual cholesterol parameters or C-reactive protein between the groups.[68] Other authors found that short-term treatment with AGE improves impaired endothelial function in men with CAD treated with aspirin and a statin.[69] In another recent pilot trial, garlic pearls were consumed with fish oil for 60 days, producing decrements in total cholesterol by 20%, low-density lipoprotein (LDL) by 21%, serum triglyceride by 37%, very LDL by 36.7%, total cholesterol: high-density lipoprotein (HDL) ratio by 23.4%. HDL increased by 5.1%.[70] This is in contrast to three studies with powdered or enteric-coated garlic products that found no effects on lipid parameters.[71–73]

Side effects of garlic odor, breath odor, and abdominal symptoms have been reported in the literature. A theoretical interaction of garlic with warfarin is based on the potential of garlic to decrease platelet aggregation and promote fibrinolysis. The selection of dose form is important to achieve the desired results. According to most herbalists, fresh preparations are significantly more effective than dried powder preparations. Suggested doses are one clove of fresh garlic per day or the equivalent (4000 mg) or 1–2 mL (300–600 mg) Aged Garlic Extract (Kyolic) or 600–900 mg of dried powder standardized to 1.3% allicin (Kwai®).

Ginkgo biloba

Ginkgo biloba leaf extract comes from the oldest living trees in the world, with fossil evidence dating back 200 million years. *Ginkgo* topped the list of best-selling herbs in the United States in 1998. It is also one of the most studied of herbs, with evidence supporting its action as an inhibitor of platelet-activating factor[74] and as a vasodilator.[75] According to the German Commission E and the World Health Organization monographs, *Ginkgo* is approved for peripheral vascular occlusive disease and post-phlebitis syndrome, as well as dementias, tinnitus, vertigo, Reynaud's disease, and acrocyanosis.[55] The evidence of its efficacy for intermittent claudication was assessed in a meta-analysis of eight randomized, double-blinded, placebo-controlled trials in humans.[76] The mean improvement in pain-free walking of the *Ginkgo* group over the placebo group was 34 m. In a head-to-head trial of *Ginkgo biloba* extract and pentoxifylline, each product caused a similar increase in pain-free walking distance and maximal walking distance.[77]

The most frequently reported adverse events are abdominal complaints, nausea, and dyspepsia. Other adverse events reported in the literature include allergic reactions, headache, dizziness, and palpitations. There are case reports of bleeding complications including subdural hematoma[78] subarachnoid hemorrhage,[79] and spontaneous hyphema associated with aspirin plus *ginkgo* use.[80] Recent randomized studies have shown that *Ginkgo* does not interfere with coagulation parameters or warfarin.[81–84] The recommended dosage is the one most studied in trials, 120 mg daily EGb 761 (Tebonin made by Schwabe).

Ginseng, american or oriental (Panax spp)

The saponins in *Panax* species act as selective calcium antagonists and enhance release of nitric oxide from endothelial cells, thus providing protection during ischemia or reperfusion[85] *Panax ginseng* also seems to have beneficial effects on lipid parameters.[86] Side effects can include nervousness, excitation, estrogenic effects, and hypoglycemic effects. A case report indicates that *Panax ginseng* decreases the pharmacological effect of loop diuretics. Despite early reports that ginseng may increase blood pressure, a recent randomized crossover trial shows that long-term ginseng use has no effect on 24-hour BP and renal function in hypertensive individuals.[87] The recommended dose is 1–2 g root (20–30 mg ginsenosides).

Ginseng, siberian (Eleutherococcus senticosus)

Animal studies show that Siberian Ginseng inhibits platelet aggregation. In early human studies, Siberian ginseng has been found to increase blood pressure in hypotensive children and promote lipid-lowering in combination with other herbs.[62] A recent randomized-controlled trial of 8 weeks of Siberian ginseng in hypertensive elders on digitalis showed improvement in social functioning but no changes in either blood pressure or digitalis levels.[88] Case-based data, however, suggests that *Eleutherococcus* can elevate digoxin levels, possibly by interfering with the laboratory test.[89] Side effects include drowsiness or nervousness. The usual dose is 2–3 g/day for up to 3 months.

Grapes (wine, juice, skins, seeds, resveratrol)

The French Paradox, that is, that people could eat a diet high in saturated fats and still have low rates of heart disease, brought to light the beneficial effects of daily intake of red wine. Many studies show the primary preventive benefits of consuming 1–2 glasses of wine.[90–92] However, wine consumption does not seem to reduce mortality in those who already have CVD[93] and alcohol has many untoward effects including many drug interactions and adverse events.

Studies on grape skin extracts have illuminated the possible mechanisms by which particular molecules may be responsible for the salutary effects of wine. Red wine and red grape skins contain numerous polyphenolic compounds, including trans-resveratrol, proanthocyanidins, and flavonoids such as quercetin, kaempferol, and catechins that act primarily as antioxidants. Resveratrol is also found in purple grape juice, mulberries, and in smaller amounts in peanuts. Grape seed extract, a by-product of wine and juice production, has also proven useful in similar ways as other grape products. The mode of action appears to be the antioxidant effect of the proanthocyanidins as demonstrated in both animal studies[94,95] and a small human study.[96]

In vitro and animal studies show that resveratrol, in addition to being an antioxidant, is anti-inflammatory, inhibits platelet aggregation, and can cause blood vessel dilation.[97] New studies in human tissue show that resveratrol induces vasodilation of small arteries, internal mammary arteries, and saphenous veins ex vivo.[98,99] Further, 600 mg of grape polyphenol extract (including resveratrol) enhances endothelial-mediated vasodilation in vivo.[100] Concord grape juice or grape seed polyphenols or can significantly lower blood pressure,[101,102] but it is important to note that grape seed polyphenols in combination with vitamin C elevate systolic blood pressure.[102]

A small human study ($n = 24$) showed that resveratrol inhibits platelet aggregation.[103] A more recent study supports this finding showing that resveratrol reduces aggregation of platelets from healthy subjects in a concentration-dependent manner.[104]

In a small, but important randomized placebo-controlled cross-over trial conducted in pre- and postmenopausal women, 36 g of a lyophilized grape powder (LGP) taken for 4 weeks significantly lowered plasma triglycerides, LDL cholesterol, and apolipoproteins B and E. In addition, cholesterol ester transfer protein activity was decreased by approximately 15% with intake of LGP ($p < 0.05$). Although LDL oxidation was not modified, whole-body oxidative stress as measured by urinary F(2)-isoprostanes was significantly reduced after LGP supplementation. LGP also decreased the levels of plasma tumor necrosis factor-alpha (TNG-α), which plays a major role in the inflammation process.[105]

Thus, evidence of beneficial alterations in five important areas: vasodilation, platelet aggregation, lipoprotein metabolism, oxidative stress, and inflammatory markers continue to accumulate for grape products. These combined effects have great promise of ameliorating risks of coronary heart disease. It is important to be aware that resveratrol is a phytoestrogen and therefore it may be best to avoid use in women with breast cancer risk. The dose for resveratrol is 200–600 mcg divided twice per day. One glass of red wine is equivalent to 640 mcg.

Guggulipid (Commiphora mukul)

In animals, guggulipid increases binding sites for LDL, thus preventing cholesterol and trigyceride elevation.[85] In humans, most of the small early studies suggested that guggulipid lowers serum total cholesterol, low-density lipoprotein (LDL), and triglycerides, as well as increases in high-density lipoprotein (HDL).[106] An early phase RCT was conducted among 103 hyperlipidemic Americans eating a typical Western diet. Subjects received either standard-dose guggulipid (1000 mg), high-dose guggulipid (2000 mg), or matching placebo three times per day for 8 weeks. Placebo lowered LDL (−5%) while guggulipid at either dose elevated LDL (+4%, +5%). There were no significant changes in total cholesterol, triglycerides, VLDL, or HDL.[107] Side effects include hypersensitivity, GI upset, headache, mild nausea, belching, and hiccups. Guggulipid may decrease propranolol and cardizem bioavailability and may have thyroid-stimulating activity. The typical dose is 100–500 mg daily.

Hawthorn (Crataegus oxycantha)

Hawthorn leaves, flowers, and berries contain pharmacologically active proanthocyanidins, bioflavonoids, and cardiotonic amines. In vitro and experimental animal studies have suggested the following modes of action of standardized *Crataegus* extracts: (1) cAMP-independent positive inotropy, (2) peripheral and coronary vasodilatation, (3) protection against ischemia-induced ventricular arrhythmias, (4) antioxidative properties, and (5) anti-inflammatory effects.

Hawthorn is traditionally used to treat CAD indirectly through its hypotensive, anti-inflammatory, and antiarrhythmic actions. Herbalists have used hawthorn as a nutritive for the myocardium, especially for patients with CAD or those at high risk for CAD. Hawthorn is usually given in moderate doses over many months to improve the function and structure of the heart. In animal and *in vitro* studies, hawthorn appears to support and prevent the destruction of the collagen-matrix in the walls of blood vessels and presumably the fibrous cap of atherosclerotic lesions.[108–110] Furthermore, in one clinical trial, hawthorn was reported to improve exercise tolerance and decrease the incidence of angina.[111] Recently an RCT showed modest improvements in diastolic blood pressure in diabetics treated with 1200 mg of *Crataegus* extract.[112]

Hawthorn has been studied more thoroughly for its effects in congestive heart failure. A meta-analysis of eight trials ($n = 632$ patients with chronic heart failure) showed that hawthorn extract was more beneficial than placebo for increasing maximal workload and decreasing pressure-heart rate product. Symptoms, such as dyspnea and fatigue, also improved significantly with hawthorn treatment. Reported adverse events included nausea, dizziness, and cardiac and GI complaints; all were mild and/or transient.[113] Furthermore, in a well-done 2-year cohort study, the three cardinal symptoms of heart failure, that is, fatigue, stress dyspnea, and palpitations, were all significantly less marked in the *Crataegus* cohort than in the comparative cohort. These favorable effects on the clinical symptoms were achieved although the patients in the *Crataegus* cohort received fewer pharmaceutical treatments than the patients in the comparative cohort (ACE-inhibitors: 36 vs. 54%, $p = 0.004$; cardiac glycosides: 18 vs. 37%, $p = 0.001$; diuretics: 49 vs. 61%, $p = 0.061$; β-blockers: 22 vs. 33%, $p = 0.052$).[114] This study intimates that in real world clinical practice, hawthorn as monotherapy or as an adjunct to pharmaceutical treatment provides improved outcomes, potentially allowing less use of other cardiac medications. This observation is important for women who often want to reduce reliance on conventional medications.

The dose range is 160–900 mg extract of flowers and leaves standardized to either procyanidins or flavonoids. Both recent research and traditional usage suggest that hawthorn takes at least 8 weeks for beneficial effects to start.

Horse chestnut seed extract (Aesculus hippocastanum)

Horse chestnut seed extract has been studied for its use in chronic venous insufficiency. Animal studies show that escins from horse chestnut inhibit vascular permeability and edema formation.[115,116] In a randomized trial of horse chestnut vs. compression stockings vs. placebo, horse chestnut and compression stockings were equal in their ability to decrease leg volume (46.7 and 43.8 mL, respectively) and both were significantly more effective than placebo (9.8 mL).[117]

A systematic review of 13 studies concluded that horse chestnut was more effective than placebo.[118] No adverse events were reported in the randomized trial.[117] The recommended dose is 250–312.5 mg dry extract two times per day in a slow release form (16–21% escin) which should deliver 100 mg escin daily.

Policicosanol

Policosanol is made from the fatty alcohols of sugar cane or beeswax. The mechanism of action is thought to be inhibition of cholesterol synthesis and increased LDL processing. Policosanol reduces LDL oxidation, platelet aggregation, endothelial damage, and smooth muscle cell proliferation.

In a meta-analysis of 29 studies of policosanol ($n = 1528$ pts on policosanol vs. 1406 pts on placebo), LDL was lowered by 23.7% versus 0.11% for placebo ($p < 0.0001$). Favorable effects on total cholesterol, HDL, and trigycerides were also noted, as well as a clinically significant decreases in the LDL:HDL ratio.[119] The relative risk for adverse effects was 0.31, comparing policosanol to placebo (CI 0.20–0.48, $p < 0.0001$). These meta-analysis results are contradicted by a recent RCT ($n = 143$) of multiple dose levels, from 10 to 80 mg daily, showing nonsignificant reduction of LDL cholesterol (–10%) that was not improved by increasing dose.[120] In animal studies, there has been no observed carcinogenesis or adverse effects on reproduction, growth, or development. The recommended dose is 12 mg daily with a range of 5–40 mg daily.[119] Product selection may be an important determinant of results in practice.

Pycnogenol (Pinus maritima)

Pycnogenol, an extract of French maritime pine bark, has been one of the best-selling herbal products in America. Pycnogenol, containing procyandins and phenolic acids, is highly bioavailable and is used for chronic venous insufficiency (CVI). In vitro and animal studies show that it acts as an antioxidant and as an ACE inhibitor.[85,121] The mechanism of action in CVI is thought to be via stabilization of the collagenous subendothelial basal membrane or scavenging free radicals. There are three small human studies for CVI that consistently show decreased pain, edema, and limb heaviness in the treatment group.[122–124]

A recent randomized-controlled trial of Pycnogenol in hypertensives showed that it significantly reduced the dose of nefidipine (N) required to control blood pressure (15 mg N vs. 21 mg N in placebo group). Biomarker analysis showed that the vasoconstrictor, endothelin-1, was decreased while the vasodilator, prostacyclin, was increased with Pycnogenol supplementation. ACE inhibition effects were not seen. Mild adverse effects included GI problems, nausea, dizziness, headache, and sleepiness.[125] The recommended dose is 100 mg Pycnogenol one to three times per day.

Terminalia bark (Terminalia arjuna)

Terminalia bark is a traditional remedy of India that has been studied for its effects in heart disease. A randomized controlled trial of 500 mg daily showed a significant decrease in total cholesterol (−9.7 +/−12.7%), and LDL cholesterol (−15.8 +/− 25.6%). In addition, lipid peroxide levels decreased significantly in the *T. arjuna* group (−29.3 +/−18.9%).[126] In another randomized, controlled crossover study in 58 men with stable angina, *T. arjuna* bark extract, 500 mg three times per day, led to improvement in clinical and treadmill exercise parameters as compared to placebo therapy. These benefits were similar to those observed with isosorbide mononitrate (40 mg/day) therapy and the extract was well tolerated.[127]

HERBS TO AVOID

Ephedra

Significant problems have been associated with the use of ephedra products for weight loss. Ephedra use may be attractive because of conventional admonishments to loose weight coupled with a paucity of effective recommendations on how to safely accomplish weight loss. Ephedra acts as a sympathomimetic, leading to increased arterial blood pressure, increased heart rate, increased oxygen consumption in heart muscle, and vasoconstriction. Recently the FDA moved to remove *Ephedra* from the United States market, but it is still available via the world wide web.

Side effects of *Ephedra* include anxiety, numbness, gastroesophageal reflux, high fever, constipation, difficulty urinating, elevated liver enzymes, and Bell's palsy. Adverse effects include heart palpitations, severe hypertension, infarction of tips of toes, chest pain, dizziness, transient ischemic attacks, brain hemorrhage, stroke, and death.

Licorice root (*Glycyrrhiza glabra*)

Powdered or finely cut licorice root is made into an infusion and used primarily for respiratory and GI problems. In addition to its anti-inflammatory actions, licorice has mineralocorticoid activity and when used over long periods and at high doses can cause hypokalemia, hypernatremia, edema, and hypertension. This can exacerbate cardiac disorders and cause pseudo-aldosteronism. In addition, deleterious herb–drug interactions are possible with pharmaceuticals commonly used for cardiovascular disease including potassium-sparing diuretics, thiazide diuretics, and digitalis.[62,85]

INTERACTIONS WITH COMMON CARDIOVASCULAR MEDICATIONS

A theoretical interaction of garlic with warfarin is based on the potential of garlic to decrease platelet aggregation and promote fibrinolysis. A case report indicates that *Panax ginseng* decreases the pharmacological effect of loop diuretics. Siberian ginseng is contraindicated in persons with hypertension or post-myocardial infraction (MI).[85] Case-based data also suggests that Siberian ginseng (*Eleutherococcus*) can elevate digoxin levels, possibly by interfering with the laboratory test.[89] Gugulipid can decreases propranolol and cardizem bioavailability.

A WOMAN'S HOLISTIC PLAN THAT INCLUDES THE USE OF HERBS

Below is a holistic plan for addressing cardiovascular disease in menopausal women. Women who present with more advanced cardiovascular disease or are experiencing severe symptoms require a more aggressive approach using procedural and/or pharmaceutical intervention along with lifestyle changes. It may be possible to phase out medications after lifestyle modifications make a clinically significant impact. For individuals with a strong family history of cardiovascular disease or other risk factors, primary prevention can be approached through nutrition, exercise, mind-body therapies, and the selected use of botanicals.

Nutrition

Encourage a diet high in fiber and antioxidant-rich foods, especially fruits and vegetables with intense colors such as melons, berries, and squashes. Encourage foods high in omega-3 fatty acids such as cold water fish (salmon, herring, sardines, etc), nuts, and flax seeds (three tablespoons finely ground per day) or flax seed oil (one tablespoon or one to two 500-mg capsules bid). Encourage the consumption of raw or very lightly cooked garlic, at least one clove every day. Putting garlic into soups, stir-fry, or sauces at the very end of cooking (last 5 minutes) keeps the majority of garlic's beneficial effects. Encourage a low-fat (especially saturated and polyunsaturated)/cholesterol-free diet. Have your patient investigate programs that teach a Mediterranean-based diet or use the Dean Ornish diet. Encourage the consumption of water, but not in the form of tea, coffee, sodas, or juice. Six to eight glasses per day depending on the person's weight and physical activity level are sufficient to keep an individual well hydrated.

Exercise

Help patients to develop an exercise program that will be flexible and enjoyable enough that they will continue to exercise for the rest of their life. Activity goals can be approached in a stepwise fashion with the final goal at 30–60 minutes/day combined with stretching before and after exercise.

Mind-body

Encourage women to start a mind-body technique that works for them. These techniques are well known for reducing stress but many women are unaware of the power of mind-body methods for controlling hot flashes as well. The simplest is "paced respiration" or slow deep breathing. This is helpful starting the moment a hot flash starts or in a situation where one might be expected. Have your patient sit quietly and inhale while counting slowly to four, then exhale while counting to four. As she exhales, she should let all the tension flow out of her body.

"Progressive muscle relaxation" is another helpful technique that can be used as a daily practice to lower stress level in general and for training to relax quickly during stress. The technique involves sequentially tensing and relaxing all the muscles in the body, achieving a deep state of relaxation. Your patients can learn the steps in progressive muscles relaxation from instructions on the web at http://www.guidetopsychology.com/pmr.htm. Books written for the lay audience, such as *The Relaxation & Stress Reduction Workbook* by Martha Davis et al. or *Stress Relief & Relaxation Techniques* by Judith Lazarus, may also be helpful.

Botanicals

Consider using one or more of the cardiovascular herbs in this chapter for lipid-lowering or symptom management. For hot flashes, consider soy isoflavones or black cohosh or one of the other herbal approaches. Be aware of estrogen effects in women with breast cancer risk. For cardiovascular health, consider garlic or grape products. Hawthorn may be useful in congestive heart failure. *Ginkgo biloba* may help with claudication, while horse chestnut is useful in peripheral vascular disease. In general, the combination of pharmaceuticals with botanicals and supplements has not been well studied. Both naturaldatabase.com and eFacts.com allow checking for known interactions. Be particularly alert to check herbs for their interaction with aspirin or warfarin.

A thoughtful approach that honors the woman's desire for a holistic or natural approach to the menopausal years when cardiovascular risk increases, can further the building of a trust relationship. Physicians who expand their knowledge base about herbs and other nonpharmacological approaches to cardiovascular disease and menopause will be rewarded with many proactive and grateful women patients.

REFERENCES

1. Writing Group for the Women's Health Initiative Investigators. Risks and benefits of estrogen plus progestin in healthy postmenopausal women. JAMA. 2002;288: 321–33.
2. Van Patten C, Olivotto I, Chambers K, et al. Effect of soy phytoestrogens on hot flashes in postmenopausal women with breast cancer: a randomized, controlled clinical trial. J Clin Oncol. 2002;20(6):1449–55.
3. Albert A, Altabre C, Baro F, et al. Beneficial effects and good tolerability of soy for menopausal symptoms. Phytomedicine. 2002;9:85–92.
4. Albertazzi P, Pansini F, Bonaccorsi G, et al. The effect of dietary soy supplementation on hot flushes. Obstet Gynecol. 1998;91(1):6–10.

5. Murkies A, Lombard C, Strauss B, et al. Dietary flour supplementation decreases post-menopausal hot flushes: effect of soy and wheat. Maturitus. 1995;21:189–95.
6. Chen Y, Ho S, Lam S, et al. Soy isoflavones have a favorable effect on bone loss in Chinese postmenopausal women with lower bone mass: a double-blind, randomized, controlled trial. J Clin Endocrinol Metab. 2003;88:4740–7.
7. Arjmandi BH, Lucas EA, Khalil DA, et al. One year soy protein supplementation has positive effects on bone formation markers but not bone density in postmenopausal women. Nutr J. 2005;4:8.
8. Gallagher JC, Satpathy R, Rafferty K, et al. The effect of soy protein isolate on bone metabolism. Menopause. 2004;11(3):290–8.
9. Kritz-Silverstain D, Von Muhlen D, Barrett-Connor E, et al. Isoflavones and cognitive function in older women: the SOy and Postmenopausal Health In Aging (SOPHIA) study. Menopause. 2003;10(3):196–202.
10. Cassidy A, Griffin B. Phyto-oestrogens: a potential role in the prevention of CHD? Proc Nutrition Society. 1999;58:193–9.
11. Lukaczer D, Liska DJ, Lerman RH, et al. Effect of a low glycemic index diet with soy protein and phytosterols on CVD risk factors in postmenopausal women. Nutrition. 2006;22(2):104–13.
12. Horn-Ross P, John E, Canchola A, et al. Phytoestrogen intake and endometrial cancer risk. J Nat Cancer Inst. 2003;95(15):1158–64.
13. Kurzer M. Phytoestrogen supplement use by women. Paper presented at NIH Dietary Supplement Use in Women: Current Status and Future Directions; January 28–29, 2002; Bethesda, MD.
14. Lemay A, Dodin S, Kadri N, et al. Flaxseed dietary supplement versus hormone replacement therapy in hypercholesterolemic menopausal women. Obst Gynecol. 2002;100(3):495–504.
15. Luca E, Wild, R, Hammond L, et al. Flaxseed improves lipid profile without altering biomarkers of bone metabolism in postmenopausal women. J Clin Endocrine Metab. 2002;87(4):1527–32.
16. Dodin S, Lemay A, Jacques H, et al. The effects of flaxseed dietary supplement on lipid profile, bone mineral density, and symptoms in menopausal women: a randomized, double-blind, wheat germ placebo-controlled clinical trial. J Clin Endocrinol Metab. 2005;90(3):1390–7.
17. Harper CR, Edwards MJ, DeFilipis AP, et al. Flaxseed oil increases the plasma concentrations of cardioprotective (n-3) fatty acids in humans. J Nutr. 2006;136(1):83–7.
18. Lehmann-Willenbrock E, Riedel H. Clinical and endocrinologic examinations about therapy of climacteric symptoms following hysterectomy with remaining ovaries. Zentralbl Gynakol. 1988;110:611–8.
19. Liske E, Wustenberg P. Therapy of climacteric complaints with cimicifuga racemosa: herbal medicine with clinically proven evidence. Menopause. 1998;5:250.
20. Stoll W. Phytopharmacon influences atrophic vaginal epithelium: double-blind study—cimicifuga vs estrogenic substances. Therapeuticum. 1987;1:23–31.
21. Warnecke G. Influence of a phytopharmaceutical on climacteric complaints. Die Meizinisch Welt. 1985;36:871–4.
22. Duker E, Kpanski L, Jarry H, et al. Effects of extracts from cimicifuga racemosa on gonadotropin release in menopausal women and ovarectomized rats. Planta Med. 1991;57:420–4.
23. Osmers R, Friede M, Liske E, et al. Efficacy and safety of isopropanolic black cohosh extract for climacteric symptoms. Obstet Gynecol. 2005;105(5 Pt 1):1074–83.

24. Vermes G, Banhidy F, Acs N. The effects of remifemin on subjective symptoms of menopause. Adv Ther. 2005;22(2):148–54.

25. Jacobson J, Troxel A, Evans J, et al. Randomized trial of black cohosh for the treatment of hot flashes among women with a history of breast cancer. J Clin Oncol. 2001;19(10):2739–45.

26. Munoz G, Pluchino S. Cimicifuga racemosa for the treatment of hot flushes in women surviving breast cancer. Maturitas. 2003;44 Suppl 1:S59–65.

27. Wuttke W, Seidlova-Wuttke D, Gorkow C. The cimicifuga preparation BNO 1055 vs. conjugated estrogens in a double-blind placebo-controlled study: effects on menopause symptoms and bone markers. Maturitas. 2003;44 Suppl 1:S67–77.

28. McKenna D, Jones K, Humphrey S, et al. Black cohosh: efficacy, safety, and use in clinical and preclinical applications. Altern Ther Health Med. 2001;7(3):93,98.

29. Pepping J. Black cohosh:Cimicifuga racemosa. Am J Health-Syst Pharm. 1999; 56(14):1400–2.

30. Borrelli F, Izzo A, Ernst E. Pharmacological effects of cimicifuga racemosa. Life Sci. 2003;73:1215–29.

31. Klein K, Janfaza M, Wong J, et al. Estrogen bioactivity in fo-ti and other herbs used for their estrogen-like effects as determined by a recombinant cell bioassay. J Clin Endocrin Metabol. 2003;88(9):4077–9.

32. Bodinet C, Freudenstin J. Influence of marketed herbal menopause preparations on MCF-7 cell proliferation. Menopause. 2004;11(3):281–9.

33. Tice J, Ettinger B, Ensrud K, et al. Phytoestrogen supplements for the treatment of hot flashes: the isoflavone clover extract (ICE) study. JAMA. 2003;290(2):207–14.

34. Baber R, Templeman C, Morton T, et al. Randomized placebo-controlled trial of an isoflavone supplement and menopausal symptoms in women. Climacteric. 1999;2:85–92.

35. Jeri A. The use of an isoflavone supplement to relieve hot flashes. Female Patient. 2002;27:35–7.

36. Knight D, Howes J, Eden J. The effect of promensil, and isoflavone extract, on menopausal symptoms. Climacteric. 1999;2:79–84.

37. van de Weijer P, Barentsen R. Isoflavones from red clover (Promensil) significantly reduce menopausal hot flush symptoms compared with placebo. Maturitas. 2002;42(3):187–93.

38. Nestle P, Pomeroy S, Kay S, et al. Isoflavones from red clover improve systemic arterial compliance but not plasma lipids in menopausal women [erratum appears in J Clin Endocrinol Metab. 1999;84(10):3647]. J Clin Endocrinol Metab. 1999;84(3):895–8.

39. Clifton-Bligh P, Baber R, Fulcher G, et al. The effect of isoflavones extracted from red clover (Rimostil) on lipid and bone metabolism. Menopause. 2001;8(4):259–65.

40. Schult TM, Ensrud KE, Blackwell T, et al. Effect of isoflavones on lipids and bone turnover markers in menopausal women. Maturitas. 2004;48(3):209–18.

41. Hidalgo LA, Chedraui PA, Morocho N, et al. The effect of red clover isoflavones on menopausal symptoms, lipids and vaginal cytology in menopausal women: a randomized, double-blind, placebo-controlled study. Gynecol Endocrinol. 2005;21(5):257–64.

42. Howes J, Bray K, Lorenz L, et al. The effects of dietary supplementation with isoflavones from red clover on cognitive function in postmenopausal women. Climacteric. 2004;7(1):70–77.

43. Atkinson C, Warren R, Sala E, et al. Red-clover-derived isoflavones and mammographic breat density: a double-blind, randomized, placebo-controlled trial [ISRCTN42940165]. Breast Cancer Res. 2004;6(3):R170–9.

44. Kronenberg F, Fugh-Berman A. complementary and alternative medicine for menopausal symptoms: a review of randomized, controlled trials. Annal Intern Med. 2002;137(10):805–13.

45. Hirata J, Swiersz L, Zell B, et al. Does dong quai have estrogenic effects in post menopausal women? Fertil Steril. 1997;68:981–6.

46. Chenoy R, Hussain S, Tayob Y, et al. Effect of oral gamolenic acid from evening primrose oil on menopausal flushing. BMJ. 1994;308(6927):501–3.

47. Kass-Annese B. Alternative therapies for menopause. Clin Obst Gynecol 2000;43(1):162–83.

48. Chopin L. Vitex agnus castus essential oil and menopausal balance: a research update. Complement Ther Nurs Midwifery. 2003;8:148–54.

49. Lucks B, Sorensen J, Veal L. Vitexagnus-castus essential oil and menopausal balance: a self-care survey. Complement Ther Nurs Midwifery. 2002;8(3):148–4.

50. Komesaroff P, Black C, Cable V, et al. Effects of wild yam extract on menopausal symptoms, lipids and sex hormones in healthy menopausal women. Climacteric. 2001;4:114–50.

51. Englisch W, et al. Efficacy of artichoke dry extract in patients with hyperlipoproteinemia. Arzneimittelforschung. 2000;50(3):260–5.

52. Lupattelli G, Marchesi S, Lombardini R, et al. Artichoke juice improves endothelial function in hyperlipemia. Life Sci. 2004;76(7):775–82.

53. Holtmann G, Adam B, Haag S, et al. Efficacy of artichoke leaf extract in the treatment of patients with functional dyspepsia: a six-week placebo-controlled, double-blind, multicentre trial. Aliment Pharmacol Ther. 2003;18(11–2):1099–105.

54. Marakis G, Walker AF, Middleton RW, et al. Artichoke leaf extract reduces mild dyspepsia in an open study. Phytomedicine. 2002 Dec;9(8):694–9.

55. Blumenthal M, Goldberg A, Gruenwald J, et al. (eds). The complete German Commission E monographs: therapeutic guide to herbal medicines. Austin (TX): American Botanical Council; 1998.

56. Marniemi J, Hakala P, Maki J, Ahotupa M. Partial resistance of low density lipoprotein to oxidation in vivo after increased intake of berries. Nutr Metab Cardiovasc Dis. 2000;10(6):331–7.

57. Hubbard GP, Wolffram S, Lovegrove JA, et al. Ingestion of quercetin inhibits platelet aggregation and essential components of the collagen-stimulated platelet activation pathway in humans. J Thromb Haemost. 2004;2(12):2138–45.

58. Sharma RA, Gescher AJ, Steward WP. Curcumin: the story so far. Eur J Cancer. 2005;41(13):1955–68.

59. Shah BH, et al. Inhibitory effect of curcumin, a food spice from turmeric, on platelet-activating factor- and arachidonic acid-mediated platelet aggregation through inhibition of thromboxane formation and Ca^{2+} signaling. Biochem Pharmacol. 1999;58(7):1167–72.

60. Ramirez-Tortosa MC, et al. Oral administration of a turmeric extract inhibits LDL oxidation and has hypocholesterolemic effects in rabbits with experimental atherosclerosis. Atherosclerosis. 1999;147(2):371–8.

61. Soni KB, Kuttan R. Effect of oral curcumin administration on serum peroxides and cholesterol levels in human volunteers. Indian J Physiol Pharmacol. 1992;36(4):273–5.

62. Blumenthal M, ed. Herbal medicine: expanded Commission E monographs. Newton (MA): Integrative Medicine Communications, 2000.

63. Gupta A, Gupta R, Lal B. Effect of Trigonella foenum-graecum (fenugreek) seeds on glycaemic control and insulin resistance in type 2 diabetes mellitus: a double blind placebo controlled study. J Assoc Physicians India. 2001a;49:1057–61.

64. Warshafsky S, Kamer RS, Sivak SL. Effect of garlic on total serum cholesterol: a meta-analysis. Ann Intern Med. 1993;119:599–605.

65. Silagy C, Neil A. Garlic as a lipid lowering agent–a meta-analysis. J Royal Coll Phys (Lond). 1994a;28(1):39–45.

66. Silagy CA, Neil HAW. A meta-analysis of the effect of garlic on blood pressure. J Hypertension. 1994b;12(4):463–8.

67. Koscielny J, et al. The anti-atherosclerotic effect of *Allium sativum*. Atherosclerosis. 1999;144(1):237–49.

68. Budoff MJ, Takasu J, Flores FR, et al. Inhibiting progression of coronary calcification using aged garlic extract in patients receiving statin therapy: a preliminary study. Prev Med. 2004;39(5):985–91.

69. Williams MJ, Sutherland WH, McCormick MP, et al. Aged garlic extract improves endothelial function in men with coronary artery disease. Phytother Res. 2005;19(4): 314–9.

70. Jeyaraj S, Shivaji G, Jeyaraj SD, et al. Effect of combined supplementation of fish oil with garlic pearls on the serum lipid profile in hypercholesterolemic subjects. Indian Heart J. 2005;57(4):327–31.

71. Tanamai J, Veeramanomai S, Indrakosas N. The efficacy of cholesterol-lowering action and side effects of garlic enteric coated tablets in man. J Med Assoc Thai. 2004;87(10):1156–61.

72. Turner B, Molgaard C, Marckmann P. Effect of garlic (Allium sativum) powder tablets on serum lipids, blood pressure and arterial stiffness in normo-lipidaemic volunteers: a randomised, double-blind, placebo-controlled trial. Br J Nutr. 2004;92(4):701–6.

73. Satitvipawee P, Rawdaree P, Indrabhakti S, et al. No effect of garlic extract supplement on serum lipid levels in hypercholesterolemic subjects. J Med Assoc Thai. 2003;86(8):750–7.

74. Reuter HD: *Ginkgo* biloba–botany, constituents, pharmacology and clinical trials. Br J Phytother. 1995;96;4:3–20.

75. Van Beek TA, Bombardelli D, Morazzoni F. *Ginkgo* biloba. L. Fitoterapia. 1998;169:195–244.

76. Pittler MH, Ernst E. *Ginkgo biloba* extract for the treatment of intermittent claudication: a meta-analysis of randomized trials. Am J Med. 2000;108:276–81.

77. Bohmer D, Kalinski S, Michaelis MH, et al. Behandlung der PAVK mit *Ginkgo*-biloba-extrakt (GBE) oder Pentoxifyllin. *Herz Kreislauf*. 1988;20:5–8; cited in Pittler MH, Ernst E. *Ginkgo biloba* extract for the treatment of intermittent claudication: a meta-analysis of randomized trials. Am J Med. 2000;108:276–81.

78. Rowin J, Lewis SL. Spontaneous bilateral subdural hematomas with chronic *Ginkgo* biloba ingestion. Neurology. 1996;46:1775–6.

79. Vale S. Subarachnoid hemorrhage associated with *Ginkgo biloba*. Lancet. 1998;352:36.

80. Rosenblatt M, Mindel J. Spontaneous hyphemia associated with the ingestion of *Gingo biloba* extract. N Engl J Med. 1997;336:1108.

81. Engelsen J, Nielsen JD, Hansen KF. Effect of Coenzyme Q10 and *Ginkgo* biloba on warfarin dosage in patients on long-term warfarin treatment. A randomized, double-blind, placebo-controlled cross-over trial. Ugeskr Laeger. 2003;165(18):1868–71.

82. Bal Dit Sollier C, Caplain H, Drouet L. No alteration in platelet function or coagulation induced by EGb761 in a controlled study. Clin Lab Haematol. 2003;25(4): 251–3.

83. Kohler S, Funk P, Kieser M. Influence of a 7-day treatment with *Ginkgo* biloba special extract EGb 761 on bleeding time and coagulation: a randomized, placebo-controlled,

double-blind study in healthy volunteers. Blood Coagul Fibrinolysis. 2004;15(4): 303–9.

84. Jiang X, Williams KM, Liauw WS, et al. Effect of *ginkgo* and ginger on the pharmacokinetics and pharmacodynamics of warfarin in healthy subjects. Br J Clin Pharmacol. 2005;59(4):425–32.

85. DerMarderosian A, ed. The review of natural products 2001, facts and comparisons. A Wolters Kluwer Co., USA, 2001.

86. Kim SH, Park KS. Effects of panax ginseng extract on lipid metabolism in humans. Pharmacol Res. 2003;48(5):511–3.

87. Stavro PM, Woo M, Leiter LA, et al. Long-term intake of North American ginseng has no effect on 24-hour blood pressure and renal function. Hypertension. 2006; 47(4):791–6.

88. Cicero AF, Derosa G, Brillante R, et al. Effects of Siberian ginseng (Eleutherococcus senticosus maxim.) on elderly quality of life: a randomized clinical trial. Arch Gerontol Geriatr Suppl. 2004;(9):69–73.

89. McRae S. Elevated serum digoxin levels in a patient taking digoxin and Siberian ginseng. CMAJ. 1996;155:293.

90. Renaud SC, Gueguen R, Siest G. Wine, beer, and mortality in middle-aged men from eastern France. Arch Intern Med. 1999;159(16):1865–70.

91. Kiechl S, Willeit J, Rungger G, et al. Alcohol consumption and atherosclerosis: what is the relation? Prospective results from the Bruneck Study. Stroke. 1998;29(5):900–7.

92. Klatsky AL, Armstrong MA, Friedman GD. Red wine, white wine, liquor, beer, and risk for coronary artery disease hospitalization. Am J Cardiol. 1997;80(4): 416–20.

93. Shaper AG, Wannamethee SG. Alcohol intake and mortality in middle aged men with diagnosed coronary heart disease. Heart. 2000;83(4):394–9.

94. Bagchi D, Bagchi M, Stohs SJ, et al. Free radicals and grape seed proanthocyanidin extract: importance in human health and disease prevention. Toxicology. 2000;148(2–3):187–97.

95. Bagchi D, Garg A, Krohn RL, et al. Oxygen free radical scavenging abilities of vitamins C and E, and a grape seed proanthocyanidin extract in vitro. Res Com Mol Pathol Pharmacol 1997;95(2):179–89.

96. Nuttall SL, Kendall MJ, Bombardelli E, et al. An evaluation of the antioxidant activity of a standardized grape seed extract, Leucoselect. J Clin Pharm Ther. 1998;23(5):385–9.

97. Fremont L. Biological effects of resveratrol. Life Sci. 2000;66(8):663–73.

98. Cruz MN, Luksha L, Logman H, et al. Acute responses to phytoestrogens in small arteries from men with coronary heart disease. Am J Physiol Heart Circ Physiol. 2006;290(5):H1969–75.

99. Rakici O, Kiziltepe U, Coskun B, et al. Effects of resveratrol on vascular tone and endothelial function of human saphenous vein and internal mammary artery. Int J Cardiol. 2005;105(2):209–15.

100. Lekakis J, Rallidis LS, Andreadou I, Vamvakou G, et al. Polyphenolic compounds from red grapes acutely improve endothelial function in patients with coronary heart disease. Eur J Cardiovasc Prev Rehabil. 2005;12(6):596–600.

101. Park YK, Kim JS, Kang MH. Concord grape juice supplementation reduces blood pressure in Korean hypertensive men: double-blind, placebo controlled intervention trial. Biofactors. 2004;22(1–4):145–7.

102. Ward NC, Hodgson JM, Croft KD, et al. The combination of vitamin C and grape-seed polyphenols increases blood pressure: a randomized, double-blind, placebo-controlled trial. J Hypertens. 2005;23(2):427–34.

103. Pace-Asciak CR, Rounova O, Hahn SE, et al. Wines and grape juices as modulators of platelet aggregation in healthy human subjects. Clinica Chimica Acta. 1996; 246(1–2):163–82.

104. Wang Z, Huang Y, Zou J, et al. Effects of red wine and wine polyphenol resveratrol on platelet aggregation in vivo and in vitro. Int J Mol Med.2002;9(1):77–9.

105. Zern TL, Wood RJ, Greene C, et al. Grape polyphenols exert a cardioprotective effect in pre- and postmenopausal women by lowering plasma lipids and reducing oxidative stress. J Nutr. 2005;135(8):1911–7.

106. Ulbricht C, Basch E, Szapary P, et al. Guggul for hyperlipidemia: a review by the Natural Standard Research Collaboration. Complement Ther Med. 2005;13(4):279–90.

107. Szapary PO, Wolfe ML, Bloedon LT, et al. Guggulipid for the treatment of hypercholesterolemia: a randomized controlled trial. JAMA. 20003;290(6):765–72.

108. Masquelier J. Pycnogenols: recent advances in the therapeutical activity of procyanidins. Natural Prod Med Agents. 1981a;1:243–256.

109. Masquelier J, Dumon MC, Dumas J. Stabilization of collagen by procyanidolic oligomers. Acta Therap. 1981b;7:101–5.

110. Tixier JM, et al: Evidence by in vivo and in vitro studies that binding of pycnogenols to elastin affects its rate of degradation by elastases. Biochem Pharmacol. 33:3933–3939, 1984.

111. Weng WL, et al. Therapeutic effects of Crataegus pinnaifida on 46 cases of angina pectoris–a double blind study. J Tradit Chin Med. 1984;4(4):293–4.

112. Walker AF, Marakis G, Simpson E, et al. Hypotensive effects of hawthorn for patients with diabetes taking prescription drugs: a randomised controlled trial. Br J Gen Pract. 2006;56(527):437–43.

113. Pittler MH, Schmidt K, Ernst E. Hawthorn extract for treating chronic heart failure: meta-analysis of randomized trials. Am J Med. 2003;114(8):665–4.

114. Habs M. Prospective, comparative cohort studies and their contribution to the benefit assessments of therapeutic options: heart failure treatment with and without Hawthorn special extract WS 1442. Forsch Komplementarmed Klass Naturheilkd. 2004;11 Suppl 1:36–9.

115. Guillaume M, Padioleau F. Veinotonic effect, vascular protection, antiinflammatory and free radical scavenging properties of horse chestnut extract. Arzneimittelforschung. 1994;44(1):25–35.

116. Matsuda H, et al. Effects of escins Ia, Ib, IIa, and IIb from horse chestnut, the seeds of Aesculus hippocastanum L., on acute inflammation in animals. Biol Pharm Bull. 1997;20(10):1092–5.

117. Diehm C, et al. Comparison of leg compression stocking and oral horse-chestnut seed extract therapy in patients with chronic venous insufficiency. Lancet. 1996;347(8997):292–4.

118. Pittler MH, Ernst E. Horse-chestnut seed extract for chronic venous insufficiency. A criteria-based systematic review. Arch Dermatol. 1998;134(11):1356–60.

119. Chen JT, Wesley R, Shamburek RD, et al. Meta-analysis of natural therapies for hyperlipidemia: plant sterols and stanols versus policosanol. Pharmacotherapy. 2005;25(2):171–83.

120. Berthold HK, Unverdorben S, Degenhardt R, et al. Effect of policosanol on lipid levels among patients with hypercholesterolemia or combined hyperlipidemia: a randomized controlled trial. JAMA. 2006;295(19):2262–9.

121. Packer L., Rimbach G, Virgili F. Antioxidant activity and biologic properties of a procyanidin-rich extract from pine (Pinus maritima) bark, pycnogenol. Free Radic Biol Med. 1999;27(5–6):704–24.

122. Sarrat L. Therapeutic approach to functional disorders of lower extremities. Bordeaux Med. 1981;14:685.

123. Arcangeli P. Pycnogenol in chronic venous insufficiency. Fitoterapia. 2000;71(3): 236–44.

124. Petrassi C, Mastromarino A, Spartera C. PYCNOGENOL in chronic venous insufficiency. Phytomedicine. 2000;7(5):383–8.

125. Liu X, Wei J, Tan F, et al. Pycnogenol, French maritime pine bark extract, improves endothelial function of hypertensive patients. Life Sci. 2004;74(7):855–62.

126. Gupta R, Singhal S, Goyle A, et al. Antioxidant and hypocholesterolaemic effects of Terminalia arjuna tree-bark powder: a randomised placebo-controlled trial. J Assoc Physicians India. 2001b;49:231–5.

127. Bharani A, Ganguli A, Mathur LK, et al. Efficacy of Terminalia arjuna in chronic stable angina: a double-blind, placebo-controlled, crossover study comparing Terminalia arjuna with isosorbide mononitrate. Indian Heart J. 2002;54(2):170–5.

CHAPTER

23

OBESITY AND WEIGHT LOSS: AN OVERVIEW OF DIET, DRUGS AND DIETARY SUPPLEMENTS

Rebecca B. Costello and Johanna T. Dwyer

INTRODUCTION: OBESITY AND CARDIOVASCULAR DISEASE RISK

Forecasting life expectancy by extrapolating from the past is like forecasting the weather on the basis of its history. Looking out the window, we see a threatening storm—obesity—that will, if unchecked, have a negative effect on life expectancy.[1]

Obesity continues to be a growing health problem in the United States and is now viewed as a chronic disease with morbid consequences. According to the Centers for Disease Control and Prevention (CDC), close to two-thirds of American adults surveyed in 1999–2002 were overweight, approximately 30% were obese (a doubling since the second National Health and Nutrition Examination Survey [NHANES II] of 1976–1980), 8% were diabetic, and 24% had characteristics of the metabolic syndrome.[2] Even though cardiovascular disease (CVD) risk factors have declined over the past 40 years irrespective of body mass index (BMI), obese individuals still have higher risk factor levels with a notable (55%) increase prevalence of diabetes (diagnosed and undiagnosed).[3] Additionally, the National Cholesterol Education Program (NCEP) Adult Treatment Panel III (ATP III) guidelines recognize overweight and obesity as major underlying risk factor for, and a direct target of intervention for, coronary heart disease (CHD),[4] and losing weight has proven benefits on established CVD risk factors. The recommended approaches for reducing overweight and obesity are contained in the National Heart, Lung and Blood Institute (NHLBI) Obesity Education Initiative guideline titled *Clinical Guidelines on the Identification, Evaluation, and Treatment of Overweight and Obesity in Adults.*[5]

Annual medical spending due to overweight and obesity (BMI >25) is reported to be $92.6 billion (9.1% of U.S. health expenditures). The indirect costs alone of overweight and obesity ($56 billion) are comparable to the economic costs of cigarette smoking. Success with lowering CVD risk in patients by addressing one risk factor enhances the likelihood of success with other risk factors. Because risk factors have additive effects on CVD, reducing more than one risk factor will have a larger and synergistic effect than focusing only on obesity. Randomized trials employing behavioral interventions for diet and physical activity have succeeded in maintaining clinically meaningful weight loss for 18 months (PREMIER), 3 years (Trials of Hypertension Prevention II), and 4 years (Diabetes Prevention Program [DPP]), which had significant and clinically beneficial effects on blood pressure, cholesterol, and diabetes. Moreover, these intervention strategies can be adapted to be feasible in routine care.

Since 73% of obese and overweight Americans have more than one treatable CVD risk factor, optimal clinical care requires an integrated approach involving both lifestyle modifications and pharmacotherapy when indicated. An integrated approach is scientifically sound, practically appealing, and efficient in clinical practice to control multiple risk factors. Whether starting a new drug, losing weight, or increasing physical activity, the basic steps are similar. They include screening for the risky behavior in question, assessing diet and dietary supplement intake, assessing physical activity and exercise, and then, based on findings, providing advice to the patient on the need for change, and a referral for counseling. Follow-up should also always be ascertained. The web sites in Table 23-1 provide additional information on how to achieve these goals.

DEFINING OVERWEIGHT AND OBESITY

Overweight refers to an excess of body weight compared to reference standards. This excess weight may come from muscle, bone, fat, and/or body water, but when it exceeds about 10% of standards the cause is usually excess adiposity, assuming that there is no abnormal hydration. Obesity refers specifically to having an abnormally high proportion of body fat compared to standards.[5]

Two surrogate measures important for assessing body fat are BMI and waist circumference. BMI, calculated as weight in kilograms divided by height in meters squared (kg/m^2) can be used to screen for both overweight and obesity in adults. It is the measurement of choice for many obesity researchers and health professionals. BMI is not gender-specific. While BMI does not directly measure body fat, it is a more accurate indicator of overweight and obesity than relying on weight for height alone, and correlates well with adipose tissue. Weight reduction with dietary treatment is in order for all patients with a BMI of 25–30, who have comorbidities and for all patients with a BMI over 30.

Waist circumference has also been used as a practical tool to evaluate fat patterning, which is associated with an increased risk of certain morbid conditions common among obese patients. This indirect measure of waist circumference at the level of the umbilicus is a rough measure of the patient's subcutaneous and

TABLE 23-1

KEY WEBSITES FOR HEALTH PROFESSIONALS ON GUIDANCE FOR MODIFYING

Cardiovascular	Risk Factors
Cholesterol (NCEP-ATP III) and hypertension (JNC7)	http://www.nhlbi.nih.gov/guidelines/index.htm
Diabetes	http://betterdiabetescare.nih.gov/ WHATclinicalmanagement.htm#resources http://www.shapeup.org/profcenter/download/ http://www.s2mw.com/aha/hodprologin.asp
Physical activity	http://dnrc.nih.gov/move/index.htm; http://www.americanheart.org/presenter.jhtml? identifier=1200013
Diet	http://www.nhlbi.nih.gov/health/public/heart/hbp/ dash/index.htm http://www.americanheart.org/presenter.jhtml? identifier=3004200
Overweight/obesity	http://www.niddk.nih.gov/health/nutrit/nutrit.htm http://win.niddk.nih.gov/publications/index.htm http://www.nhlbi.nih.gov/guidelines/obesity/ ob_gdlns.htm http://www.nhlbi.nih.gov/health/public/heart/ obesity/lose_wt/profmats.htm

mesenteric fat in the abdomen. It is helpful to take this circumference before, during, and after treatment for weight reduction. A high waist circumference is associated with an increased risk for Type II diabetes, dyslipidemia, hypertension, and CVD in patients with a BMI between 25 and 34.9. Men and women are at an increased relative risk for disease if they have a waist circumference greater than 40 in and 35 in, respectively, as outlined in Table 23-2.

A variety of other factors such as smoking, high blood pressure, sedentary lifestyle, and comorbidities further add to the risks that decrease quality of life and increase morbidity and mortality associated with an elevated BMI and/or waist circumference that indicates overweight or obesity.

Detailed information on the classification and assessment of obesity and an obesity treatment algorithm is provided in the *Practical Guide to the Identification, Evaluation and Treatment of Overweight and Obesity in Adults.*[5] It provides step-by-step guidance for assessing overweight and obesity; it does not reflect the overall evaluation of other conditions and diseases. Additional guidance for cholesterol disorders and hypertension are described in NCEP-ATP III[4] and the Seventh

TABLE 23-2

CLASSIFICATION OF OVERWEIGHT AND OBESITY BY BMI AND WAIST CIRCUMFERENCE AND ASSOCIATED DISEASE RISKS[5]

| | BMI (kg/m^2) | Obesity Class | Disease Risk* Relative to Normal Weight and Waist Circumference | |
			Men ≤102 cm (≤40 in) Women ≤ 88 cm (≤35 in)	>102 cm (>40 in) >88 cm (>35 in)
Underweight	<18.5		—	—
Normal*	18.5–24.9		—	—
Overweight	25.0–29.9		Increased	High
Obesity	30.0–34.9	I	High	Very high
	35.0–39.9	II	Very high	Very high
Extreme obesity	≥40	III	Extremely high	Extremely high

*National Institutes of Health. Clinical guidelines on the identification, evaluation, and treatment of overweight and obesity in adults—the evidence report. Obes Res. 1998;6 Suppl 2:51S–209S. [PMID: 9813653.] [PubMed-indexed for MEDLINE.] Accessed at http://www.nhlbi.nih.gov/guidelines/obesity/ob-glns.pdf

Report of the Joint National Committee on Prevention, Detection, Evaluation, and Treatment of High Blood Pressure (JNC7).[6]

Patients for whom weight-loss therapy is not appropriate include most pregnant or lactating women, children, and adolescents if they are without benefit of guidance by a knowledgeable physician, persons with serious uncontrolled psychiatric illness, and patients who have a serious illness and/or eating disorder where calorie restriction would be contraindicated. Therapy is also not appropriate if the patient indicates that he or she is not willing to participate. Attempting to treat patients who do not want assistance is rarely effective.

CLINICAL ASSESSMENT OF THE OVERWEIGHT OR OBESE PATIENT

The treatment algorithm in Figure 23-1 will help guide the clinician in performing an examination of the overweight and/or obese patient.

Key questions to ask in obtaining a medical history

(http://Endotext.com/obesity/obesity13/obesity13.htm)

- Medical history, risk factors, and established complications from obesity—inquire about snoring and daytime somnolence

Treatment algorithm*

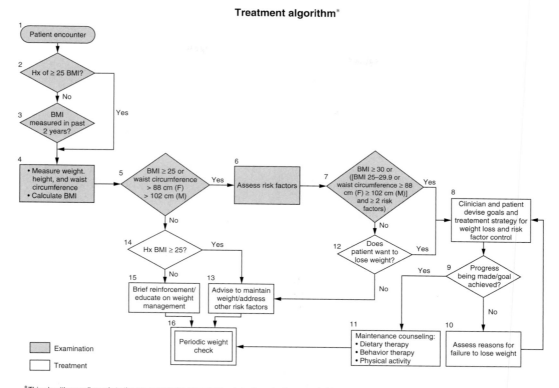

*This algorithm applies only to the assessment for overweight and obesity and subsequent decisions based on that assessment for other conditions and diseases that the physician may wish to do.

FIGURE 23-1   *Treatment algorithm for assessment of overweight and obesity. (With permission from National Institutes of Health. Clinical guidelines on the identification, evaluation, and treatment of overweight and obesity in adults—the evidence report. Obes Res. 1998;6 Suppl 2:51S–209S. [PMID: 9813653.] [PubMed-indexed for MEDLINE.] Accessed at http://www.nhlbi.nih.gov/guidelines/ obesity/ob-glns.pdf*

- Body weight history (pattern and landmarks for weight gain: puberty, employment, marriage, pregnancies, age at menopause, injuries, and disabilities
- History of previous treatment(s) for obesity
- Family history of obesity and related risk factors (i.e., Type II diabetes, hypertension, premature CHD, and gallstones)
- Diet history including usual eating pattern and alcohol intake
- Activity and lifestyle including type, frequency, and pattern of exercise, note any physical limitations
- Relevant social history including cigarette smoking
- Drug history—drugs associated with weight gain (e.g., phenothiazides, tricyclic antidepressants, anticonvulsants, lithium, anabolic and glucocorticoid steroids) as well as drugs associated with weight loss

(e.g., diuretics, anorectics, dietary supplements, and herbal products containing stimulants)

- In women, menstrual history and status (irregular menses associated with polycystic ovary syndrome)

Key clinical examination features

In particular, the clinician should pay attention to identifying and defining coexisting cardiovascular risk factors such as hypertension, evidence of cardiac valvular disease, pulmonary hypertension, cor pulmonale, or congestive cardiac failure. The clinician should document if physical signs of hyperlipidemia, thyroid disease, or ophthalmic evidence for diabetes or hypertension exists. Initial laboratory investigations should include fasting blood glucose, fasting lipid profile, strip test for urine glucose and protein, and free thyroxine and thyroid-stimulating hormone (TSH). Further discussion of these features can be found at http://Endotext.com/obesity/.

DIETARY MODIFICATIONS TO TREAT OBESITY

As reviewed in the *Clinical Guidelines on the Identification, Evaluation, and Treatment of Overweight and Obesity in Adults*,[5] randomized controlled trials evaluating the effectiveness of diets provide strong and consistent evidence that an average weight loss of 8% of initial body weight can be obtained over 3–12 months with a low-calorie diet and that this weight-loss effects a decrease in abdominal fat. Lower fat diets with targeted caloric reduction were found to promote greater weight loss than lower fat diets alone.

Evidence-based reviews of successful weight-control techniques increasingly emphasize the importance of individualized multidisciplinary care, a health-outcomes focus, realistic goal setting, and making permanent lifestyle change. The approach to setting goals and treating obese patients must be non-judgmental and focused on an acceptable weight for good health outcomes rather than solely on body weight. Definitions of success should be patient-specific. Even if weight is not lost, the reduction of risk factors can be achieved and translated into improved health.

Very low calorie diet plans

Very low calorie diets (VLCDs) or "protein-supplemented modified fasts" that provide less than 800 and often less than 500 calories/day are used in weight reduction. These diets may pose risks of nutrient inadequacy and be unsafe if they are not formulated appropriately. Because the metabolic effects of VLCDs are considerable, they are presumably safest when prescribed, dispensed, and monitored under a physician's direction as a part of a comprehensive weight reduction program. The safety and efficacy of VLCDs have been reviewed and reasonable recommendations for their use have been provided. Careful physician monitoring is essential with these regimens; patients should not embark upon them on their own because the metabolic risks are considerable. VLCDs usually require supplementation, fortification, or special formulations of foods with certain micronutrients, electrolytes, and other nutrients since so little food is supplied. Protein needs may rise when energy is severely restricted because dietary as well as bodily protein stores may be used to maintain blood glucose levels, especially after the body's limited endogenous carbohydrate stores have been exhausted. Depending on the VLCD plan and its formulation, the need for nutrient supplements and/or electrolytes may vary, and should be frequently evaluated—particularly for patients on potassium-sparing diuretics, digoxin, and other hypertensive medications. Nevertheless, adverse events may still occur. Also, medications often need adjustment on such regimes.

The Institute of Medicine of the National Academies reports that dietary intakes of potassium on usual American diets are approximately 2.9–3.2 g/day in adults, considerably below the adequate intake of 4.7 g/day and extremely hypocaloric, VLCDs are probably often even lower. Fruits and vegetables, which are especially rich in potassium and other nutrients, are generally very limited on VLCDs. Therefore potassium intakes may be inadequate. Also, when dietary intake is reduced, the kidney is inefficient in conserving potassium, and hypokalemia (serum potassium concentration <3.5 mmol/L) may result. Signs and symptoms of hypokalemia include cardiac arrhythmias, muscle weakness, and glucose intolerance. Moderate potassium deficiency may also occur without hypokalemia. Individuals on VLCDs are therefore often prescribed potassium supplements. Risks of hyperkalemia also may result from self-medication with potassium supplements. In contrast, the risks of excessive amounts of potassium from consuming ordinary foods on weight-reduction diets are minimal among those with normal kidney function.

Some VLCDs rely on commercially available formula foods (e.g. *Optifast* a very low calorie, protein-supplemented modified fast available through physicians and *Slim-Fast*, an over-the-counter formulated product), and are generally formulated to include vitamins and minerals in amounts approximating the recommended dietary allowances (RDAs) or adequate intakes (AIs) if consumed in recommended amounts. VLCD plans based on ordinary foods usually include recommendations for specific supplements to ensure that needs for vitamins, minerals, electrolytes, and other nutrients are met so that the combination of foods plus supplements achieve adequate and recommended intakes. As noted previously, for safety reasons, VLCDs should be followed under a physician's direction. Information on the safety and efficacy of VLCDs and recommendations for their use is available.[7]

Low-calorie diet plans

Low-calorie diets (LCDs) of 1200–1500 calories/day are designed to create a caloric deficit of about 500 calories a day for adult women and to promote weight loss of about 1 lb/week. A 10% reduction in body weight reduces disease risk factors. A reasonable time to achieve a 10% reduction in body weight is within about 6 months of therapy. Another way of expressing attainable goals is through a reduction in BMI units. A BMI unit is approximately 10–15 lb depending on an individual's height and weight, so a decrease in 2 BMI units over 6 months is reasonable. Reductions of this magnitude decrease risk factors and thus result in "healthier" weights.

Reducing diets, even lower in calories than LCDs (e.g., 800–1200 calories), cause more rapid weight loss but are often even more limited in micronutrients. Such reducing diets often consist of foods that are commonly available in grocery stores. It may be difficult to achieve RDA levels for certain nutrients such as iron, calcium, and vitamin B_6. The lower the diet is in calories, the greater the probability that some nutrients may fall short. Options for achieving recommended intake levels include addition of several servings of foods rich in the specific nutrient, use of fortified foods or commercially prepared meal-replacement products that are relatively high in nutrients for the calories they provide, a single nutrient supplement, and/or a multivitamin/mineral supplement. For individuals who already consume adequate intakes of most nutrients from food sources, there is no recognized health benefit from consuming higher levels, and they may be at risk of excessive intakes, particularly if they exceed the tolerable upper intake levels (ULs). The dietary reference intakes (DRIs) encompass a set of four intake levels, including the ULs, and are available online at the National Academies web site (www.iom.edu/cms/3708.aspx).

Meal replacements

A partial meal replacement (PMR) plan that prescribes one or two portioned-controlled, vitamin/mineral-fortified meal replacements along with traditional reduced calorie meals or snacks may offer additional versatility and utility to the LCD approaches described above. A PMR includes one or more meals replaced by a commercially available, calorie-reduced product(s) that is fortified with vitamins and minerals taken together with at least one daily meal consisting of regular foods. Calorie content should remain in the 800–1600 calorie/day range. There are limited data on randomized controlled trials and these trials have used the same commercial product. A meta- and pooling analysis from six studies (a total of 249 PMR-treated subjects and 238 control subjects with a mean BMI of 31.l) concluded that utilizing PMR plans for weight management can safely and effectively produce significant sustainable weight loss and improve weight-related risk factors of disease.[8] In this analysis, the intervention group replaced two meals per day with liquid PMRs during the weight-loss phase and one meal per day with a liquid PMR in the weight-maintenance phase. Greater weight losses were demonstrated in the PMR group (e.g., about 2.5 kg at 3 months and 2.4 kg at 1 year) compared to controls. However, it is important to note that at the 1-year evaluation, 64% of subjects in the control group had dropped out compared to 47% of the subjects in the PMR group. Overall weight loss in the control group was about 4% and in the PMR group 7–8% at 1 year, with significant

reductions in cardiovascular risk factors. Diabetic subjects e
ies achieved a significant weight loss, but the differences
between the PMR and control groups. Results of more re
evaluating PMR interventions for weight loss were simila

TIPS FOR BRINGING ABOUT WEIGHT CHANGE THROUGH DIETARY INTERVENTIONS:[11]

- Small steps work.
  Focus on small achievable goals that are individualized for patients to gain energy balance in their everyday life.
- Use biomarkers.
  Monitor progress and adherence to dietary/lifestyle modification through clinical laboratory or biomarker assessment, such as blood cholesterol levels or glycated hemoglobin.
- Tap into motivators.
  Identify and tap into a patient's primary motivator as this will greatly increase the ability to induce and sustain behavioral change. Insist upon personal responsibility as a component of treatment strategies.
- Focus on real foods.
  People don't eat nutrients, they eat foods. Provide recommendations for healthy eating plans.
- Recognize and teach the concept of nutrient density.
  Foods with a high-energy density or high calorie per unit of weight may foster obesity.
- Teach portion size.
  Consumers need to be re-educated on what a healthy portion size is and how it has come to be distorted in our on-the-go convenience packaged food world.
- Involve the family.
  Support and encouragement from those close to the patient will also dramatically improve success.
- Sustain and maintain weight loss.
  Incorporate a flexible, individualized, multidisciplinary approach through diet, exercise, and self-monitoring tools, such as dietary intake and physical activity records.

As weight maintenance becomes a major challenge, long-term monitoring and encouragement to maintain weight loss requires regular clinical visits, group meetings, or encouragement via telephone or e-mail.

TABLE 23-3

GUIDELINES FOR COMPOSITION OF HEALTHFUL WEIGHT-CONTROL PLANS

Carbohydrate	VLCD: > 50g/day LCD: > 100g/day
Protein	VLCD: 1.5 g/kg body wt. (>65–70 g/day) LCD: 1.0 g/kg body wt.
Fat	<30% dietary energy from total fat <10% saturated fat <10% polyunsaturated fat <15% monounsaturated fat
Cholesterol	<300 mg/day
Fiber	20–30 g/day
Water	Eight glasses (~2 quarts or 2 L) More needed with exercise and/or heat
Vitamins/minerals	Supplements desirable on diets < 1200 kcal/day to levels specified in the DRIs, with special emphasis on iron, calcium, and folic acid for women of reproductive age
Sodium chloride	<1000 mmol/day (approx. 6 g/day)
Calcium	1500–2000 mg/day
Alcohol	Minimal to none

http://endotext.com/obesity/obesity18/obesity18.htm

The composition of the reducing diet influences nutritional status and the composition of the weight that is lost. Recommendations for healthful weight-control plans are outlined in Table 23-3 and discussed in detail in several excellent resources.[12]

PHARMACOLOGICAL MEASURES TO TREAT OBESITY

Antiobesity drugs may have a role—along with a hypocaloric diet, physical activity, and behavior therapy—in weight reduction in patients whose condition is refractory to nonpharmacological measures and for the maintenance of weight loss as well. Drug therapy is indicated in patients with a BMI >30 but may also be considered for those with a BMI of 27–30 if comorbidities are present or in heavier patients without comorbidities, who have been unsuccessful with dietary measures alone. These drugs can also improve other CVD risk factors such as glycemic control and lipid levels. They should be used only in the context of a treatment program that includes diet, physical activity changes, and behavior therapy. Drugs currently used to treat obesity are classified as centrally acting appetite suppressants (sibutramine, fluoxetine, phentermine, diethylpropion, bupropion, and topiramate) and drugs that affect nutrient partitioning (orlistat). Sibutramine and orlistat are the only two prescription drugs currently approved for long-term use in weight reduction. Both drugs bring about modest weight loss and somewhat improved CVD risk factor profiles. Patients who are likely to respond to drugs do so within the first month of therapy, and if they fail to lose about 5 lb in the first month the drug is unlikely to be effective. In some cases, the magnitude of weight loss is not as great as it might be with intensive lifestyle interventions, but patient adherence to intensive lifestyle interventions may not be good. It is not known if these drugs reduce the risk of cardiovascular events, and each has some adverse effects.

Sibutramine

Sibutramine is a prescription drug approved for short-term use by the U.S. Food and Drug Administration (FDA). Another centrally acting compound for obesity was dexfenfluramine, which was removed from the market in 1997 due to increased incidence of pulmonary hypertension and valvular heart disease. Safety concerns have been raised by Health Canada and several European countries regarding significant adverse events. Sibutramine is contraindicated in persons with coronary artery disease, congestive heart failure, arrhythmias, stroke, or inadequately controlled hypertension and in those receiving psychiatric medications. Common side effects of sibutramine include dry mouth, constipation, and insomnia and more rarely palpitations and increased blood pressure.

Orlistat

Orlistat is a gastrointestinal-tract lipase inhibitor that decreases intestinal fat absorption by up to 30%. It only works on fat in the food consumed. It is generally well tolerated, has a good safety profile, and has been shown to produce clinically meaningful and sustained decreases in weight and BMI when combined with other lifestyle interventions in nondiabetics as well as diabetics.[13] Orlistat treatment has been associated with lower levels of fat-soluble vitamins in plasma, although limited data exist regarding the frequency and magnitude of this effect. Because malabsorption is involved, the drug includes fat-soluble vitamins to replace those losses. Additional information is available for health-care professionals at: http://win.niddk.nih.gov/publications/prescription.htm#meds.

Current state of drug therapy

A recent review and meta-analysis of pharmacological and surgical treatments for obesity in adults, adolescents, and children concluded that sibutramine, orlistat, phentermne, diethylpropion, bupropion, fluoxetine, and topiramate all promote weight loss at 6 and/or 12 months when given in conjunction with dietary modifications.[14] The report reviewed the evidence of these treatments on adults, adolescents, and children. While no drug promoted more weight loss than another, a modest weight loss was documented (less than 5 kg at 1 year). Side effects were also documented for all drugs. A similar systematic review evaluating trials of weight loss found a 4.3 kg greater weight loss with sibutramine (taken at 10–20 mg/day) and a 2.7 kg greater weight loss in patients who used orlistat (120 mg, 3 times/day) compared to placebo at 1 year. More subjects in the orlistat and sibutramine groups achieved 5% and 10% weight losses than those in the placebo group.[15] A recent meta-analysis evaluated the efficacy of pharmacotherapy for weight loss in adults with Type II diabetes mellitus and found that fluoxetine, orlistat, and sibutramine can produce significant but modest weight loss over 26–52 weeks with improvements in glycated hemoglobin.[16]

The scientific literature is devoid of studies that examine the effectiveness of pharmacotherapy *combined* with a comprehensive lifestyle or behavioral modification program. Just recently, such a study was published evaluating lifestyle modification plus medication for weight loss in obese subjects. In this 1-year randomized study, treatment with a lifestyle modification program of diet, exercise, and behavioral therapy when used in combination with sibutramine resulted in significantly greater weight loss among obese adults than treatment with the medication alone (an average of more than 26 lb compared to 11 lb).[17] Further work is needed to examine whether the combination of lifestyle modification (e.g., a hypocaloric diet, exercise/physical activity, and behavioral modification) and pharmacotherapy improves the efficacy of drug therapy, and whether such combinations are synergistic or additive and what dosage schedules and sequencing of the two interventions are optimal.

DIETARY SUPPLEMENTS FOR WEIGHT LOSS

The majority of Americans are on a mission to combat their weight. According to a recent survey by the Natural Marketing Institute, 59% of the general population is managing weight for health or appearance. Of this 59%, approximately 26% had used weight-loss products in the past year. About 18% stated they had used an over-the-counter medication, 21% had used a prescription medication, and 11% had tried weight-loss supplements in the past year to lose weight.[18]

A large number of dietary supplements are marketed today with claims that they offer a safe, natural, and rapid means to weight loss. FDA regulates dietary supplements under a different set of regulations than those covering "conventional" foods and drug products (http://www.cfsan.fda.gov).

Data collected from the CDC's Behavioral Risk Factor Surveillance System (1996–1998) demonstrated that 7% of those surveyed were using nonprescription weight-loss products (an estimated 17.2 million Americans), 2% were taking phenylpropanolamine (5 million), and 1% were taking ephedra (2.5 million).[19] In 1998, observational data collected from poison control centers revealed that 14% of callers reported weight loss as the intended use for the suspected product causing an adverse reaction.[20]

However, for most weight-loss supplements, little scientific evidence to date supports their efficacy. Although there have been studies on specific ingredients, the research has often been of short duration, involved small numbers of subjects, or used study approaches that limited the usefulness of their findings. There have been few comprehensive reviews or long-term studies of efficacy. Searching the Natural Medicines Comprehensive Database (www.naturaldatabase.com),[21] we identified 61 individual dietary supplements and 10 proprietary products with purported weight-loss effects.

Dietary supplements have been proposed as being useful for stimulating or enhancing weight loss by altering body functions. The supposed mechanisms of action vary, depending on the ingredient. Some are claimed to have anorectic effects and decrease food intake, others to bring about metabolic changes that increase energy output and cause weight loss. A number of common dietary supplements purported to act by increasing energy expenditure include ephedra, bitter orange, guarana, and caffeine. Typically these supplements are not consumed as single ingredient supplements and occur in various mixtures and formulations.

Botanical weight-loss supplements

EPHEDRA (EPHEDRA SINICA) OR MA HUANG

One of the most well-known supplements for weight loss is ephedra or ma huang (*Ephedra sinica*), which was the staple of many weight-loss product formulations. The principle alkaloid constituents are ephedrine, pseudoephedrine and sometimes small amounts of phenylpropanolamine. Ephedrine and pseudoephedrine are both non-selective alpha- and beta-receptor agonists. While shown to be moderately effective for weight loss in a few small clinical studies, a systematic review of the literature[22] along with a large series of adverse-event reports have highlighted the potential dangers of this botanical ingredient. Its use has fallen dramatically since the FDA removed it from the market in April 2004. Ephedra-containing supplements were banned on the grounds that they present "a significant or unreasonable risk of illness or injury when used according to its labeling or under ordinary conditions of use." Other botanicals typically formulated in combination with ephedra (such as guarana and caffeine, see Table 23-4.) have made efficacy and safety evaluations of ephedra difficult.

TABLE 23-4

STIMULANT HERBAL BLENDS CONTAINING CAFFEINE

Green or black tea
Guarana
Kola nut (cola)
Cacao (cocoa)
Coffee
Yerba mate (Paraguay tea, ilex)

Recent placebo-controlled studies have shown that single doses of an ephedra- and caffeine-containing dietary supplements were responsible for a clinically significant prolonged QT corrected for heart rate (QTc) and elevated blood-pressure response.[23] Ephedra in combination with guarana produced persistent increases in heart rate and blood pressure with unfavorable actions on postprandial glucose concentrations and serum potassium concentrations. Such effects could be detrimental in persons with hypertension, atherosclerosis, or glucose intolerance—conditions strongly associated with obesity.[24]

BITTER ORANGE (CITRUS AURANTIUM)

A newer botanical touted for weight loss is bitter orange or *Citrus aurantium*, which may also prove to be equally as problematic as ephedra. It is also known as Seville orange, sour orange, green orange, neroli oil, and kijitsu. The alkaloids present in *Citrus aurantium* include isomers of synephrine with selective α- and β-agonist activity shown to stimulate lipolysis, increase basal metabolic rate (BMR), and oxidation of fat. Weight loss has been reported in two clinical trials and increased thermogenesis reported in three. A recent meta-analysis[25] reviewed the literature and found one 6-week randomized, placebo-controlled trial involving 23 healthy subjects with a BMI >25 suitable for analysis. Subjects were randomized to one of three groups to receive: (1) an herbal mixture containing 975 mg *Citrus aurantium* (6% synephrine alkaloids), 900 mg St. John's wort (3% hypericum), and 528 mg caffeine or (2) a maltodextrin placebo, or (3) nothing (the control group). All subjects received dietary counseling and participated in an exercise program. Clinically significant changes were not seen for weight, percent body fat, fat mass, and BMR. Overall, the systematic review found no evidence that *Citrus aurantium* is effective for weight loss. There is confusion in the literature as to which synephrine alkaloids are present in *Citrus aurantium*, thus making determination of safety and efficacy difficult.[26] The synephrine in bitter-orange products may increase blood pressure and therefore would be contraindicated in individuals with hypertension, CVD, or wide-angle glaucoma. Bitter orange is typically sold as a standardized extract containing 1–6% synephrine. Higher amounts of synephrine in dietary supplements may suggest adulteration with purified synephrine.

GARCINIA CAMBOGIA

One of the fastest growing botanicals in market sales has been *Garcinia cambogia*, containing hydroxycitrate (HCA). The plant grows in Southeast Asia where it is used as a seasoning in Thai and other Asian cuisines. As an antiobesity agent, it is purported to reduce appetite and decrease fatty acid synthesis, thereby reducing body weight. HCA has been evaluated in numerous randomized, controlled clinical trials where it has demonstrated equivocal results. Early trials with HCA alone or in combination with other ingredients in subjects on restricted diets showed increased weight loss. The most rigorous study to date was a 12-week randomized controlled trial in 135 men and women utilizing 1500 mg/day of HCA vs. placebo in combination with a low-energy, high-fiber diet. Both groups lost weight and percent fat mass, but there was no difference between the groups in amount of weight or fat lost. Product labels for HCA may refer to the fruit of *Garcinia cambogia* or the active compound. HCA represents up to 16% of the weight of the dried fruit and typically 50% of the extract. HCA is considered safe, but no data from long-term studies are available.

GREEN TEA POLYPHENOLS

Green tea polyphenols, such as epigallocatechin gallate (EGCG), have thermogenic properties and promote fat oxidation beyond that explained by the caffeine content of green tea. Two small studies in men found very slight increases in metabolism. A recent double-blind, randomized trial in 46 female subjects (mean BMI 27.7) consuming a low-energy diet plus three capsules of green tea extract or placebo were evaluated during a weight-loss and weight maintenance period of 87 days.[27] Together, supplements of the extract and a low-energy diet had no sustained effect on free fatty acids, triglycerides, β-hydroxybutrate, glucose, or total cholesterol levels.

Nonbotanical supplements for weight loss

Aside from botanical supplements, calcium, chromium, conjugated linoleic acid (CLA), and chitosan supplements have been purported to offer some promise of efficacy with a low-side effect profile, but the data are just beginning to emerge on these supplements.

CONJUGATED LINOLEIC ACID

Conjugated linoleic acid (CLA), found naturally in milk and meat products, is produced in the rumen of animals and also from sunflower and safflower oil. CLA is believed to increase metabolic rate and alter body composition by increasing lean-tissue deposition and decreasing fat deposition. Consistent and convincing effects of CLA on body composition have been documented in several animal models, but reduction in body weight or adipose-tissue mass has not been consistently demonstrated in human studies. CLA-induced changes have been linked to increased lipolysis in adipocytes and enhanced fatty acid oxidation in both adiopocytes and skeletal muscle cells.[28]

There are 28 different types of CLA. As a weight-loss product, it is an isoform of CLA, specifically the *trans*-10, *cis*-12 isomer, that is of interest. Effects in humans are unclear though animal studies suggest that CLA may increase fat oxidation and decrease triglyceride uptake in adipose tissue. In a randomized-controlled trial, 60 obese men with metabolic syndrome were given one of three interventions: a mixture of CLA; the *trans*-10, *cis*-12 isomer; or a placebo for 12 weeks for the intention of weight loss. The findings were not promising. There was no change in body weight or BMI, and there was an increase in parameters of oxidative stress, as measured by vitamin E levels, and an increase in inflammatory biomarkers. In this study, CLA was also associated with worsening of insulin resistance. Data for 24 months of supplementation are now available showing good compliance with CLA therapy (3.4 g/day in the triglyceride form) and a 6–8% reduction in body fat mass compared to baseline, while maintaining lean body mass.[29] Noted however were higher levels of LP(a) and an increase in biomarkers associated with inflammation and CVD risk. More clinical studies in humans are needed to better understand the effects of CLAs, found naturally in dairy and meat, on weight loss and other aspects of health.

CALCIUM

Growing evidence suggests a relationship between increased calcium intake and reduction in body weight. The impact of calcium intake on weight loss or prevention of weight gain has been demonstrated across the age span, in Caucasians and African-Americans, and in both men and women. Epidemiologic data as well as clinical data demonstrate that dairy products exert a substantially greater effect on both fat loss and fat distribution compared to an equivalent amount of supplemental calcium.[30] The postulated mechanism for calcium's action is the suppression of parathyroid hormone and 1,25 dihydroxyvitamin D3 to inhibit fat production and promote lipolysis in the adipocytes. However, in human trials there is inconsistency in results. In one small study, increasing amounts of dietary calcium through high consumption of dairy products augmented weight and fat loss on reducing diets. In a larger multicenter study of close to 100 overweight adults on hypocaloric diets by the same research group, high calcium intakes of 1400 mg/day offered no significant-benefits on weight loss or body composition compared to a lower-calcium diet (600 mg/day). On the other hand, a high dairy diet with three servings of milk and milk products per day providing 1400 mg calcium augmented weight loss and fat loss.

In another study by a different research group working on this same issue, calcium supplementation did not increase weight loss in a randomized, double-blind, placebo-controlled weight-loss intervention with adult women,[31] nor did another randomized, controlled trial find an effect on weight loss. The positive results are limited to small studies, and therefore it is not yet firmly established that either calcium or dairy foods enhance weight loss combined with low-calorie diets. No safety problems were identified under the conditions of use of calcium in these studies. More clinical trials with larger numbers of subjects are needed to clarify these observations. Within the past year, work has extended to post and premenopausal women. So far, the results suggest that calcium intakes may need to be in excess of usual intakes to maintain bone during weight loss. The potential benefits of calcium supplements on weight loss remain disputed and more work is needed.

In the Coronary Artery Risk Development in Young Adults (CARDIA) study, increased dairy consumption showed a strong inverse association with the 10-year cumulative incidence of obesity and insulin resistance syndrome. The odds of obesity, abnormal glucose homeostasis, insulin resistance syndrome, and increased blood pressure were 20% lower with each additional serving of dairy product.

CHITOSAN

Chitosan, derived from the exoskeletons of crustaceans, is purported to work by binding and thereby blocking the absorption the fats. A meta-analysis of clinical trials suggested a slight additional weight loss associated with chitosan versus placebo when coupled with an energy-restricted diet. However, in a more recent double-blind randomized trial, the same investigators[32] found no clinically significant reduction in weight when overweight volunteers following their typical diet were given 1000 mg/day of chitosan for 28 days. Vitamin K levels increased in the chitosan group and while there we no serious adverse events, more adverse effects were noted. Caution is noted because chitosan's binding to fat could mean that fat-soluble vitamins in the diet might need to be replaced. A more recent 24-week randomized, controlled clinical trial in 250 overweight and obese adults confirmed a lack of effect on body weight, blood cholesterol, and glucose measures on 3 g chitosan per day compared to placebo.[33]. Additionally, chitosan had no effect on fecal fat excretion, suggesting that it does not bind fat in the intestine. This study was the largest trial of chitosan to date, with the largest number of follow-up visits and the most outcome measures. It casts further doubt on the efficacy of chitosan for weight loss. Nausea, constipation, and flatulence have also been cited as potential side effects.

CHROMIUM

Chromium is a cofactor for insulin and has been evaluated for its effect on carbohydrate, protein, and lipid metabolism. Reported effects of chromium supplementation include an increase in BMR and lean body mass, a decrease in percentage body fat, and decreased blood insulin levels. The most extensively used form of chromium is chromium picolinate. Data from clinical trials regarding chromium's effect on weight loss are mixed. A review of 24 studies that examined the effects of 200–1000 mcg/day of chromium picolinate on body mass or composition found no significant benefits. A meta-analysis that included data from 10 double-blind, randomized, controlled trials noted a reduction of 1.1–1.2 kg over 6 to 14 weeks in overweight subjects, but these differences were small.[34] Earlier, safety concerns regarding the toxicity of chromium picolinate have been removed with more through reviews, including human study data. Few serious adverse effects have been linked to high intakes of chromium, so the Institute of Medicine has not established a tolerable upper intake level (UL) for this mineral. In 2004, chromium picolinate received a qualified health claim from the FDA for its possible benefits in lowering blood glucose levels. This supplement will likely become more popular in patients seeking to reduce their CVD risk factors beyond weight loss.

APPLICATIONS: LOCATING RELIABLE INFORMATION ON DIETARY SUPPLEMENTS

Recent studies and observations suggest that some dietary supplements may interact with other over-the-counter and prescription drugs that individuals may be taking for weight reduction and, thereby, alter drug effectiveness. In addition, these dietary supplements may interact with foods and other supplements, so reliable sources should be consulted when providing advice on weight reduction. Among the list of weight-loss supplements that should be avoided by patients with CVD are ephedra and combination products containing ephedra (herbal "phen-fen"), guarana, germander, botanicals used as weak diuretics (juniper, goldenrod, parsley), botanicals used as laxatives (plantago as plantain or psyllium), and so-called dieter's teas (containing ingredients such as aloe, buckthorn, cascara, castor oil, rhubarb root, or other herbal laxatives). Health professionals can find reliable information about dietary supplements and fact sheets for themselves and consumers online at the NIH Office of Dietary Supplements website: http://ods.od.nih.gov/ (Table 23-5). Nutrient-containing dietary supplements are helpful for achieving nutrient adequacy on hypocaloric diets. Because there is no demonstrated nutritional need for the ingredients in botanical and other supplements that are marketed for weight loss, and because their benefits remain largely unproven, clinicians need to be alert to the potential safety concerns associated with their use.

Health professionals should ask patients who are trying to lose weight about what dietary supplements and medications they are taking. Any interactions should be identified and communicated to the physician and the patient. The research base for these products is woefully inadequate, given the extent of their use. Until the evidence base on dietary supplements yields compelling data, physicians should continue to recommend a healthy lifestyle that includes regular physical activity and a balanced diet.

TABLE 23-5

WEB SITES PROVIDING INFORMATION ON DIETARY SUPPLEMENTS

NIH Office of Dietary Supplements	http://ods.od.nih.gov
IBIDS Bibliographic Database	http://grande.nal.usda.gov/ibids/index.php
NIH National Library of Medicine, PUBMED	http://www.ncbi.nlm.nih.gov/entrez/ query.fcgi?DB=pubmed
FDA Center for Food Safety and Applied Nutrition	http://www.cfsan.fda.gov/~dms/supplmnt.html
American Botanical Council	http://www.herbalgram.org/
Natural Medicines Comprehensive Database (by subscription)	http://www.naturaldatabase.com
Micromedex (by subscription)	www.micromedex.com

REFERENCES

1. Olshansky SJ. http://www.nia.nih.gov/NewsAndEvents/PressReleases/ PR20050316 Obesity.htm
2. Ford ES, Giles WH, Dietz WH. Prevalence of the metabolic syndrome among US adults. Findings from the Third National Health and Nutrition Examination Survey. JAMA. 2002;287:356–9. [PMID: 11790215.] [PubMed-indexed for MEDLINE.]
3. Gregg EW, Cheng YJ, Cadwell BL, et al. Secular trends in cardiovascular disease risk factors according to body mass index in US adults. JAMA. 2005;293:1868–74. [PMID: 15840861.] [PubMed-indexed for MEDLINE.]
4. Executive Summary of the Third Report of the National Cholesterol Education Program (NCEP). Expert Panel on Detection, Evaluation, and Treatment of High Blood Cholesterol in Adults (Adult Treatment Panel III). JAMA. 2001;285:2486–97. [PMID: 11368702] [PubMed-indexed for MEDLINE.]
5. National Institutes of Health. Clinical guidelines on the identification, evaluation, and treatment of overweight and obesity in adults—the evidence report. Obes Res. 1998;6 Suppl 2:51S–209S. [PMID: 9813653.] [PubMed-indexed for MEDLINE.] Accessed at http://www.nhlbi.nih.gov/guidelines/obesity/ob-home.htm
6. The Seventh Report of the Joint National Committee on Prevention, Detection, Evaluation, and Treatment of High Blood Pressure. National Heart, Lung, and Blood Institute. NIH Publication No. 04-5230, 2004.
7. Lowe, MR. Self-regulation of energy intake in the prevention and treatment of obesity: is it feasible? Obes Res. 2003;11 Supplement: 44S–59S. [PMID: 14569037.] [PubMed-indexed for MEDLINE.]
8. Heymsfield SB, van Mierlo CAJ, van der Knapp HCM, Heo M, Frier HI, et al. Weight management using a meal replacement strategy: meta and pooling analysis from six studies. Int J Obes Relat Metab Disord. 2003;27:537–49. [PMID: 12704397.] [PubMed-indexed for MEDLINE.]
9. Allison DB, Gadbury G, Schwartz LG, et al. A randomized controlled clinical trial of a novel soy-based meal replacement formula for weight loss among obese individuals. Eur J Clin Nutr. 2003;57:514–22. [PMID: 12700612.]
10. Vander Wal JS, Waller SM, Klurfeld DM, et al. Effect of a post-dinner snack and partial meal replacement program on weight loss. Int J Food Sci Nutr. 2006;57:97–106. [PMID: 16849118.]
11. Hoolihan L. The role of education and tailored intervention in preventing and treating overweight. Nutr Today. 2005;40:224–231.
12. Augustin J. Web-based resources for weight loss. Nutr Clin Care. 2001;4:272–3; http://endotext.com/obesity; and, the American Heart Association. No fad diet: a personal plan for healthy weight loss.
13. Torgerson J, Hauptman J, Boldrin MN, Sjostrom L. XENical in the prevention of diabetes in obese subjects (XENDOS) study: a randomized study of orlistat as an adjunct to lifestyle changes for the prevention of type 2 diabetes in obese patients. Diabetes Care. 2004;27:155–61. [PMID: 14693982.] [PubMed-indexed for MEDLINE.]
14. Shekelle PG, Morton SC, Maglione M, et al. Pharmacological and surgical treatment of obesity. Evid Rep Technol Assess. 2004 Jul;103:1–6. [PMID: 15526396.] [PubMed-indexed for MEDLINE] http://www.ahrq.gov/clinic/epcsums/obesphsum.htm
15. Padwal R, Li SK, Lau DC. Long-term pharmacotherapy for obesity and overweight. Cochrane Database Syst Rev. 2004;3:CD004094. [PMID: 15266516.] [PubMed-indexed for MEDLINE.]

16. Norris SL, Zhang X, Avenell A, et al. Efficacy of pharmacotherapy for weight loss in adults with type 2 diabetes mellitus. Arch Intern Med. 2004;164:1395–404. [PMID: 15249348.] [PubMed-indexed for MEDLINE.]

17. Wadden TA, Berkowitz RI, Womble LG, et al. Randomized trial of lifestyle modification and pharmacotherapy for obesity. New Eng J Med. 2005;353:2111–120. [PMID: 16291981.] [PubMed-indexed for MEDLINE.]

18. The Health & Wellness Trends Database. The Natural Marketing Institute, 2005.

19. Blanck HM, Khan LK, Serdula MK. Use of nonprescription weight loss products: results from a multistate survey. JAMA. 2001;286:930–5. [PMID: 11509057.] [PubMed-indexed for MEDLINE.]

20. Palmer ME, Haller C, McKinney PE, et al. Adverse events associated with dietary supplements: an observational study. Lancet. 2003;36:101–6. [PMID: 12531576.] [PubMed-indexed for MEDLINE.]

21. Natural Medicines Comprehensive Database. Accessed on December 20, 2005. (www.naturaldatabase.com).

22. Shekelle PG, Hardy ML, Morton SC, et al. Efficacy and safety of ephedra and ephedrine for weight loss and athletic performance: a meta-analysis. JAMA. 2003;289:1537–45. [PMID: 12672771.] [PubMed-indexed for MEDLINE.]

23. McBride BF, Karapanos AK, Krudysz A, Kluger J, Coleman GI, White CM. Electrocardiographic and hemodynamic effects of a multicomponent dietary supplement containing ephedra and caffeine: a randomized controlled trial. JAMA. 2004;291:216–21. [PMID: 14722148.] [PubMed-indexed for MEDLINE.]

24. Haller CA, Jacob P, Benowitz NL. Short-term metabolic and hemodynamic effects of ephedra and guarana combinations. Clin Pharmacol Ther. 2005;77:560–71. [PMID: 15961987.] [PubMed-indexed for MEDLINE.]

25. Bent S, Padula A, Neuhaus J. Safety and efficacy of citrus aurantium for weight loss. Am J Cardiol. 2004;94:1359–61. [PMID: 15541270.] [PubMed-indexed for MEDLINE.]

26. Allison DB, Cutter G, Poehlman ET, Moore DR, Barnes S. Exactly which synephrine alkaloids does Citrus aurantium (bitter orange) contain? Int J Obes. 2005;29:443–6. [PMID: 15700046.] [PubMed-indexed for MEDLINE.]

27. Diepvens K, Kovacs EM, Vogels N, Westerterp-Plantenga MS. Metabolic effects of green tea and of phases of weight loss. Physiol Behav. 2006;87:185–91. Epub 2005 Nov. 7. [PMID: 16277999.] [PubMed-in process.]

28. Larsen TM, Toubro S, Astrup A. Efficacy and safety of dietary supplements containing CLA for the treatment of obesity: evidence from animal and human studies. J Lipid Res. 2003;44:2234–41. Epub 2003 Aug. [PMID: 12923219.] [PubMed-indexed for MEDLINE.]

29. Gaullier JM, Halse J, Hoye K, et al. Supplementation with conjugated linoleic acid for 24 months is well tolerated by and reduces body fat mass in healthy, overweight humans. J Nutr. 2005;135:778–84. [PMID: 15795434.] [PubMed-indexed for MEDLINE.]

30. Parikh SJ, Yanovski JA. Calcium intake and adiposity. Am J Clin Nutr. 2003;77:281–7. [PMID: 12540383.] [PubMed-indexed for MEDLINE.]

31. Shapses SA, Heshka S, Heymsfield SB. Effect of calcium supplementation on weight and fat loss in women. J Clin Endocrinol Metab. 2004 Feb; 89:632–7. [PMID: 14764774.] [PubMed-indexed for MEDLINE.]

32. Pittler MH, Ernst E. Dietary supplements for body-weight reduction: a systematic review. Am J Clin Nutr. 2004;79:529–36. [PMID: 15051593.] [PubMed - indexed for MEDLINE]

33. Mhurchu CN, Poppitt SD, McGill AT,; et al. The effect of the dietary supplement, Chitosan, on body weight: a randomized controlled trial in 250 overweight and obese adults. Int J Obes Metab Disord. 2004;28:1149–1156. PMID: 15311218 [PubMed-indexed for MEDLINE.]
34. Pittler MH, Stevinson C, Ernst E. Chromium picolinate for reducing body weight: Meta-analysis of randomized trials. Int J Obes Metab Disrod. 2003;27:522–9. [PMID: 12664086.] [PubMed-indexed for MEDLINE.]

CHAPTER

24

COMPLEMENTARY AND ALTERNATIVE MEDICINE AND CARDIAC SURGERY

Steven F. Bolling, Martinus T. Spoor and Sara L. Warber

INTRODUCTION

Complementary and alternative medicine (CAM) therapies have been utilized far longer than conventional medicine.[1] However, while it is hard to define what precisely CAM is, it is only in the last decade that surveys of the widespread and increasing CAM use have brought the attention of the health-care community, employers, and insurers to the pervasiveness of these therapies. In 1998 Eisenberg reported that 43% of Americans used at least one form of CAM therapy[2] and that there had been a 25% increase in users and a 43% increase in visits to CAM practitioners since 1990.[1] About 18% of patients taking prescription drugs were also using herbal remedies, and the estimated market for CAM therapy was $21 billion annually. More recently, another survey showed that in 2001, more than 50% of Americans were using CAM therapies.[3] An estimated 600 million visits per year were made to CAM practitioners, with an estimated market of $30 billion annually. In that survey, the estimated market for herbal remedies was $10 billion, growing at 20–30% per year.

The use of CAM is not only for primary care diseases but, as shown by a study of 376 consecutive patients undergoing cardiac surgery at Columbia Presbyterian Medical Center in New York, many cardiac surgery patients use some form of CAM but do not discuss its use with their physicians.[4] Among patients surveyed, 75% admitted the use of alternative medical therapy (44% without prayers and vitamins), but only 17% had discussed CAM use with their cardiac physicians, and 48% did not want to discuss it with any physicians. Thus, it is increasingly important for cardiac practitioners to gain familiarity with various forms of CAM and to specifically elicit and document a history of CAM use from patients. Those patients undergoing cardiac surgery may have important interactions with their CAM practices and these should be accounted for and understood. CAM practices are highly prevalent and cardiac practitioners need to acknowledge and be familiar with their use. The most common CAM practices that cardiac surgeons need to understand are generally grouped into mind-body therapies and vitamin/herbal supplements.

MIND-BODY THERAPIES

The use of these therapies before, during, and after cardiac surgery may occur in roughly 50% of patients undergoing surgery. Cardiac surgeons need to be aware of the rationale of their use. Depression is common among patients with heart disease and cardiac surgery, and is associated with adverse outcomes and increased long-term mortality. In addition, the cost of treating cardiac patients with mild to moderate depression is 41% higher in the first year following a major cardiac event, including surgery.[5] Type A behavior is thought to predispose to heart disease. Hostility and anger are associated with increased risk of acute coronary events, as are anxiety, panic symptoms, and perhaps, vital exhaustion.[6] Social isolation and lack of social support are more powerful risk factors than some traditional risk factors like smoking.[7] The autonomic nervous system is sensitive to thoughts and emotions, with negative reactions creating disorder and imbalance in the ANS and positive feelings, such as appreciation, creating order and balance.[8] In addition, chronic stress elevates basal cortisol and impairs the body's ability to respond to acute stressors and can precipitate poor healing and recovery following surgery. Thus many mind-body therapies have potential utility following or in conjunction with cardiac surgery.

Meditation, massage, hypnosis, biofeedback, Yoga, Qi Gong, Tai Chi, religious practice, guided imagery, cognitive-behavior treatment, and music therapy have been looked at as possible mind-body interventions for cardiac surgery. Transcendental meditation decreases basal cortisol and improves carotid atherosclerosis, a surrogate marker for coronary artery disease.[9] Hypnosis and biofeedback have been shown to decrease both heart rate and high blood pressure. Yoga, which includes focused control of the mind, breath, and body, decreases sympathetic tone, improves blood pressure, decreases heart rate, and decreases oxygen requirement without affecting work. Qi Gong, a traditional Chinese practice of breathing, meditation, and movement, has beneficial effects on hypertension, depression, anxiety, and CAD. Tai Chi, another mind, breath, and movement discipline improves exercise endurance, reduces stress, and enhances positive mood. Cognitive-behavioral treatment has been applied to reducing risk factors such as obesity, blood pressure, exercise, and type A behavior. Music therapy, that is, singing, playing instruments, and listening to music has the ability to directly alter heart rate, stress levels, anxiety among heart patients. Each of these approaches potentially brings the mind, spirit, and emotions into "balance" with the body, thus enhancing a variety of mechanisms that promote optimal health. Finally and specifically, religious practice, belief patterns, and the related social support appear to play a positive role in various aspects of recovery from cardiac surgery, and guided imagery during cardiac surgery, as shown by Tusek et al, has been shown to enhance recovery and limit postoperative length of stay.[10–18]

Furthermore, acupuncture has been extensively used in Western countries for the treatment of numerous conditions, including chronic pain, postoperative pain, asthma, drug addiction, headache, nausea, osteoarthritis, fibromyalgia, allergies, and gastrointestinal (GI) motility disorders. However, data on the use of acupuncture for the treatment of cardiovascular disease are currently limited. In Russia and in China, acupuncture has been used for the treatment of hypertension, congestive heart failure, and myocardial ischemia. However, these uses have not yet been tested in randomized clinical trials. In spontaneously hypertensive rats, acupuncture like electrical stimulation activates central opioid pathways, which leads to a decrease in sympathetic activity and in blood pressure. Thus, there appears to be a pharmacological basis for the use of acupuncture in essential hypertension and in other conditions such as congestive heart failure, in which sympathetic activation plays an important role. An NIH-sponsored randomized clinical trial is currently recruiting patients with hypertension to determine the effectiveness of acupuncture in essential hypertension.

Finally, mind-body therapies may not be entirely free of complications. Vertebral artery occlusion, acute cerebellar infarction, and acute medullary infarction have been reported in people practicing yoga. Acute psychosis has been associated with Qi Gong practice.[19] Psychological problems may emerge during other mind-body work and in addition, the philosophy underlying meditation, yoga, Tai Chi, or Qi Gong may conflict with the belief systems of some individuals.[20]

VITAMIN/HERBAL SUPPLEMENTS

A herb is a plant or part of a plant that produces and contains chemical substances that can exert a biological or pharmacological effect. According to the Dietary Supplement Health and Education Act of 1994, herbal remedies or botanicals are currently not regulated by the U.S. Food and Drug Administration if sold as dietary supplements. Therefore, they are not regulated for purity, potency, standardization, and formulation. The lack of regulation for potency and composition implies that there might be significant batch-to-batch variability and that there are often many active ingredients in the same preparation. The current regulations allow marketing with statements explaining their reported effect on the structure or function of the human body or the role in promoting general well-being, but not for diagnosis, treatment, cure, or prevention of diseases. Table 24-1 lists the many common herbal remedies used for cardiovascular care, some of which are more extensively discussed in the text. However, cardiac surgeons should be aware of the use of all vitamin and herbals by the patients and the possible underlying rationale of their use. In this way, the surgeon helps the patient in being open with his surgeon, without fear of censure and is able to discuss use or discontinuation with the patient in the perioperative period.

HERBAL PRODUCTS AND ORTHOMOLECULAR THERAPIES COMMONLY USED IN CARDIOVASCULAR CARE

Herbal Product	Active Compound	Mechanism of Action	Indication	Clinical Evidence
Garlic	Allicin	Inhibition of platelet aggregation, antilipemic effect, antihypertensive effect	Hypertension Hypercholesterolemia	Limited
Soy protein	Soy protein	Phytoestrogenic effect, decreased cholesterol absorption	Hypercholesterolemia	Limited
Cholestin (red rice yeast)	Statin compounds	Inhibition of HMG—CoA reductase	Hypercholesterolemia	Supportive
Guggul gum	Gugulipid	Cholesterol lowering	Hypercholesterolemia	Supportive
Ginkgo biloba	Ginkgo flavone glycosides and terpenoids	Antiplatelet effect, antioxidant effect, vasodilatation (NO mediated)	Dementia Cognitive dysfunction	Supportive
Hawthorn	Poliphenolic compounds (flavonoids and glycosides) and triterpene acids	Positive inotropic effect, vasodilatation, antioxidant, and anti-inflammatory effects	Congestive heart failure	Study currently ongoing

Coenzyme Q10	Coenzyme Q10	Antioxidant effect (obligatory component of mitochondrial electron transport chain)	Congestive heart failure CAD	None
Vitamin E	-	Antioxidant effect on lipoprotein metabolism, antiplatelet effect	Prevention of CAD	None
Vitamin C	-	Antioxidant effect	Prevention of CAD	None
Vitamin A	-	Antioxidant effect	Prevention of CAD	None
Lutein		Antioxidant effect	Prevention of CAD	Animal data
Folic acid	-	Pivotal role in DNA synthesis	Prevention of CAD Prevention of restenosis after percutaneous coronary intervention	Supportive

Vitamin/herbal supplements used by patients prior to cardiac surgery

ARGININE

Arginine is a semi-essential amino acid that is synthesized in the liver and kidneys. During periods of physical or emotional stress, the endogenous production of arginine is insufficient and dietary sources of arginine are needed to avoid a relative deficiency. L-Arginine is the precursor to endothelium-derived nitric oxide (NO) and appears to enhance NO production when taken as a supplement. In animal studies, L-arginine has been found to prevent the formation of endothelial lesions, prevent restenosis following PTCA, and to ameliorate ischemic and reperfusion injury during acute myocardial infarctions (MIs). However, in human studies, there are side effects of diarrhea, constipation, nausea, vomiting, and headache. Furthermore, patients who have renal or hepatic failure or who are using potassium-sparring diuretics should avoid L-arginine supplementation, since it can lead to hyperkalemia. Oral L-arginine supplementation may increase the frequency of herpes simplex outbreak.

ARTICHOKE LEAF (CYNARA SCOLYMUS)

Animal studies have shown that artichoke leaf inhibits cholesterol synthesis. In humans, this results in a 10% improvement in total cholesterol, 17% improvement in low-density lipoprotein (LDL) cholesterol compared to placebo.[21]

CURCUMIN (CURCUMA LONGA)

In vitro studies show that curcumin inhibits platelet aggregation.[22] In rabbits and in humans it also decreases lipid peroxidation and lipid levels, thus possibly protecting against both atherogenesis and thrombotic sequelae.[23,24]

COENZYME Q10 (UBIQUINONE)

Coenzyme Q10 (CoQ10), also known as ubiquinone, is a powerful antioxidant. CoQ10 is a mitochondrial coenzyme that is present in every cell, and it is derived by endogenous synthesis from acetyl-coenzyme A (acetyl CoA) and phenylalanine. The most common medicinal use of CoQ10 is for systolic congestive heart failure. CoQ10 is also used for the treatment of coronary artery disease, diastolic heart failure, and hypertension and to prevent myocardial toxic effects of chemotherapeutic agents.[25] The rationale for use of CoQ10 for congestive heart failure is related to the fact that heart failure is characterized by chronic myocardial energy depletion and increased oxidative stress. Because CoQ10 is an obligatory component of the electron transport chain, and because it is essential for adenosine triphosphate generation during oxidative phosphorylation, dietary supplement could facilitate adenosine triphosphate generation and restore myocardial energy deposits. In addition, it has been proposed that, as a potent lipid-soluble antioxidant, CoQ10 can act as free radical scavenger, thus counteracting the increased oxidative stress that characterizes congestive heart failure. Finally, a membrane-stabilizing property may also have a role in preventing arrhythmic death. More than 30 studies that have suggested that

CoQ10 can improve symptoms, quality of life, left ventricular function, and prognosis of patients with systolic congestive heart failure. Unfortunately, these studies have been limited by small sample size, lack of controls, suboptimal study design (no randomization or blinding), and inadequate measures of left ventricle systolic function. More recently, Watson et al.[26] reported the result of a double-blind, randomized trial of 30 patients with congestive heart failure, who had an ejection fraction of less than 35%. CoQ10, at a dose of 33 mg three times daily, or placebo was administered for 3 months. There were no significant differences in congestive heart failure-related quality of life and no improvement in left ventricular ejection fraction despite a more than twofold increase in serum levels of CoQ10. In addition, no changes in baseline left ventricular ejection fraction, peak exercise oxygen consumption, or exercise duration were reported from another double-blind placebo-controlled clinical trial in which 55 patients were randomly assigned to receive either placebo or CoQ10 at a dose of 200 mg daily and were monitored for 6 months.[21] Thus, according to the results of these two well-designed randomized clinical trials, it does not appear that CoQ10 is effective in the treatment of congestive heart failure.

Folic acid

The term *folate* was coined by Mitchell and coworkers in 1994 after its isolation from leafy vegetables. *Folic acid* refers to the synthetic form of this vitamin. The folate-cobalamin (vitamin B_{12}) interaction plays a pivotal role for the normal synthesis of purines, pyrimidines, and deoxyribonucleic acid. Folate deficiency has been unquestionably associated in a causative relationship with the development of neural tube defects and of megaloblastic anemia, and folic acid supplementation has been shown in randomized clinical trials to reduce the incidence of neural tube defects by up to 70%.[27] In addition, there is now substantial evidence linking a low intake of folic acid to an increased risk of cancer and of coronary artery disease. The relationship between folate and risk of coronary disease is further strengthened by the identification of high homocysteine levels as a risk factor for coronary artery disease. High folate intake has been shown to be associated with lower homocysteine levels.[28] In addition, randomized clinical trials have shown that folic acid administration in patients with high pretreatment homocysteine levels results in a 25% reduction of plasma homocysteine levels. The addition of vitamin B_{12} results in an additional 7% reduction.[29] The absolute reduction is related to pretreatment homocysteine levels; higher reductions are observed in patients with higher levels. The current recommended daily allowance (RDA) of folate is 400 µg/day. This dose is adequate for reducing plasma homocysteine levels in most patients, but higher doses might be required. Thus, daily dosages of folate and of 0.5 mg of vitamin B_{12} have been suggested for patients with persistently elevated homocysteine levels.[30] Because the estimated daily intake of folate with the average diet is 200 µg/day, routine folate supplementation with at least the RDA appears advisable.

More recently, high plasma homocysteine levels have been found to be associated with a higher risk of restenosis after coronary angioplasty.[31] As a follow-up of this finding, a randomized placebo-controlled clinical trial showed that administration of a combination of folic acid (1 mg/day), vitamin B_{12} (400 μg/day), and pyridoxine (10 mg/day) significantly reduced homocysteine levels, and decreased restenosis and the need of target lesion revascularization in patients undergoing percutaneous transluminal angioplasty.[32] While current evidence supports the link between hyperhomocysteinemia and endothelial cell damage, the progression toward cardiovascular disease is unclear. Currently, randomized clinical trials, in patients given vitamin B_6, B_{12}, and folate with resultant lower serum levels of homocysteine have little effect on CAD.[33,34]

FENUGREEK SEED (TRIGONELLA FOENUM-GRAECUM)

Fenugreek seed has hypoglycemic effects when studied in rats and dogs. Glycoxidation is thought to be one of the mechanisms contributing to oxidized LDL and atherogenesis. There is a single study in human diabetics that reports decreased cholesterol when taking fenugreek seed.[35]

GARLIC

The medicinal use of garlic (*Allium sativum*) dates back to early Egyptian times, and has been advocated for the treatment and prevention of several diseases. The active ingredient is allicin, an odorous sulfurous compound that has been shown to exert several pharmacological effects, including inhibitions of platelet aggregation (possibly irreversible), lowering of cholesterol and triglyceride levels, and lowering of blood pressure.

In animal models, garlic has an antiatherosclerotic effect, as evidenced by a reduction of the development of new atheromatous lesions and a slowing in the progression of existing lesions. Garlic is currently available as fresh cloves, extracts, powders, and tablets. Several studies have suggested that at least 12 garlic clove per day[19,20] is required for a pharmacological effect. Dried powders and tablets appear to be more practical formulations, but doses of the active ingredient are often inadequate. Several studies have assessed the effect of garlic on serum lipids and blood pressure control. Two recent meta-analyses showed that garlic administration resulted in a 9–12% reduction in total cholesterol, a modest reduction in triglyceride levels, and no significant changes in high-density lipoprotein levels.[19,20] A meta-analysis of eight antihypertensive trials showed on average an Il-mm Hg reduction in systolic blood pressure and a 6.S-mm Hg reduction in diastolic blood pressure.[36] Another well-designed randomized clinical trial evaluating the effect of garlic on claudication secondary to peripheral vascular disease showed no significant effect on pain-free walking distance or on anklelbrachial index. In yet another double-blind, randomized, placebo-controlled clinical trial evaluating the effect of garlic oil on serum lipoprotein levels and potential mechanisms of action, no significant effects on serum lipoproteins, cholesterol absorption, or cholesterol synthesis were identified.[37] Variation in the concentration of the active compound in formulations may explain some of the differences between the results of clinical trials. The most common adverse effects of garlic are on the GI system and include flatulence, esophageal pain, and abdominal pain. Significant interaction between garlic and an antiretroviral agent has been reported. This interaction results in marked reduction of blood levels of the anti-human immunodeficiency virus (HIV) drug saquinavir in patients taking garlic supplements.[38]

GINKGO BILOBA

Ginkgo biloba has been used for memory loss and to improve circulation. The EGB 761 extract of ginkgo biloba is highly standardized, and it is currently widely used in Europe. There are at least three active compounds in ginkgo biloba: ginkgo flavone, glycosides, and terpenoids. Ginkgo biloba has an antiplatelet and antioxidant effect, it reduces platelet-activating factors, and it reduces production of thromboxane A2.[39] It has also been shown to enhance endothelial cell-derived NO through either an increase in NO synthase activity or a decrease breakdown of NO mediated by its antioxidant effect. Ginkgo biloba has been approved in Europe for treatment of dementia. In a study involving 202 patients, ginkgo biloba was found to decrease the Alzheimer's Disease Assessment Scale-Cognitive subscale score better than did placebo.[34] There were no significant differences in the incidence of adverse reactions.

Overall, ginkgo biloba is considered a safe supplement; the most common adverse effects are headache and gastrointestinal discomfort. However, cases of subdural hematomas and bleeding have been described.[33,40,41] It is currently believed that the increase in bleeding risk is due to ginkgo Ii de B, an important inhibitor of platelet-activating factor. Thus, the use of ginkgo biloba is currently not recommended for patients receiving anticoagulants, aspirin, or nonsteroidal anti-inflammatory agents or for patients undergoing surgical procedures.

GINSENG, AMERICAN OR ORIENTAL (PANAX SPP)

The saponins in *Panax* species act as selective calcium antagonists and enhance release of NO from endothelial cells, thus providing protection during ischemia or reperfusion.[42] Side effects can include nervousness, excitation, estrogenic effects, and hypoglycemic effects. A case report indicates that *Panax ginseng* decreases the pharmacological effect of loop diuretics. Animal studies show that Siberian Ginseng inhibits platelet aggregation. In human studies, it has been found to increase blood pressure in hypotensive children and promote lipid lowering in combination with other herbs.[35] Side effects include drowsiness or nervousness in people with hypertension or post-MI.[42] Case-based data suggests that Siberian Ginseng (Eleutherococcus) can elevate digoxin levels, possibly by interfering with the laboratory test.[43]

GRAPES (WINE, JUICE, SKINS, SEEDS, RESVERATROL)

The French paradox, that is, that people could eat a diet high in saturated fats and still have low rates of heart disease, brought to light the beneficial effects of daily intake of red wine. Many studies show the primary preventive benefits of consuming 1–2 glasses of wine.[44,45] However, wine consumption does not seem to reduce mortality in those who already have cardiovascular disease (CVD)[46] and alcohol has many untoward effects including many drug interactions and adverse events. Studies on grape skin extracts have illuminated the possible mechanisms by which particular molecules may be responsible for the salutary effects of wine. Red wine and red grape skins contain numerous polyphenolic compounds, including trans-resveratrol, proanthocyanidins, and flavonoids such as quercetin, kaempferol, and catechins that act primarily as antioxidants. Resveratrol is also found in purple grape juice, mulberries, and in smaller amounts in peanuts. In vitro and animal studies show that resveratrol, in addition to being an antioxidant, is anti-inflammatory, inhibits platelet aggregation, and can cause blood vessel dilation.[47,48] A single small study ($n = 24$) in humans shows that resveratrol inhibits platelet aggregation.[49] Grape seed extract has also proven useful in similar ways as other grape products. The mode of action appears to be the antioxidant effect of the proanthocyanidins as demonstrated in both animal studies[50,51] and a small human study.[52] Resveratrol has estrogenic effects which may agonize or antagonize estrogen receptors, therefore it is best to avoid use in persons with hormone-sensitive conditions.

GUGULIPID (COMMIPHORA MUKUL)

Gugulipid is an extract from the natural resin (gum guggula) of the mukul myrrh tree. It has been used in India to lower cholesterol, and it has been evaluated in well-designed clinical trials performed in India.[53-55] These studies have shown that gugulipid administration results in a reduction of total cholesterol levels ranging from 11% to 22% and a reduction of triglyceride levels ranging from 12% to 25%. One study showed a 12% reduction of LDL. Gugulipid may cause GI tract upset, headache, mild nausea, belching and hiccups, decreased propranolol and cardizem bioavailability.

HAWTHORN (CRATAEGUS)

The use of hawthorn as a cardiac medication can be traced back to Roman physicians in the first century AD. Since then, it has been used for the treatment of congestive heart failure. Hawthorn is derived from a small, fruit-bearing plant. The active components include two groups of polyphenolic derivatives that are present in the leaf and the flower, and, at a lower concentration, in the berries. The polyphenolic compounds include flavonoids and their glycoside and oligomeric proanthocyanidins. Triterpene acids are additional active components.[56] The pharmacological effects of hawthorn include a positive inotropic effect, coronary and peripheral vasodilation and antioxidant and anti-inflammatory effects, resulting in an overall cardioprotective activity. Hawthorn has been evaluated in several clinical trials enrolling a total of 1,500 patients. In these studies, administration of hawthorn was found to improve exercise efficiency, to increase duration of exercise to anaerobic threshold, to increase left ventricular function, and to result in beneficial hemodynamic changes, which include a decrease of systemic blood pressure, a decrease in heart rate, an increase in cardiac output, a decrease in pulmonary artery pressure and pulmonary wedge pressure, and an overall decrease in systemic vascular resistance. These studies are limited in that some were unblinded and uncontrolled, they were largely limited to New York Heart Association Class II patients, and background therapy usually included only diuretics and possibly digoxin. The place of hawthorn in the contemporary management of chronic congestive heart failure is being investigated in two ongoing randomized, placebo-controlled clinical trials, both using *Crataegus* special extract WS 1442 (Willmar Schwabe Pharmaceuticals, Karlsruhe, Germany).

LUTEIN

Lutein is a carotenoid found in dark green leafy vegetables and in egg yolks. In one study, an inverse relationship was found between lutein concentration and progression of intima-media thickness of the carotid artery in 480 middle-aged men and women who were monitored for 18 months.[52] In that study, just one portion of dark green leafy vegetables a day increased plasma concentration of lutein to the highest level. In vitro experiments showed inhibition by lutein of LDL-induced migration of monocytes in arterial walls, and in apolipoprotein E-null and in LDL receptor-null mice, addition of lutein in the diet decreased the development of atherosclerotic lesions.[52] Although, as in other observational studies, a direct causal relationship between lutein levels and the observed progression of intima-media thickness cannot be inferred, these results are promising and support the need for further investigation of carotenoids other than β-carotene in the prevention of atherosclerotic vascular disease.

RED YEAST RICE (MONASCUS PURPUREUS) EXTRACTS

Cholestin is a fermented product of rice on which red yeast is grown, and it has been used for centuries in China. It contains starch, proteins, fiber, and at least eight statin compounds that function as 3-hydroxy-3-methylglutaryl coenzyme A (HMG-CoA) reductase inhibitors. Chinese studies have shown that total cholesterol reduction after cholestin administration varies from 11% to 32%. A more recent randomized clinical trial showed a 15% reduction in total cholesterol and a 22% reduction in LDL cholesterol.[57] Two human studies document lower LDL, total cholesterol, and trigycerides in the red yeast rice group.[32,58] A single study found red yeast as effective as its analog, simvastatin (Zocor).[59] Because cholestin contains several statin-like compounds, its use requires the same precautions as with prescription statins. Side effects may include anaphylaxis following inhalation, gastritis, abdominal discomfort, elevated liver enzymes, heartburn, flatulence, and dizziness. Theoretically, similar reactions may occur like HMG-CoA reductase inhibitor (statin) drugs.

SOY

Soy protein has been shown to be effective in lowering cholesterol through a decrease of cholesterol absorption, a decrease in bile reabsorption in the gut, and a phytoestrogenic effect. A meta-analysis of 22 trials showed a 9% decrease in total cholesterol levels, a 13% decrease in LDL levels, and a 10% decrease in triglyceride levels.[60] A more recent study has shown that the lipid-lowering effect is present both in normocholesterolemic and in hypercholesterolemic men.

VITAMIN E

Vitamin E includes at least eight compounds, of which alpha-tocopherol is the most active. The potential beneficial effect of alpha-tocopherol on the risk of coronary artery disease is related to its antioxidant effect on the metabolism of LDL. In addition, vitamin E has an antiplatelet effect,[22] and it inhibits smooth muscle cell proliferation.[23] Available dietary supplements contain 200–800 IV, a dose that is significantly higher than the current RDA of 30 IV and significantly higher than the dose that could be achieved with diet alone. The data concerning the effect of vitamin E on the risk of coronary artery disease are conflicting; some studies show a beneficial effect, and some studies show no effect. Part of the conflicting results might be related to dosing, to study design, to duration of clinical follow-up, and to its use for "primary prevention" versus "secondary prevention." In the Nurses' Health Study, women in the fifth quintile of daily intake diet of vitamin E supplements had significant reductions in age- and smoking-adjusted risk of major adverse cardiac events, including MI and cardiovascular death (relative risk, 0.66; 95% confidence interval, 0.50 to 0.87). The median dose of vitamin E in this group was 208 IU/day, and the total follow-up time was 679,485 person-years.[24] In another large prospective study of 39,910 men with 139,883 person-years of follow-up, men in the highest quintile had a significant reduction in major adverse cardiac events in comparison with men in the lowest quintile of dietary vitamin E intake (relative risk, 0.60; 95% confidence interval, 0.44 to 0.81).[35] Both studies evaluated patients who were free of cardiovascular disease at the time of the enrollment. A third nonrandomized prospective study also showed an inverse relationship between dietary intake of vitamin E and the risk of death from coronary disease in 34,486 postmenopausal women, from lowest quintile of less than 5.68 IU/day to the highest quintile of >35.59 IU/day. In that study, no additional benefit from vitamin E supplement was identified. However, no information was available on the duration of dietary supplements use, and only 12.9% of women reported a supplemental intake of more than 100 IU/day.[61]

Several randomized controlled clinical trials have evaluated the use of vitamin E for secondary prevention. In the Heart Outcome Prevention Evaluation, patients with existing coronary artery disease or at high risk of coronary events because of a history of diabetes and other risk factors were randomly assigned to receive placebo or to vitamin E, 400 IU/day, and to ramipril or matching placebo. Treatment with vitamin E for a mean of 4.5 years did not result in a reduction of cardiovascular events.[62] Also, no significant effect of vitamin E supplement on the incidence of major cardiac events was reported by the Gruppo Italiano per 10 Studio della Sopravvivenza nell'Infarto Miocardico.[44] However, in that study, a reduction in deaths from cardiac causes was observed. The Cambridge Heart Antioxidant Study randomly assigned 2002 patients with coronary atherosclerosis to receive either vitamin E (400 or 800 IU/day) or placebo.[63] At a median follow-up of 1.4 years, there was a significant reduction in the incidence of nonfatal MI in the vitamin E recipients in comparison with the placebo recipients (relative risk, 0.53), but there was no significant difference in rates of mortality from cardiovascular causes. A small number of events and differences in baseline clinical characteristics were potential limitations of that study. In another randomized clinical trial of primary prevention, no significant effects were observed in patients at high risk.[42] In summary, although vitamin E, particularly long-term high dietary intake of vitamin E, might have a role in primary prevention of coronary artery disease, current available data do not support use of vitamin E supplements for secondary prevention.

VITAMIN C

Available data do not support the use of vitamin C supplements for the prevention of coronary artery disease.[43] Some studies have suggested an inverse relationship between dietary intake of vitamin C and the risk of coronary disease and of stomach cancer. Except for one study that did not adjust for supplemental intake of vitamin E, no study has so far shown a benefit from higher dietary or supplemental intake. Tissue saturation at high level of intake may explain the lack of effect observed with supplements.[64] The current recommended dietary allowance is 60 mg/day.

VITAMIN A AND CAROTENOIDS

The generic term *vitamin A* is used to denote a family of fat-soluble compounds that have the same biological properties as retinol, the most active form of vitamin A. The observation that vitamin A content in plants varies with the degree of pigmentation led to the discovery of carotenoids. The group of carotenoids includes β-carotene, α-carotene, lycopene, lutein, and zeaxanthin. β-Carotene and α-carotene are important sources of vitamin A; the other carotenoids cannot be converted into retinol but nonetheless have important antioxidant effects. Vitamin A plays an essential role in the function of the retina, has an antioxidant effect, and regulates cell differentiation. In view of these effects, several investigators have assessed the relationship between vitamin A intake and the risks of cancer and coronary artery disease. Unfortunately, although observational studies have suggested an inverse relationship between carotenoid intake and the risk of coronary artery disease,[45] randomized clinical trials have consistently failed to demonstrate a beneficial effect of supplemental doses of β-carotene on the risk of cancer or of coronary artery disease.[46–50] It has been suggested that this discrepancy between observational studies and clinical trials might be due to the fact that clinical trials have used β-carotene as a supplement, but the effect of dietary intake of vitamin A might be attributable to other carotenoids.[43, 51]

ADVERSE EFFECTS OF HERBALS WITH CARDIAC SURGERY

Many medicinal herbs have biologically active compounds that can have toxic effects and can interact with commonly used drugs. As stated before, herbal supplements are currently not regulated for purity, potency, standardization, and formulation. Thus, there might be significant variability in efficacy between different manufacturers but also within batches from the same manufacturer.[59] Labeling of products may also not reflect their content. For example, cases of nephrotoxicity from a weight loss preparation initially attributed to fang-ji (*Stephania tetrandra*) were later found to be caused by the presence in the preparation of guang-fang-ji (*Aristolochiafangchi*), a herb that contains a known nephrotoxin. The confusion in that case was attributed to the similarity between the two names.[65] The importance of variability among products has been well documented by a study of St. John's wort products that was commissioned by the *Los Angeles Times*.[66] The result of the study showed that there were significant differences between the potency of the product and the claims on labels. Other potential problems related to herbal products include contamination with heavy metals in several Asian herbal products and the addition of pharmaceutical compounds, including caffeine, acetaminophen, indomethacin, hydrochlorothiazide, and prednisolone to proprietary "herbal" Chinese products.[59,67] Herbal products are not regulated for significant variability in efficacy between different manufacturers and within batches from the same manufacturer.

Specific herbals to avoid perioperatively with cardiac surgery

EPHEDRA

Significant problems have been associated with the use of ephedra products for weight loss. Ephedra acts as a sympathomimetic, leading to increased arterial blood pressure, increased heart rate, increased oxygen consumption in heart muscle, and vasoconstriction.

DANDELION

This herb is prototypical of potassium-wasting herbs, of which there are numerous anecdotal and other reports.

LICORICE ROOT (GLYCYRRHIZA GLABRA)

Powdered or finely cut licorice root is made into an infusion and used primarily for respiratory and GI problems. In addition to its anti-inflammatory actions, licorice has mineralocorticoid activity and when used over long periods and at high doses can cause hypokalemia, hypernatremia, edema, and hypertension. This can exacerbate cardiac disorders and cause pseudo-aldosteronism. In addition, deleterious herb–drug interactions are possible with pharmaceuticals commonly used for cardiovascular disease including potassium-sparing diuretics, thiazide diuretics, and digitalis.[35,42]

PRO AND ANTICOAGULANT HERBAL EFFECTS

Lastly and most importantly for cardiac surgeons, over 40 different herbs have anticoagulant effects of their own and thus could increase the risk of adverse bleeding events (See Table 24-2). Other popular herbs are associated with decreased activity of warfarin (See Table 24-3). In all persons taking aspirin or warfarin, it is imperative to inquire about the use of plant-based medicines. There are numerous pocket guides available of herb–drug pharmacological interactions, which should be used by cardiac health-care practitioners. In conclusion, it is beholden on the cardiac health-care provider to be aware of and familiar with all the CAM therapies utilized by our patients. Only in this way, will the best patient outcome be insured.

T A B L E 2 4 - 2

HERBS WITH ANTICOAGULANT EFFECTS COULD INCREASE THE RISK OF ADVERSE BLEEDING EVENTS

Drug	Herbal Product	Effect	Evidence
Aspirin	Ginkgo biloba	Increased risk of bleeding	Case report
	Feverfew	Possible increased risk of bleeding	Theoretical
	Red clover		
Warfarin	Vitamin E-containing herbs (e.g., sunflower seeds)	Increased risk of bleeding due to vitamin E interference with vitamin K-dependent clotting factors	Case reports and controlled study
	Danshen	Increased risk of bleeding	Case reports
	Devil's claw		
	Dong quai		
	Ginkgo biloba		
	Papain		
	Quinine		
	Angelica root	Possible increased risk of bleeding	Theoretical
	Anise		
	Arnica flower		
	Asafoetida		
	Borage seed oil		
	Bromelain		
	Celery		
	Chamomile		
	Clove		
	Fenugreek		
	Feverfew		
	Garlic		
	Ginger		
	Horse chestnut		

TABLE 24-3

OTHER POPULAR HERBS ASSOCIATED WITH DECREASED ACTIVITY OF WARFARIN

Drug	Herbal Product	Effect	Evidence
Warfarin	Vitamin K-containing herbs (e.g., alfalfa, green tea)	Decreased anticoagulant activity due to potentiation of vitamin K-dependent clotting factors	Case reports
	Ginseng St. John's wort Ubiquinone (Coenzyme Q10)	Decreased anticoagulant activity	Case reports

REFERENCES

1. Eisenberg DM, Kessler RC, Foster C, Norlock FE, Calkins DR, Delbanco TL. Unconventional medicine in the United States. Prevalence, costs, and patterns of use. New Eng J Med. 1993 Jan 28;328(4):246–52.
2. Eisenberg DM, Davis RB, Ettner SL, Appel S, Wilkey S, Van Rompay M, et al. Trends in alternative medicine use in the United States, 1990–1997: results of a follow-up national survey. JAMA. 1998 Nov 11;280(18):1569–75.
3. Hager M. Chairman 2005 summary of the conference Education of Health Professionals in Complementaryl Alternative Medicine. Paper presented at: Josiah Macy, Jr. Foundation, New York; 2001.
4. Liu EH, Turner LM, Lin SX, Klaus L, Choi LY, Whitworth J, et al. Use of alternative medicine by patients undergoing cardiac surgery. J Thorac Cardiovasc Surg. 2000 Aug;120(2):335–41.
5. Hemingway H, Marmot M. Evidence based cardiology: psychosocial factors in the aetiology and prognosis of coronary heart disease. Systematic review of prospective cohort studies. (Clinical research ed.) BMJ. 1999 May 29;318(7196):1460–7.
6. Grunbaum JA, Vernon SW, Clasen CM. The association between anger and hostility and risk factors for coronary heart disease in children and adolescents: a review. Ann Behav Med. 1997 Spring;19(2):179–89.
7. Linden W, Stossel C, Maurice J. Psychosocial interventions for patients with coronary artery disease: a meta-analysis. Arch Intern Med. 1996 Apr 8;156(7):745–52.
8. Luskin FM, Newell KA, Griffith M, Holmes M, Telles S, Marvasti FF, et al. A review of mind-body therapies in the treatment of cardiovascular disease. Part 1: Implications for the elderly. Altern Ther Health Med. 1998 May;4(3):46–61.
9. van Tulder MW, Koes BW, Bouter LM. Conservative treatment of acute and chronic nonspecific low back pain. A systematic review of randomized controlled trials of the most common interventions. Spine. 1997 Sep 15;22(18):2128–56.

10. Ai AL, Peterson C, Tice TN, Bolling SF, Koenig HG. Faith-based and secular pathways to hope and optimism subconstructs in middle-aged and older cardiac patients. J Health Psychol. May 2004;9(3):435–450.

11. Ai AL, Peterson C, Gillespie B, Bolling SF, Jessup MG, Behling BA, et al. Designing clinical trials on energy healing: ancient art encounters medical science. Altern Ther Health Med. 2001 Jul–Aug;7(4):83–90.

12. Ai AL, Peterson C, Dunkle RE, Saunders DG, Bolling SF, Buchtel HA. How gender affects psychological adjustment one year after coronary artery bypass graft surgery. Women Health. 1997;26(4):45–65.

13. Ai AL, Peterson C, Bolling SF, Koenig H. Private prayer and optimism in middle-aged and older patients awaiting cardiac surgery. Gerontologist. 2002 Feb;42(1):70–81.

14. Ai AL, Peterson C, Bolling SF. Psychological recovery from coronary artery bypass graft surgery: the use of complementary therapies. J Altern Complement Med. 1997 Winter;3(4):343–53.

15. Ai AL, Kronfol Z, Seymour E, Bolling SF. Effects of mood state and psychosocial functioning on plasma Interleukin-6 in adult patients before cardiac surgery. Int J Psychiat Med. 2005;35(4):363–76.

16. Ai AL, Dunkle RE, Peterson C, Saunders DG, Bolling SF. Self-care and psychosocial adjustment of patients following cardiac surgery. Soc Work Health Care. 1998;27(3):75–95.

17. Ai AL, Dunkle RE, Peterson C, Bolling SF. The role of private prayer in psychological recovery among midlife and aged patients following cardiac surgery. Gerontologist. 1998 Oct;38(5):591–601.

18. Ai AL, Bolling SF. The use of complementary and alternative therapies among middle-aged and older cardiac patients. Am J Med Qual. 2002 Jan–Feb;17(1):21–7.

19. Warshafsky S, Kamer RS, Sivak SL. Effect of garlic on total serum cholesterol. A meta-analysis. Annals Intern Med. 1993 Oct 1;119(7 Pt 1):599–605.

20. Silagy C, Neil A. Garlic as a lipid lowering agent—a meta-analysis. J R Coll Physicians Lond. 1994 Jan–Feb;28(1):39–45.

21. Khatta M, Alexander BS, Krichten CM, Fisher ML, Freudenberger R, Robinson SW, et al. The effect of coenzyme Q10 in patients with congestive heart failure. Annals Intern Med. 2000 Apr 18;132(8):636–640.

22. Calzada C, Bruckdorfer KR, Rice-Evans CA. The influence of antioxidant nutrients on platelet function in healthy volunteers. Atherosclerosis. 1997 Jan 3;128(1):97–105.

23. Boscoboinik D, Szewczyk A, Hensey C, Azzi A. Inhibition of cell proliferation by alpha-tocopherol. Role of protein kinase C. J Biol Chem. 1991 Apr 5;266(10):6188–94.

24. Stampfer MJ, Hennekens CH, Manson JE, Colditz GA, Rosner B, Willett WC. Vitamin E consumption and the risk of coronary disease in women. New Eng J Med. 1993 May 20;328(20):1444–9.

25. Tran MT, Mitchell TM, Kennedy DT, Giles JT. Role of coenzyme Q10 in chronic heart failure, angina, and hypertension. Pharmacotherapy. 2001 Jul;21(7):797–806.

26. Watson PS, Scalia GM, Galbraith A, Burstow DJ, Bett N, Aroney CN. Lack of effect of coenzyme Q on left ventricular function in patients with congestive heart failure. J Am Coll Cardiol. 1999 May;33(6):1549–52.

27. Wald, N. Prevention of neural tube defects: results of the Medical Research Council Vitamin Study. MRC Vitamin Study Research Group. Lancet. 1991 Jul 20;338(8760):131–7.

28. Jacques PF, Selhub J, Bostom AG, Wilson PW, Rosenberg IH. The effect of folic acid fortification on plasma folate and total homocysteine concentrations. New Eng J Med. 1999 May 13;340(19):1449–54.

29. Homocysteine Lowering Trialists' Collaboration. Lowering blood homocysteine with folic acid based supplements: meta-analysis of randomised trials. (Clinical research ed.) BMJ. 1998 Mar 21;316(7135):894–98.

30. Tice JA, Ross E, Coxson PG, Rosenberg I, Weinstein MC, Hunink MG, et al. Cost-effectiveness of vitamin therapy to lower plasma homocysteine levels for the prevention of coronary heart disease: effect of grain fortification and beyond. JAMA. 2001 Aug 22–29;286(8):936–43.

31. Schnyder G, Roffi M, Flammer Y, Pin R, Hess OM. Association of plasma homocysteine with restenosis after percutaneous coronary angioplasty. Eur Heart J. 2002 May;23(9):726–33.

32. Schnyder G, Roffi M, Pin R, Flammer Y, Lange H, Eberli FR, et al. Decreased rate of coronary restenosis after lowering of plasma homocysteine levels. New Eng J Med. 2001 Nov 29;345(22):1593–600.

33. Rowin J, Lewis SL. Spontaneous bilateral subdural hematomas associated with chronic Ginkgo biloba ingestion. Neurology. 1996 Jun;46(6):1775–6.

34. Le Bars PL, Katz MM, Berman N, Itil TM, Freedman AM, Schatzberg AF. A placebo-controlled, double-blind, randomized trial of an extract of Ginkgo biloba for dementia. North American EGb Study Group. JAMA. 1997 Oct 22–29;278(16):1327–32.

35. Rimm EB, Stampfer MJ, Ascherio A, Giovannucci E, Colditz GA, Willett WC. Vitamin E consumption and the risk of coronary heart disease in men. New Eng J Med. 1993 May 20;328(20):1450–6.

36. Silagy CA, Neil HA. A meta-analysis of the effect of garlic on blood pressure. J Hyperten. 1994 Apr;12(4):463–8.

37. Berthold HK, Sudhop T, von Bergmann K. Effect of a garlic oil preparation on serum lipoproteins and cholesterol metabolism: a randomized controlled trial. JAMA. 1998 Jun 17;279(23):1900–02.

38. Piscitelli SC, Burstein AH, Welden N, Gallicano KD, Falloon J. The effect of garlic supplements on the pharmacokinetics of saquinavir. Clin Infect Dis. 2002 Jan 15; 34(2):234–8.

39. Chung KF, Dent G, McCusker M, Guinot P, Page CP, Barnes PJ. Effect of a ginkgolide mixture (BN 52063) in antagonising skin and platelet responses to platelet activating factor in man. Lancet. 1987 Jan 31;1(8527):248–51.

40. Vale S. Subarachnoid haemorrhage associated with Ginkgo biloba. Lancet. 1998 Jul 4;352(9121):36.

41. Benjamin J, Muir T, Briggs K, Pentland B. A case of cerebral haemorrhage—can Ginkgo biloba be implicated? Postgrad Med J. 2001 Feb;77(904):112–3.

42. de Gaetano G. Low-dose aspirin and vitamin E in people at cardiovascular risk: a randomised trial in general practice. Collaborative Group of the Primary Prevention Project. Lancet. 2001 Jan 13;357(9250):89–95.

43. Rimm EB, Stampfer MJ. Antioxidants for vascular disease. Med Clin North Am. 2000 Jan;84(1):239–49.

44. Gruppo Italiano per lo Studio della Sopravvivenza nell'Infarto miocardico. Dietary supplementation with n-3 polyunsaturated fatty acids and vitamin E after myocardial infarction: results of the GISSI-prevenzione trial. Lancet. 1999 Aug 7; 354(9177):447–55.

45. Kritchevsky SB. Beta-Carotene, carotenoids and the prevention of coronary heart disease. J Nutr. 1999 Jan;129(1):5–8.

46. Greenberg ER, Baron JA, Karagas MR, Stukel TA, Nierenberg DW, Stevens MM, et al. Mortality associated with low plasma concentration of beta carotene and the effect of oral supplementation. JAMA. 1996 Mar 6;275(9):699–703.

47. Hennekens CH, Buring JE, Manson JE, Stampfer M, Rosner B, Cook NR, et al. Lack of effect of long-term supplementation with beta carotene on the incidence of malignant neoplasms and cardiovascular disease. New Eng J Med. 1996 May 2;334(18):1145–9.

48. Omenn GS, Goodman GE, Thornquist MD, Balmes J, Cullen MR, Glass A, et al. Effects of a combination of beta carotene and vitamin A on lung cancer and cardiovascular disease. New Eng J Med. 1996 May 2;334(18):1150–55.

49. Malila N, Virtamo J, Virtanen M, Pietinen P, Albanes D, Teppo L. Dietary and serum alpha-tocopherol, beta-carotene and retinol, and risk for colorectal cancer in male smokers. Eur J Clin Nutr. 2002 Jul;56(7):615–21.

50. The Alpha-Tocopherol, Beta Carotene Cancer Prevention Study Group. The effect of vitamin E and beta carotene on the incidence of lung cancer and other cancers in male smokers. New Eng J Med. 1994 Apr 14;330(15):1029–35.

51. Kohlmeier L, Kark JD, Gomez-Gracia E, Martin BC, Steck SE, Kardinaal AF, et al. Lycopene and myocardial infarction risk in the EURAMIC Study. Am J Epidemiol. 1997 Oct 15;146(8):618–26.

52. Dwyer JH, Navab M, Dwyer KM, Hassan K, Sun P, Shircore A, et al. Oxygenated carotenoid lutein and progression of early atherosclerosis: the Los Angeles atherosclerosis study. Circulation. 2001 Jun 19;103(24):2922–7.

53. Agarwal RC, Singh SP, Saran RK, Das SK, Sinha N, Asthana OP, et al. Clinical trial of gugulipid—a new hypolipidemic agent of plant origin in primary hyperlipidemia. Indian J Med Res. 1986 Dec;84:626–34.

54. Singh RB, Niaz MA, Ghosh S. Hypolipidemic and antioxidant effects of Commiphora mukul as an adjunct to dietary therapy in patients with hypercholesterolemia. Cardiovasc Drugs Ther. 1994 Aug;8(4):659–64.

55. Verma SK, Bordia A. Effect of Commiphora mukul (gum guggulu) in patients of hyperlipidemia with special reference to HDL-cholesterol. Indian J Med Res. 1988 Apr; 87:356–60.

56. Rigelsky JM, Sweet BV. Hawthorn: pharmacology and therapeutic uses. Am J Health Syst Pharm. 2002 Mar 1;59(5):417–22.

57. Heber D, Yip I, Ashley JM, Elashoff DA, Elashoff RM, Go VL. Cholesterol-lowering effects of a proprietary Chinese red-yeast-rice dietary supplement. Am J Clin Nutr. 1999 Feb;69(2):231–6.

58. Clarke NE, Clarke CN, Mosher RE. The in vivo dissolution of metastatic calcium; an approach to atherosclerosis. Am J Med Sci. 1955 Feb;229(2):142–9.

59. Fugh-Berman A. Herb-drug interactions. Lancet. 2000 Jan 8;355(9198):134–8.

60. Anderson JW, Johnstone BM, Cook-Newell ME. Meta-analysis of the effects of soy protein intake on serum lipids. New Eng J Med. 1995 Aug 3;333(5):276–82.

61. Kushi LH, Folsom AR, Prineas RJ, Mink PJ, Wu Y, Bostick RM. Dietary antioxidant vitamins and death from coronary heart disease in postmenopausal women. New Eng J Med. 1996 May 2;334(18):1156–62.

62. Yusuf S, Dagenais G, Pogue J, Bosch J, Sleight P. Vitamin E supplementation and cardiovascular events in high-risk patients. The Heart Outcomes Prevention Evaluation Study Investigators. New Eng J Med. 2000 Jan 20;342(3):154–60.

63. Stephens NG, Parsons A, Schofield PM, Kelly F, Cheeseman K, Mitchinson MJ. Randomised controlled trial of vitamin E in patients with coronary disease: Cambridge Heart Antioxidant Study (CHAOS). Lancet. 1996 Mar 23;347(9004):781–6.

64. Monsen ER. Dietary reference intakes for the antioxidant nutrients: vitamin C, vitamin E, selenium, and carotenoids. J Am Diet Assoc. 2000 Jun;100(6):637–40.

65. But PP. Herbal poisoning caused by adulterants or erroneous substitutes. J Trop Med Hyg. 1994 Dec;97(6):371–4.

66. Monmaney T. Remedy's U.S. sales zoom, but quality control lags. St. John's wort: regulatory vacuum leaves doubt about potency, effects of herb used for depression. Los Angeles Times. Aug 31, 1998.

67. Huang WF, Wen KC, Hsiao ML. Adulteration by synthetic therapeutic substances of traditional Chinese medicines in Taiwan. J Clin Pharmacol. 1997 Apr;37(4): 344–50.

CHAPTER

25

CHRONIC HEART FAILURE: AN INTEGRATIVE APPROACH TO ALTERNATIVE AND COMPLEMENTARY THERAPIES

Michael S. Cuffe

INTRODUCTION

Over the past 30 years, the understanding and treatment of chronic heart failure is itself a story of the success of alternatives to conventional practice. In the 1980s, heart failure was believed to be understood as fully a "pump" problem; laying out a course that still stimulates the search for compounds with "safe" positive inotropic properties. Contrary to that conventional wisdom, β-blockers (themselves negative inotropes) have moved from a contraindicated therapy to a core biologically based therapy for the disease. Exercise and stress reduction therapies are currently receiving substantial attention. Heart failure also provides nearly the strongest foundation to consider herbal therapies in modern medicine; over 100 years ago extracts of the foxglove plant, now recognized to contain the cardiac glycoside digoxin, was the first modern effective therapy for heart failure and its use continues today. The story of the cardiac glycoside digitalis also highlights important lessons for the modern consideration of alternative herbal therapies: the necessity of pharmaceutical standardization through bioassays, the required understanding of active components and bioavailability, and the further need for these to guide efficacy and safety trials. Unfortunately much of the herbal therapy literature remains lacking in one or more of these principles, but some conclusions can be drawn toward the therapy of heart failure.

Notwithstanding developing possibilities, the treatment of heart failure is rooted very firmly in traditional Western medicine. There are few illnesses that have as robust an evidence base supporting the beneficial effects of traditional pharmaceutical therapies on disease progression, symptoms, and mortality. Yet even with these traditional therapies, heart failure remains a major public health problem in the United States, affecting over 5 million adults, and the most common reason for hospitalization among Medicare patients.[1] This increasing heart failure burden is due to many factors, notably (1) the aging of the American population base, (2) the increasing prevalence of heart failure risk factors such as coronary artery disease and diabetes, and (3) the very effective available cardiovascular therapies which extend patients' lives to later experience, or to live with heart failure. The development of new therapies, and examination of complimentary therapies, deserves our attention to improve the lives and functioning of these patients.

PATHOPHYSIOLOGY

Heart failure is a syndrome with multiple causes but common symptoms, signs, and clinical progression. Left ventricular dysfunction may occur in the setting of acute myocardial injury (infarction or myocarditis), but is more often insidious in onset. The causes of heart failure are many, though some precipitating injury is a common underlying theme (Table 25-1). Often left ventricular dysfunction is idiopathic in nature, defying extensive evaluation to exclude reversible causes, and some third of these idiopathic cases may represent a familial genetic predisposition. Patients with heart failure initially experience dyspnea, fatigue, and/or reduced exercise tolerance. These symptoms, as well as physical signs are caused by either, or both, reduced cardiac output due to systolic dysfunction, or a cardiac output maintained only in the presence of elevated cardiac filling pressures (diastolic dysfunction) (Table 25-2). In both cases, activation of the renin-angiotensin system and adrenergic nervous system occur, and symptoms typically progress. The former causes sodium and volume retention, eventually contributing to symptoms. Symptoms are classified by means of the New York Heart

TABLE 25-1

CAUSES OF CHRONIC HEART FAILURE

Hypertension	Congenital heart abnormalities
Ischemic coronary disease	Diabetes mellitus
Valvular heart disease	Sustained tachyarrhythmias
Alcohol abuse	Thyroid disorders
Chemotherapeutic agents (doxorubicin)	Disorders of metabolism
Myocarditis (viral or idiopathic)	Peripartum state
Chronic anemia	Toxic exposures

TABLE 25-2

SIGNS AND SYMPTOMS OF CHRONIC HEART FAILURE

Symptoms	Clinical Signs
Dyspnea	Pulmonary rales or effusion
Fatigue/exercise intolerance	Elevated jugular venous pulsation
Orthopnea	Peripheral edema
Swelling in the feet, ankles, or legs	Ascites
Cough	S3 or S4 cardiac gallop
Palpitations	Tachycardia

Association (NYHA) Class (Table 25-3), long used to guide therapeutic clinical trials of pharmaceutical agents, which have typically evaluated patients with Class II and III symptoms.[2]

When one considers chronic heart failure, differentiation between systolic and diastolic is necessary. Diastolic heart failure is the result of diastolic dysfunction, or impairment of the relaxation and filling phase of the cardiac cycle; the result of which is elevated cardiac filling pressures and often reduced peak cardiac output. Systolic heart failure results from impaired systolic heart function, and the outcome of which is reduced rest and exercise cardiac output, also eventually with elevation of cardiac filling pressures. In fact, these two mechanisms often occur together, though our randomized evidence base best supports the treatment of systolic heart failure. Studies do suggest a benefit of standard therapies in patients experiencing diastolic heart failure symptoms, though morbid outcomes are less common in this group.[3,4] The body's

TABLE 25-3

NEW YORK HEART ASSOCIATION (NYHA) HEART FAILURE SYMPTOM CLASSES

Class I	Asymptomatic LV dysfunction
Class II	Symptoms with ordinary activity, mild limitations
Class III	Symptoms with minimal activity, marked limitation
Class IV	Symptoms with any activity or at rest

TABLE 25-4

AMERICAN HEART ASSOCIATION/AMERICAN COLLEGE OF CARDIOLOGY HEART FAILURE STAGES

Stage A	Patients at risk for heart failure and LV dysfunction but with neither structural heart disease nor symptoms
Stage B	Patients at risk for heart failure with current structural heart disease but without symptoms of heart failure
Stage C	Patients with current or prior symptoms of heart failure as well as underlying structural heart disease
Stage D	Patients with advanced structural heart disease and marked symptoms of heart failure at rest despite maximal medical therapy and who require specialized interventions

response to reduced cardiac output of either cause is neurohormonal.[5] Elevation of naturally occurring catecholamines, as well as salt- and water-retaining mechanisms, initially act to increase cardiac output. The sympathetic nervous system activation results in tachycardia, vasoconstriction, and furthers myocardial injury through increased myocardial workload, oxygen consumption, and direct effects. As the heart failure progresses, diuretic and natiuretic hormones such as brain natiuretic peptide (BNP) elevate in response to myocardial stretch and overload. Neurohormonal output continues to rise, volume retention and catecholamine stimulus further exacerbate myocardial stress; a vicious circle of increasing myocardial oxygen demand, arrhythmias, and continued worsening of left ventricular dysfunction is created. The American College of Cardiology and American Heart Association guidelines on heart failure, last updated in 2005, describe this progression from patients at risk to symptomatic heart failure by the use of heart failure stages[6] (Table 25-4). It is in this setting then that the potent pharmacological neurohormonal blocking agents are proven effective.

PHARMACEUTICAL AGENTS

There is overwhelming evidence of the benefit and safety of standard Western pharmaceuticals approaches. A brief review is appropriate here; however, the guidelines on the treatment of heart failure from the American College of Cardiology and American Heart Association represent the best single resource.

These guidelines, last updated in late 2005, outline the appropriate evaluation and therapy for all patients suffering from heart failure.[6] Traditionally, first among these agents are inhibitors of angiotensin-converting enzyme (ACE), proven in randomized trials across the spectrum of heart failure from prevention in the asymptomatic state to the most severe heart failure. Countless studies have demonstrated their efficacy in reducing symptom progression, improving left ventricular dysfunction, all-cause mortality, hospitalization, and overall quality of life. ACE inhibitors now form the foundation by which all patients, including those at risk of heart failure, should be treated. Though patients were generally undertreated with appropriate agents in the past, today undertreatment occurs in underdosing or through late initiation in patients at risk of heart failure. ACE inhibitors are safe and usually well-tolerated when initiated and titrated toward the maximum doses demonstrated in clinical trials to be effective.[7,8] The most common side effect, occurring in some 5% of treated patients, is a persistent cough that resolves upon discontinuation. In patients intolerant to ACE inhibitors due to cough or other effects, substitution with an angiotensin receptor blocker (ARB) is appropriate.

ARBs became available in the late 1990s and were once on pace to fully replace ACE inhibitors. Despite the improved side effect profile (cough) with this class, trials of direct comparison to ACE inhibitors provided mixed results. However, several direct comparison studies, particularly in the post-myocardial patient, and as an alternative for ACE-inhibitor-intolerant patients, have demonstrated substantial efficacy or equivalence.[6,9,10] Though ACE inhibitors remain the first choice, intolerant patients or those who are experiencing progression of their heart failure despite standard therapy should be considered candidates for ARB therapy.

Historically contraindicated in heart failure due to concerns about negative inotropic properties, β-blockers now have as solid a treatment foundation as ACE inhibitors. Clinical trials of β-blockers in the modern post-myocardial infraction (MI) setting have demonstrated mortality benefit in all patients, including those with symptomatic and asymptomatic left ventricular dysfunction.[11-13] β-Blockers as a group describe agents with β_1-adrenergic receptor, β_2-adrenergic receptor, and/or α-adrenergic receptor activity. The clinical trials of β-blockade have had discordant results with the "class" leading to guidelines from the American professional societies that call for treatment with a small subset of proven therapies.[6] These include only carvedilol, metoprolol succinate, and bisoprolol. In fact, this clinical setting has given us the unique COMET trial proving the superiority of one active β-blocking agent (carvedilol) over another (metoprolol tartrate).[14] Today's guidelines recommend the treatment of all patients at risk for or with left ventricular dysfunction except those in cardiogenic shock. Further, initiation with β-blocker as a single agent may be preferable to single-agent ACE inhibitor. As with many "blocking" agents, patients and physicians should be counseled against abrupt discontinuation as adrenergic rebound can itself exacerbate symptoms of heart failure.

Digoxin, a digitalis cardiac glycoside first identified as a herbal extract of digitalis purpurea (common or purple foxglove plant), continues to have a role in heart failure. As a historic standard of treatment, with efficacy first proven in drug-withdrawal studies, it was late in our understanding that a definitive and prospective trail was attempted. The DIG studied eventually allowed us to place this therapy in its defined role: at low doses and serum levels, typically 0.125 mg daily, digitalis improves symptoms and reduces hospitalization in symptomatic patients.[4] Although standard, its renal clearance form the body means caution must be used in the elderly and those with renal insufficiency. Even as a nutritional supplement, cardiac glycoside-containing compounds have no role in the treatment of asymptomatic patients.

Two aldosterone antagonists have proven efficacious in symptomatic heart failure patients. Aldactone improves mortality and morbidity in NYHA Class III and IV patients, while epleronone has a proven similar effect in patients with post-MI left ventricular dysfunction.[15,16] At the present, studies are not available to guide the use of aldosterone antagonists in the broader heart failure segment. As it is rare to find a class that provides benefit in the mildest disease form (epleronone), and the most advanced disease state (aldactone), without benefit between, many cardiologists are now considering earlier treatment of Stage B and C patients with aldosterone antagonists. Certainly, such a decision to treat has a sound physiological basis given our neurohormonal understanding of heart failure, but caution as well is advised as hyperkalemia can easily occur and treatment requires close monitoring.

When combined with standard ACE-inhibitor and β-blocker therapy, diuretics are a mainstay of symptomatic volume overload states. Their use, however, should be tertiary; early initiation and intravascular dehydration can lead to underutilization of other therapies. The dose used should be minimized to control symptoms. Larger doses in some studies have been associated with increased mortality, even when controlling for other factors.[17]

Other pharmacological therapies, such as antiarrhythmic drugs and anticoagulants have no general role in the treatment of heart failure but rather should be used with caution in select populations. Antiarrhythmic agents, including amiodarone, should be used only when indicated to treat arrhythmias. Coumadin, aspirin, or other anticoagulants should be employed as indicated only when concomitant atrial fibrillation or thrombotic disorders are present.[6]

SURGICAL AND DEVICE APPROACHES

Revascularization, particularly surgical revascularization, is paramount when the underlying cause of heart failure is active ischemic coronary artery disease. Similarly, in patients for whom acute or chronic valvular disease precipitates heart failure, surgical correction may provide a means to return left ventricular function and eliminate symptoms.

Implantable Cardiac Defibrillators (ICD) are now well established to improve mortality in all patients, and are indicated in all patients with systolic heart failure, ejection fraction ≤35%.[18] When combined with biventricular pacing for patients with intrinsic conduction disturbances and ventricular dysynchrony, symptom improvement is also noted.[19] However, ICD placement is not appropriate for all patients. Those with a new diagnosis of nonischemic cardiomyopathy should wait several months to exclude spontaneous improvement.[6] In the post-MI patient, 6 or more weeks should pass before elective placement is considered.[20] Finally, patient understanding of benefit and risk is paramount. The benefit of ICD placement is of substantially improved mortality; however, inappropriate ICD shocks, the risk of ICD infection, the need to forego future magnetic resonance imaging, or simply intolerable awareness of the implant must all be considered by patient and caregiver before *informed* consent is achieved.

Enhanced external counterpulsation (EECP) involves paired inflatable pressure cuffs applied to the calves, lower thighs, and upper thighs with electrocardiogram triggered sequential inflation at the start of diastole. EECP, through retrograde increased diastolic coronary flow and reduced preload, is proven to be beneficial in chronic anginal patients; its use in heart failure has been experimental. A recent study of 187 heart failure patients treated with EECP for 7 weeks demonstrated modest improvements in NYHA heart failure Class and exercise duration, but no changes in peak oxygen consumption, suggesting possible placebo effect.[21] EECP currently remains controversial as a primary therapy for heart failure and best individually tailored to patient need.

SHARED APPROACHES

Lifestyle

As soon as heart failure is recognized, lifestyle modification should begin concomitant with pharmaceutical therapy. Adequate instruction, disease education, and family involvement are vital to reinforce changes particularly around diet. Because heart failure results in sodium and subsequently water retention, restricting dietary sodium intake is vitally important.[22] The typical Western diet contains more than 4 g of dietary sodium, but for heart failure patients, restriction to less than 2 g daily is advised. Diet recommendations need to be individually tailored taking into account ethnic preferences, with a reduced sodium goal. Less commonly, fluid restriction may be advised in cases of severe heart failure, but even for typical patients moderation in fluid intake is appropriate. Water and sodium retention is most easily assessed by weight. The patients should weigh themselves daily, so that they and their care team can become familiar with weight fluctuations and how they relate to their volume state and symptoms.

As heart failure is often caused by, or complicated by ischemic coronary disease, elimination of tobacco products, moderation or elimination of alcohol (a direct cardiac toxin), and reduced dietary fat intake are all appropriate. Weight loss, is of course, recommended for obese patients.[6]

Rest, previously encouraged for most cardiac patients, is now understood to lead to physical deconditioning, and thus worsened symptoms of fatigue and reduced exercise tolerance. In several controlled trials, aerobic exercise training has been shown to be beneficial in improving functional capacity and measures of quality of life.[23–25] Recent literature reviews concluded that short-term improvement in exercise capacity is well supported, but that the longer term effects impact on quality of life, and appropriateness in advanced heart failure were less certain.[26] One review evaluating mortality suggested benefit, concluding safety in stable patients was well established.[27] Most exercise studies include a formal exercise guidance program involving progressive training 3–5 times per week, for several months, achieving workloads of up to 70% maximal effort. Though the impact on long-term mortality and hospitalization is not conclusive, the largest and likely definitive assessment of structured exercise is currently underway; the National Institutes of Health (NIH)-funded HF-ACTION trial will evaluate the long-term impact of aerobic training on mortality and hospitalization in 3000 patients. Pending these results, current guidelines do recommend exercise training for all stable heart failure patients.[6]

The support of community and spiritual life can never be underestimated; this is particularly true in heart failure. Social isolation and depression are highly prevalent in patients with heart disease generally, and typically predictive of adverse outcomes.[28] Similar studies of heart failure patients, often more elderly than a general cardiology population, have documented rates of depression symptoms in the range of 30–50%, with strong correlations to worsened clinical outcomes including mortality.[29–32] Social isolation is also prevalent, related to depression, and similarly predictive of poor outcomes even when controlling for depression.[33–34] Though interventions to address social isolation are few, the literature of support groups common to other end-of-life ailments provides insight. Further, a multidisciplinary approach, involving frequent patient contact, education, and many types of caregivers, has proven successful in the management of heart failure.[35] Such comprehensive disease management programs, with appropriate end-of-life planning, are now considered standard when available.[6]

An integrative approach

Integrative medicine combines mainstream medical therapies and complementary or alternative medicine (CAM) therapies for which there is scientific evidence of safety and effectiveness. The prevalence of CAM therapy use in the heart failure population has not been well studied. One survey suggested nearly one-third of patients with heart failure use biologically based supplements for their illnesses.[36] Though conventional medical therapy must remain central in the care of patients with heart failure, the symptoms of heart failure differ among individuals, and are dynamic over the course of illness. A care team, which includes patient and loved ones, should assist in understanding and guiding pharmaceutical, lifestyle, and the best combination of alternative medicines.

BIOLOGICALLY BASED THERAPIES

Biologically based therapies use substances found in nature such as herbs and vitamins, typically employing them as dietary supplements. A wide-range of such therapies have been evaluated in the treatment of heart failure; small trials created support for several biological therapies, notably hawthorn, coenzyme Q10 (CoQ10), and L-carnitine, but more definitive studies have been disappointing. In no case do these therapies provide an appropriate substitute for the well-proven pharmaceutical basis of treatment.

Vitamin supplements

Overall there is no convincing evidence to demonstrate vitamin supplements as an effective alternative therapy for treating or preventing heart failure. There is some suggestion of benefit to a few agents outlined below, such as CoQ10 and L-carnitine, but there are also cautionary tales. L-Arginine, an amino acid supplement with solid physiological rationale for benefit increased mortality in a large randomized experience.[37] A large placebo-controlled, randomized study of vitamin E (400 international units) in nearly 10,000 patients with vascular disease or diabetes found no clear evidence of benefit after 7 years.[38] Importantly, those taking vitamin E actually experienced a 13% increased risk of heart failure. The NIH released the results of a 2005 State-of-the-Science conference on multivitamin/mineral supplements and disease prevention.[39] In the NIH summary, leaders call for more study, randomized-controlled trials, and FDA oversight of the field; suggesting further that lack of available efficacy or safety data didn't allow firm recommendations at present other than caution.[39] These and other results emphasize the need to study vitamins and other natural supplements, particular in populations with heart failure, prior to recommending their standard use.

L-Carnitine

L-Carnitine, a compound derived from the amino acid lysine, is found widely in meats, legumes, and dairy products. It plays a key role in skeletal and myocardial muscle utilization of glucose and fatty acids. Primary carnitine deficiency, an inherited disorder of early childhood, is a condition which prevents the body from using fatty acids for energy that presents with many symptoms including a cardiomyopathy.[41,42] In patients with heart failure, studies have documented higher plasma and urinary carnitine levels, but lower myocardial free carnitine.[42] This role, the contribution of skeletal muscle to heart failure symptomatology, and animal studies suggesting reduced apoptosis of skeletal muscle with carnitine supplementation has led to human supplementation studies.[43] Historic and more recent small human studies have suggested improved left ventricular remodeling, ejection fraction, and tissue levels with longer term carnitine supplementation (typically up to 3 g daily).[44,45] The largest and most definitive studies of safety and efficacy have provided continued optimism. About 80 patients with moderate to severe heart failure supplemented with 2 g daily or placebo were followed first for 3 months; at that time, small hemodynamic improvements were noted and the study was unblinded. After open supplementation was continued for 3 years, a substantial mortality benefit was noted despite the small number of events (3% vs. 18%).[46]

The largest experience, the Carnitine Ecocardiografia Digitalizzata Infarto Miocardico (CEDIM) trial, randomized 472 patients within 24 hours after first infarction to L-carnitine supplement (5 days intravenous therapy followed by 2 g three times a day for 1 year) or placebo.[47] Substantial improvements in left venticular parameters (end-systolic and end-diastolic volumes) were sustained at 3, 6, and 12 months in L-carntine-treated patients. Though not powered on clinical endpoints, a trend toward clinical improvement was noted. The CEDIM II trial, a planned 4000-patient mortality trial of similar carnitine therapy, was terminated early due to poor enrollment but nonetheless enrolled 2330 post-MI patients.[48] A small early reduction was noted in 5-day mortality, but was not sustained at 6 months (carnitine 9.2% vs. placebo 10.5% rate of death plus heart failure, $p = 0.27$).[48] Overall, dietary supplementation with L-carnitine has a well founded metabolic hypothesis, and studies suggest some benefit. The largest trials to date support a modest benefit on clinical endpoints with no apparent safety concerns; complimenting standard therapies with L-carnitine supplementation 3–6 g daily is reasonable.

L-Arginine

Many forms of direct and indirect vasodilatation have been investigated in chronic heart failure. As heart failure progresses, vascular endothelium-dependent vasodilatation becomes impaired. The role of nitric oxide has come to be understood as among the most potent endothelium-derived vascular-relaxing factors. The amino acid L-arginine is a potentially attractive supplement as it is the substrate by which nitric oxide synthase creates nitric oxide, and its vascular availability is known to be impacted in heart failure.[49–51] The use of L-arginine has been studied both as an oral supplement, as well as investigated as an intravenous therapy. When given intravenously over 1 hour, L-arginine resulted in a substantial increase in nitric oxide production, and was associated with favorably increased cardiac output, stroke volume, and reduced vascular resistance.[52,53] Blood pressure was also substantially reduced. Hemodynamics returned to normal within 1 hour, but such studies prompt the consideration of long-term therapeutic effect with oral supplementation. Unfortunately, there is little data available to support long-term oral administration. The most robust study to date involved 153 patients randomized to 3 g three times daily after first MI. No change was seen after 6 months of therapy in vascular resistance, ejection fraction, or other parameters. However, the study was terminated by the data and safety monitoring committee when an increased mortality rate was noted (8.6% vs. 0%), in the group receiving L-arginine supplementation.[54] Therefore at this point, the chronic use of L-arginine showed be viewed with great caution in cardiac patients, particularly those with ischemic coronary disease.

Coenzyme Q10 (CoQ10 or ubiquinone)

Among alternative approaches to heart failure, dietary supplementation with CoQ10 has received perhaps the most attention in the traditional medical literature. CoQ10 was first described in the 1957 by Frederick Crane, PhD, and shortly thereafter Peter D. Mitchell, PhD, deciphered CoQ10's role in cellular energy production. In the 1970s it received approval for the treatment of heart failure in Japan. Since that time there has been a host of small studies, evaluating both hemodynamic and clinical endpoints, but with mixed efficacy results. Some small well-controlled studies have failed to suggest an effect,[55,56] while others demonstrated benefit on important hemodynamic markers.[57] CoQ10 is vital to mitochondrial energy production, is an endogenous antioxidant present in LDL cholesterol, and has been demonstrated to be depleted in many cardiac conditions.[58] Treatment with 3-hydroxy-3-methyl-glutaryl (HMG)-CoA reductase inhibitors further depletes CoQ10 in a dose-dependent manner.[59] The documented depletion of CoQ10 in general cardiac diseases and cardiomyopathy patients, its biochemical role, and the availability of an oral supplement provide the perfect circumstances for its evaluation as a complementary therapy.[60,61]

A recent review of the available literature suggested primarily minor benefits on left ventricular ejection fraction and end diastolic volume, though these are important surrogates for clinical endpoints.[62] As importantly CoQ10 has been shown to be safe in these smaller studies with a low incidence of side effects.[62] Given the progressive depletion of CoQ10, it was hypothesized by Berman that maximal benefit might be observed in the most severely ill patients. A small randomized trial of 32 end-stage heart failure patients awaiting transplant resulted in improved NYHA Class and exercise tolerance after treatment with 60 mg/day.[63] One of the larger contemporary studies of CoQ10 supplementation randomized 55 advanced heart failure patients to 200 mg/day or placebo. After 6 months, no change was found in ejection fraction, symptoms, or exercise duration.[64] Contemporary experience is important to the evaluation of CoQ10 as effective background pharmacological therapy gas evolved substantially over the past 30 years. Nonetheless, this study was criticized on the basis of both dose and concomitant use of β-blockers (the latter purported to compromise CoQ10 efficacy).[65] It is, therefore, important to highlight the conclusive data demonstrating β-blockers' positive impact on heart failure morbidity and mortality. Overall, CoQ10 supplementation appears safe at doses from 100 to 200 mg/day, with possible benefit, particularly in the most advanced patients complimenting standard therapy.

Herbal therapies

Herbs have been used as medicines since human civilization; many important modern cardiac therapies (aspirin, paclitaxel, and digoxin) are the result of rigorous scientific evaluation and purification of plant derivatives. Despite their widespread use, and the wide variety of plant extracts that contain cardiac glycosides, only one phytomedicine, hawthorn, has been the subject of substantial recent evaluation in the clinical setting of heart failure.[66]

Hawthorn (crataegus extract, or extract WS 1442)

Crataegus extract has received substantial attention in the treatment of heart failure. The small hawthorn tree, typically crataegus laevigata or monogyna, found in Europe, North America, and East Asia has long had a role in native medicine. An extract of the hawthorn leaf and flower, of standard methodology, is the subject of current phytomedicine. This extract (WS 1442), contains no cardiac glycosides but rather two groups of pharmaceutically active compounds: flavonoids and oligomeric proanthocyanidins. Several large reviews summarize its effects of mild positive inotropy similar to digitalis glycosides, antioxidant, and vasodilatation, the latter possibly via ACE inhibition.[67] This preparation is approved by the German Commission E (on herbal therapies) for the treatment of heart failure at doses of 300–900 mg daily.[68] A 2003 meta-analysis of available studies (8 trials in 632 patients) concluded small benefit in exercise capacity and symptoms when compared with placebo, as well as infrequent mild side effects.[69]

More recent experiences include a similarly small positive effect on exercise tolerance with Hawthorn berry extract.[70] Some of the larger studies to date with WS 1442 standard extract have also demonstrated improvements in symptoms. A nonrandomized matched cohort study of 260 patients over 2 years documented improved fatigue and dyspnea.[71] A dose-ranging randomized trial of 1800 mg, 900 mg, or placebo showed a favorable side effect profile and improved exercise workload and symptoms with active therapy.[72] These experiences, however, suffered from methodological limitations. The most robust trial to date, HERB-CHF (Hawthorne Extract Randomized Blinded Chronic Heart Failure trial), was a randomized, double-blind, placebo-controlled experience in 120 heart failure patients. WS 1442 was used at a standard dose of 450 mg twice daily; at 6 months no effect was found in symptoms, walk distance, or standard quality of life scales. A small improvement was noted in left ventricular ejection fraction, but the authors concluded evidence remained lacking for symptom benefit.[73] Overall, hawthorn has a more substantial evidence base for tolerability and mild symptom efficacy than any other herbal therapy. Use is clearly appropriate to consider as a complimentary therapy, guided in large part by patient and provider preference.

Other nutritional approaches

There are various other nutritional therapies that have been considered in the treatment of heart failure. Diets high in fish oils, which contain marine polyunsaturated fatty acids, are associated with lower cardiovascular mortality in general populations. Further, the addition of fish oil to diet can reduce cardiovascular mortality post-infarction. Fish oil supplements are therefore very appropriate to consider in heart failure patients, and in small studies have been shown to reduce markers of the neurohormonal activation typical of heart failure.[74-76]

Disorders of skeletal muscle may contribute to fatigue and other limiting symptoms in heart failure. Short-term creatine supplementation can increase body weight and muscle strength, but no effect on overall symptoms or other disease markers has been demonstrated in heart failure.[77]

Dietary supplements with natural stimulant properties should be avoided in patients with heart failure. Kava kava, ma huang, ephedra, and other biologically based therapies, often used for weight loss, can increase blood pressure, heart rate, and myocardial demand.

MANIPULATIVE AND BODY-BASED METHODS

Manipulative and body-based practices focus on therapies designed to impact the structures and systems of the body, including the bones, joints, soft tissues, and circulatory system. In heart failure, few of these therapies have data supporting their effective use; some limited experiences are available to guide our choices. The two most common body-based methods, massage therapy and chiropracty, have no identified role in the treatment of heart failure. It remains important for body-based practitioners to be able to recognize the signs of heart failure;[78] patients with heart failure symptoms may choose to visit nontraditional practitioners, at which point early referral for assessment and pharmacological therapy is vital.

Hydrotherapy

As chronic heart failure is characterized by systemic vasoconstriction, the possibility of nonpharmacological peripheral vasodilatation as therapy has been suggested. Hydrotherapy includes external warm water immersion (40–60°C, for short periods of 10–15 minutes) or exercise in a temperature-controlled swimming pool (typical around 33–35°C). Some hydrotherapy regimens also include the use of brief intermittent cold water exposures, in hopes of producing more prolonged peripheral vasodilatation. Studies of the efficacy of such regimens are few, but some small experiences have demonstrated temporary improvements in hemodynamic parameters such as increased cardiac index, and a reduction in pulmonary capillary wedge pressure, cardiac dimensions, and vascular resistance.[79] Other experiences have recorded improved quality of life compared to control subjects.[80] In all recorded small experiences, whether combined with exercise or at rest, hydrotherapy appears well tolerated.[79–82]

Energy therapies

Energy therapies describe efforts to positively affect the energy fields that supposedly envelope the human body, or employ alternative uses of electromagnetic fields. Some forms of energy therapy manipulate these purported biofields by applying pressure and/or manipulating the body by placing the hands in these fields. Examples include Reiki (in person or at a distance), which employs spiritual energy to assist healing processes, therapeutic touch, and some forms of spirituality. Apart from rare case reports in the peer review literature, little is known regarding these therapies and their specific impact on patients with heart failure. Distant prayer has been the subject of more considerable study; however the largest studies of cardiac patients have failed to demonstrate effect.[83,84] As no health detriment has been demonstrated, the use of energy therapies should be individualized based on patient preference.

MIND-BODY INTERVENTIONS

Mind-body interventions include a variety of techniques designed to enhance the mind's capacity to affect bodily function and affect perceived symptoms. Due to heart failure's activated neurohormonal state and the ability of meditation, support, and mindfulness to positively impact adrenergic activation, mind-body interventions present a particularly attractive path to better health. Potential therapies range from widely accepted patient support groups and meditation, to prayer, mental healing, and therapies that use creative outlets. Most mind-body interventions have been demonstrated in small experiences to improve quality of life and are recommended when individually tailored to patient and caregiver preference.

Meditation/relaxation training

Heart failure is a chronic disease associated with substantial early mortality and end-of-life decision making. As such, anxiety is extremely prevalent and closely associated with depression and poor outcomes.[85,86] Similar to efforts to reduce anxiety and impact disease outcomes in hypertension, reducing anxiety symptoms alone is fitting and relaxation interventions have been shown to have beneficial impact for heart failure patients. Support groups and relaxation response/meditation training can contribute to improvements in physical and emotional quality of life.[87,88] One small study of meditation added to optimal medical therapy over 12 weeks reduced biochemical markers of sympathetic activation and improved standard measures of quality of life.[89] Together with providing the comfort of social support, some form of relaxation therapy is appropriate for all willing heart failure patients.

Respiratory training and therapies

Patients with heart failure have a high incidence of anxiety, dyspnea, and breathing disorders such as sleep apnea. Therapies targeted toward directly improving the sensation of dyspnea, or toward improving oxygenation hold some promise. Evidence supports acute hemodynamic improvements with continuous airway pressure, and for those patients with central sleep apnea may improve outcomes of heart failure.[90,91] Taught controlled breathing, or yoga-derived type respiration, can improve perceptions of dyspnea and improve exercise tolerance.[92] Inspiratory muscle training (IMT), may also be beneficial as patients with heart failure may have reduced endurance of respiratory muscles contributing to exercise intolerance.[92,93] IMT, usually over 8–12 weeks, has been shown in several experiences to increase 6-minute walk distance, functional capacity, and measures of quality of life,[94,95] though not all experiences have been able to demonstrate positive impact.[96]

Biofeedback

Biofeedback relaxation techniques are often used to treat condition associated with increased sympathetic nervous activity, such as heart failure. In one study with skin-temperature biofeedback, single session training during invasive hemodynamic monitoring, slight improvements in respiratory rate, systemic vascular resistance, and increased skin temperature were all noted. Such evidence suggests that biofeedback is a viable means toward assisting relaxation training for heart failure patients.[97]

Tai Chi/yoga

Few studies have begun to explore Tai Chi mind-body movement therapy or yoga in patients with heart failure. Though experience is limited, the few pilots or descriptive experiences suggest positive trends in quality of life and safety for selected patients.[98,99] One well designed, small randomized in optimally medically treated heart failure patients explored twice weekly Tai Chi training for 12 weeks. Training resulted in substantially improved quality of life, exercise tolerance measured by 6-minute walk distance, and even improved (reduced) B-type natriuretic peptide levels, an important biochemical marker of disease severity and outcome.[100] Tai Chi and similar training is appropriate and likely beneficial for capable individuals experiencing heart failure.

Spirituality

Spiritual care is an integral part of palliative care; spiritual expression an important dimension of quality of life. For patients experiencing new or progressing heart failure, as with any life-threatening condition, a period of religious struggle may result.[101,102] Described stages of struggle include (1) regret over past actions, (2) search for present meaning, and (3) search for hope and reclaiming optimism.[103] Compared with patients with diabetes, or those hospitalized for cancer, heart failure patients experienced even greater religious struggle, and this struggle was further associated with increased depressive symptoms and emotional distress.[104] In one analysis, spirituality predicted nearly one-quarter of variance in global quality of life.[105] In this light, patients and family may benefit from special care givers trained to facilitate religious coping; most health-care professionals lack the time and experience necessary to recognize and address religious struggle. Trained advanced practice nurses in the context of disease management programs may optimally meet this need. Complementing special carers, screening for religious practice and personal importance may be useful to identify patients with ongoing spiritual needs and struggle.[106]

CONCLUSION AND COMMENT

We are faced with a large and growing burden of heart failure. This epidemic of heart failure is manifest in symptoms, untimely mortality, caregiver burden, and society's financial burden. There is a large and robust evidence base for pharmacological and other Western medical therapies in large part because of the extremely poor outcome experienced by these patients, and therefore the ease of conducting robust clinical trials. To demonstrate efficacy and safety, the gold standard is the placebo-controlled randomized trial. In heart failure, there is a small but growing evidence base for many alternative medical therapies suggesting their appropriate complement to proven effective Western standards. Unfortunately, and as in the case in many other disease states, few alternative therapies have been adequately investigated to conclude either safety or efficacy. This is particularly disappointing given the long and positive history of herbal extracts and alternative hypotheses impacting our understanding and treatment of patients experiencing heart failure. The burden of this disease remains large despite the advancements we have recognized; it is hoped that further robust evaluation of complimentary therapies will continue to identify opportunities for caregivers to positively and safely impact our patients.

REFERENCES

1. American Heart Association. Heart and stroke statistical update. Dallas (TX): American Heart Association; 2004.
2. Williams JF, Bristow MR, Fowler MB, et al. Guidelines for the evaluation and management of heart failure: report of the American College of Cardiology/American Heart Association Task Force on Practice Guidelines (Committee on Evaluation and Management of Heart Failure). Circulation. 1995;92:2764–84 [PMID: 7586389.]
3. Cleland JG, Tendera M, Adamus J, Freemantle N, Polonski L, Taylor J. The perindopril in elderly people with chronic heart failure (PEP-CHF) study. Eur Heart J. 2006 Sep 8; [Epub ahead of print] [PMID: 16963472.]
4. The Digitalis Investigation Group. The effect of digoxin on mortality and morbidity in patients with heart failure. N Engl J Med. 1997;336(8):525–33 [PMID: 9036306.]
5. Packer M. The neurohormonal hypothesis: a theory to explain the mechanism of disease progression in heart failure. J Am Coll Cardiol. 1992;20:248–54. [PMID: 1351488.]
6. Hunt SA, Abraham WT, Chin MH, et al. ACC/AHA 2005 guideline ipdate for the diagnosis and management of chronic heart failure in the adult: a report of the American College of Cardiology/American Heart Association Task Force on Practice Guidelines (Writing Committee to Update the 2001 Guidelines for the Evaluation and Management of Heart Failure): developed in collaboration with the American College of Chest Physicians and the International Society for Heart and Lung Transplantation: endorsed by the Heart Rhythm Society. Circulation. 2005;112:1853–87. [PMID: 16168273.]

7. SOLVD Investigators. Effect of enalapril on survival in patients with reduced left ventricular ejection fractions and congestive heart failure. N Engl J Med. 1991;325:293–302. [PMID: 2057034.]

8. The CONSENSUS Trial Study Group. Effects of enalapril on mortality in severe congestive heart failure. N Engl J Med. 1987;316:1429–35. [PMID: 2883575.]

9. Pfeffer MA, McMurray JJ, Velazquez EJ, et al. Valsartan, captopril, or both in myocardial infarction complicated by heart failure, left ventricular dysfunction, or both. N Engl J Med. 2003 Nov 13;349(20):1893–906. Epub 2003 Nov 10. Erratum in: N Engl J Med. 2004 Jan 8;350(2):203. [PMID: 14610160.]

10. Cohn JN, Tognoni G; Valsartan Heart Failure Trial Investigators. A randomized trial of the angiotensin-receptor blocker valsartan in chronic heart failure. N Eng J Med. 2001;345(23):1667–75. [PMID: 11759645.]

11. Hjalmarson A, Goldstein S, Fagerberg B, et al. Effects of controlled-release metoprolol on total mortality, hospitalizations, and well-being in patients with heart failure: the Metoprolol CR/XL Randomized Intervention Trial in congestive heart failure (MERIT-HF). MERIT-HF Study Group. JAMA. 2000 Mar 8;283(10):1295–302. [PMID: 10714728.]

12. Krum H, Roecker EB, Mohacsi P, et al. Effects of initiating carvedilol in patients with severe chronic heart failure: results from the COPERNICUS Study. JAMA. 2003 Feb 12;289(6):712–8. [PMID: 12585949.]

13. Dargie HJ. Effect of carvedilol on outcome after myocardial infarction in patients with left-ventricular dysfunction: the CAPRICORN randomised trial. Lancet. 2001 May 5;357(9266):1385–90. [PMID: 11356434.]

14. Poole-Wilson PA, Swedberg K, Cleland JG, et al. Comparison of carvedilol and metoprolol on clinical outcomes in patients with chronic heart failure in the carvedilol or metoprolol European trial (COMET): randomised controlled trial. Lancet. 2003;362(9377):7–13. [PMID: 12853193.]

15. The RALES Investigators. Effectiveness of spironolactone added to an angiotensin-converting enzyme inhibitor and a loop diuretic for severe chronic congestive heart failure (the Randomized Aldactone Evaluation Study [RALES]). Am J Cardiol. 1996;78:902–7. [PMID: 8888663.]

16. Pitt B, White H, Nicolau J, et al. Eplerenone reduces mortality 30 days after randomization following acute myocardial infarction in patients with left ventricular systolic dysfunction and heart failure. J Am Coll Cardiol. 2005;46(3):425–31. [PMID: 16053953.]

17. Eshaghian S, Horwich TB, Fonorow GC. Relation of loop diuretic dose to mortality in advanced heart failure. Am J Cardiol. 2006;97(12):1759–64. [PMID: 16765130.]

18. Bardy GH, Lee KL, Mark DB, et al. Amiodarone or an implantable cardioverter-defibrillator for congestive heart failure. N Engl J Med. 2005;352(3):225–37. [PMID: 15659722.]

19. Young JB, Abraham WT, Smith AL. Combined cardiac resynchronization and implantable cardioversion defibrillation in advanced chronic heart failure: the MIRACLE ICD Trial. JAMA. 2003;289(20):2685–94. [PMID: 12771115.]

20. Hohnloser SH, Kuck KH, Dorian P, et al. Prophylactic use of an implantable cardioverter-defibrillator after acute myocardial infarction. N Engl J Med. 2004;351(24):2481–8. [PMID: 15590950.]

21. Feldman AM, Silver MA, Francis GS, et al. Enhanced external counterpulsation improves exercise tolerance in patients with chronic heart failure. J Am Coll Cardiol. 2006;48:1198–205. [PMID: 16979005.]

22. American Heart Association Nutrition Committee. Diet and lifestyle recommendations revision 2006: a scientific statement from the American Heart Association Nutrition Committee. Circulation. 2006;114(1):82–96. [PMID: 16785338.]

23. Piepoli MF, Flather M, Coats AJ. Overview of studies of exercise training in chronic heart failure: the need for a prospective randomized multicentre European trial. Eur Heart J. 1998;19:830–41. [PMID: 9651706.]

24. Keteyian SJ, Levine AB, Brawner CA, et al. Exercise training in patients with heart failure: a randomized, controlled trial. Ann Intern Med. 1996;124(12):1051–7. [PMID: 8633818.]

25. Belardinelli R, Georgiou D, Cianci G, Purcaro A. Randomized controlled trial of long-term moderate exercise training in chronic heart failure: effects of functional capacity, quality of life, and clinical outcome. Circulation. 1999;99(9):1173–82. [PMID: 10069785.]

26. Rees K, Taylor RS, Singh S, Coats AJ, Ebrahim S. Exercise based rehabilitation for heart failure. Cochrane Database Syst Rev. 2004;(3):CD003331. [PMID: 15266480.]

27. Piepoli MF, Davos C, Francis DP, Coats AJ; ExTraMATCH Collaborative. Exercise training meta-analysis of trials in patients with chronic heart failure (ExTraMATCH). BMJ. 2004;328(7433):189. [PMID: 14729656.]

28. Horsten M, Mittleman MA, Wamala SP, Schenck-Gustafsson K, Orth-Gomer K. Depressive symptoms and lack of social integration in relation to prognosis of CHD in middle-aged women. Eur Heart J. 2000;21(13):1072–80. [PMID: 10843825.]

29. Vaccarino V, Kasl SV, Abramson J, Krumholz HM. Depressive symptoms and risk of functional decline and death in patients with heart failure. J Am Coll Cardiol. 2001;38(1):199–205. [PMID: 11451275.]

30. Rumsfeld JS, Havranek E, Masoudi FA, et al. Depressive symptoms are the strongest predictors of short term declines in health status in patients with heart failure. J Am Coll Cardiol. 2003;42(10):1811–17. [PMID: 14642693.]

31. Gottleib S, Khatta M, Friedmann E, et al. The influence of age, gender, and race on the prevalence of depression in heart failure patients. J Am Coll Cardiol. 2004;43(9):1542–9. [PMID: 15120809.]

32. Jiang W, Alexander J, Christopher E, et al. Relationship of depression to increased risk of mortality and rehospitalizatoin in patients with congestive heart failure. Arch Intern Med. 2001;161:1849–56. [PMID: 11493126.]

33. Moser DK, Worster PL. Effect of psychosocial factors on physiologic outcomes in patients with heart failure. J Cardiovasc Nurs. 2000;14(4):106–15. [PMID: 10902107.]

34. Murberg TA, Bru E. Social relationships and mortality in patients with congestive heart failure. J Psychosom Res. 2001;51(3):521–7. [PMID: 11602222.]

35. Rich MW, Beckham V, Wittenberg C, et al. A multidisciplinary intervention to prevent the readmission of elderly patients with congestive heart failure. N Engl J Med. 1995;333(18):1190–5. [PMID 7565975.]

36. Zick S, Blume A, Aaronson K. The prevalence and pattern of complementary and alternative supplement use in individuals with congestive heart failure. J Card Failure. 2005;11(8):586–9. [PMID: 16230260.]

37. Schulman SP, Becker LC, Kass DA, et al. L-arginine therapy in acute myocardial infarction. JAMA. 2006;295(1):58–64. [PMID: 16391217.]

38. Lonn E, Bosch J, Yusuf S, et al. Effects of long term vitamin E supplementation on cardiovascular events and cancer: a randomized controlled trial. JAMA. 2005;293(11):1338–47. [PMID: 15769967.]

39. NIH State of the Science Panel. National Institutes of Health state-of-the-science conference statement: multivitamin/mineral supplements and chronic disease prevention. Ann Intern Med. 2006;145:364–71. [PMID: 16880453.]

40. Longo N, Amat di San Filippo C, Pasquali M. Disorders of carnitine transport and the carnitine cycle. Am J Med Genet C Semin Med Genet. 2006;142(2):77–85. [PMID: 16602102.]

41. Hou JW. Primary systemic carnitine deficiency presentation as recurrent Reye-like syndrome and dilated cardiomyopathy. Chang Gung. 2002;25(12):832–7. [PMID: 12635840.]

42. El-Aroussy W, Rizk A, Mayhoub G, Aleem SA, El-Tobgy S, Mokhtar MS. Plasma carnitine levels as a marker of impaired left ventricular functions. Mol Cell Biochem. 2000;213(1–2):37–41. [PMID: 11129956.]

43. Vescovo G, Ravara B, Gobbo V, et al. L-Carnitine: a potential treatment for blocking apoptosis and preventing skeletal muscle myopathy in heart failure. Am J Physiol Cell Physiol. 2002;283:C802–10. [PMID: 12176737.]

44. Masumura Y, Kobayashi A, Yamasaki N. Myocardial free carnitine and fatty acylcarnitine levels in patients with chronic heart failure. Jpn Circ J. 1990;54(12):1471–6. [PMID: 2077143.]

45. Romagnoli GF, Naso A, Carraro G, Lidestri V. Beneficial effects of L-carnitine in dialysis patients with impaired left ventricular function: an observational study. Curr Med Res Opin. 2002;18(3):172–5. [PMID: 12094827.]

46. Jeejeebhoy F, Keith M, Freeman M, et al. Nutritional supplementation with MyoVive repletes essential cardiac myocyte nutrients and reduces left ventricular size in patients with left ventricular dysfunction. Am Heart J. 2002;143(6):1092–100. [PMID: 12075268.]

47. Colonna P, Iliceto S. Myocardial infarction and left ventricular remodeling: results of the CEDIM trial. Am Heart J. 2000;139 (2 pt 3):S124–30. [PMID: 10650326.]

48. Tarantini G, Scrutinio D, Bruzzi P, Boni L, Rizzon P, Iliceto S. Metabolic treatment with L-Carnitine in acute anterior ST segment elevation myocardial infarction: a randomized trial. Cardiology. 2006;106:215–23. [PMID: 16685128.]

49. Kaye DM, Parnell MM, Ahlers BA. Reduced myocardial and systemic L-arginine uptake in heart failure. Circ Res. 2002;91(12):1198–203. [PMID: 12480822.]

50. Bauersachs J, Schafer A. Endothelial dysfunction in heart failure: mechanism and therapeutic approaches. Curr Vasc Pharm. 2004;2(2):115–24. [PMID: 15320512.]

51. Mendes Ribeiro AC, Brunini TM, Ellory JC, et al. Abnormalities in L-arginine transport and nitric oxide biosynthesis in chronic renal and heart failure. Cardiovasc Res. 2001;49(4):697–712. [PMID: 11230969.]

52. Koifman B, Wollman Y, Bogomolny N, et al. Improvement of cardiac performance by intravenous infusion of L-arginine in patients with moderate congestive heart failure. JACC. 1995;26(5):1251–6. [PMID: 7594039.]

53. Bocchi EA, Vilella De Moraes AV, Esteves-Filho A, et al. L-arginine reduces heart rate and improves hemodynamics in severe congestive heart failure. Clin Cardiol. 2000;23(3):205–10. [PMID: 10761810.]

54. Schulman SP, Becker LC, Kass DA, et al. L-Arginine therapy in acute myocardial infarction. JAMA. 2006;295:58–64. [PMID: 16391217.]

55. Weant KA, Smith KM. The role of coenzyme Q10 in heart failure. Ann Pharmacother. 2005;39(9):1522–6. [PMID: 16046484.]

56. Watson PS, Scalia GM, Galbraith A, Burstow DJ, Bett N, Aroney CN. Lack of effect of Coenzyme Q on left ventricular function in patients with congestive heart failure. J Am Coll Cardiol. 1999;33(6):1549–52. [PMID: 10334422.]

57. Soja AM, Mortensen SA. Treatment of congestive heart failure with coenzyme Q10 illuminated by meta-analyses of clinical trials. Mol Aspects Med. 1997;18 Suppl: S159–68. [PMID: 9266518.]

58. Sarter B. Coenzyme Q10 and cardiovascular disease: a review. J Cardiovasc Nurs. 2002;16(4):9–20. [PMID: 12597259.]

59. Langsjoen PH, Langsjoen AM. The clinical use of HMG CoA-reductace inhibitors and the associated depletion of coenzyme Q10: a review of animal and human publications. Biofactors. 2003;18(1–4):101–11. [PMID: 14695925.]

60. Folkers K, Vadhanavikit S, Mortenson SA. Biochemical reational and myocardial tissue data on the effective therapy of cardiomyopathy with coenzyme Q10. Proc Natl Acad Sci. 1985;82(3):901–4. [PMID: 3856239.]

61. Folkers K, Littarru GP, Ho L, Runge TM, Havanonda S, Cooley D. Evidence for a deficiency of coenzyme Q10 in human heart disease. Int Z Vitaminforsch. 1972;40(3):380–90. [PMID: 5450999.]

62. Weant KA, Smith KM. The role of coenzyme Q10 in heart failure. Ann Pharmacother. 2005;39(9):1522–6. [PMID: 16046484.]

63. Bernam M, Erman A, Ben-Gal T, et al. Coenzyme Q10 in patients with end-stage heart failure awaiting cardiac transplantation: a randomized, placebo-controlled study. Clin Cardiol. 2004;27(5):295–9. [PMID: 15188947.]

64. Khatta M, Alexander BS, Krichten CM, et al. The effect of coenzyme Q10 in patients with congestive heart failure. Ann Intern Med. 2000;132(8):636–40. [PMID: 10766682.]

65. Sinatra ST. Coenzyme Q10 and congestive heart failure. Ann Intern Med. 2000;133(9):745–6. [PMID: 11074911.]

66. Mashour NH, Lin GI, Frishman WH. Herbal medicine for the treatment of cardiovascular disease: clinical considerations. Arch Intern Med. 1998;158: 2225–34. [PMID: 9818802.]

67. Fong HH, Bauman JL. Hawthorne. J Cardiovasc Nurs. 2002;16(4):1–8 [PMID: 12597258.]

68. Steinhoff B. [The pharmacopoeia and Commission E of the ESCOP and the WHO. Hawthorn in the view of the monographs]. Pharm Unserer Zeit. 2005;34(1):14–21. German. [PMID: 15700790.]

69. Pittler MH, Schmidt K, Ernst E. Hawthorn extract for treating chronic heart failure: meta-analysis of randomized trials. Am J Med. 2003;114(8):665–74. [PMID: 12798455.]

70. Degenring FH, Suter A, Weber M, Saller R. A randomized double blind clinical trial of a standardized extract of fresh Crataegus berries (Crataegisan) in the treatment of patients with congestive heart failure NYHA II. Phytomed. 2003;10(5): 363–9. [PMID: 12833999.]

71. Habs M. Prospective, comparative cohort studies and their contribution to the benefit assessments of therapeutic options: heart failure treatment with and without hawthorn special extract WS 1442. Forsch Komplementarmed Klass Naturheilkd. 2004;11 Suppl 1:36–9. [PMID: 15353901.]

72. Tauchert M. Efficacy and safety of crataegus extract WS 1442 in comparison with placebo in patients with chronic stable New York Heart Association class-III heart failure. Am Heart J. 2002;143:910–5. [PMID: 12040357.]

73. Lalukota K, Cleland JG, Ingle L, Clark AL, Coletta AP. Clinical trials update from the Heart Failure Society of America: EMOTE, HERB-CHF, BEST genetic substudy and RHYTHM-ICD. Eur J Heart Fail. 2004;6(7):953–5. [PMID: 15556058.]

74. Mehra MR, Lavie CJ, Ventura HO, et al. Fish oils produce anti-inflammatory effects and improve body weight in severe heart failure. J Heart Lung Transplant. 2006;25(7):834–8. [PMID: 16818127.]

75. Witte KK, Clark AL. Fish oils-adjuvant therapy in chronic heart failure. Eur J Cardiovasc Prev Rehab. 2004;11(4):267–74. [PMID: 15292759.]

76. McCarty MF. Fish oil and other nutritional adjuvants for treatment of congestive heart failure. Med Hypotheses. 1996;46(4):400–6. [PMID: 8733172.]

77. Kuethe F, Krack A, Richartz BM, et al. Creatine supplementation improves muscle strength in patients with congestive heart failure. Pharmazie. 2006;61(3):218–22. [PMID: 16599263.]

78. Osterhouse MD, Kettner NW, Boesch R. Congestive heart failure: a review and case report from a chiropractic teaching clinic. J Manipulative Physiol Ther. 2005;28(5):356–64. [PMID: 15965412.]

79. Tei C, Horikiri Y, Park JC, et al. Acute hemodynamic improvement by thermal vasodilatation in congestive heart failure. Circulation. 1995;91(10):2582–90. [PMID: 7743620.]

80. Michalsen A, Ludtke R, Buhring M, Spahn G, Langhorst J, Dobos GJ. Thermal hydrotherapy improves quality of life and hemodynamic function in patients with chronic heart failure. Am Heart J. 2003;146(4):728–33. [PMID: 14564334.]

81. Cider A, Schaufelberger M, Sunnerhagen KS, Andersson B. Hydrotherapy—a new approach to improve function in the older patient with chronic heart failure. Eur J Heart Failure. 2003;5(4):527–35. [PMID: 12921815.]

82. Cider A, Sunnerhagen KS, Schaufelberger M, Andersson B. Cardiorespiratory effects of warm water immersion in elderly patients with chronic heart failure. Clin Physiol Funct Imag. 2005;25(6):313–7. [PMID: 16268981.]

83. Benson H, Dusek JA, Sherwood JB, et al. Study of the therapeutic effects of intercessory prayer (STEP) in cardiac bypass patients: a multicenter randomized trail of uncertainty and certainty of receiving intercessory prayer. Am Heart J. 2006;151(4):934–42. [PMID: 16569567.]

84. Krucoff MW, Crater SW, Gallup D, et al. Music, imagery, touch and prayer as adjuncts to interventional cardiac care: the monitoring and actualization of noetic trainings (MANTRA) II randomised study. Lancet. 2005;366:211–17. [PMID: 16023511.]

85. Konstam V, Moser DK, De Jong MJ. Depression and anxiety in heart failure. J Card Failure. 2005;11(6):455–63. [PMID: 16105637.]

86. Jiang W, Kuchibhatla M, Cuffe MS, et al. Prognostic value of anxiety and depression in patients with chronic heart failure. Circulation. 2004;110(22):3452–6. [PMID: 15557372.]

87. Chang BH, Jones D, Hendricks A, Boehmer U, Locastro JS, SLawsky M. Relaxation response for veterans affairs patients with congestive heart failure: results from a qualitative study within a clinical trial. Prev Card. 2004;7(2):64–70. [PMID: 15133373.]

88. Cuffe MS. The results of the SEARCH study. Mindful meditation, education, and support group therapy in chronic heart failure. Personal communication.

89. Curiati JA, Bocchi E, Freire JO, et al. Meditation reduces sympathetic activation and improves the quality of life in elderly patients with optimally treated heart failure: a prospective randomized study. J Altern Compliment Med. 2005;11(3):465–72. [PMID: 15992231.]

90. Sin DD, Logan AG, Fitzgerald FS, Liu PP, Bradley TD. Effects of continuous positive airway pressure on cardiovascular outcomes in patients with and without Cheyne-Stokes respiration. Circulation. 2000;102:61–6. [PMID: 10880416.]

91. Obenza-Nisheme E, Liu LC, Coulter TD, Gassler JP, Dinner DS, Milles RM. Heart failure and sleep-related breathing disorders. Cardiol Rev. 2000;8(4):191–201. [PMID: 11174895.]

92. Bernardi L. Modifying breathing patterns in chronic heart failure. Eur Heart J. 1999; 20(2):83–4. [PMID: 10099900.]

93. McConnell AK. Inspiratory muscle training for managing breathlessness. Nurs Pract. 2005;20:60–3. [PMID: 20009086500.] (CINAHL).

94. Dall'Ago P, Chiappa GR, Guths H, Stein R, Ribeiro JP. Inspiratory muscle training in patients with heart failure and inspiratory muscle weakness: a randomized trial. J Am Coll Card. 2006;47(4):757–63. [PMID: 16487841.]

95. Laoutaris I, Dritsas A, Brown MD, Manginas A, Alivizatos PA, Cokkinos DV. Inspiratory muscle training using an incremental endurance test alleviates dyspnea and improves functional status in patients with chronic heart failure. Eur J Cardiovasc Prev Rehab. 2004;11(6):489–96. [PMID: 15580060.]

96. Johnson PH, Cowley AJ, Kinnear WJ. A randomized controlled trail of inspiratory muscle training in stable chronic heart failure. Eur Heart J. 1998;19(8):1249–53. [PMID: 9740347.]

97. Moser DK, Dracup K, Woo MA, Stevenson LW. Voluntary control of vascular tone by using skin-temperature biofeedback-relaxation in patients with advanced heart failure. Altern Ther Health Med. 1997;3(1):51–9. [PMID: 8997805.]

98. Fontana JA, Colella C, Baas LS, Ghazi F. Tai chi chih as an intervention for heart failure. Nurs Clin North Am. 2000;35(4):1031–46. [PMID: 11072287.]

99. Sherman KJ. Heart failure patients improve quality of life and exercise capacity with tai chi. Focus Altern Complement Ther. 2005;10(1):50–1. [PMID: 2005110915.] (CINAHL).

100. Yeh GY, Wood MJ, Lorell BH, et al. Effects of tai chi mind-body movement therapy on functional status and exercise capacity in patients with chronic heart failure: a randomized controlled trial. Am J Med. 2004;117(8):611–2. [PMID: 15465501.]

101. Murray SA, Kendall M, Boyd K, Worth A, Benton TF. Exploring the spiritual needs of people dying of lung cancer or heart failure: a prospective qualitative interview study of patients and their carers. Palliat Med. 2004;18(1):39–45. [PMID: 14982206.]

102. Oates L. Providing spiritual care in end-stage cardiac failure. Int J Palliat Nurs. 2004;10(10):485–90. [PMID: 15577708.]

103. Westlak C, Dracup K. Role of spirituality in adjustment of patients with advanced heart failure. Prog Cardiovasc Nurs. 2001;16(3):119–25. [PMID: 11464434.]

104. Fitchett G, Murphy PE, Kim J, Gibbons JL, Cameron JR, Davis JA. Religious struggle: prevalence, correlates and mental health risks in diabetic, congestive heart failure, and oncology patients. Int J Psychiatry Med. 2004;34(2):179–96. [PMID: 15387401.]

105. Beery TA, Baas LS, Fowler C, Allen G. Spirituality in persons with heart failure. J Holist Nurs. 2002;20(1):5–25. [PMID:11898688.]

106. Kub JE, Nolan MT, Hughes MT, et al. Religious importance and practices of patients with a life-threatening illness: implications for screening protocols. Appl Nurs Res. 2003;16(3):196–200. [PMID: 12931334.]

26

MANAGEMENT OF COMMON PROBLEMS IN CARDIOVASCULAR CARE, SUDDEN DEATH AND ARRHYTHMIAS

Brian Olshansky and Mina Chung

INTRODUCTION

Cardiac arrhythmias are slow (brady), fast (tachy), dissociated (atria from ventricles), or irregular (ectopy, atrial fibrillation, and others) heart rhythm disturbances that may be related to changes in autonomic tone, or to an underlying structural or electrical problem of the heart. Common arrhythmias include atrial and ventricular premature beats, sinus bradycardia, AV blocks, supraventricular tachycardia, nonsustained ventricular tachycardia, and atrial fibrillation. Potentially highly symptomatic arrhythmias include atrial fibrillation, supraventricular tachycardia(s), sinus bradycardia (and pauses), atrioventricular (AV) block, and ventricular tachycardia. Potentially life-threatening arrhythmias include sustained ventricular tachycardia and ventricular fibrillation that can cause cardiac arrest and death. It is particularly important to identify and treat patients who are at risk for these life-threatening ventricular arrhythmias.

Cardiac arrhythmia management is diverse and potentially complex. Outcomes depend on the rhythm abnormality identified, the arrhythmia etiology, presence or absence of underlying cardiovascular disease or genetic abnormality, and/or the severity, frequency, and impact of the associated symptoms. A review of the entire management of cardiac arrhythmias is beyond the scope of this chapter, encompasses the practice of clinical cardiac electrophysiology, and has been reviewed extensively elsewhere. This chapter will focus on treatment of common and potentially life-threatening arrhythmias using an integrative approach and address issues regarding risk reduction of sudden cardiac death due to a cardiac arrhythmia.

WHY TREAT CARDIAC ARRHYTHMIAS?

There are multiple reasons to evaluate and treat arrhythmias: (1) to eliminate ongoing symptoms, (2) to prevent imminent death and hemodynamic collapse, and (3) to reduce the long-term risk of serious morbidity and mortality. A rhythm curiosity, by itself, is not a reason to treat with any therapy unless one of these three mentioned issues is at stake. No known therapy can prevent death, but several approaches can lower the risk and can extend meaningful life to varying degrees. In some instances, the standard antiarrhythmic drug treatments available are more dangerous than a non-life-threatening condition itself, and therefore, should be used cautiously; it is often best to leave some specific non-life-threatening rhythm disturbances alone. With life-threatening arrhythmias, however, it is critical to identify patients at risk and to reduce their risk using evidence-based therapies.

SYMPTOMS DUE TO ARRHYTHMIAS

Symptoms from cardiac arrhythmias are a key reason to treat, but it is important to recognize that many of the symptoms from cardiac arrhythmias are nonspecific and may *not* be worth treating. Common symptoms include a variety of palpitations, episodes of dizziness or lightheadedness, chronic fatigue, dyspnea, chest discomfort consistent with angina, loss of energy, weakness, or other nonspecific symptoms attributable to many causes rather than cardiac arrhythmias alone. However, symptoms can range from an occasional "flip-flop" palpitation of the heart to cardiac arrest.

Since symptoms attributable to arrhythmias can be nonspecific, it becomes important to correlate the symptom to an arrhythmia temporally and to identify whether or not an arrhythmia is actually the cause for the symptom. For example, in a patient who has frequent ventricular ectopic beats, symptoms of palpitations may occur with ventricular ectopic beats but may occur also during times when there are no ventricular ectopic beats. Similarly, patients with atrial fibrillation can be symptomatic when they are in sinus rhythm and be asymptomatic when they are in atrial fibrillation. Some specific symptoms deserve attention:

Palpitations

Palpitations are common and may be due to a wide range of causes, but palpitations are among the most common complaints in patients who have arrhythmias. Palpitations can be intermittent, sustained, rapid, regular or irregular, and even unrelated to an arrhythmia. Catecholamine excess alone can cause a sensation of palpitations without an arrhythmia even being present.[1]

Many causes of palpitations are unrelated to a specific arrhythmia. They may be due to anxiety, alcohol intake, stimulants (cocaine, methamphetamine, pseudoephedrine, drinks containing caffeine, theobromine, or theophylline), poor sleep (or irregular sleep cycle), and several over-the-counter supplements and remedies (including decongestants, cold remedies, ginkgo biloba, ephedra, ginseng, guarana, horny goat weed, yohimbine, and others). Hormonal changes can lead to palpitations as can thyroid hormone excess.

Palpitations can be a somatization of a psychiatric disorder and not be related to a specific cardiac arrhythmia.[2,3,4] One study reported that up to half of those complaining of palpitations referred for Holter monitoring have a psychiatric disorder[5] or high sensitivity to bodily sensations.[3] Nevertheless, careful evaluation of palpitations is important to rule out organic disease, as about 40% will be due to a cardiac cause.

Palpitations may occur in patients with arrhythmias, yet not be related to a rhythm disturbance. In a study of 1454 elderly patients (aged 60–94 years), 8.3% had palpitations. Arrhythmias, predominantly conduction abnormalities and sinus bradycardia, were found in 12.6%.[6] The prevalence of palpitations was similar in those with and without arrhythmias. In another study of 518 patients who had 24-hour electrocardiographic recordings, 34% had their typical symptoms at a time when the electrocardiogram was normal.[7]

Only rarely are palpitations the result of a life-threatening process, although they can be associated with, or represent, manifestations of underlying ventricular dysfunction or other structural heart disease. Palpitations in a patient with heart disease, especially coronary artery disease, should raise suspicions that the palpitations are due to an arrhythmia.

Syncope

Transient abrupt loss of consciousness can be due to a sudden change (increase or decrease) in heart rate. Brady- and tachyarrhythmias can initiate sudden loss of consciousness. Associated symptoms such as dizziness, lightheadedness, near syncope, "pre-syncope," fatigue, apparent seizure disorder, collapse, and even coma can be due to an arrhythmic cause. Syncope is not necessarily due to an arrhythmia; the list of non-arrhythmogenic causes is extensive, but includes cardiac outflow tract obstruction (e.g., aortic stenosis, hypertrophic obstructive cardiomyopathy), pulmonary embolism, seizures, and global cerebral ischemia. One common form of syncope is caused by transient autonomic fluctuations that can involve secondary heart rhythm changes (neurocardiogenic syncope), most commonly marked sinus bradycardia, sinus arrest/pauses, and/or AV block or vasodilatory changes. Syncope, in the presence of underlying structural heart disease, especially if there is impairment in left ventricular function, a positive electrophysiology study,[8] and/or the presence of a bundle branch block, can be a premonitory symptom indicating risk for sudden cardiac death.[9–12]

Nonspecific symptoms

Arrhythmias can present as several often difficult to diagnose and nonspecific symptoms. Symptoms can be overlooked or misinterpreted. It may be hard to associate an arrhythmia with a symptom. The presence of ventricular bigeminy, for example, can lead to effective impairment in cardiac output, reduction in stroke volume, and even tachycardia-induced cardiomyopathy.[13] This can cause slow, pounding palpitations with an effective pulse of one-half the actual heart rate (including the ventricular ectopic beats), dyspnea, heart failure, or fatigue. A transient or chronic bradycardia can lead to fatigue as well, but it can be difficult to correlate a rhythm disturbance with a symptom. Similarly, various tachycardias, ectopic rhythm disturbances, and atrioventricular dissociation can lead to significant symptoms mimicked by other medical conditions such as angina or congestive heart failure. It becomes important to correlate the symptom with the arrhythmia. Otherwise, the treatment directed at a specific rhythm disturbance may have little impact on the ultimate outcome of the patients and on the symptom itself.

EVALUATION OF ARRHYTHMIAS

The first steps in the evaluation and treatment of a cardiac arrhythmia or symptoms due to a cardiac arrhythmia are proper diagnosis and risk assessment. To achieve the proper diagnosis, a history involving all aspects of the symptoms and careful risk assessment is crucial. For the patient's peace of mind and for appropriate treatment, a series of tests is often required. The tests can begin simply by an electrocardiogram or a monitor recording during an episode of symptoms. For a patient with palpitations, it makes most sense to know what the diagnosis is from the start before prescribing a medication or instituting an invasive test such as electrophysiological testing. Evaluation may include ambulatory monitors, including a Holter monitor, external loop recorder (or implantable loop recorder), echocardiography to evaluate for structural heart disease, and/or exercise testing, which may ultimately indicate a need to proceed to invasive testing, including cardiac catheterization or electrophysiological testing.

For risk assessment, aside from knowledge of patient risk factors and symptoms, tests that can have prognostic value include measurement of the left ventricular ejection fraction, exercise testing, a variety of noninvasive tests including T-wave alternans, Holter monitoring, heart rate variability, signal-averaged electrocardiography, measurements of spectral turbulence, and other tests which fall in and out of favor. The role of invasive electrophysiological tests as a prognosticator has recently become less useful in some cases, with the results of large multicenter studies that have demonstrated benefits of defibrillator implantation in patients identified to be at high risk by noninvasive tests of ventricular function and certain clinical characteristics.

SUDDEN CARDIAC DEATH—A POSSIBLE MANIFESTATION OF A MALIGNANT ARRHYTHMIA

Sudden, generally out of hospital, cardiac death remains one of the most common causes for death in the United States and throughout the world. It is perhaps second only to cancer as the most common form of death in the United States, with over

330,000 individuals dying from this cause annually. Accurate statistical epidemiological data concerning this problem is challenging to acquire, but it is likely that:

1. Sudden cardiac death occurs at an average of about 60 years of age, is unexpected, and often heartbreaking.

2. Death often occurs without warning even in patients and individuals who have never had a diagnosis of heart disease made.

3. Death for the average individual occurs at home except for patients with serious underlying structural heart disease and in that case, death occurs commonly in the hospital.

4. While effective cardiopulmonary resuscitation and early defibrillation on the scene may be lifesaving, it is rare for a patient to be resuscitated effectively. In major metropolitan areas, survival is poor (<5%). Most die before they reach the hospital.

5. Sudden cardiac death is most common in the elderly but can occur at any age.

6. The great majority of those who died from sudden cardiac death have underlying structural heart disease. In the United States, coronary artery disease is the most common etiology, followed by dilated cardiomyopathy due to an idiopathic cause. Valvular heart disease, hypertrophic cardiomyopathy, various congenital abnormalities, and various congenital "channelopathies" may also be responsible.

7. Many of those who have out-of-hospital cardiac arrest die from ventricular fibrillation, yet the fibrillation and correction of this rhythm does not necessarily ensure good long-term outcome in all patient populations, especially those with severe underlying structural heart disease or an acute myocardial infarction, for example. It is generally accepted that ventricular fibrillation or hemodynamically intolerable ventricular tachycardia is responsible for the majority of patients who have sudden cardiac arrest.[14] There are several caveats concerning this, however. Despite extensive research and better understanding of the medical conditions that can result in a sudden cardiac death, very little is known about the mechanisms responsible for and the best treatments of this challenging problem.

Although some episodes of ventricular fibrillation are an end-stage manifestation of a serious uncorrectable cardiac abnormality,[15] prevention of cardiac death in patients without such end-stage disease may be achievable with implantation of an implantable cardioverter-defibrillator (ICD). Ventricular fibrillation could be rare event that, if effectively treated early, and prevented from occurring again or treated with prompt automatic defibrillation from an ICD, could be associated with an excellent long-term outcome. An example of this is a patient who is young and has long QT syndrome (or one of several genetic based "channelopathies") and has an occasional episode of ventricular fibrillation treated with an ICD. For a healthy individual with this specific medical problem, ventricular fibrillation causing sudden cardiac death would not necessarily be an end-stage event for which a healer should throw in the towel.

Despite the frequency with which sudden cardiac death occurs, the general population is often not as fearful of this problem as it is of other medical problems that cause death (such as cancer). This is potentially understandable since, of all the causes of death, a sudden painless death has appeal over a painful death involving prolonged suffering. A clinician, who considers an ICD to prevent sudden cardiac death must realize that implantation of such a device may be trading one issue for another. A circumspect view must include the best interests of the patient, the underlying medical conditions, and the chance that the ICD can reduce the risk of death to allow for a productive and potentially happy life. The prevention of sudden death may also be preferable to many patients and their families, as the emotional impact of a sudden loss without time for preparation may be less desired by many.

Arrhythmia management using complementary and alternative medicine (CAM) approaches have not been well substantiated through controlled clinical trials. These will be crucial to understand the roles of CAM therapies. Nevertheless, several adjunctive CAM interventions may affect long-term outcomes and could be used in conjunction with standard measures that have been established as effective in improving long-term survival. A few specific adjunctive CAM practices are based on solid information showing improvement in outcomes. Further, standard therapies given to reduce the risk of death may incur adverse effects that could be counteracted by a CAM intervention.

RISK ASSESSMENT—WHO WILL DIE SUDDENLY?

No one risk factor is robust enough to determine who will die suddenly and when this may happen. Any risk factor must be considered based on its sensitivity, specificity, and predictive accuracy in the general population to help discern if an individual with various risk factors is at high enough risk to warrant an extensive assessment and interventional therapy. Any specific therapy that may reduce the risk of sudden cardiac death may not eliminate or reduce overall mortality and may have extensive risks. Reduction in total (not arrhythmic) mortality, improvement in symptoms, and enhancement of quality of life are keys issues in risk assessment and risk reduction.

In the general population, sudden cardiac death is associated with a variety of epidemiological factors such as smoking,[16–18] hypertension,[19] high cholesterol,[20] diabetes,[16,21] obesity,[22] renal failure,[23] positive family history for atherosclerotic cardiovascular disease,[24] depression,[25,26] sedentary lifestyle,[27] inflammatory markers (such as high sensitivity C-reactive protein),[28] use of hormone replacement therapy in women[29–31], and age[32] but these risk factors can vary by the population evaluated.[32,33] The risk factor list is extensive and includes some rather unlikely suspects (including rheumatoid arthritis,[34] psychological stress,[35] marital stress,[36] or seizure disorder[37]).

A high-fat and low-omega-3 fat diet may be associated with risk for sudden cardiac death, whereas a lifestyle change with a diet low in calories, high in omega-3 fats[38] and alcohol (e.g., red wine[39]), or a Mediterranean diet[40,41] is associated with a better outcome[42-46], although data conflict.[47] Even chronic exposure to diesel fumes[48,49] and noise[50] have been reported affect risk for cardiovascular mortality. No one factor alone is highly predictive of outcome and even combinations of these risk factors are not accurate enough to determine who will and who will not die of a sudden cardiac arrhythmic event or a cardiac arrest.

Similarly, no one test can predict which patient will or will not die. Electrophysiological testing, for example, as well as tests that are more noninvasive including T-wave alternans testing, heart rate variability,[51] and signal average electrocardiography can predict, to some extent, who will and who will not die.[52] The presence of nonsustained ventricular tachycardia or premature ventricular complexes (PVCs) may increase risk but not to a large enough extent to use this as a measure of who requires an exercise evaluation or aggressive treatment.[53] Not one of these tests, however, is considered an effective approach to distinguish outcomes of the patients with a high degree of accuracy and even with a negative result, it is likely that if any risk exists, many patients will opt for a surefire approach to reduce the risk to as close to zero as possible. This has led to proliferation of ICD implants. Nevertheless, the benefits of ICDs in reducing mortality has been demonstrated in multiple randomized multicenter trials in select high-risk populations, including general populations of heart failure and coronary disease patients.

Where we are now in terms of general risk assessment for the average patient regarding sudden cardiac death includes determination of the presence of an impaired left ventricular ejection fraction (with increasing risk as the ejection fraction becomes more impaired), symptomatic congestive heart failure, and in such patients a QRS complex that exceeds 120 ms. The presence of coronary artery disease increases the risk of sudden cardiac death. Patients who have significant impairment of ventricular function and these indicators should be considered for ICD implantation.

Unfortunately, the average individual who dies suddenly (and presumably of a ventricular arrhythmia) has not been seen by a doctor and death may not be easily predicted even with a complete evaluation, since many who die suddenly have no symptoms beforehand and have no obvious markers of risk.[54] Risk stratification of the overall population is challenging and impractical. The best long-term approach for an individual without an identified cardiovascular problem is to attempt to reduce the risk by preventive measures (proper diet and exercise).

TREATMENT OF CARDIAC ARRHYTHMIAS

Standard (allopathic) therapies

There is a wide range of accepted medical therapies available for cardiac arrhythmia treatment. The management of cardiac arrhythmias using standard therapeutic approaches has generally been widely researched. This is important since the randomized, controlled clinical trials regarding cardiac arrhythmias often have shown paradoxical or surprising results. For example, the Cardiac Arrhythmia Suppression Trial (CAST)[55] highlighted that use of antiarrhythmic drugs that suppress ventricular ectopic beats in patients with coronary artery disease after myocardial infarction had an unexpected paradoxical effect on survival. For several types of the antiarrhythmic therapies used (i.e., ablation for supraventricular tachycardia, for example), no placebo-controlled, double-blinded, randomized, controlled trials were or could be undertaken, yet the success of ablation is so compelling (greater than 95% for most standard supraventricular tachycardias) that such a trial was not necessary.

MEDICATIONS

Class I and class III antiarrhythmic drugs can suppress cardiac arrhythmias to improve symptoms, reduce ICD activations, and improve hemodynamics. Beta-adrenergic blockers, calcium channel antagonists, and digoxin can control the rate of atrial fibrillation. No antiarrhythmic drug class, except β-blockers have been shown to reduce the risk of sudden cardiac death. Medications including statins, β-adrenergic blockers, and angiotensin-converting enzyme inhibitors can reduce the risk of atrial fibrillation and sudden death.

ABLATION

Ablation is an invasive procedure in which cold (cryoablation) or heat energy (radiofrequency) is delivered directly to the myocardium to eliminate the tissue responsible for tachyarrhythmias. Ablation for supraventricular tachycardia can be highly successful (in >95% for standard forms or supraventricular tachycardia) and can be performed at low risk and with excellent outcomes. Ablation techniques have also emerged to help eliminate episodes of atrial fibrillation with improving technology, but proof of long-term efficacy is still wanting. Ablation is also used to create complete heart block to allow for rate control in atrial flutter or fibrillation, but requires implantation of a permanent pacemaker. Therefore, ablation can be used for complete cure or palliation of rhythm disturbances. Ablation may also be used for certain ventricular arrhythmias and may be causative in some forms of these arrhythmias in normal hearts or adjunctive in patients with reduced ventricular function, where an ICD may also be indicated.

DEVICES

Recent, extensive research has shown potential benefits of implantable antiarrhythmic device therapy to improve symptoms, reduce risk of heart failure, and improve overall prognosis. Pacemakers are effective in preventing symptomatic bradycardias that may be due to sinus node dysfunction or AV block. ICDs are often used now to prevent recurrent episodes of life-threatening ventricular tachycardia and ventricular fibrillation in patients with structural heart disease. They are also indicated for prophylaxis of sudden death in patients with congestive heart failure, coronary disease with significant left ventricular dysfunction after myocardial infarction, or an electrophysiology study positive for significant inducible sustained ventricular arrhythmias, congenital disorders at high risk for sudden death, and other specific conditions.[56] No therapy equals that of the ICD to reduce risk in a population at high risk of sudden cardiac death.

Biventricular or cardiac resynchronization devices are pacemakers or ICDs used to coordinate activation of left and right ventricles in patients with underlying wide QRS complexes and congestive heart failure with use of left ventricular pacing. These devices may not only reduce the risk of sudden death but they may also substantially improve cardiac function, cardiac output, and symptoms related to congestive heart failure.

CAM therapies

CAM therapies involve a wide range of approaches to attempt to reduce symptomatic arrhythmias, to improve understanding and acceptance of an arrhythmia, if benign, and to attempt to improve long-term prognosis by reducing or modulating risk factors including arrhythmic events. Although investigation continues, little research supports the great majority of CAM techniques and modalities used to suppress arrhythmias and improve long-term outcomes. Nevertheless, several specific therapies, such as the use of omega-3 fatty acids, may improve the prognosis of patients at risk for arrhythmias or arrhythmic death.

THE MEANING RESPONSE

This is actually not a CAM therapy, but it is a crucial aspect of medicine[57–59] and becomes highlighted with the use of CAM modalities. This aspect of medical therapy involves the patient. The patient, who understands what is going on with respect to a disease and understands how a therapy may work to prevent a problem will have a better grasp on the medical condition and can become involved in his/her own medical care.[58,60,61] Moreover, the meaning response allows the patient to understand what may be the risks and benefits of treatment as well as the risks of the condition itself. An informed and educated patient can be more compliant and understanding of the medical conditions so that the medical condition is now mastered by the patient rather than the other way around. For example, benign palpitations due to ventricular ectopic activity may not require therapy at all if the patient understands the benign nature of the condition and recognizes that it is something that does not specifically need to be treated.

HERBAL SUPPLEMENTS

Many drugs used to treat arrhythmias were derived from herbs. Examples include quinidine (a stereoisomer of quinine from cinchona bark), amiodarone from Khellin (originally from the herb ammi visnaga), lidocaine, digoxin (from foxglove), warfarin, and others. Some herbal remedies not developed as drugs appear to have antiarrhythmic effects but the data are not sufficient to recommend any of these herbal supplements for general use in patients. Some may act as a supplement provided it does not increase risk. For the great majority of these herbs, the risk and the benefit of the supplement is not known. Moreover, interactions with conventional medications that may be required for therapy may not be well studied for most herbs. Presently, the uses of most herbal therapies used for arrhythmia reduction are not well founded and cannot be routinely advised. What follows is a review of reputed effects of various herbs. However, their effectiveness and safety has not been established enough to recommend their use.

Several Chinese herbs (e.g., xin bao, ci zhu wan, bu xin dan, yu zhu, and mai dong) may be antiarrhythmic. Symptomatic ventricular premature beats treated with mai dong improved symptoms in 80% of 84 in one report with no side effects.[62] In a study of 87 patients with sick sinus syndrome, xin bao reportedly improved symptoms of sick sinus syndrome, such as dizziness, palpitations, and chest pressure.[63]

Similarly, ginkgo biloba may reduce ventricular premature beats and even reperfusion-associated ventricular fibrillation.[64] Angelica and gingko biloba may have a protective influence during myocardial ischemia and reperfusion.[65] In a rat model, the incidence of ventricular premature beats and the total incidence of arrhythmia were greatly reduced.[66]

Suppression of ischemia-reperfusion induced ventricular arrhythmias has been observed with Fissistigma glaucescens (inhibits sodium and I to channel activity)[67] and Ciwujia[68] (Acanthopanax senticosus) extract. Lappaconitine inhibits tetrodotoxin-sensitive, voltage-dependent sodium channels in atria.[69] Garlic[70,71] may reduce reperfusion-induced arrhythmia, suppress premature ventricular contractions and ventricular tachycardia in ouabain-toxic dogs and suppress ectopic left atrial rhythms in rats.[72]

Agrimony, celery, hawthorn, and ginger may be beta-blockers. Corkwood may be anticholinergic. Stephania tetrandra root is a calcium channel blocker[73] as is Rhynchophylline,[74] tetrandrine (a T- and L-type calcium channel blocker),[75] and taxine.[76]

Crataegus (hawthorn) may reduce ischemia-induced ventricular arrhythmias[77,78] and prolong effective refractory periods.[79] In a study of 1011 patients with NYHA stage II congestive heart failure, crataegus improved ejection fraction,[80] slowed resting pulse, improved exercise tolerance, fatigue, palpitations, and exercise-induced dyspnea. Fewer arrhythmias and ventricular extrasystoles at maximum exercise were reported.

Hawthorn has been used to treat atrial fibrillation and it might affect ischemic ventricular arrhythmias.[77] A dose of 160–900 mg of the water ethanol extract is used. Hawthorn contains hyperoside (vitexin, rhamnose) rutin, and oligomeric procyanidins. Hawthorn berry has bathmotropic and dromotropic effects that are ascribed to the flavonoids present. It is unclear exactly where this herb works, but it might affect the sodium-potassium ATPase pump similar to digoxin or act as a phosphodiesterase inhibitor.

Japanese studies on indole alkaloids from uncaria rhynchophylla and amsonia elliptica contain hirsutine, hirsuteine, rhynchophylline, isorhynchophylline, and dihydrocorynantheine.[81] These and β-yohimbine isolated from amsonia elliptica have shown potential benefit for aconitine-induced arrhythmias in mice and ouabain-induced arrhythmias in guinea pigs.[81] Uncaria rhynchophylla and amsonia elliptica contain indole alkaloids with similar antiarrhythmic potency to indole alkaloids in the antiarrhythmic ajmaline, an antiarrhythmic drug (no longer available), also an indole alkaloid. Hirsutine and dihydrocory-nantheine affects action potentials of the sinoatrial node, the atria and the ventricles.

Ciwujia (acanthopanax senticosus harms), used for athletic performance and weight loss, may have antiarrhythmic effects. Ciwujia, studied in isolated rat hearts with transient coronary occlusion reduced reperfusion-induced ventricular fibrillation and ventricular tachycardia.[82] Ciwujia may reduce the incidence of malignant arrhythmias.[83]

Licorice root may have antiarrhythmic properties.[84] Zhigancao (prepared licorice) injection can antagonize arrhythmias induced by chloroform, catecholamines, aconitine, strophanthine K and barium chloride. It may slow the heart rate, prolong P-R and Q-T intervals, and antagonize the positive chronotropic response induced by catecholamines. Another component of licorice, sodium 18 beta-glycyrrhetate strongly counteracts arrhythmias induced by chloroform, lengthens the appearance time of arrhythmia induced by $CaCl_2$, slightly retards the heart rate of rats and rabbits, and partly antagonizes the acceleration effect of isoproterenol on rabbit hearts. The clinical significance of these experimental findings is unclear.[85]

Motherwort[86] contains bufenolide, glycosides (stachydirine), and alkaloids bufenolide. It may decrease palpitations due to a mild beta-blocking effect. No randomized, controlled trial has been performed.

Khellin (ammi visnaga) has significant antiarrhythmic effects. In the 1950s, Khella, derived from ammi visnaga, was used to treat angina. It has also been used by naturopaths to decrease palpitations. Khella is the original substance from which the antiarrhythmic, amiodarone, was derived.[87–90]

Eleutherococcus (Siberian ginseng) may be antiarrhythmic. Siberian ginseng can cause an apparent increase in digoxin levels.[91] It is unclear whether this is a false serum elevation, if ginseng converts to digoxin in vivo, or whether ginseng alters the metabolism of digoxin. Panax notoginseng (pseudoginseng) can prolong the sinus node recovery time, AV Wenckebach conduction cycle length, ventricular effective refractory period, and ventricular action potential durations, and increase ventricular fibrillation threshold in dogs.[92]

Rhodiola has shown some antiarrhythmic effects[93] in a rat model of adrenaline and $CaCl_2$-induced arrhythmias. The antiarrhythmic effect of the Rhodiola may be due to activation of the opioid system and stimulation of kappa-opioid receptors.[94] Rhodiola rosea may affect arrhythmia reduction by activating the opioid system.[95] Rhodiola may affect intracellular calcium handling[96] but may exacerbate palpitations in some instances.

Berberine may have an antiarrhythmic effect and help reduce ectopy and mortality in patients with congestive heart failure secondary to ischemic or idiopathic dilated cardiomyopathy.[97] A placebo-controlled study of 1.2–2.0 g/day of berberine in 156 patients with heart failure and ventricular ectopy and/or non-sustained ventricular tachycardia reported that berberine use was associated with significantly greater increase in left ventricular ejection fraction, exercise capacity, improvement in dyspnea-fatigue index, decrease in frequency and complexity of

PVCs, and decreased mortality (mean follow-up 24 months). No proarrhythmia was observed. The authors concluded that barberine improved quality of life, PVC frequency, and mortality in these patients with congestive heart failure. Other data also support a potential antiarrhythmic effect of this and similar herbal products.[98–101]

Potential adverse effects of herbs   Herbs can exacerbate arrhythmias. Ma huang, from the Chinese ephedra plant, contains catecholamines including ephedrine, which can initiate ectopic rhythm disturbances.[102] Ephedra (ma huang) can trigger potentially life-threatening arrhythmias and precipitate death.[102] Previously taken off the market, ma huang is available again and is often combined with stimulants that can further exacerbate arrhythmias, hypertension, and ischemia.[103,104] Aconite (wolfsbane) may initiate fatal arrhythmias.[105] Broom and Sparteine may be antiarrhythmic but both are considered unsafe.[106] Veratrum (hellebore) may precipitate bradycardia, AV dissociation, and hypotension by the Bezold-Jarisch reflex.[73,107,108] Agnus castus, black cohosh, cola, yerba maté, St. John's Wort, aniseed, capsicum, parsley, and vervain contain sympathomimetics and should be used with caution although little data indicate they are harmful.[109,110] Herbal preparations (drinks) contain caffeine as guarana or cola nut and may be combined with glucuronolactone and taurine, for example. These combinations may provide for a greater degree of alertness without adverse effects, but large studies have not been undertaken to assess arrhythmic or other risk.[111–113] It has been suggested that ambertose, ginkgo biloba, and other commonly used substances may exacerbate or even cause arrhythmias. Drug information centers may be helpful to provide correct, up-to-date information should questions arise.[111–114] In fact, very little is known about the risk-benefit ratio of most of the herbal products. They simply have not been extensively tested.

Several herbs containing cardiac glycosides can potentiate the effect of digoxin, and elevate, or falsely elevate, digoxin levels. Hawthorn, Kyushu, licorice, plantain, and uzara root are examples. Siberian ginseng may interact with the digoxin assay, causing an apparent increase in digoxin levels.[91] Oleander even in small amounts can be toxic.[115] Yellow oleander (Thevetia peruviana) poisoning is manifest by high serum cardiac glycoside levels and AV conduction defects.[116,117] Herbal oleander (Nerium oleander) leaf tea has been associated with elevated digoxin levels, arrhythmias, and hyperkalemia.[118,119]

NONHERBAL SUPPLEMENTS

Omega-3 fatty acids   These appear beneficial for patients with coronary artery disease but data conflict regarding the extent of benefit. Of all the antiarrhythmic supplements, omega-3 fatty acids are associated with the largest amount of supportive data and are well worth considering as routine supplements to standard therapies for those at risk of cardiac arrhythmias and potentially even the general population. Omega-3 fats appear to reduce total and sudden death cardiac mortality, reduce ventricular arrhythmias, and may improve outcomes in patients with atrial fibrillation. They reduce heart rate.[120] Conversely, trans fats and high levels of omega-6 fatty acids[121] are associated with adverse cardiovascular outcomes. Omega-3 fatty acids appear to have a direct effect on a variety of myocardial channels that can affect arrhythmias.[122–127] Specifically, omega-3 fatty acids appear to have an effect on calcium and potassium channels.[127]

A prospective, randomized, double-blind, placebo-controlled trial of fish (cod liver) oil versus placebo sunflower seed oil, involving 79 patients with frequent premature ventricular complexes without overt structural heart disease, showed fish oil reduced PVCs by >70% in 44% of patients versus 15% in the placebo group.[128] However, data conflict.[129]

The Lyon Diet study, the GISSI-Prevenzione trial, and the Physician's Health study have all shown a benefit to the use of fish oil. The Diet and Reinfarction Trial (DART) randomized 2033 men after myocardial infarction to receive advice on one of three diet strategies: (1) reduction in fat intake to 30% of total energy and increase in ratio of polyunsaturated to saturated fat; (2) increase in fatty fish intake to at least two 200–400 g portions of fatty fish weekly or 1.5 g fish oil capsules; or (3) increase in cereal fiber to 18 g daily.[130] The fatty fish advice group had a 29% reduction in 2-year all-cause mortality compared to those who did not receive this advice.

The GISSI-Prevenzione trial of 1,1324 patients surviving recent (≤3 months) myocardial infarction were assigned N-3 polyunsaturated fatty acids (PUFA) 1 g daily, vitamin E 300 mg daily, both or none.[131] Patients treated with N-3 PUFA had a 20% decrease in total mortality and 45% reduction in sudden death.

The Physicians' Health Study[46,132] reported that dietary fish and N-3 PUFA intakes were associated with a lower risk of sudden death among 20,551 U.S. male physicians completing a baseline questionnaire regarding fish consumption. Dietary fish intake was associated with a reduced risk of sudden death and total mortality. The threshold for the effect appeared to be at one fish meal per week. The multivariate relative risk of sudden death was 0.48 (52% lower risk) in males who consumed fish at least once per week compared with men who had fish less than monthly. A lower risk of sudden death was also seen when analyzed by any intake of N-3 PUFA.

Besides the large-scale studies noted above, other clinical studies have also reported significant reductions in sudden cardiac death from N-3 PUFA.[133–136] Omega-3 PUFA also increased heart rate variability in survivors of myocardial infarction randomized to fish oil or olive oil.[137,138] A primary beneficial effect of fish consumption and N-3 PUFA intake may be via a reduction in the risk of fatal arrhythmias.

These findings motivated trials of omega-3 fatty acids for the prevention of recurrent ventricular arrhythmias in patients with ICDs. Many of these patients can have malignant ventricular arrhythmias leading to shocks from their device. The aim of these studies was to decrease the number of shocks. In a randomized, double-blind, placebo-controlled study by Raitt,[139] 200 patients with ICDs and a recent episode of sustained ventricular tachycardia or fibrillation were randomly treated with 1.8 g/day of fish oil (72% omega-3 PUFAs), or placebo. This study reported that recurrent ventricular tachycardia and fibrillation episodes were *more* common in patients randomized to the fish oil supplement, concluding that fish oil supplementation did not reduce the risk of ventricular tachycardia and ventricular fibrillation and might have been proarrhythmic in some patients.

In contrast, fish oil was effective in the FAAT Trial, a randomized, placebo-controlled trial of 3 g of fish oil compared to cod-scented olive oil, studying the incidence of recurrent ventricular arrhythmias/shocks in patients who have ICDs.[140] Also, in the Study On Omega-3 Fatty Acids and Ventricular Arrhythmia (SOFA), which was presented in September, 2005,[141] patients with ICDs were also randomized in double-blind fashion to treatment with fish oil (2 g/day) or placebo oil (n = 273 in each group) for up to 12 months. The primary endpoint of life-threatening arrhythmias or death at 12 months did not differ between groups, but in a subgroup with prior myocardial infarction, there was a trend toward a benefit in survival free of ventricular tachycardia and ventricular fibrillation, and there were no apparent safety concerns in the fish oil group. The latter study suggests that omega-3 fatty acids may be more beneficial for ischemic rather than nonischemic arrhythmias. Indeed, in animal studies, omega-3 PUFA have been demonstrated to decrease vulnerability to ventricular fibrillation induced by coronary occlusion or reperfusion. Animal models have demonstrated the arrhythmogenic effects of long-chain saturated fatty acids and the antiarrhythmic effects of N-3 PUFA.[142]

Tuna fish oil supplementation reduced ventricular fibrillation during coronary artery occlusion and reperfusion in rats.[143] In marmosets-fed diets supplemented with PUFA-rich tuna fish oil or sunflower seed oil, PUFA increased ventricular fibrillation threshold (that is, the ease of inducibility of ventricular fibrillation) and a low incidence of sustained fibrillation after acute myocardial ischemia induced by coronary artery occlusion.[144] In a dog model of sudden cardiac death with balloon inflation of the left circumflex coronary artery during treadmill exercise 1 month after surgically induced large anterior wall myocardial infarction, N-3 PUFA were antiarrhythmic.[123,145] Ischemic-induced ventricular fibrillation was prevented in up to 87% of dogs by intravenous administration of the purified N-3 PUFA, DHA, or EPA.

Arrhythmogenicity of fatty acids appears highly dependent upon N-3 versus N-6 subtype. The N-6 fatty acids, particularly linoleic acid, can be elongated and desaturated to arachidonic acid, and then oxygenated via cyclooxygenase to two-series prostaglandins and thromboxane, which have been shown to be arrhythmogenic, except for prostacyclin.[146,147] In contrast, none of the three-series cyclooxygenase products of EPA were shown to be arrhythmogenic and in fact N3 fatty acids appeared protective.

Omega-3 fatty acids have also been studied in the prevention of atrial arrhythmias. In a study in patients with dual-chamber pacemakers, which have diagnostic capabilities of storing frequency of atrial fibrillation episodes, 40 patients with paroxysmal atrial tachyarrhythmias recorded on pacemaker interrogation were treated with omega-3 supplements (1 g/day).[148] After 4 months of treatment, pacemakers were reevaluated and treatment stopped with reevaluation after another 4 months. The authors concluded that omega-3 fatty acids reduced the burden of atrial tachyarrhythmias in these patients.

In another study by Calo,[149] N-3 PUFAs reduced the incidence of postoperative atrial fibrillation occurring after coronary bypass graft surgery. In this prospective, randomized, open-label trial of 160 patients undergoing elective bypass surgery, N-3 PUFAs (2 g/day beginning 5 days before surgery) was associated with reduction in postoperative atrial fibrillation (15.2% versus 33.3%, $p = 0.013$).

The data on fish oil on arrhythmias and improving outcomes in patients with heart disease is extensive.[150,151] While the data in some cases conflict, fish oil is associated with improved autonomic influences,[152–154] reduction in atrial fibrillation,[155] reduction in risk of all-cause mortality, reduction in symptomatic ventricular ectopy, and reduction in depression.[38]

Omega-3 fatty acids are available in a variety of forms, not only fish oil.[156] A variety of plant oils can be metabolized into omega-3 fatty acids, including flax seed oil, which also has other potential benefits,[157] including those on mood. As omega-3 fatty acids can improve mood, they may also have an autonomic effect that can decrease the sensation of arrhythmias or decrease arrhythmias all together. However, it should be noted that metabolism of N-3 PUFAs from plant sources to DHA or EPA is very inefficient. The main source of DHA or EPA in our diets is from fish.

Coenzyme Q10 Coenzyme Q10 may have a small effect on reducing premature ventricular depolarizations in patients with diabetes or hypertension[158] and may reduce atrial fibrillation. Coenzyme Q10 at a dose of 100–300 mg a day may decrease episodes of atrial fibrillation by an unknown mechanism. Coenzyme Q10 can also have an effect on ventricular and atrial ectopy.[159]

Carnitine Carnitine has been reported to be antiarrhythmic and improve outcomes in patients with cardiomyopathy. L-Carnitine, a dose of 3 g a day or more, may improve mitochondrial function, left ventricular function, and may prevent some atrial and ventricular arrhythmias. Several small, randomized, controlled trials of carnitine have shown a reduction in risk for sudden cardiac death and total death in patients with cardiomyopathy. The mechanism is not clear but it might be that carnitine improves mitochondrial function and myocardial function due to this.[160–163] Carnitine may prove to be a promising therapy for ischemia or reperfusion-induced arrhythmias. Carnitine has been reported to decrease the incidence of supraventricular and ventricular arrhythmias during hemodialysis.[164] In a cat model, thresholds for electrically induced atrial fibrillation were reduced by 100 mg/kg intravenous carnitine.[165] Another study reported a reduction in ventricular extrasystoles in hypertensive patients treated with oral L-carnitine 2 g/day.[166] There are no known adverse effects of carnitine.

Carnitine supplements may have specific benefit in some genetic defects of fatty acid metabolism, particularly in defects of long-chain fatty acid transport across the inner mitochondrial membrane or other defects in which intermediary metabolites of fatty acids, such as long-chain acylcarnitines, accumulate and are arrhythmogenic.[167]

Potassium   Potassium supplementation is extraordinarily important especially if a patient is taking drugs that are lowering their potassium levels. Potassium has been implicated for all types of rhythm disturbances and potassium deficiencies can lead to torsades de pointes. It is clear that anyone who is at risk with long QT syndrome and specifically drugs that lower potassium may need potassium supplementation. This can also be done though potassium in the diet including fruits and vegetables that contain high potassium levels.

Selenium   Deficiency of selenium can cause heart problems including arrhythmias. There are no good data, however, to suggest that low selenium levels, that are supplemented, will improve arrhythmia status.[168]

Calcium and Magnesium   Approximately 1 g a day each of a salt (magnesium sulfate, for example), has been associated with a decrease in arrhythmias. Magnesium can decrease triggered activity and can slow conduction in the AV node. Magnesium may suppress symptomatic arrhythmias but data supporting a real benefit are scarce. Magnesium supplementation given to patients in congestive heart failure in a double blind, placebo-controlled trial showed improvements in arrhythmias. Individuals taking 3.2 g/day of magnesium chloride equivalent to 384 mg/day of elemental magnesium had between 23–52% occurrences of specific arrhythmias in a 6-week follow-up period.[169]

Although many studies have reported that magnesium supplementation decreased arrhythmias after cardiac surgery,[170,171] myocardial infarction,[172–176] or heart failure.[169,177,178] Other studies have produced disappointing results.[179–181] In Fourth International Study of Infarct Survival (ISIS-4), 58,050 patients with suspected acute myocardial infarction were randomized to oral captopril versus placebo, oral mononitrate versus placebo, and 24 hours of intravenous magnesium (8 mmol followed by 72 mmol) versus open control.[182] Magnesium failed to reduce mortality. Nevertheless, subsequent studies have suggested that early, rather than later, intravenous magnesium may be beneficial.[183–185]

Copper and Zinc   Three cases have been reported in which ventricular premature beats decreased after copper supplementation at a dose of 4 mg per day.[186] However, zinc worsened arrhythmias, and extra zinc can lead to copper deficiency. However, there is a potential problem with copper, as high copper levels can lead to atherosclerosis.

VITAMINS

Vitamin D   A long-standing case of sick sinus syndrome was reported to resolve with supplementation of 800 units per day of vitamin D.[187] However, it is not clear that vitamin D was the cause for this change.

Vitamin C   In a pilot study for the prevention of postoperative atrial fibrillation, vitamin C was associated with a reduction in postoperative atrial fibrillation (16.3% incidence of atrial fibrillation versus 34.9% in age- and gender-matched controls),[188] but in a larger trial vitamin C did not appear to have benefit.

Vitamin E   Despite initial data suggesting benefit, vitamin E has been a lesson in the use of supplements. Large-scale studies have been disappointing[189–191] and a meta-analysis indicates potential harm from supplementation. This is especially true in those patients taking statin drugs.

POTENTIAL HARMFUL EFFECTS OF NONHERBAL SUPPLEMENTS

Some nonherbal supplements may be toxic. Cesium is one example. In one of the most dramatic instances of supplement-induced proarrhythmia, Saliba[192] reported a case of a patient presenting with cardiac arrest due to torsades de pointes. It was discovered that the patient was using a cesium supplement, being used for cancer prevention. Cesium is a well-recognized potassium channel blocker that is used in experimental animal models to provoke prolongation action potential duration, early afterdepolarizations, QT prolongation, and torsades de pointes. This case highlights the potential life-threatening danger of some supplements.

Mind-body therapies

Various forms of psychological stress have been known to affect hemodynamics, cardiovascular responses, autonomic fluctuations, syncope, myocardial ischemia, and even sudden death.[193,194] It is not completely clear if the stress is the direct predictor or if specific individuals who are likely to experience high stress are also more likely to experience cardiac arrest. There does appear to be a tacit relationship, however, between the presence of psychological stress and various arrhythmias, including PVCs, supraventricular tachycardia, ventricular tachycardia, and ventricular fibrillation. There also appears to be a relationship between mortality and psychological stress. It would make sense that reduction of stress may be associated with improved outcomes. This has never been tested carefully but there appears to be a relationship between blood pressure and meditation, for example. There even appears to be some suggestion that meditation may affect regression of atherosclerosis.

Autonomic variations can occur with a variety of different lifestyle interventions, including acupuncture, meditation, and other mind/body issues.[195–197] The influence can be profound and may occur by several potential mechanisms: (1) change in autonomic function, (2) a placebo effect, (3) a direct effect on the rhythm, (4) a change in perception of the importance of the arrhythmias to the patient, (5) shifting of the attention from the arrhythmia to some other issue.

Biofeedback can decrease the number, frequency, and severity of the palpitations related to arrhythmias. Effect of biofeedback have been known for some time.[198–202] Another issue is simple one, of developing an awareness that a patient can learn to identify a rhythm disturbance as not potentially a noxious experience. The interpretation of the severity of the rhythm disturbance will amplify the severity of the affects on symptoms. By having a patient face the problem, it can actually become an issue of empowerment so that the patient can improve their perception of the arrhythmia and its implications. Ultimately, properly used psychosocial therapy can reduce the risk of death.[203]

Acupuncture has direct effects on the autonomic nervous system and can decrease rhythm disturbances.

Meditation has been associated with decreased risk factors of sudden death in high-risk patients[204–213] and may reduce the risk of ventricular fibrillation Meditation may affect the autonomic nervous system in a beneficial way.[214] It may also change the perception of the arrhythmia for those who have a benign cause for their problem.

Meditation and relaxation techniques may be also useful for individuals who have an implantable cardioverter defibrillator for life-threatening rhythm disturbances. If the device is activated frequently, it can cause tremendous grief. Meditation and relaxation techniques can improve outcomes in such patients. These techniques may also allow for better patient acceptance of the shocks.

Relaxation appears to have a positive benefit. For those who do have knowledge of medications, for years, physicians have used benzodiazepines to treat rhythm disturbances such as atrial fibrillation and supraventricular tachycardia. If a patient comes into an emergency room with such an arrhythmia and is allowed to relax, the rhythm will often stop spontaneously.

DOES THE STATE OF MIND INFLUENCE OUTCOMES?

It is likely that the state of mind will affect outcomes. There appears to be a relationship between depression and adverse cardiovascular outcomes including sudden cardiac death in patients with cardiovascular disease. The issue is which came first, severe disease causing the depression or depression exacerbating the disease? The answer to this question is not yet known. Epidemiological data support the idea that optimism is associated with better long-term outcomes for patients in several studies.[215,216] Lack of optimism can be associated with dietary indiscretion.[217] On the other hand, there are data that conflict with this, including data in terminal cancer patients demonstrating that optimism has no beneficial effect. Indeed, optimism may have an adverse affect in select situations or be no better than pessimism.[218] False hope may have a negative impact.[219] Pessimism or realism may also have a benefit regarding cardiovascular outcomes.[220,221]

Jim Collins in his book *Good to Great* pointed out the Stockdale Paradox in which survival in a North Vietnamese prisoner of war camp in Vietnam occurred importantly with and due to a lack of optimism. Much has yet to be learned about the impact of hope, optimism, and despair and pessimism with regard to cardiovascular outcomes. It does appear, however, that it is best for a physician to have an optimistic attitude that reflects realistically the issues regarding the patient.

Stress reduction techniques encompass a wide variety of modalities. While cardiovascular responses can be affected, data that demonstrate long-term benefit of these therapies to improve cardiovascular risk reduce arrhythmic events, improve quality-of-life, and enhance outcomes over and above standard therapies has yet to be shown. Nevertheless, there are some specific situations in which mind-body therapies may serve a role. In patients who received ICD implants but then undergo multiple ICD shocks, the stress of this series of shocking events could be devastating and may influence the patient's interpretation of the benefits of the therapy. Stress reduction may have specific advantages in this situation.

Another example would be patients who have neurocardiogenic syncope under times of severe psychological distress. Although not tested, it would make sense that stress reduction may improve outcomes by reducing the risk of stress-induced syncopal events. Many cardiac arrhythmias, particularly ischemic-induced ventricular tachyarrhythmias, exercise-induced ventricular tachycardias, and episodes of supraventricular tachycardias are frequently catecholamine generated and stress induced. Reduction of stress may allow for fewer episodes of both life-threatening and non-life-threatening but highly symptomatic episodes.

ENERGY MEDICINE

While there are some data to demonstrate benefits of energy medicine healing, little substantial data document the benefits of an energy medicine approach to reduce the risk of cardiac arrest or arrhythmic events in patients. If a patient is so inclined to undergo such a therapeutic intervention, they may derive some placebo benefit or perhaps a real benefit but there is little data to support the idea that energy medicine healing would be appropriate to reduce the risk of sudden cardiac death.

ACUPUNCTURE

Acupuncture may have a role in readjusting the autonomic nervous system especially in patients who have autonomic evidence for catecholamine excess. Acupuncture may serve a role in patients who have syncope or in those who have congestive heart failure. There are little data to support the use of acupuncture to reduce arrhythmic episodes.

EXERCISE

Exercise and physical exertion can be the trigger of a variety of arrhythmias. Maintaining excellent physical health through exercise, however, will decrease effects of the sympathetic nervous system on the heart and the heart rhythm and improve outcomes in almost all circumstances. The sympathetic nervous system often plays a major role in serious and benign atrial and ventricular arrhythmias. Exercise performed regularly with enhancement of aerobic capacity will decrease sensitivity to catecholamines, decrease circulating catecholamine levels, decrease sympathetic nervous system tone, and enhance vagal tone. All of these may increase heart rate variability, which may decrease the risk for sudden death and decrease the potential for catecholamine-initiated or sympathetically initiated atrial and ventricular arrhythmias.

Exercise can also modulate other potential rhythm disturbances such as sinus tachycardia. Especially in young women, inappropriate sinus tachycardia and postural orthostatic tachycardia syndrome are potential problems.[222] Inappropriate sinus tachycardia is a condition when the sinus node appears to be hyperactive; the cause for this is not completely known. It might be, in part, related to abnormal sympathetic nervous system stimulation, but it could also be an intrinsic problem with the sinus node. Increasing exercise will decrease the potential for this problem. Inappropriate sinus tachycardia may develop after a viral syndrome. Exercise will downregulate the sympathetic nervous system and lower catecholamine levels. By several mechanisms, it can lower heart rate.

Exercise appears to be beneficial in treating many arrhythmias but it must be used with caution, as it is a double-edged sword. For patients with malignant arrhythmias, use of exercise therapy must be discussed with a qualified physician who is knowledgeable about the risks, benefits, and methods of monitoring the patient.

A patient who can be compliant with a stringent exercise program may derive substantial benefit with regard to arrhythmia that are stress induced or catecholamine induced. This could apply to patients who have sinus node abnormalities, sinoatrial reentry tachycardia, supraventricular tachycardia from various causes, and ventricular tachycardia associated with the possibility of sudden cardiac death. Exercise programs, properly delivered, provide substantial benefit and should be undertaken even in patients who can be treated with standard medical approaches. Exercise can improve the quality of life and the extent to which the patient may live. Exercise often has greater benefit in a social setting such as the cardiac rehabilitation facility. In addition, in such a facility, the patient will more likely have a controlled prescribed exercise approach rather than a random undisciplined approach.

DIET

Diet has been underemphasized in the treatment and reduction of arrhythmic events in patients who have symptomatic arrhythmias or are at risk for sudden cardiac death. On the other hand, various foods and food products can increase catecholamine effects and can trigger cardiac arrhythmias. Examples of this are effects of caffeine and alcohol on atrial and ventricular arrhythmias and potential deleterious effects of 18-2 trans fatty acids versus the beneficial effects of fish oil. Diet affects obesity, glucose intolerance, cholesterol levels, and other medical issues that could further exacerbate arrhythmic events.

There may even be some foods that act as triggers and patients will often provide some evidence for this: in some patients, alcohol is one of the major triggers for atrial fibrillation and ventricular ectopy.[223–226] Caffeine is frequently another trigger for ectopic beats.[227,228] Conversely, it is important to recognize that restriction of alcohol and caffeine may have no effect on arrhythmias in some patients. If this is the case, restriction will be of no benefit and may adversely influence the patient's lifestyle. Specific food allergies can trigger a reaction causing palpitations. Trans fats, particularly of the 18-2 type (found in doughnuts, fried foods, and artificial cheese such as in processed pizza), has been associated with cardiac arrest.[229] Omega-3 fats improve outcomes.[146] Fat balance appears to have an effect on cardiovascular health.[230]

The effects of diet on the autonomic nervous system are complex. Several foods will increase sympathetic nervous system tone. High levels of sodium also increase the effects of catecholamines. Electrolytes can influence ventricular ectopy.[169,186,231–234] Eating a large diet that causes bloating and is difficult to digest can alternatively increase vagal tone, which may also enhance the problem of rhythm disturbances. Bloating from excessively fatty, fried, or poorly digestible foods and other foods with which a patient is not accustomed can create a sensation of palpitations.

It may turn out that caffeine, theophylline, or theobromine present in coffee, tea, or chocolate may be inciting factors or that they may have a positive benefit.[235-239] Trial and error with these food substances is worthwhile, but there is no particular reason to try to eliminate all these foods if they do not have an effect on the arrhythmia. Patients may complain that a specific food triggers a rhythm disturbance by an unknown mechanism. This is not that uncommon and it is even possible it will be related to some type of allergic reaction or other related issue.

Diet and anticoagulation   The diet becomes very important in arrhythmia management, especially in patients who require anticoagulation for atrial fibrillation or other arrhythmias. If the diet changes markedly and, due to this, there are significant alterations in vitamin K levels, there will be tremendous fluctuation in the prothrombin time. A balanced diet low in fat, high in roughage that will lead to a moderate level of blood sugar and as little stress as possible on the GI tract may improve arrhythmias.

LIFESTYLE

Lifestyle has a major impact on arrhythmias.[240-243] Cigarette smoking and other forms of nicotine have no potential benefit and may be harmful for any individual.[242,244] Its use can exacerbate risk of sudden death, malignant and benign arrhythmias of all types. Alcohol, while it may have a beneficial effect on cardiovascular mortality, myocardial infarction, and cholesterol has no benefit for any arrhythmia. The combination of alcohol and nicotine is even more likely to trigger an arrhythmia. Frequently alcohol is used in combination with caffeine and cigarettes. Cigarettes may trigger a variety of rhythm disturbances including cardiac arrest by several potential mechanisms. If possible, it is best to try to eliminate smoking under any circumstance. The differences between the different types of alcohol are unclear in terms of their ability to trigger rhythm disturbances. It appears that all alcohol can trigger arrhythmias and it is not clear that a specific type of alcohol, whether it is wine or hard liquor, has a greater propensity to do this.

Specific arrhythmia management

DESCRIPTION: ECTOPIC BEATS–NOT DUE TO OR ASSOCIATED WITH A MALIGNANT CAUSE

Atrial ectopic beats can trigger atrial fibrillation and supraventricular tachycardias. If this occurs, treatments listed below do not apply. Ventricular ectopic beats can be associated with risk of cardiac arrest, cardiomyopathy, and structural heart disease. These comments do not apply for these situations. The *goal* is to reduce symptoms or their impact.

Symptomatic atrial and ventricular ectopy can be an important issue in clinical practice for several reasons:

1. There are no good, safe, medical therapies.[245-257] With the possible exception of beta-adrenergic blockers, drugs that are used to suppress atrial ectopy may have a small but definite risk for "proarrhythmia," which could

increase the risk for sudden death, increase the severity of the arrhythmias, and/or lead to a variety of other serious complications.

2. The problem can be highly symptomatic and concerning to the patient. It can have a tremendous impact on the quality of life.

3. The degree of symptoms from benign arrhythmias varies tremendously and those with highly symptomatic arrhythmias may require a variety of types of therapeutic interventions, which can range from drug therapy to radiofrequency catheter ablation approaches.

Atrial premature depolarizations can be frequent and occasionally symptomatic, although not usually associated with significant risk. Conventional treatment generally includes reassurance, avoidance of precipitating factors (e.g., caffeine, sympathomimetic agents), and occasionally beta blockers or calcium channel blockers.

Isolated premature ventricular depolarizations are not associated with significant risk in patients without structural heart disease, but frequent or complex premature ventricular complexes can be markers for potential increased risk in those with structural heart disease. Conventional treatment of isolated, symptomatic premature complexes generally includes assessment of risk if there is structural heart disease or risk factors, avoidance of precipitating factors (e.g., caffeine, sympathomimetic agents), and reassurance with occasional beta blockers or rarely other antiarrhythmic agents for persistently symptomatic patients. Electrophysiology study with mapping and catheter ablation of focally originating premature ventricular complexes or tachycardias also has been performed for frequent and refractory symptoms.

TREATMENT APPROACHES FOR ECTOPIC BEATS

The meaning response: For patients who have benign atrial and ventricular ectopic activity and who have symptoms, it is often necessary, and important, to describe to the patient the meaning of these rhythm disturbances. If a patient understands that ectopic activity is associated with specific symptoms but that the symptoms will not necessarily indicate the presence of more progressive symptoms such as syncope or congestive heart failure and that the ectopic beats will not lead to sudden arrhythmic cardiac death or death at all, this may be the only treatment the patient requires.

Manipulative and body-based methods: No specific manipulative and body-based therapies are recommended. Meditation or stress reduction techniques may help the acceptance of ectopic beats. Reduction in stress may also improve outcomes by reducing catecholamine-generated ectopic activity.

Energy therapies, acupuncture, mind-body interventions: There is no specific advantage of using these approaches for ectopic beats.

Exercise: An exercise program may suppress frequent ectopic beats especially if they are related to catecholamine excess or are triggered by catecholamines. The exercise program could be used in conjunction with a beta adrenergic-blocking drug. It might take several months before a response is seen.

Diet and lifestyle: If it appears that frequent ectopic beats and other arrhythmias may be generated by changes in or poor sleep patterns, use of nonprescription drugs such as over-the-counter or illicit drugs, and use of caffeine, then modification of these triggers should be advised. A diet that is well-balanced, high in roughage, low in saturated fat and trans fat, and high in omega-3 fats may reduce ectopic activity.

Supplements: Several supplements have been tried for ectopic activity but no supplement has been well documented to have beneficial effects except for perhaps one: fish oil. Omega-3 fatty acids appear to reduce the risk of ventricular ectopic activity in symptomatic patients. Magnesium appears to be safe but there is no specific compelling evidence to indicate that magnesium would be effective in this population. There are little data to support the use of carnitine or coenzyme Q10.

BIOLOGICALLY BASED TREATMENTS

Medical therapy: It is important to limit therapy to those patients who highly symptomatic, since the risk of the therapy may outweigh the benefit in most situations.

Ablation: A patient who may benefit is one who has ventricular bigeminy or such frequent PVCs that they cause a tachycardia-induced cardiomyopathy, or one in whom the PVCs cause life-style learning symptoms refractory to non-invasive or medical therapies.

SINUS BRADYCARDIA, ASYSTOLE, SINUS PAUSES

Sinus bradycardia, which generally is defined as sinus rates of less than 60 beats/minute, is common in young, healthy adults (especially in athletes), with normal rates during sleep falling to as low as 35–50 beats/minute. It usually is benign, but it can be associated with diseases, such as hypothyroidism, vagal stimulation, increased intracranial pressure, MI, and drugs, such as beta blockers (including those used for glaucoma), calcium channel blockers, amiodarone, clonidine, lithium, and parasympathomimetic drugs. Treatment often is unnecessary if the patient is asymptomatic. Patients with chronic bradycardia or chronotropic incompetence and symptoms of congestive heart failure or low cardiac output, however, may benefit from permanent pacing. Sinus pauses or arrest may result from degenerative changes of the sinus node, acute MI, excessive vagal tone or stimuli, digitalis toxicity, sleep apnea, or stroke. Symptomatic or very long pauses may require permanent pacing.

ATRIAL FIBRILLATION

An extensive literature and multiple, randomized, controlled clinical trials address rate versus rhythm control and the use of anticoagulation. This discussion is far beyond the scope of this chapter and available in many references and texts. The *goal* is to reduce symptoms, improve functionality, and reduce the sequelae of atrial fibrillation. In some cases, the triggers for atrial fibrillation can be known but this is rare. While there are known precipitants of atrial fibrillation, including acute illness otherwise, there are no well-described precipitants in the population of patients at large. No specific recommendations can be made with regard to restriction of specific dietary or exercise-related concerns.

The meaning response   It is important to describe to the patients the implications of atrial fibrillation, the outcomes of atrial fibrillation, the importance of reduction in symptoms, and the risks and benefits of medications.

SUMMARY

Arrhythmia management is complex and multifaceted. The treatment depends on the arrhythmia, its implications, the symptoms, and the effect that it has on the patient. This is especially important if the arrhythmias are potentially life threatening. If not, an approach to improve outcomes should involve change in lifestyle and exercise.

Dietary changes may be useful. If this is not enough, mind-body effects can be substantial. Several herbal preparations may influence the presence of an arrhythmia and some supplements, such as Ma huang, can worsen an arrhythmia or even create a new, life-threatening one. In some instances, treatment will require invasive testing and treatment with antiarrhythmic drugs, ablation or implantation of a pacemaker, or a defibrillator to prevent serious symptoms or cardiac arrest. No CAM approach can substitute for a pacemaker and/or an implantable defibrillator if it is indicated.

For patient with symptomatic ectopy/PVCs

- Determine the severity of the symptoms and their relation to the arrhythmia.
- Assess underlying conditions
- Determine the risk to the patient.
- For benign ectopy, discuss the risks of drug therapy and suggest alternatives.
- Eliminate dietary triggers.
- Mind-body interventions. Meditation. Provide patient a careful understanding of the condition and its nature. Patients who understand will be able to tolerate the arrhythmia better. Reassure the patient (if this is in order).
- Determine relation to exercise; suggest an exercise program.
- Suggest omega-3 fatty acids.
- Drug therapy only if resistant to above.
  - Beta-blockade titrated upwards
  - Occasionally, calcium channel blockers will be effective

- Antiarrhythmic drugs with caution (if no structural heart disease, flecainide, propafenone, sotalol first choice then amiodarone but only in resistant, highly symptomatic cases
- Ablative therapy

For patients with paroxysmal atrial fibrillation

- Correlate symptoms with arrhythmia. Determine presence of underlying conditions, including hyperthyroidism.
- Assess risk to the patient and need for rate control, anticoagulation, maintenance of sinus rhythm.
- Determine triggers, if possible. If a relationship: eliminate caffeine, alcohol, and any potential offending drug.
- If at hight, consider changes in diet (no large meals causing gastric distension).
- If exercise related, consider the exercise program.
- Mind-body interventions. Relaxation techniques. Counsel patient and educate about disease process.
- Drug therapy.
  - Beta blockade (to control rhythm and rate)
  - Calcium channel blockade (to control rate)
  - Antiarrhythmic drugs depend on the patient and the conditions
  - Antithrombiotic therapy
- Nonpharmacological intervention
  - Ablation/isolation around pulmonary veins
  - Ablation of the AV node with a pacemaker (remains in AF)
  - Ablation of other inciting arrhythmia

REFERENCES

1. Rosano GM, Rillo M, Leonardo F, Pappone C, Chierchia SL. Palpitations: what is the mechanism, and when should we treat them? Int J Fertil Womens Med. 1997;42:94–100.
2. Barsky AJ. Palpitations, arrhythmias, and awareness of cardiac activity. Ann Intern Med. 2001;134:832–7.
3. Barsky AJ, Ahern DK, Bailey ED, Delamater BA. Predictors of persistent palpitations and continued medical utilization. J Fam Pract. 1996;42:465–72.
4. Weber BE, Kapoor WN. Evaluation and outcomes of patients with palpitations. Am J Med. 1996;100:138–48.
5. Barsky AJ, Cleary PD, Coeytaux RR, Ruskin JN. Psychiatric disorders in medical outpatients complaining of palpitations. J Gen Intern Med. 1994;9:306–13.
6. Lok NS, Lau CP: Prevalence of palpitations, cardiac arrhythmias and their associated risk factors in ambulant elderly. Int J Cardiol. 1996;54:231–6.

7. Zeldis SM, Levine BJ, Michelson EL, Morganroth J. Cardiovascular complaints. Correlation with cardiac arrhythmias on 24-hour electrocardiographic monitoring. Chest. 1980;78:456–61.

8. Steinberg JS, Beckman K, Greene HL, et al. Follow-up of patients with unexplained syncope and inducible ventricular tachyarrhythmias: analysis of the AVID registry and an AVID substudy. Antiarrhythmics versus implantable defibrillators. J Cardiovasc Electrophysiol. 2001;12:996–1001.

9. Nerheim P, Olshansky B. Syncope. Curr Treat Options Cardiovasc Med. 2001;3: 299–310.

10. Olshansky B. Syncope evaluation at a crossroad: for which patients? Circulation. 2001;104:7–8.

11. Goldschlager N, Epstein AE, Grubb BP, et al. Etiologic considerations in the patient with syncope and an apparently normal heart. Arch Intern Med. 2003;163:151–62.

12. Olshansky B. For whom does the bell toll? J Cardiovasc Electrophysiol. 2001;12: 1002–3.

13. Nerheim P, Birger-Botkin S, Piracha L, Olshansky B. Heart failure and sudden death in patients with tachycardia-induced cardiomyopathy and recurrent tachycardia. Circulation. 2004;110:247–52.

14. Zipes DP. Epidemiology and mechanisms of sudden cardiac death. Can J Cardiol. 2005;21 Suppl A:37–40.

15. Viskin S, Halkin A, Olgin JE. Treatable causes of sudden death: not really "treatable" or not really the cause? J Am Coll Cardiol. 2001;38:1725–7.

16. Simons LA, Simons J, McCallum J, Friedlander Y. Impact of smoking, diabetes and hypertension on survival time in the elderly: the Dubbo Study. Med J Aust. 2005;182:219–22.

17. Lind P, Engstrom G, Stavenow L, Janzon L, Lindgarde F, Hedblad B. Risk of myocardial infarction and stroke in smokers is related to plasma levels of inflammation-sensitive proteins. Arterioscler Thromb Vasc Biol. 2004;24:577–82.

18. Goldenberg I, Jonas M, Tenenbaum A, et al. Current smoking, smoking cessation, and the risk of sudden cardiac death in patients with coronary artery disease. Arch Intern Med. 2003;163:2301–5.

19. Tin LL, Beevers DG, Lip GY. Hypertension, left ventricular hypertrophy, and sudden death. Curr Cardiol Rep. 2002;4:449–57.

20. De Sutter J, Firsovaite V, Tavernier R. Prevention of sudden death in patients with coronary artery disease: do lipid-lowering drugs play a role? Prev Cardiol. 2002;5: 177–82.

21. Rosenberg DE, Jabbour SA, Goldstein BJ. Insulin resistance, diabetes and cardiovascular risk: approaches to treatment. Diabetes Obes Metab. 2005;7:642–53.

22. Chen Z, Yang G, Zhou M, et al. Body mass index and mortality from ischaemic heart disease in a lean population: 10 year prospective study of 220,000 adult men. Int J Epidemiol. 2005;35(1):141–50.

23. Varma R, Garrick R, McClung J, Frishman WH. Chronic renal dysfunction as an independent risk factor for the development of cardiovascular disease. Cardiol Rev. 2005;13:98–107.

24. Arking DE, Chugh SS, Chakravarti A, Spooner PM. Genomics in sudden cardiac death. Circ Res. 2004;94:712–23.

25. Grace SL, Abbey SE, Kapral MK, Fang J, Nolan RP, Stewart DE. Effect of depression on five-year mortality after an acute coronary syndrome. Am J Cardiol. 2005; 96:1179–85.

26. Glassman AH, O'Connor CM, Califf RM, et al. Sertraline treatment of major depression in patients with acute MI or unstable angina. JAMA. 2002;288:701–9.

27. Franco OH, de Laet C, Peeters A, Jonker J, Mackenbach J, Nusselder W. Effects of physical activity on life expectancy with cardiovascular disease. Arch Intern Med. 2005;165:2355–60.

28. Albert CM, Ma J, Rifai N, Stampfer MJ, Ridker PM. Prospective study of C-reactive protein, homocysteine, and plasma lipid levels as predictors of sudden cardiac death. Circulation. 2002;105:2595–9.

29. Grady D, Herrington D, Bittner V, et al. Cardiovascular disease outcomes during 6.8 years of hormone therapy: Heart and Estrogen/progestin Replacement Study follow-up (HERS II). JAMA. 2002;288:49–57.

30. Nelson HD, Humphrey LL, Nygren P, Teutsch SM, Allan JD. Postmenopausal hormone replacement therapy: scientific review. JAMA. 2002;288:872–81.

31. Beral V, Banks E, Reeves G. Evidence from randomised trials on the long-term effects of hormone replacement therapy. Lancet. 2002;360:942–4.

32. Menotti A, Lanti M, Nedeljkovic S, Nissinen A, Kafatos A, Kromhout D. The relationship of age, blood pressure, serum cholesterol and smoking habits with the risk of typical and atypical coronary heart disease death in the European cohorts of the Seven Countries Study. Int J Cardiol. 2006;106:157–63.

33. Woodward M, Huxley H, Lam TH, Barzi F, Lawes CM, Ueshima H. A comparison of the associations between risk factors and cardiovascular disease in Asia and Australasia. Eur J Cardiovasc Prev Rehabil. 2005;12:484–91.

34. Maradit-Kremers H, Crowson CS, Nicola PJ, et al. Increased unrecognized coronary heart disease and sudden deaths in rheumatoid arthritis: a population-based cohort study. Arthritis Rheum. 2005;52:402–11.

35. Pignalberi C, Ricci R, Santini M. [Psychological stress and sudden death]. Ital Heart J Suppl. 2002;3:1011–21.

36. Orth-Gomer K, Wamala SP, Horsten M, Schenck-Gustafsson K, Schneiderman N, Mittleman MA. Marital stress worsens prognosis in women with coronary heart disease: The Stockholm Female Coronary Risk Study. JAMA. 2000;284:3008–14.

37. Stollberger C, Finsterer J. Cardiorespiratory findings in sudden unexplained/unexpected death in epilepsy (SUDEP). Epilepsy Res. 2004;59:51–60.

38. Mozaffarian D, Ascherio A, Hu FB, et al. Interplay between different polyunsaturated fatty acids and risk of coronary heart disease in men. Circulation. 2005;111:157–64.

39. Diebolt M, Bucher B, Andriantsitohaina R. Wine polyphenols decrease blood pressure, improve NO vasodilatation, and induce gene expression. Hypertension. 2001;38:159–65.

40. de Lorgeril M, Salen P. Suitability of the Mediterranean-style diet in the modern world. Asia Pac J Clin Nutr. 2005;14:S78–83.

41. de Lorgeril M, Salen P, Paillard F. Diet and medication for heart protection in secondary prevention of coronary heart disease. New concepts. Nutr Metab Cardiovasc Dis. 2000;10:216–22.

42. Hu FB, Cho E, Rexrode KM, Albert CM, Manson JE. Fish and long-chain omega-3 fatty acid intake and risk of coronary heart disease and total mortality in diabetic women. Circulation. 2003;107:1852–7.

43. da Luz PL, Coimbra SR. Wine, alcohol and atherosclerosis: clinical evidences and mechanisms. Braz J Med Biol Res. 2004;37:1275–95.

44. Sands SA, Reid KJ, Windsor SL, Harris WS. The impact of age, body mass index, and fish intake on the EPA and DHA content of human erythrocytes. Lipids. 2005;40:343–7.

45. Sdringola S, Nakagawa K, Nakagawa Y, et al. Combined intense lifestyle and pharmacologic lipid treatment further reduce coronary events and myocardial perfusion abnormalities compared with usual-care cholesterol-lowering drugs in coronary artery disease. J Am Coll Cardiol. 2003;41:263–72.

46. Albert CM, Campos H, Stampfer MJ, et al. Blood levels of long-chain n-3 fatty acids and the risk of sudden death. N Engl J Med. 2002;346:1113–8.

47. Spies CD, Sander M, Stangl K, et al. Effects of alcohol on the heart. Curr Opin Crit Care. 2001;7:337–43.

48. Yamawaki H, Iwai N. Mechanisms underlying nano-sized air-pollution-mediated progression of atherosclerosis. Circ J. 2006;70:129–40.

49. Sydbom A, Blomberg A, Parnia S, Stenfors N, Sandstrom T, Dahlen SE. Health effects of diesel exhaust emissions. Eur Respir J. 2001;17:733–46.

50. Willich SN, Wegscheider K, Stallmann M, Keil T. Noise burden and the risk of myocardial infarction. Eur Heart J. 2005;27(3):276–82.

51. Nolan RP, Kamath MV, Floras JS, et al. Heart rate variability biofeedback as a behavioral neurocardiac intervention to enhance vagal heart rate control. Am Heart J. 2005;149:1137.

52. Iravanian S, Arshad A, Steinberg JS. Role of electrophysiologic studies, signal-averaged electrocardiography, heart rate variability, T-wave alternans, and loop recorders for risk stratification of ventricular arrhythmias. Am J Geriatr Cardiol. 2005;14:16–9.

53. Grimm W, Christ M, Maisch B. Long runs of non-sustained ventricular tachycardia on 24-hour ambulatory electrocardiogram predict major arrhythmic events in patients with idiopathic dilated cardiomyopathy. Pacing Clin Electrophysiol. 2005; 28 Suppl 1:S207–10.

54. Huikuri HV, Castellanos A, Myerburg RJ. Sudden death due to cardiac arrhythmias. N Engl J Med. 2001;345:1473–82.

55. The Cardiac Arrhythmia Suppression Trial (CAST) Investigators. Preliminary report: effect of encainide and flecainide on mortality in a randomized trial of arrhythmia suppression after myocardial infarction. N Engl J Med. 1989;321: 406–12.

56. Bardy GH, Lee KL, Mark DB, et al. Amiodarone or an implantable cardioverter-defibrillator for congestive heart failure. N Engl J Med. 2005;352:225–37.

57. Moerman DE, Jonas WB. Deconstructing the placebo effect and finding the meaning response. Ann Intern Med. 2002;136:471–6.

58. Brody HB, Brody D. Placebo and health-II. Three perspectives on the placebo response: expectancy, conditioning, and meaning. Adv Mind Body Med. 2000; 16:216–32.

59. Thompson WG. Placebos: a review of the placebo response. Am J Gastroenterol. 2000;95:1637–43.

60. Walach H, Jonas WB. Placebo research: the evidence base for harnessing self-healing capacities. J Altern Complement Med. 2004;10 Suppl 1:S103–12.

61. Moerman DE. The meaning response and the ethics of avoiding placebos. Eval Health Prof. 2002;25:399–409.

62. Wang Q, Zhang B. Research design and statistical methods in Chinese medical journals. JAMA. 1998;280:283–5.

63. Chen ZY. [Use of xin bao in the treatment of 87 patients with sick sinus syndrome]. Zhong Xi Yi Jie He Za Zhi. 1990;10:529–31, 516.

64. Lo HM, Lin FY, Tseng CD, Chiang FT, Hsu KL, Tseng YZ. Effect of EGb 761, a ginkgo biloba extract, on early arrhythmia induced by coronary occlusion and reperfusion in dogs. J Formos Med Assoc. 1994;93:592–7.

65. Shen J, Wang J, Zhao B, Hou J, Gao T, Xin W. Effects of EGb 761 on nitric oxide and oxygen free radicals, myocardial damage and arrhythmia in ischemia-reperfusion injury in vivo. Biochim Biophys Acta. 1998;1406:228–36.

66. Zhuang XX. [Protective effect of Angelica injection on arrhythmia during myocardial ischemia reperfusion in rat]. Zhong Xi Yi Jie He Za Zhi. 1991;11:360–1, 326.

67. Chang CC, Acharfi S, Wu MH, et al. A novel SCN5A mutation manifests as a malignant form of long QT syndrome with perinatal onset of tachycardia/bradycardia. Cardiovasc Res. 2004;64:268–78.

68. Sun XD, Li JM, Tian LJ, Wang YP, Yu YF, Zhang KY. [Effect of berberine on slow inward ionic current in guinea pig ventricular papillary muscle]. Zhongguo Yao Li Xue Bao. 1989;10:130–4.

69. Heubach JF, Schule A. Cardiac effects of lappaconitine and N-deacetyllappaconitine, two diterpenoid alkaloids from plants of the Aconitum and Delphinium species. Planta Med. 1998;64:22–6.

70. Rietz B, Belagyi J, Torok B, Jacob R. The radical scavenging ability of garlic examined in various models. Boll Chim Farm. 1995;134:69–76.

71. Martin N, Bardisa L, Pantoja C, Vargas M, Quezada P, Valenzuela J. Anti-arrhythmic profile of a garlic dialysate assayed in dogs and isolated atrial preparations. J Ethnopharmacol. 1994;43:1–8.

72. Alonso A, Martinez-Gonzalez MA, Serrano-Martinez M. [Fish omega-3 fatty acids and risk of coronary heart disease]. Med Clin (Barc). 2003;121:28–35.

73. King VF, Garcia ML, Himmel D, Reuben JP, Lam YK, Pan JX, Han GQ, Kaczorowski GJ. Interaction of tetrandrine with slowly inactivating calcium channels. Characterization of calcium channel modulation by an alkaloid of Chinese medicinal herb origin. J Biol Chem. 1988;263:2238–44.

74. Wang XL, Zhang LM, Hua Z: Blocking effect of rhynchophylline on calcium channels in isolated rat ventricular myocytes. Zhongguo Yao Li Xue Bao. 1994;15:115–8.

75. Zhang M, Huang YH, Li A, Yang ZC: Effects of tetrandrine on functions and ultrastructure of alveolar macrophages in smoke inhalation-injured rabbits. Zhngguo Yao Li Xue Bao. 1993;14:529–32.

76. Tekol Y, Gogusten B. Comparative determination of the cardioselectivity of taxine and verapamil in the isolated aorta, atrium and jejunum preparations of rabbits. Arzneimittelforschung. 1999;49:673–8.

77. Garjani A, Nazemiyeh H, Maleki N, Valizadeh H. Effects of extracts from flowering tops of Crataegus meyeri A. Pojark. on ischaemic arrhythmias in anaesthetized rats. Phytother Res. 2000;14:428–31.

78. al Makdessi S, Sweidan H, Dietz K, Jacob R. Protective effect of Crataegus oxyacantha against reperfusion arrhythmias after global no-flow ischemia in the rat heart. Basic Res Cardiol. 1999;94:71–7.

79. Popping S, Rose H, Ionescu I, Fischer Y, Kammermeier H. Effect of a hawthorn extract on contraction and energy turnover of isolated rat cardiomyocytes. Arzneimittelforschung. 1995;45:1157–61.

80. Tauchert M, Gildor A, Lipinski J. [High-dose Crataegus extract WS 1442 in the treatment of NYHA stage II heart failure]. Herz. 1999;24:465–74; discussion 475.

81. Ozaki Y. [Pharmacological studies of indole alkaloids obtained from domestic plants, Uncaria rhynchophylla Miq. and Amsonia elliptica Roem. et Schult]. Nippon Yakurigaku Zasshi. 1989;94:17–26.

82. Tian BJ, Gao TL, Song ZL: [Effects of ciwujia (Acanthopanax senticosus Harms) on reperfusion-induced arrhythmia and action potential alterations in the isolated rat heart]. Zhongguo Zhong Yao Za Zhi. 1989;14:493–95.

83. Tian BJ, Gao TL, Song ZL. [Effects of ciwujia (Acanthopanax senticosus Harms) on reperfusion-induced arrhythmia and action potential alterations in the isolated rat heart]. Zhongguo Zhong Yao Za Zhi. 1989;14:493–5, 508, 512.

84. Chen R, Yuan C. [Experimental anti-arrhythmic effects of zhigancao (prepared licorice) injection]. Zhongguo Zhong Yao Za Zhi. 1991;16:617–9 (inside back cover).

85. Klepser TB, Klepser ME. Unsafe and potentially safe herbal therapies. Am J Health Syst Pharm. 1999;56:125–38; quiz 139–41.

86. Xia YX. The inhibitory effect of Motherwort extract on pulsating myocardial cells in vitro. J Tradit Chin Med. 1983;3:185–8.

87. Balbaa SI, Zaki AY, Abdel-Wahab SM. A micro-method for the estimation of khellin in presence of other constituents of Ammi visnaga fruits. Planta Med. 1968;16:329–34.

88. Chen M, Stohs SJ, Staba EJ. The biosynthesis of visnagin from 2-14C-acetate by Ammi visnaga suspension cultures and the metabolism of 14C-visnagin and 14C-khellin by A. visnaga and A. majus. Lloydia. 1969;32:339–46.

89. Chen M, Stohs SJ, Staba EJ. The biosynthesis of radioactive khellin and visnagin from C14-acetate by Ammi visnaga plants. Planta Med. 1969;17:319–27.

90. Rauwald HW, Brehm O, Odenthal KP. The involvement of a Ca^{2+} channel blocking mode of action in the pharmacology of Ammi visnaga fruits. Planta Med. 1994;60:101–5.

91. McRae S. Elevated serum digoxin levels in a patient taking digoxin and Siberian ginseng. CMAJ. 1996;155:293–5.

92. Lin MC, Nahin R, Gershwin ME, Longhurst JC, Wu KK. State of complementary and alternative medicine in cardiovascular, lung, and blood research: executive summary of a workshop. Circulation. 2001;103:2038–41.

93. Maimeskulova LA, Maslov LN. [The anti-arrhythmia action of an extract of Rhodiola rosea and of n-tyrosol in models of experimental arrhythmias]. Eksp Klin Farmakol. 1998;61:37–40.

94. Maimeskulova LA, Maslov LN, Lishmanov Iu B, Krasnov EA. [The participation of the mu-, delta- and kappa-opioid receptors in the realization of the anti-arrhythmia effect of Rhodiola rosea]. Eksp Klin Farmakol. 1997;60:38–9.

95. Lishmanov Iu B, Maslova LV, Maslov LN, Dan'shina EN. [The anti-arrhythmia effect of Rhodiola rosea and its possible mechanism]. Biull Eksp Biol Med. 1993;116:175–6.

96. Zhang WS, Zhu LQ, Niu FL, Deng RC, Ma CX. [Protective effects of salidroside on injury induced by hypoxia/hypoglycemia in cultured neurons]. Zhongguo Zhong Yao Za Zhi. 2004;29:459–62.

97. Zeng XH, Zeng XJ, Li YY. Efficacy and safety of berberine for congestive heart failure secondary to ischemic or idiopathic dilated cardiomyopathy. Am J Cardiol. 2003;92:173–6.

98. Guo ZB, Fu JG. [Progress of cardiovascular pharmacologic study on berbamine]. Zhongguo Zhong Xi Yi Jie He Za Zhi. 2005;25:765–8.

99. Lau CW, Yao XQ, Chen ZY, Ko WH, Huang Y. Cardiovascular actions of berberine. Cardiovasc Drug Rev. 2001;19:234–44.

100. Wang YX, Zheng YM, Zhou XB. Inhibitory effects of berberine on ATP-sensitive K^+ channels in cardiac myocytes. Eur J Pharmacol. 1996;316:307–15.

101. Huang W. [Ventricular tachyarrhythmias treated with berberine]. Zhonghua Xin Xue Guan Bing Za Zhi. 1990;18:155–6, 190.

102. Haller CA, Benowitz NL. Adverse cardiovascular and central nervous system events associated with dietary supplements containing ephedra alkaloids. N Engl J Med. 2000;343:1833–8.

103. Zahn KA, Li RL, Purssell RA. Cardiovascular toxicity after ingestion of "herbal ecstacy." J Emerg Med. 1999;17:289–91.

104. Yates KM, O'Connor A, Horsley CA. "Herbal Ecstasy": a case series of adverse reactions. N Z Med J. 2000;113:315–7.

105. Guha S, Dawn B, Dutta G, Chakraborty T, Pain S. Bradycardia, reversible pan-conduction defect and syncope following self-medication with a homeopathic medicine. Cardiology. 1999;91:268–71.

106. Pugsley MK, Saint DA, Hayes E, Berlin KD, Walker MJ. The cardiac electrophysiological effects of sparteine and its analogue BRB-I-28 in the rat. Eur J Pharmacol. 1995;294:319–27.

107. Giles TD, Sander GE. Comparative cardiovascular responses to intravenous capsaicin, phenyldiguanide, veratrum alkaloids and enkephalins in the conscious dog. J Auton Pharmacol. 1986;6:1–7.

108. Jaffe AM, Gephardt D, Courtemanche L. Poisoning due to ingestion of Veratrum viride (false hellebore). J Emerg Med. 1990;8:161–7.

109. Pittler MH, Schmidt K, Ernst E. Adverse events of herbal food supplements for body weight reduction: systematic review. Obes Rev. 2005;6:93–111.

110. Min B, McBride BF, Kardas MJ, et al. Electrocardiographic effects of an ephedrafree, multicomponent weight-loss supplement in healthy volunteers. Pharmacotherapy. 2005;25:654–9.

111. Warburton DM, Bersellini E, Sweeney E. An evaluation of a caffeinated taurine drink on mood, memory and information processing in healthy volunteers without caffeine abstinence. Psychopharmacology (Berl). 2001;158:322–8.

112. Reyner LA, Horne JA. Efficacy of a "functional energy drink" in counteracting driver sleepiness. Physiol Behav. 2002;75:331–5.

113. Alford C, Cox H, Wescott R. The effects of red bull energy drink on human performance and mood. Amino Acids. 2001;21:139–50.

114. Shields KM, McQueen CE, Bryant PJ. National survey of dietary supplement resources at drug information centers. J Am Pharm Assoc (Wash DC). 2004;44:36–40.

115. Szabuniewicz M, McCrady JD, Camp BJ. Treatment of experimentally induced oleander poisoning. Arch Int Pharmacodyn Ther. 1971;189:12–21.

116. Eddleston M, Ariaratnam CA, Sjostrom L, et al. Acute yellow oleander (Thevetia peruviana) poisoning: cardiac arrhythmias, electrolyte disturbances, and serum cardiac glycoside concentrations on presentation to hospital. Heart. 2000;83:301–6.

117. Nishioka Sde A, Resende ES. Transitory complete atrioventricular block associated to ingestion of Nerium oleander. Rev Assoc Med Bras. 1995;41:60–2.

118. Osterloh J, Herold S, Pond S. Oleander interference in the digoxin radioimmunoassay in a fatal ingestion. JAMA. 1982;247:1596–7.

119. Haynes BE, Bessen HA, Wightman WD. Oleander tea: herbal draught of death. Ann Emerg Med. 1985;14:350–3.

120. Mozaffarian D, Geelen A, Brouwer IA, Geleijnse JM, Zock PL, Katan MB. Effect of fish oil on heart rate in humans: a meta-analysis of randomized controlled trials. Circulation. 2005;112:1945–52.

121. Berry EM. Who's afraid of n-6 polyunsaturated fatty acids? Methodological considerations for assessing whether they are harmful. Nutr Metab Cardiovasc Dis. 2001;11:181–8.

122. Billman GE, Hallaq H, Leaf A. Prevention of ischemia-induced ventricular fibrillation by omega-3 fatty acids. Proc Natl Acad Sci USA. 1994;91:4427–30.

123. Billman GE, Kang JX, Leaf A. Prevention of sudden cardiac death by dietary pure omega-3 polyunsaturated fatty acids in dogs. Circulation. 1999;99:2452–7.

124. Xiao YF, Ke Q, Chen Y, Morgan JP, Leaf A. Inhibitory effect of n-3 fish oil fatty acids on cardiac Na^+/Ca^{2+} exchange currents in HEK293t cells. Biochem Biophys Res Commun. 2004;321:116–23.

125. Kang JX, Leaf A. Prevention of fatal cardiac arrhythmias by polyunsaturated fatty acids. Am J Clin Nutr. 2000;71:202S–7S.

126. Leaf A, Xiao YF, Kang JX, Billman GE. Prevention of sudden cardiac death by n-3 polyunsaturated fatty acids. Pharmacol Ther. 2003;98:355–77.

127. Hallaq H, Smith TW, Leaf A. Modulation of dihydropyridine-sensitive calcium channels in heart cells by fish oil fatty acids. Proc Natl Acad Sci USA. 1992;89: 1760–4.

128. Sellmayer A, Witzgall H, Lorenz RL, Weber PC. Effects of dietary fish oil on ventricular premature complexes. Am J Cardiol. 1995;76:974–7.

129. Geelen A, Brouwer IA, Schouten EG, Maan AC, Katan MB, Zock PL. Effects of n-3 fatty acids from fish on premature ventricular complexes and heart rate in humans. Am J Clin Nutr. 2005;81:416–20.

130. Burr ML, Fehily AM, Gilbert JF, et al. Effects of changes in fat, fish, and fibre intakes on death and myocardial reinfarction: diet and reinfarction trial (DART). Lancet. 1989;2:757–61.

131. Gruppo Italiano per lo Studio della Sopravvivenza nell'Infarto miocardico. Dietary supplementation with n-3 polyunsaturated fatty acids and vitamin E after myocardial infarction: results of the GISSI-Prevenzione trial. Lancet. 1999;354: 447–55.

132. Albert CM, Hennekens CH, O'Donnell CJ, et al. Fish consumption and risk of sudden cardiac death. JAMA. 1998;279:23–8.

133. Siscovick DS, Lemaitre RN, Mozaffarian D. The fish story: a diet-heart hypothesis with clinical implications: n-3 polyunsaturated fatty acids, myocardial vulnerability, and sudden death. Circulation. 2003;107:2632–4.

134. Singh RB, Niaz MA, Sharma JP, Kumar R, Rastogi V, Moshiri M. Randomized, double-blind, placebo-controlled trial of fish oil and mustard oil in patients with suspected acute myocardial infarction: the Indian experiment of infarct survival-4. Cardiovasc Drugs Ther. 1997;11:485–91.

134. de Lorgeril M, Salen P, Martin JL, Monjaud I, Boucher P, Mamelle N. Mediterranean dietary pattern in a randomized trial: prolonged survival and possible reduced cancer rate. Arch Intern Med. 1998;158:1181–7.

136. De Lorgeril M, Salen P. Use and misuse of dietary fatty acids for the prevention and treatment of coronary heart disease. Reprod Nutr Dev. 2004;44:283–8.

137. Hoffmann GF, Athanassopoulos S, Burlina AB, et al. Clinical course, early diagnosis, treatment, and prevention of disease in glutaryl-CoA dehydrogenase deficiency. Neuropediatrics. 1996;27:115–23.

138. Christensen JH, Gustenhoff P, Korup E, et al. [n-3 polyunsaturated fatty acids, heart rate variability and ventricular arrhythmias in post-AMI-patients. A clinical controlled trial]. Ugeskr Laeger. 1997;159:5525–9.

139. Raitt MH, Connor WE, Morris C, et al. Fish oil supplementation and risk of ventricular tachycardia and ventricular fibrillation in patients with implantable defibrillators: a randomized controlled trial. JAMA. 2005;293:2884–91.

140. Leaf A, Albert CM, Josephson M, et al. Prevention of fatal arrhythmias in high-risk subjects by fish oil n-3 fatty acid intake. Circulation. 2005;112:2762–8.

141. Brouwer IA, Zock PL, Wever EF, et al. Rationale and design of a randomised controlled clinical trial on supplemental intake of n-3 fatty acids and incidence of cardiac arrhythmia: SOFA. Eur J Clin Nutr. 2003;57:1323–30.

142. Murnaghan MF. Effect of fatty acids on the ventricular arrhythmia threshold in the isolated heart of the rabbit. Br J Pharmacol. 1981;73:909–15.

143. McLennan PL, Abeywardena MY, Charnock JS. Dietary fish oil prevents ventricular fibrillation following coronary artery occlusion and reperfusion. Am Heart J. 1988;116:709–17.

144. McLennan PL, Bridle TM, Abeywardena MY, Charnock JS. Dietary lipid modulation of ventricular fibrillation threshold in the marmoset monkey. Am Heart J. 1992;123:1555–61.

145. Billman GE, Kang JX, Leaf A. Prevention of ischemia-induced cardiac sudden death by n-3 polyunsaturated fatty acids in dogs. Lipids. 1997;32:1161–8.

146. Leaf A. Diet and sudden cardiac death. J Nutr Health Aging. 2001;5:173–8.

146. Li Y, Kang JX, Leaf A. Differential effects of various eicosanoids on the production or prevention of arrhythmias in cultured neonatal rat cardiac myocytes. Prostaglandins. 1997;54:511–30.

148. Biscione F, Totteri A, De Vita A, Lo Bianco F, Altamura G. [Effect of omega-3 fatty acids on the prevention of atrial arrhythmias]. Ital Heart J Suppl. 2005;6:53–9.

149. Calo L, Bianconi L, Colivicchi F, et al. N-3 Fatty acids for the prevention of atrial fibrillation after coronary artery bypass surgery: a randomized, controlled trial. J Am Coll Cardiol. 2005;45:1723–8.

150. Chung MK. Vitamins, supplements, herbal medicines, and arrhythmias. Cardiol Rev. 2004;12:73–84.

151. Holub DJ, Holub BJ. Omega-3 fatty acids from fish oils and cardiovascular disease. Mol Cell Biochem. 2004;263:217–25.

152. Christensen JH. n-3 fatty acids and the risk of sudden cardiac death. Emphasis on heart rate variability. Dan Med Bull. 2003;50:347–67.

153. Monahan KD, Wilson TE, Ray CA. Omega-3 fatty acid supplementation augments sympathetic nerve activity responses to physiological stressors in humans. Hypertension. 2004;44:732–8.

154. Holguin F, Tellez-Rojo MM, Lazo M, et al. Cardiac autonomic changes associated with fish oil vs soy oil supplementation in the elderly. Chest. 2005;127:1102–7.

155. Mozaffarian D, Psaty BM, Rimm EB, et al. Fish intake and risk of incident atrial fibrillation. Circulation. 2004;110:368–73.

156. Platt R. Current concepts in optimum nutrition for cardiovascular disease. Prev Cardiol. 2000;3:83–7.

157. Ander BP, Weber AR, Rampersad PP, Gilchrist JS, Pierce GN, Lukas A. Dietary flaxseed protects against ventricular fibrillation induced by ischemia-reperfusion in normal and hypercholesterolemic Rabbits. J Nutr. 2004;134:3250–6.

158. Fujioka T, Sakamoto Y, Mimura G. Clinical study of cardiac arrhythmias using a 24-hour continuous electrocardiographic recorder (5th report)—antiarrhythmic action of coenzyme Q10 in diabetics. Tohoku J Exp Med. 1983;141 Suppl:453–63.

159. Langsjoen PH, Langsjoen AM. Overview of the use of CoQ10 in cardiovascular disease. Biofactors. 1999;9:273–84.

160. Lango R, Smolenski RT, Rogowski J, et al. Propionyl-L-carnitine improves hemo-dynamics and metabolic markers of cardiac perfusion during coronary surgery in diabetic patients. Cardiovasc Drugs Ther. 2005;19:267–75.

161. Lango R, Smolenski RT, Narkiewicz M, Suchorzewska J, Lysiak-Szydlowska W. Influence of L-carnitine and its derivatives on myocardial metabolism and function in ischemic heart disease and during cardiopulmonary bypass. Cardiovasc Res. 2001;51:21–9.

162. Arsenian MA. Carnitine and its derivatives in cardiovascular disease. Prog Cardiovasc Dis. 1997;40:265–86.

163. Mondillo S, Faglia S, D'Aprile N, et al. [Therapy of arrhythmia induced by myocardial ischemia. Association of L-carnitine, propafenone and mexiletine]. Clin Ter. 1995;146:769–74.

164. Takimoto M, Sakurai T, Kodama K, et al. [Protective effect of CoQ 10 adminis-tration on cardial toxicity in FAC therapy]. Gan To Kagaku Ryoho. 1982;9:116–21.

165. DiPalma JR, Ritchie DM, McMichael RF. Cardiovascular and antiarrhythmic effects of carnitine. Arch Int Pharmacodyn Ther. 1975;217:246–50.

166. Digiesi V, Palchetti R, Cantini F. [The benefits of L-carnitine therapy in essential arterial hypertension with diabetes mellitus type II.] Minerva Med. 1989;80: 227–31.

167. Bonnet D, Martin D, Pascale De L, et al. Arrhythmias and conduction defects as presenting symptoms of fatty acid oxidation disorders in children. Circulation. 1999;100:2248–53.

168. Lehr D. A possible beneficial effect of selenium administration in antiarrhythmic therapy. J Am Coll Nutr. 1994;13:496–8.

169. Bashir Y, Sneddon JF, Staunton HA, et al. Effects of long-term oral magnesium chloride replacement in congestive heart failure secondary to coronary artery dis-ease. Am J Cardiol. 1993;72:1156–62.

170. Maslow AD, Regan MM, Heindle S, Panzica P, Cohn WE, Johnson RG. Postoperative atrial tachyarrhythmias in patients undergoing coronary artery bypass graft surgery without cardiopulmonary bypass: a role for intraoperative magnesium supplementation. J Cardiothorac Vasc Anesth. 2000;14:524–30.

171. Speziale G, Ruvolo G, Fattouch K, et al. Arrhythmia prophylaxis after coronary artery bypass grafting: regimens of magnesium sulfate administration. Thorac Cardiovasc Surg. 2000;48:22–6.

172. Raghu C, Peddeswara Rao P, Seshagiri Rao D. Protective effect of intravenous magnesium in acute myocardial infarction following thrombolytic therapy. Int J Cardiol. 1999;71:209–15.

173. Gyamlani G, Parikh C, Kulkarni AG. Benefits of magnesium in acute myocardial infarction: timing is crucial. Am Heart J. 2000;139:703.

174. Singh RB, Singh NK, Niaz MA, Sharma JP. Effect of treatment with magnesium and potassium on mortality and reinfarction rate of patients with suspected acute myocardial infarction. Int J Clin Pharmacol Ther. 1996;34:219–25.

175. Bhargava B, Chandra S, Agarwal VV, Kaul U, Vashishth S, Wasir HS. Adjunctive magnesium infusion therapy in acute myocardial infarction. Int J Cardiol. 1995;52: 95–9.

176. Shechter M, Hod H, Chouraqui P, Kaplinsky E, Rabinowitz B. Magnesium therapy in acute myocardial infarction when patients are not candidates for thrombolytic therapy. Am J Cardiol. 1995;75:321–3.

177. Ceremuzynski L, Gebalska J, Wolk R, Makowska E. Hypomagnesemia in heart failure with ventricular arrhythmias. Beneficial effects of magnesium supplementation. J Intern Med. 2000;247:78–86.

178. Parikka H, Toivonen L, Verkkala K, Jarvinen A, Nieminen MS. Ventricular arrhythmia suppression by magnesium treatment after coronary artery bypass surgery. Int J Angiol. 1999;8:165–70.

179. Steinberger HA, Hanson CW, III. Outcome-based justification for implementing new point-of-care tests: there is no difference between magnesium replacement based on ionized magnesium and total magnesium as a predictor of development of arrhythmias in the postoperative cardiac surgical patient. Clin Lab Manage Rev. 1998;12:87–90.

180. Ziegelstein RC, Hilbe JM, French WJ, Antman EM, Chandra-Strobos N. Magnesium use in the treatment of acute myocardial infarction in the United States (observations from the Second National Registry of Myocardial Infarction). Am J Cardiol. 2001;87:7–10.

181. Santoro GM, Antoniucci D, Bolognese L, et al. A randomized study of intravenous magnesium in acute myocardial infarction treated with direct coronary angioplasty. Am Heart J. 2000;140:891–7.

182. ISIS-4 (Fourth International Study of Infarct Survival) Collaborative Group. ISIS-4: a randomised factorial trial assessing early oral captopril, oral mononitrate, and intravenous magnesium sulphate in 58,050 patients with suspected acute myocardial infarction. Lancet. 1995;345:669–85.

183. Barsky AJ, Delamater BA, Clancy SA, Antman EM, Ahern DK. Somatized psychiatric disorder presenting as palpitations. Arch Intern Med. 1996;156:1102–8.

184. Shechter M, Hod H, Rabinowitz B, Boyko V, Chouraqui P. Long-term outcome of intravenous magnesium therapy in thrombolysis-ineligible acute myocardial infarction patients. Cardiology. 2003;99:205–10.

185. Seelig MS. Consequences of magnesium deficiency on the enhancement of stress reactions; preventive and therapeutic implications (a review). J Am Coll Nutr. 1994;13:429–46.

186. Spencer JC. Direct relationship between the body's copper/zinc ratio, ventricular premature beats, and sudden coronary death. Am J Clin Nutr. 1979;32:1184–5.

187. Kessel L. Sick sinus syndrome cured by ... vitamin D? Geriatrics. 1990;45: 83–5.

188. Carnes CA, Chung MK, Nakayama T, et al. Ascorbate attenuates atrial pacing-induced peroxynitrite formation and electrical remodeling and decreases the incidence of postoperative atrial fibrillation. Circ Res. 2001;89:E32–8.

189. Marchioli R, Schweiger C, Levantesi G, Tavazzi L, Valagussa F. Antioxidant vitamins and prevention of cardiovascular disease: epidemiological and clinical trial data. Lipids. 2001;36 Suppl:S53–63.

190. Stephens NG, Parsons A, Schofield PM, Kelly F, Cheeseman K, Mitchinson MJ. Randomised controlled trial of vitamin E in patients with coronary disease: Cambridge Heart Antioxidant Study (CHAOS). Lancet. 1996;347:781–6.

191. Virtamo J, Rapola JM, Ripatti S, et al. Effect of vitamin E and beta carotene on the incidence of primary nonfatal myocardial infarction and fatal coronary heart disease. Arch Intern Med. 1998;158:668–75.

192. Saliba W, Erdogan O, Niebauer M. Polymorphic ventricular tachycardia in a woman taking cesium chloride. Pacing Clin Electrophysiol. 2001;24:515–7.

193. Lown B, DeSilva RA. Roles of psychologic stress and autonomic nervous system changes in provocation of ventricular premature complexes. Am J Cardiol. 1978;41:979–85.

194. Engel GL. Psychologic stress, vasodepressor (vasovagal) syncope, and sudden death. Ann Intern Med. 1978;89:403–12.

195. Zamarra JW, Schneider RH, Besseghini I, Robinson DK, Salerno JW. Usefulness of the transcendental meditation program in the treatment of patients with coronary artery disease. Am J Cardiol. 1996;77:867–70.

196. Alexander CN, Schneider RH, Staggers F, et al. Trial of stress reduction for hypertension in older African Americans. II. Sex and risk subgroup analysis. Hypertension. 1996;28:228–37.

197. Schneider RH, Alexander CN, Staggers F, et al. A randomized controlled trial of stress reduction in African Americans treated for hypertension for over one year. Am J Hypertens. 2005;18:88–98.

198. Weiss T. Biofeedback training for cardiovascular dysfunctions. Med Clin North Am. 1977;61:913–28.

199. Johnston D. Clinical applications of biofeedback. Br J Hosp Med. 1978;20:561–6.

200. Silver BV, Blanchard EB. Biofeedback and relaxation training in the treatment of psychophysiological disorders: or are the machines really necessary? J Behav Med. 1978;1:217–39.

201. Janssen K. Treatment of sinus tachycardia with heart-rate feedback. J Behav Med. 1983;6:109–14.

202. Vaitl D. ["One need not be a fakir or guru." Biofeedback as an interdisciplinary research technic]. Fortschr Med. 1984;102:541–4.

203. Cowan MJ, Pike KC, Budzynski HK. Psychosocial nursing therapy following sudden cardiac arrest: impact on two-year survival. Nurs Res. 2001;50:68–76.

204. Walton KG, Schneider RH, Nidich S. Review of controlled research on the transcendental meditation program and cardiovascular disease. Risk factors, morbidity, and mortality. Cardiol Rev. 2004;12:262–6.

205. Walton KG, Fields JZ, Levitsky DK, Harris DA, Pugh ND, Schneider RH. Lowering cortisol and CVD risk in postmenopausal women: a pilot study using the Transcendental Meditation program. Ann NY Acad Sci. 2004;1032:211–5.

206. Singh RB, Pella D, Otsuka K, Halberg F, Cornelissen G. New insights into circadian aspects of health and disease. J Assoc Physicians India. 2002;50:1416–25.

207. Singh RB, Cornelissen G, Weydahl A, et al. Circadian heart rate and blood pressure variability considered for research and patient care. Int J Cardiol. 2003;87:9–28; discussion 29–30.

208. Schneider RH, Alexander CN, Staggers F, et al. Long-term effects of stress reduction on mortality in persons > or = 55 years of age with systemic hypertension. Am J Cardiol. 2005;95:1060–4.

209. Neki NS, Singh RB, Rastogi SS. How brain influences neuro-cardiovascular dysfunction. J Assoc Physicians India. 2004;52:223–30.

210. Mamtani R, Mamtani R. Ayurveda and yoga in cardiovascular diseases. Cardiol Rev. 2005;13:155–62.

211. Kim DH, Moon YS, Kim HS, et al. Effect of Zen meditation on serum nitric oxide activity and lipid peroxidation. Prog Neuropsychopharmacol Biol Psychiatry. 2005; 29:327–31.

212. Bijlani RL, Vempati RP, Yadav RK, et al. A brief but comprehensive lifestyle education program based on yoga reduces risk factors for cardiovascular disease and diabetes mellitus. J Altern Complement Med. 2005;11:267–74.

213. Barnes VA, Treiber FA, Davis H. Impact of transcendental meditation on cardiovascular function at rest and during acute stress in adolescents with high normal blood pressure. J Psychosom Res. 2001;51:597–5.

214. Cysarz D, Bussing A. Cardiorespiratory synchronization during Zen meditation. Eur J Appl Physiol. 2005;95(1):88–95.

215. Maruta T, Colligan RC, Malinchoc M, Offord KP. Optimists vs pessimists: survival rate among medical patients over a 30-year period. Mayo Clin Proc. 2000;75: 140–3.

216. Steele A, Wade TD. The contribution of optimism and quality of life to depression in an acute coronary syndrome population. Eur J Cardiovasc Nurs. 2004;3: 231–7.

217. Kelloniemi H, Ek E, Laitinen J. Optimism, dietary habits, body mass index and smoking among young Finnish adults. Appetite. 2005;45:169–76.

218. Segerstrom SC. Optimism and immunity: do positive thoughts always lead to positive effects? Brain Behav Immun. 2005;19:195–200.

219. Ruddick W. Hope and deception. Bioethics. 1999;13:343–57.

220. Gibson B, Sanbonmatsu DM. Optimism, pessimism, and gambling: the downside of optimism. Pers Soc Psychol Bull. 2004;30:149–60.

221. Lovallo D, Kahneman D. Delusions of success. How optimism undermines executives' decisions. Harv Bus Rev. 2003;81:56–63, 117.

222. Shen WK, Low PA, Jahangir A, et al. Is sinus node modification appropriate for inappropriate sinus tachycardia with features of postural orthostatic tachycardia syndrome? Pacing Clin Electrophysiol. 2001;24:217–30.

223. Koskinen P, Kupari M. Alcohol consumption of patients with supraventricular tachyarrhythmias other than atrial fibrillation. Alcohol Alcohol. 1991;26: 199–206.

224. Koskinen P, Kupari M. Alcohol and cardiac arrhythmias. BMJ. 1992;304:1394–5.

225. Koskinen P, Kupari M, Leinonen H, Luomanmaki K. Alcohol and new onset atrial fibrillation: a case-control study of a current series. Br Heart J. 1987;57: 468–73.

226. Rigou DG, Pichel G, Fasah L. [Ventricular arrhythmia in young university students without evidence of heart disease]. Medicina (B Aires). 1990;50:47–51.

227. Dobmeyer DJ, Stine RA, Leier CV, Greenberg R, Schaal SF. The arrhythmogenic effects of caffeine in human beings. N Engl J Med. 1983;308:814–6.

228. Donnerstein RL, Zhu D, Samson R, Bender AM, Goldberg SJ. Acute effects of caffeine ingestion on signal-averaged electrocardiograms. Am Heart J. 1998;136:643–6.

229. Lemaitre RN, King IB, Raghunathan TE, et al. Cell membrane trans-fatty acids and the risk of primary cardiac arrest. Circulation. 2002;105:697–701.

230. Renaud S, Lanzmann-Petithory D. Dietary fats and coronary heart disease pathogenesis. Curr Atheroscler Rep. 2002;4:419–24.

231. Lehr D. A possible beneficial effect of selenium administration in antiarrhythmic therapy. J Am Coll Nutr. 1994;13:496–8.

232. Lumme JA, Jounela AJ. The effect of potassium and potassium plus magnesium supplementation on ventricular extrasystoles in mild hypertensives treated with hydrochlorothiazide. Int J Cardiol. 1989;25:93–7.

233. Tsuji H, Venditti FJ, Jr., Evans JC, Larson MG, Levy D. The associations of levels of serum potassium and magnesium with ventricular premature complexes (the Framingham Heart Study). Am J Cardiol. 1994;74:232–5.

234. Hardarson T, Kristinsson A, Skuladottir G, Asvaldsdottir H, Snorrason SP. Cod liver oil does not reduce ventricular extrasystoles after myocardial infarction. J Intern Med. 1989;226:33–7.

235. Mehta A, Jain AC, Mehta MC, Billie M. Caffeine and cardiac arrhythmias. An experimental study in dogs with review of literature. Acta Cardiol. 1997;52:273–83.

236. Chou T. Wake up and smell the coffee. Caffeine, coffee, and the medical consequences. West J Med. 1992;157:544–53.

237. Newcombe PF, Renton KW, Rautaharju PM, Spencer CA, Montague TJ. High-dose caffeine and cardiac rate and rhythm in normal subjects. Chest. 1988;94:90–4.

238. Myers MG, Harris L. High dose caffeine and ventricular arrhythmias. Can J Cardiol. 1990;6:95–8.

239. Prineas RJ, Jacobs DR, Jr., Crow RS, Blackburn H. Coffee, tea and VPB. J Chronic Dis. 1980;33:67–72.

240. Lochen ML, Rasmussen K. Palpitations and lifestyle: impact of depression and self-rated health. The Nordland Health Study. Scand J Soc Med. 1996;24 :140–4.

241. Lochen ML. The Tromso Study: associations between self-reported arrhythmia, psychological conditions, and lifestyle. Scand J Prim Health Care. 1991;9 :265–70.

242. Hinkle LE, Jr., Thaler HT, Merke DP, Renier-Berg D, Morton NE. The risk factors for arrhythmic death in a sample of men followed for 20 years. Am J Epidemiol. 1988;127:500–15.

243. Albert CM, Manson JE, Cook NR, Ajani UA, Gaziano JM, Hennekens CH. Moderate alcohol consumption and the risk of sudden cardiac death among US male physicians. Circulation. 1999;100:944–50.

244. McCarty MF. Fish oil may be an antidote for the cardiovascular risk of smoking. Med Hypotheses. 1996;46:337–47.

245. Slater W, Lampert S, Podrid PJ, Lown B. Clinical predictors of arrhythmia worsening by antiarrhythmic drugs. Am J Cardiol. 1988;61:349–53.

246. Podrid PJ, Lampert S, Graboys TB, Blatt CM, Lown B. Aggravation of arrhythmia by antiarrhythmic drugs—incidence and predictors. Am J Cardiol. 1987;59:38E–44E.

247. Levy S. Torsades de pointes. A clearly defined syndrome or an electrocardiographic curiosity? Int J Cardiol. 1985;7:421–7.

248. Roden DM, Woosley RL, Primm RK. Incidence and clinical features of the quinidine-associated long QT syndrome: implications for patient care. Am Heart J. 1986;111:1088–93.

249. The Cardiac Arrhythmia Suppression Trial II Investigators. Effect of the antiarrhythmic agent moricizine on survival after myocardial infarction. N Engl J Med. 1992;327:227–33.

250. Velebit V, Podrid P, Lown B, Cohen BH, Graboys TB. Aggravation and provocation of ventricular arrhythmias by antiarrhythmic drugs. Circulation. 1982;65: 886–94.

251. The Task Force of the Working Group on Arrhythmias of the European Society of Cardiology. The "Sicilian Gambit". A new approach to the classification of antiarrhythmic drugs based on their actions on arrhythmogenic mechanisms. Eur Heart J. 1991;12:1112–31.

252. Pratt CM, Camm AJ, Cooper W, et al. Mortality in the Survival With Oral D-sotalol (SWORD) trial: why did patients die? Am J Cardiol. 1998;81:869–76.

253. Camm AJ, Karam R, Pratt CM. The azimilide post-infarct survival evaluation (ALIVE) trial. Am J Cardiol. 1998;81:35D–9D.

254. Boutitie F, Boissel JP, Connolly SJ, et al. Amiodarone interaction with beta-blockers: analysis of the merged EMIAT (European Myocardial Infarct Amiodarone Trial) and CAMIAT (Canadian Amiodarone Myocardial Infarction Trial) databases. The EMIAT and CAMIAT Investigators. Circulation. 1999; 99:2268–75.

255. Janse MJ, Malik M, Camm AJ, Julian DG, Frangin GA, Schwartz PJ. Identification of post acute myocardial infarction patients with potential benefit from prophylactic treatment with amiodarone. A substudy of EMIAT (the European Myocardial Infarct Amiodarone Trial). Eur Heart J. 1998;19:85–95.
256. Julian DG, Camm AJ, Frangin G, et al. Randomised trial of effect of amiodarone on mortality in patients with left-ventricular dysfunction after recent myocardial infarction: EMIAT. European Myocardial Infarct Amiodarone Trial Investigators. Lancet. 1997;349:667–74.
257. Cairns JA, Connolly SJ, Roberts R, Gent M. Randomised trial of outcome after myocardial infarction in patients with frequent or repetitive ventricular premature depolarisations: CAMIAT. Canadian Amiodarone Myocardial Infarction Arrhythmia Trial Investigators. Lancet. 1997;349:675–82.

27

AGING: THE ENVIRONMENT REFLECTS HUMANITY

John H. K. Vogel

Many things can be said about aging and how we may influence it, but, perhaps realizing the most important thing in your life is your relationship with your heart, your family, and the air you breathe.

Immortality—what is that? It is interesting that the Hawaiians are not concerned about dying or immortality because they believe we live on both sides. In promoting aging with grace, style, love, many things are helpful. Music is perhaps one of the most powerful as it is all about the balance of human emotion and elevating consciousness (Santana). Perhaps even more important, however, is listening. To develop the trust, the love, the feeling of safety that is so important between us is the power of listening. It is only through listening to our friends, our loved ones, and our patients, that we can engage their trust. When a friend or patient is able to talk to you and has a feeling that you are truly listening, trust begins. When trust develops between you, it results in a feeling of being safe together, truly a powerful thing. The most rewarding sensation as a physician is to have a patient place his hand on your arm and say—I feel safe with you doctor, whatever you want to do, I will do.

Many things have been written about aging. I think a most powerful book on aging is called, *Healthy Aging*, by Dr Andrew Weil.[1] Dr Weil details an easy-to-implement anti-inflammatory diet that will protect the immune system and aid your body in resisting and adapting to the changes that time brings. He provides extensive practical advice on exercise; preventive health care; stress management; physical, mental, and emotional flexibility; and spiritual enhancement—all of which can help you achieve and maintain the best health throughout the life-long process of aging.

His 12-point program for helping follows:

1. Eat an anti-inflammatory diet.
2. Use dietary supplements wisely to support the body's defenses and natural healing power.

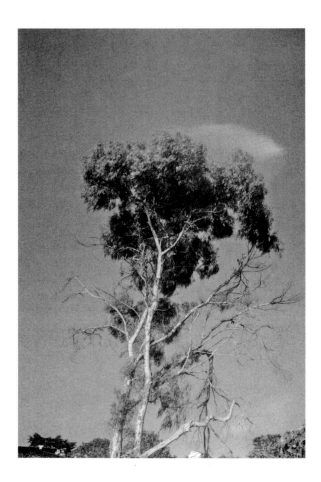

3. Use preventive medicine intelligently: know your risks of age-related disease, get appropriate diagnostic and screening tests and immunizations, and treat problems (like elevated blood pressure and cholesterol) in the early stages.

4. Get regular physical activity throughout life.

5. Get adequate rest and sleep.

6. Learn and practice methods of stress reduction.

7. Exercise your mind as well as your body.

8. Maintain social and intellectual connections as you go through life.

9. Be flexible in mind and body: learn to adapt to losses and let go of behaviors no longer appropriate for your age.

10. Think about and try to discover for yourself the benefits of aging.

11. Do not deny the reality of aging or put energy into trying to stop it. Use the experience of aging as a stimulus for spiritual awakening and growth.

12. Keep an ongoing record of the lessons you have learned, the wisdom you have gained, and the values you hold. At critical points in your life, read this over, add to it, revise it, and share it with people you care about.

Dr Robert A. Vogel has also provided a very helpful prospective on how to age successfully.[2] The steps he emphasized include:

1. Eat less.
2. Exercise more.
3. Don't smoke.
4. Slow down your heart rate.
5. Procreate later.
6. Take a statin.
7. One drink per day.
8. Get good genes.
9. Enjoy yourself, have a dog, but have fewer kids and cats.

The importance of diet cannot be overemphasized. An important effect of high-fat meals is a marked reduction in flow-mediated dilatation in normal subjects as compared to a low-fat meal.[3] Clearly as pointed out by Tsevat,[4] obesity has a profound effect on survival. In addition, cardiovascular disease, smoking, and cancer have large impacts on survival, although obesity actually is a greater risk than cancer but less than smoking or cardiovascular disease. The tragedy of obesity is the frightening increase in its frequency, particularly over the last 5–6 years.[5]

Physical activity has profound beneficial effects. It has been shown that increased physical activity can improve flow-mediated vasodilatation in older age as well as younger, considerably more so than seen in the sedentary elderly person.[6] From a practical standpoint, daily walking in the elderly reduces cardiovascular risks substantially, and heavy exertion is even more beneficial particularly if it is performed five to seven times weekly.[7] Smoking remains a popular habit but a devastating one. Again, in looking at endothelial function, smoking just one cigarette almost eliminates normal flow-mediated vasodilatation.[8] Death from preventable causes in the United States in 2000 was led by tobacco use.[9] It is very important to note that even if one is obese, one can dramatically reduce their risk with exercising and being fit.[10] Of note is that heart rate is very important, and the lower one's heart rate, the better one's life expectancy. This has been shown very nicely in animals.[11]

Of note is that experimental studies in monkeys, when sinoatrial (SA) nodal ablation was performed, the extent of atherosclerosis was markedly reduced, again, indicating the benefit of a lower heart rate.[12] An unrecognized benefit of delayed reproduction, that is, procreating later, is also a prolongation of survival, at least as shown in flies.[13] Genes are important as we all know in observing our patients and families that we care for. Clearly, endothelial progenitor cells are important in survival. In this regard, the importance of statins is clear in that it has been shown that with statins, progenitor cell senescence is markedly reduced.[14] Statins have also been shown to reduce dementia.[15] In the Physicians Health Study, it has been shown that the simple use of aspirin has reduced the relative risk of myocardial infarction according to C-reactive protein quartiles.[16] Alcohol has enjoyed wide popularity as a method for extending survival. Modest alcohol consumption has been shown to reduce C-reactive protein in amounts of 1–1$\frac{1}{2}$ glasses (4–6 oz) barring any contraindications to alcohol.[17]

The Hard Cider House Rules, based on research, indicate 1–1$\frac{1}{2}$ drinks daily, drinking what you like on a regular basis, not episodically, with meals and, most importantly, responsibly, reduce mortality. However, all-cause mortality starts to rise when one goes to 2 drinks daily. Most importantly, reducing stress and enjoying yourself are powerful in affecting one's survival. Paramount in this regard is the quality of one's marriage. A bad marriage results in earlier death, particularly if one has heart failure.[18] Pets are important, and it has been shown that pets have an affect on one's relative cardiovascular disease risk. Dogs are particularly powerful in this regard whereas cats are not.[19] R. Vogel suggests: enjoy yourself, have a dog but have few kids and cats. In summary, to implement the tender loving care (TLC) for your heart program, consider switching to diet drinks, stuff your stomach (salads and soups), smaller food portions, smarter snacks, specific foods (sterols, fiber, nuts, soy, omega-3), exercise—10,000 steps daily, strength exercises, stretching, smoking cessation, and most important—stress reduction, but don't forget the dogs.[12]

REFERENCES

1. Weil A. Healthy aging. New York, Alfred A Knopf: 2005. www.aaknopf.com
2. Vogel RA. 15-minute lifestyle modification: the TLC for your heart program. The 20th Annular Cardiovascular Conference At Hawaii; 2005.
3. Vogel RA, Corretti MC, Plotnick GD. Effect of a high-fat meal on endothelial function in healthy subjects. Am J Cardiol. 1997 Feb 1;79(3):350–4.
4. Tsevat J, Weinstein MC, Williams LW, Tosteson AN, Goldman L. Expected gains in life expectancy from various coronary heart disease risk factor modifications. Circulation. 1991 Apr;83(4):1194–201.
5. Mokdad AH, Serdula MK, Dietz WH, Bowman BA, Marks JS, Koplan JP. The spead of the obesity epidemic in the United States, 1991–1998. JAMA. 1999 Oct 27; 282(16):1519–22.
6. DeSouza C, et al. Regular aerobic exercise prevents and restores age-related declines in endothelium-dependent vasodilation in healthy men. Circulation. 2000;102:1351.
7. Hakim AA, et al. Effects of walking on coronary heart disease in elderly men: the Honolulu Heart Program. Circulation. 1999;100:9.
8. Lekakis JP, et al. Endotheliai dysfunction after cigarette smoking. Insights on duration of the phenomenon and development of tolerance (abstr). Circulation. 1997;96:1–355.
9. Mokdad AH, et al, Actual causes of death in the United States, 2000. JAMA. 2004; 291:1238.
10. Lee CD, et al. Cardiorespiratory fitness, body composition, and all-cause and cardiovascular disease mortality in men. Am J Clin Nutr. 1999;69:373.

11. Levine HE. Rest heart rate and life expectancy. JACC. 1997;30:1104.
12. Beere TA, Glagov S, Zarins CK. Retarding effect of lowered heart rate on coronary atherosclerosis. Science. 1984 Oct 12;2226(4671):180–2.
13. Rose MR. Can human aging be postponed? Sci Am. 1999 Dec;281(6):106–11.
14. Assmus B, Urbich C, Alcher A, Hofmann WK, Haendeler J, Rossig L, Spyridopoulos I, Zeiher AM, Dimmeler S. HMG-CoA reductase inhibitors reduce senescence and increase proliferation of endothelial progenitor cells via regulation of cell cycle regulatory genes. Circ Res. 2003 May 16;92(9):1049–55. Epub 2003 Apr 3.
15. Jick H, et al. Statins and the risk of dementia. Lancet. 2000;356:1627.
16. Ridker PM, Cushman M, Stampfer MJ, Tracy RP, Hennekens CH. Inflammation, aspirin, and the risk of cardiovascular disease in apparently healthy men. N Engl J Med. 1997 Apr 3;336(14):973–9.
17. Imhof A, et al. Antiinflammatory effects of moderate alcohol consumption: a link to mortality. Eur Heart J. 2000;21:497.
18. Coyne J, Rohrbaugh MJ, Shoham V, Sonnega JS, Nicklas JM, Cranford JA. Prognostic importance of marital quality for survival of congestive heart failure. Am J Cardiol. 2001 Sep 1;88(5):526–9.
19. Lawlor DA, Emberson JR, Ebrahim S, Whincup PH, Wannamethee SG, Walkekr M, Smith GD. British Women's Heart and Health Study; British Regional Heart Study. Is the association between parity and coronary heart disease due to biological effects of pregnancy or adverse lifestyle risk factors associated with child-rearing? Findings from the British Women's Heart and Health Study and the British Regional Heart Study. Circulation. 2003 Mar 11;107(9):1260–4.

28

END-OF-LIFE CARE: HOSPICE FOR THE HEART

John H K. Vogel and Julie H. Webster

"Always Beginning
Always Ending
Never Beginning
Never Ending,
Sunsets,
Like Life."

—Jack of Hearts

The scientific advances in cardiovascular medicine have provided millions of patients diagnosed with coronary disease extended lives. Our advances in the last 25 years have included wondrous life-saving drugs for the acute myocardial infraction (MI), devices that have opened otherwise critically closed arteries,

surgery to bypass with only a "keyhole" incision, heart valves, and devices that protect the electrical vulnerability of the heart and can prevent sudden death.

Patients and their families often struggle with facing end-of-life planning. Too often, the patient is in the final or terminal stages of their disease process when this subject is approached. Many chronic cardiovascular disease processes have a high mortality rate and can be a source of considerable torment.

But has our medical community, just as gregariously, sought to learn and understand how to manage these same patients when they have end-stage heart failure, chronic reversible angina, palliative medical treatment, and are faced with dying? End-of-life discussion must be initiated when treatment focus has changed from curative to palliative.[1] Our patients expect and deserve the same expertise and quality of medical care from us when they are nearing death as they did during their acute event.

Increased public awareness is changing the way America talks about and plans for care at the end of life. The media has increased this awareness by sharing many personal struggles with dying over the news stations, airwaves, and Internet.[2] Although these have generated much heated public debates, they have also started the end-of-life discussion in many households. Many organizations, including churches, synagogues, hospices, hospitals, doctor and law offices, and social service agencies are distributing documents to help people plan for themselves and have those delicate discussions with their aging parents.

Today, there are developed methods, tools, and approaches that can provide a more positive "end-of-life" experience for our patient, but they, too, require learning and implementing into our daily practice so that we become as effective in treating end of life as we are at diagnosing heart disease.

The every other day planning process begins with patient education. In addition to their personal beliefs, cultural influences, and personal wishes and desires, patients need guided discussion with health-care providers to maneuver through the very complex system of health care options for end-of-life care including maximal fine-tuning medically and stress reduction.[3] A good beginning starts with a discussion. Patients may be able to thoughtfully review what their personal wishes and desires are with help from available published services.

The *Five Wishes* document helps you express how you want to be treated if you are seriously ill and unable to speak for yourself. It is unique among all other living will and health agent forms because it looks to all of a person's needs: medical, personal, emotional, and spiritual. *Five Wishes* also encourages discussing your wishes with your family and physician.

Five Wishes lets your family and doctors know:

1. Which person you want to make health care decisions for you when you can't make them.
2. The kind of medical treatment you want or don't want.
3. How comfortable you want to be.
4. How you want people to treat you.
5. What you want your loved ones to know.

Five Wishes was introduced and originally distributed with support from a generous grant by The Robert Wood Johnson Foundation, the nation's largest philanthropy devoted exclusively to health and health care.[4] (http://fivewishes.org)

Physicians are often the source of information to whom patients turn. The discussion about end-of-life decisions often involves advanced medical procedures that need to be discussed with a physician so that all the details can be accurately explained and doubts clarified. Every medical decision involving end-of-life care is unique and specific for the patient. Therefore, even the best documents are not going to include all case scenarios and answer all hypothetical situations, although most of them can be covered. Most advance directives documents, for obvious reasons, are just too simplistic. It is crucial then for physicians to have these discussions with patients so that the physician can better assess their patient's level of comfort with aggressive measures and act upon that if necessary.

Specific physician education on end-of-life treatment is available through national programs. The EPEC Project (Education in Palliative and End-Of-Life Care) was developed by the American Medical Association and funded by a grant from The Robert Wood Johnson Foundation. It is designed to educate all U.S. Physicians on the essentially clinical competencies required to provide quality end-of-life care. At the heart of the project is a core curriculum that provides physicians with the basic knowledge and skills needed to appropriately care for dying patients.[5]

In an effort to improve communication on the subject of death and dying, many institutions have implemented a team approach to managing cardiovascular disease processes.[6] Disease management programs have the ability to follow patients closely and establish trusting relationships with the patient and family. Team members often have the uninterrupted time and appropriate learning environments to approach end-of-life discussions.[7] These teams are multidisciplinary and include initiation of end-of-life discussion and planning on initial visits. A palliative care coordinator is an ideal member of the team. Palliative care, as described by the Institute of Medicine, "seeks to prevent, relieve, reduce or soothe the symptoms of disease or disorder without effecting a cure...Palliative care in this broad sense is not restricted to those who are dying or those enrolled in hospice programs."[8]

PALLIATIVE CARE STORY

Mr S, an 82-year-old gentleman with a history of recurrent decompensated heart rate secondary to ischemic cardiomyopathy, was referred to the outpatient heart failure resource center for comprehensive management. He was hospitalized four times in the past 6 months for decompensated heart failure. He presented with severe fatigue, dyspnea at rest, and swelling of his lower extremities.

He shared his accounts and experiences of past hospitalizations which he intently wanted to avoid in the future. He was successfully treated with intravenous (IV) diuretics in the clinic to relieve his fluid overload. During his treatment, opportunity arose to further discuss his medical care options. Much time was spent with him and his wife, educating them on his medical plan of care. This included optimization of his heart failure medications, symptom management, assessment of his functional status, quality of life, and their individual educational needs.

Upon initial assessment, he revealed he did have a living will that he and his wife created 10 years ago. At the time it was executed, Mr S was not faced with the diagnosis of end-stage heart failure. He openly discussed plans and treatment options available with the health-care team.

Over the next few months, his symptoms were well managed. As time progressed, his kidneys began to fail and he was unable to maintain an adequate blood pressure to support the metabolic demands of this body. He was brought back to the clinic for diuresis and inotropic infusion, which he responded to very well. At this time, the patient and his wife met with the palliative care team and rewrote his living will to express his wishes for future treatment, clearly expressing his desire to not return to the hospital and to let "nature take its course." He wanted to die with dignity and declined further supportive intravenous infusion. His health rapidly deteriorated. His wife realized his level of physical care required him to be transferred into an inpatient hospice center. He continued to deteriorate and became weaker and weaker. He remained there comfortably for 3 weeks until he passed away. He died peacefully with his wife and family at his side.

"End-of-Life," "Palliative Care," or "Hospice," are all terms that reflect a time in which the medical team and patient have agreed to move beyond treating and curing, but to improving the inevitable "end of a life."[7] The medical teams implementing this care should be as equally prepared as they are in the act of "saving a life." There is one certainty, every individual faces death. The disease state, the event, or the duration of the process is uncertain. But death is certain. Are our medical professionals as "skill for skill" matched to aiding patients and their families in the "art of dying" as we are in the "act of saving a life?" Educational resources are not meeting the needs of our professionals by providing continuing education on this critical topic. Our educational growth in this field must begin to equal the advances in cardiovascular invasive technology. Medical professionals and the cardiovascular patients they treat are in desperate need for long overdue educational efforts on the subject that will face them all—"Heart Hospice."[9]

REFERENCES

1. Tyree TL, Long CO, Greenberg EA. Nurse practitioners and end-of-life care: beliefs, practices, and perceptions. J Hosp Palliat Nurs. 2005;7:45–51.
2. Rogene Fisher. Planning for dying wishes. http://abcnews.go.com/Health/LegalCenter/story?id=594830 & page=1. 2005 Mar 21:1–3.
3. http://www.critical-conditions.org. Critical conditions. Accessed on May 12, 2005.
4. Available at http://fivewishes.org. Aging with dignity. Five Wishes. Accessed on November 14, 2005.

5. http://www.epec.net/EPEC/Webpages/about.cfm. The EPEC™ Project, Education in Palliative and End-of-Life-Care. Accessed on January 30, 2006.
6. Selecky PA, Eliasson AH, Hall RI, Schneider RF, Varkey B, et al. Palliative and end-of-life care for patients with cardiopulmonary diseases. Chest. 2005;128:3599–610.
7. Stewart S, McMurray JJV. Palliative care for heart failure—time to move beyond treating and curing to improving the end of life. BMJ. 2002;325:915–6.
8. Field MJ, Cassel CK, eds. Committee on care at the end of life, Institute of Medicine. Approaching death: improving care at the end of life. Washington DC, National Academy Presence; 1997: p. 31.
9. Conti Richard C, Vogel H. K. Heart Hospice. Clin Cardiol. 2006;29:187–188.

29

PRESENCE, HEALING, AND HEALERS: AN INTRODUCTION TO MINDFULNESS, MEDITATION, AND ITS RELEVANCE TO STRESS REDUCTION AND HEALTH FOR PATIENTS, PHYSICIANS AND HEALTH-CARE PROFESSIONALS

Jeffrey Brantley, Martin J. Sullivan, Suzanne W. Crater and Mitchell W. Krucoff

INTRODUCTION

Is there a significant relationship between being present with attention and awareness—being *mindful*—and better health?

Can a person become a powerful partner in their own healing process through the activity and discipline of paying closer attention to the inner and outer experiences of daily living?

Could the stress and burnout felt by health-care providers be impacted by systematic applications of mindfulness in the daily routine?

There is currently a growing popular and medical interest in the role of meditation in promoting health and healing. Mindfulness meditation is a way of paying attention that focuses upon present moment inner and outer experience in a friendly, nonjudging, and accepting way. Mindfulness differs significantly from other methods of meditation studied by Western medicine in that it emphasizes nonconceptual presence, and inclusive, allowing attention rather than a narrow and concentrated focus of attention.

Over the past 25–30 years, a body of research has grown regarding the application of various methods of meditation to medical conditions. Mindfulness meditation has been applied largely through the vehicle of mindfulness-based stress reduction (MBSR), and benefits have been reported in a number of different diagnostic groups, but relatively little in the field of cardiology. Among the conditions reported to benefit from mindfulness practice have included depression, anxiety, chronic pain, chronic stress, ability to cope with chronic illness, and overall mood disturbance.

Relatively recent literature in the field of cardiology has investigated the links between specific psychosocial factors and diseases of the cardiovascular system. The psychosocial factors that have been most studied are: depression, anxiety, personality and character traits, social isolation and lack of social support, acute and chronic stress, and coping style.

An extensive recent literature now establishes that psychosocial factors play a significant role in the pathogenesis of coronary artery disease (CAD). Less research exists regarding psychosocial factors and congestive heart failure (CHF); however, it does appear that depression, level of social support, and style of coping are important factors related to morbidity and mortality.

Reviews of the research literature in mindfulness meditation and in the psychological factors contributing to morbidity and mortality in heart diseases are similar in the conclusions that much more research is needed. Yet, from what is already known, an important question arises: *Is it possible that training in meditation, and the practice of mindfulness may directly and positively influence some or most of the critical psychosocial factors that impact upon CAD, CHF, and possibly other diseases of the cardiovascular system?*

In reflecting on the reported benefits of mindfulness training for patient populations, especially in the areas of stress reduction and improved coping and quality of life, a second question arises. *Is it possible that training and practice of mindfulness by busy health care professionals, including physicians, could have a positive impact on subjective quality of life, and even upon clinical effectiveness?*

This chapter aims to provide the reader with an introduction to mindfulness and meditation from a historical and clinical perspective. It also aims to link these two through existing research findings in other areas of medicine, and to suggest the possibility that evidence now exists to suggest that mindfulness practice may benefit not only patients, but may also help physicians and other busy health-care professionals cope more effectively with the tremendous demands of practicing modern day medicine.

MINDFULNESS AND MEDITATION

Mindfulness is a nonconceptual knowing/awareness that arises as one pays attention on purpose in an open, nonjudging, and accepting way to the details of experience—inner and outer—moment-by-moment (Kabat-Zinn, 2003).[1] Mindfulness is a capacity available to any human being who elects to develop it. Mechanisms by which being mindful can positively impact clinical conditions are poorly understood, yet are also the subject of intense current interest among psychologists and clinicians (Bishop, Lau, Shapiro, et. al. 2004).[2]

Although mindfulness occurs spontaneously and naturally, development of mindfulness can be explicitly cultivated through *meditation*, which is an activity of directing attention in a particular way for a particular purpose. Meditation practiced to cultivate mindfulness has been the primary vehicle for the introduction and application of mindfulness in clinical settings in Western medicine since 1979 (Baer, 2003).[3]

Meditation practices have existed since ancient times and in diverse cultures. They have historically been the vehicles for profound personal healing and transformation. In the last 25–30 years, they have become one of the most widely practiced of the mind-body therapies in Western medicine.

Either in their organized religious/spiritual contexts, or in more modern behavioral medicine applications, one of the primary purposes of meditation is to shift the perspective of the meditator. Practicing meditation, one becomes a more detached observer of mental, emotional, and physical experience, and this can lead to awareness of unconscious habits and distortions and to transformation from such insight. In contrast to many cognitive-behavioral techniques, meditation involves the application and regulation of *attention*, rather than the management or control of thoughts, beliefs, or other cognitive processes (Hayes and Feldman, 2004).[4]

Any form of meditation is a "hands-on" activity. It is learned and understood only through direct experience. Meditation requires repeated practice, and, usually, the guidance of an experienced teacher. This kind of *experiential learning* is essential if an individual is to benefit from any method of meditation, including mindfulness meditation.

HOW MINDFULNESS CAME TO WESTERN MEDICINE

Mindfulness practices taught in current Western therapeutic contexts have their origins in traditional Buddhist meditation. Mindfulness is the foundation where the diverse forms of Buddhist meditation practice meet and grow. It is found in the Theravada tradition of the countries of Southeast Asia, the Mahayana schools of Japan, Korea, China, and Vietnam, and the Vajrayana tradition of Tibetan Buddhism.

In 1979, Jon Kabat-Zinn, PhD, and his colleagues at the University of Massachusetts Medical Center in Worcester began offering a program in mindfulness training to patients referred to their clinic. They sought to make mindfulness available, through meditation practice, in a nonsectarian way focused on stress reduction and health enhancement, which did not depend upon any particular spiritual or religious context. The program and the application of mindfulness meditation in medical patients was conceived as a vehicle through which people could begin to assume a degree of responsibility for their own well-being, and could realize a greater level of health through the cultivation of the inner capacity to be present and more deeply aware of life, moment-by-moment (Kabat-Zinn, 2003).[1]

In this program, which came to be known as MBSR, participants attended a weekly class made up of people with a wide variety of illnesses and stress-related conditions. In the class, they were taught a number of meditation practices aimed at developing mindfulness and relaxation, and encouraged to practice formal meditation at home for an hour daily, and also to practice being more "mindful" informally in the activities and situations of daily life. Typically, the class would extend for a period of 8 weeks, and also included participation in a day-long session of intensive practice (the Day of Mindfulness) near the end of the course.

Since 1979, literally thousands of people have completed MBSR programs, large numbers of health-care providers have been exposed to mindfulness practice, and over 200 clinics, hospitals, and individuals in the United States and abroad were offering stress reduction programs based on mindfulness training. In addition, media attention has come to this use of mindfulness, and Kabat-Zinn and the MBSR program at University of Massachusetts were featured in the best-selling book and PBS documentary by Bill Moyers, *Healing and the Mind*.

Medical literature has reflected the interest in applying mindfulness meditation in differing clinical settings. Literature reviews, and meta-analysis reflect a diverse methodology which ranges from descriptive and observational studies to those utilizing a randomized wait-list control design. Such findings are typical of an emerging discipline, yet, despite variations in research methodology, reviewers have concluded that mindfulness practice, especially as taught in the MBSR model, may help a broad range of individuals cope with both clinical and nonclinical problems (Baer, 2003; Grossman, P., Niemann, L., et. al., 2004).[3,5]

A wide variety of clinical benefits have been noted using the MBSR model. For example, benefits have been reported for stress reduction and quality of life; generalized anxiety disorder, panic disorder, and panic disorder with agoraphobia; relapsing depression; chronic pain; mood disturbance and function in cancer; fibromyalgia; eating disorders; and psoriasis (Baer, 2003; Kabat-Zinn, 2003).[1,3]

In a pilot study of women with heart disease (Tacon, McComb, et. al., 2003),[6] the subjects, who participated in an MBSR program were found to have significantly reduced anxiety, improved ability to express negative feelings, and less reactive coping behaviors than their matched controls.

Using MBSR practices as a foundation, Segal, Williams, and Teasdale (2002)[7] developed a unique approach to treating depression that combines mindfulness with cognitive behavioral therapy. They named this approach Mindfulness-Based Cognitive Therapy for Depression (MBCT).

Separate from mindfulness as taught in MBSR programs, Marsha Linehan developed a cognitive behavioral approach for treatment of borderline personality disorder (BPD) that involved core skills of mindfulness. In her multifaceted approach, known as Dialectical Behavior Therapy (DBT), Linehan defined mindfulness training—with its emphasis on a nonjudging observation of experience—as a core skill for all DBT clients. Dean Ornish, MD, developed a program for reversing heart disease that included daily meditation practice. This approach encouraged a variety of methods of meditation, including mindfulness. In this approach, meditation was combined with other stress management skills, dietary change, exercise, smoking cessation, and enhanced communication skills.

APPROACHING LIFE MINDFULLY

As more and more medical and psychological applications of mindfulness appear, there is a risk of losing sight of the larger context from which meditation practices like mindfulness developed. There are important and unique qualities and characteristics of mindfulness *as a meditation practice* that should be noted. These may be summarized briefly as follows. First, mindfulness is not just another "technique" or "method" to be used in times of stress and illness. As it is taught in the MBSR model, mindfulness is most effective when one makes it a part of daily life, indeed makes it a way of being in one's life. This reflects a commitment on the part of the individual to reside as best they can moment-by-moment in awareness with openness, and a spacious friendly attitude as they "pay attention on purpose" (Kabat-Zinn, 2003).[1] Such a way of being means working compassionately with one's failures to be present and aware, as well as with the painful and unpleasant experiences that arise. This commitment to being more mindful in life—toward all experience—can be a doorway to healing and transformation.

Secondly, it is important to note that the reference to "practice" in the context of mindfulness meditation does not mean "rehearsal." When practicing mindfulness, one is not preparing for some performance to occur at a later time. Rather, practice in this context means making the commitment to being more present right now, in this moment. Each time one does that, he or she is actually embodying the orientation of calm and open, nonjudging awareness.

Finally, a personal meditation practice should be part of the life of anyone who undertakes to teach mindfulness meditation. The ancient origins of mindfulness as a meditation practice emphasize the necessity of making the practice a part of one's own life. This means bringing the same commitment to meditation practice in one's own life and work as one asks for in the students one teaches. Segal, Williams, and Teasdale (2002)[7] noted in some detail the importance of group leaders being grounded in a personal practice of mindfulness meditation before leading groups in their approach, known as MBCT.

For physicians or other health-care providers, who wish their patients to use mindfulness yet do not have a personal practice from which to teach mindfulness, a reasonable choice might be to send the patient to a good mindfulness meditation teacher, or to a well-established program in MBSR.

HEALING THE HEALER

Stress is not limited to patients. The stress inherent in health care negatively impacts health-care professionals in many ways (Shapiro, S.L., Astin, J.A., et. al. 2005).[8] Physicians are not immune to stress. There is evidence that physicians are growing less satisfied with professional life, and that many feel that their family and personal lives have suffered because of their professional demands

(Spickard, A.J., Jr., Gabbe, S.G., and Christensen, J.F., 2002).[9] For any health-care provider, including physicians, satisfaction with one's work directly affects patient satisfaction and outcomes. Over 100 years ago, Sir William Osler encouraged physicians to: work today without worrying about yesterday or tomorrow; live by the Golden Rule with colleagues and patients; cultivate equanimity (composure, patience, imperturbability), and to recognize that the physician's heart is the most important aspect of practice (Silverman, M.E., Murray, T.J., and Bryan, C.S. 2003).[10]

Self-care may be thought of as learning to be aware of one's own needs, to recognize when stress is mounting, and to have effective skills for managing stress and its consequences. These things are vital if one is to maintain professional satisfaction and personal and family health.

Unfortunately, the training most physicians have received has not empowered them to manage their own stress effectively. Indeed, by mid-career (if not sooner), the momentum of working while fatigued and emotionally exhausted is often the norm. Any ideas about self-care have been submerged or not reinforced in a culture that awards esteem and recognition by peers for hard work and placing others before self-care (Spickard, A.J., Jr., Gabbe, S.G., and Christensen, J.F., 2002).[9]

Stress, from whatever source, impacts on individual health-care providers. In its extreme, stress can lead to *burnout*. Maslach and Leither describe burnout as a measure of the dislocation between what people are doing versus what they are expected to do (Spickard, A.J., Jr., Gabbe, S.G., and Christensen, J.F. 2002).[9] Burnout spreads gradually over time, and represents an erosion of will, values, and spirit. For health-care providers, symptoms of burnout can lead to a downward spiral of error, more burnout, and increasing distress and dissatisfaction.

Preventing burnout is a responsibility for individuals, and for the organizations in which they work. Crucial values to promote the sense of well-being have been identified as: cultivating elements of personal renewal, developing emotional self-awareness, maintaining connection with social support systems, and having an on-going sense of mastery and meaning in one's work.

COULD PRACTICING MINDFULNESS BENEFIT THE HEALER?

In addition to clinical studies with patients reporting a wide range of benefits in reducing stress and symptoms such as pain, sleep disturbance, anxiety, and depression, there are also reports of mindfulness training specifically for health care providers.

Shapiro and colleagues (2005)[8] reported reduced stress, increased quality of life, and increased self-compassion in a group of health care professionals who completed an 8-week MBSR intervention.

Beddoe and Murphy (2004)[11] reported significantly reduced anxiety, and improved sense of well-being and coping in a group of baccalaureate nursing students who completed an 8-week MBSR course.

Cohen-Katz, J. and colleagues (2004)[12] reported in a three-part series, benefits of MBSR on nurse stress and burnout.

Rozenzweig, S. and colleagues (2003)[13] reported results of an MBSR intervention with 140 second-year medical students. They found significantly lower scores in total mood disturbance, tension-anxiety, confusion-bewilderment, fatigue-inertia, and vigor-activity in the students who practiced mindfulness compared with students in a control group who did not.

PRACTICING MINDFULNESS

One does not have to wait for an 8-week MBSR course or go to a mountain top to practice mindfulness. The key element is a willingness to pay attention to one's own experience as it happens—here—in the present moment.

In one of the author's experience (JB), a simple phrase clarifies the understanding of mindfulness practice, and also offers a simple instruction to guide practice. The phrase is: *relax—pay attention—allow*.

"Relax" means to stop, soften, and let go of trying to change anything or to make anything happen. In mindfulness meditation practice, this is often called practicing *being* instead of doing.

"Pay attention" means to turn attention and the resulting awareness to direct experience (not thoughts about the experience) and receive it. Attention does not mean to have more thoughts about anything. It does mean to open, attend, and recognize when each experience happens at each sense gate. Thus attention here leads to directly *feeling* sensations, *hearing* sound vibrations, *seeing* sights, *smelling* odors, *tasting* tastes, and just listening (not adding to) thoughts happening in the mind.

"Allow" means to not interfere with whatever comes into awareness. The practice of mindfulness is to bring attention and to accurately reflect what happens, while allowing it to unfold naturally. This means especially not being caught in habits of judging, or commenting on what is happening. Rather, it is good mindfulness practice to simply notice when there is judging or commentary and to allow that as a form of thinking, without adding more to it.

What follows are two examples of simple mindfulness practices. The first is a basic practice, awareness of breathing that can be used in any circumstance to establish mindfulness and to connect more fully with the present moment. The second example here is a specific application of mindfulness useful in a busy cardiac catheterization lab.

AWARENESS OF BREATHING

- In any situation, for any length of time comfortable to you, make the decision to become more mindful by bringing nonjudging, allowing attention to your breath. You can do this practice for just a breath or two at times, or more breaths, up to a "formal" practice of 30 minutes or more at a time.

- Turn your attention on purpose to the direct physical sensations of your breath. No need to control the breath, just let yourself feel and receive the sensations as they unfold. If it helps, you may want to close your eyes as you practice.
- Let your attention rest, and return (whenever your mind wanders) to the place in your body—tip of the nose, abdomen, chest, for example—where it is easiest for you to actually feel the breath come and go.
- As you direct a kind and welcoming attention to each breath sensation, you could set down all of your burdens for the time of this meditation. It is not necessary to make anything happen, or to become anything else during the time of the meditation.
- When you notice that your attention has wandered off of the breath sensations, you have NOT done anything wrong. You have merely noticed the tendency of your mind to wander. Practice kindness and patience for yourself as you kindly and firmly bring attention back to the direct sensation of your breath.
- As you practice, feeling each breath, noticing the wandering mind, being kind with yourself, returning attention to the next breath, let the meditation support you. Rest and let attention notice the changing patterns of the breath and body. As attention becomes steadier, move it closer and notice the qualities of each component of breath, noticing the beginning, the middle, and the end of the in-breath, the out-breath, and even the space between the breaths. Notice how each breath is precious and unique.
- End your meditation by shifting the focus off of the breath, opening your eyes, and moving gently.

CONCLUSION

Mindfulness is a basic human capacity for nonjudging, nonconceptual awareness of present moment experience, both inner and outer. Mindfulness has been systematically developed through meditation methods for thousands of years by human beings interested in spiritual transformation. In the past 25–30 years, mindfulness meditation practices (in addition to other methods of meditation) have been applied in a variety of Western medical settings as complements to treatment.

The traditional goals of meditation, including development of qualities of attention, awareness, kindness, compassion, and a deeper sense of the mystery of human experience, have not been well linked to experimental measures. What connections there may be between such traditional goals and the power of meditation practices, including mindfulness, to benefit patients in contemporary health-care settings remains to be systematically explored.

REFERENCES

1. Kabat-Zinn J. Mindfulness-based interventions in context: past, present, and future. Clin Psychol Sci Pract. 2003;10(2):144–56.
2. Bishop S, Lau M, Shapiro S, Carlson L, Anderson ND, Carmody J, et al. Mindfulness: a proposed operational definition. Clin Psychol Sci Pract. 2004;11(3):230–41.
3. Baer R. Mindfulness training as a clinical intervention:a conceptual and empirical review. Clin Psychol Sci Pract. 2003:10(2);125–42.
4. Hayes A., Feldman G. Clarifying the construct of mindfulness in the context of emotion regulation and the process of change in therapy. Clin Psychol Sci Pract. 2004;11(3):255–62.
5. Grossman P, Niemann L, Schmidt S, Walach H. Mindfulness-based stress reduction and health benefits. A meta-analysis. J Psychosom Res. 2004;57(1):35–43.
6. Tacon AM, McComb J, Caldera Y, Randolph P. Mindfulness meditation, anxiety reduction, and heart disease: a pilot study. Fam Community Health. 2003;26(1):25–33.
7. Segal ZV, Williams JMG, Teasdale J. Mindfulness-based cognitive therapy for depression: a new approach to preventing relapse. New York: Guilford Press; 2002.
8. Shapiro SL, Astin JA, Bishop SR, Cordova M. Mindfulness-based stress reduction for health care professionals: results from a randomized trial. Int J Stress Manage. 2005;12(2):164–76.
9. Spickard AJ, Jr, Gabbe SG, Christensen JF. Mid-career burnout in generalist and specialist physicians. JAMA. 2002;288(12):1447–50.
10. Silverman ME, Murray TJ, Bryan CS. The quotable osler. Philadelphia (PA): The American College of Physicians; 2003.
11. Beddoe AE, Murphy SO. Does mindfulness decrease stress and foster empathy among nursing students? J Nurs Educ. 2004;43(7):305–12.
12. Cohen-Katz J, Wiley SD, Capuano T, Baker DM, Shapiro S. The effects of mindfulness-based stress reduction on nurse stress and burnout: a quantitative and qualitative study. Holist Nurs Pract. 2004;18(6):302–8.
13. Rosenzweig S, Reibel DK, Greeson JM, Brainard GC, Hojat M. Mindfulness-based stress reduction lowers psychological distress in medical students. Teach Learn Med. 2003;15(2):88–92.

P A R T

6

APPENDIX

REFERENCE SOURCES FOR INFORMATION ON DIETARY SUPPLEMENTS AND HERBAL MEDICINES

Rebecca B. Costello

MONOGRAPHS ONLINE
American Herbal Pharmacopeia and Therapeutic Compendium (AHP) Scotts Valley, CA **Web site**: http://www.herbal-ahp.org **Description:** The American Herbal Pharmacopoeia began developing qualitative and therapeutic monographs in 1994, and intends to produce 300 monographs on botanicals, including many of the Ayurvedic, Chinese, and Western herbs most frequently used in the United States.

The Complete German Commission E Monographs: Therapeutic Guide to Herbal Medicines
Mark Blumenthal, German Federal Institute for Drugs and Medical Devices
  Commission E, American Botanical Council, Integrative Medicine Communications, Werner R. Busse, J. Klein, Robert Rister (editors)
Siegrid
  Klein, Chance Riggins
Austin, TX: American Botanical Council
Boston, MA: Integrative Medicine Communications, 1998. 685 pp.
ISBN: 096555550X
Web site: www.herbalgram.org
Description: The German government's Commission E findings regarding the approved uses, contraindications, side effects, dosage, drug interactions, and other therapeutic effects of 300 herbs and phytomedicines.

Health Canada. Natural Health Products Compendium of Monographs Natural Health Products Directorate, Health Canada, 2003. **Web site:** http://www.hc-sc.gc.ca/dhp-mps/prodnatur/applications/ licen-prod/monograph/index_e.html

Description: The Health Canada Natural Health Products Directorate developed the Compendium of Monographs as a tool for the timely and efficient evaluation of the safety and efficacy of many commonly used medicinal ingredients that comprise natural health products.

WHO Monographs on Selected Medicinal Plants, Volume 1
World Health Organization. Geneva, Switzerland, 1999. 295 pp.
ISBN: 92 4154517 8
Web site: http://www.who.org.
Description: Provides scientific information on the safety, efficacy, and quality control/quality assurance of widely used medicinal plants.

BOOKS AND PUBLICATIONS

The Health Professionals Guide to Popular Dietary Supplements, 2nd edition
American Dietetic Association/Allison Sarubin Fragakis
From the Joint Working Group on Dietary Supplements, 2003. 552 pp.
Web site: http://www.eatright.org/cps/rde/xchg/ada/hs.xsl/3926_1351_ ENU_ HTML.htm
ISBN: 0880911735
Description: More than 80 popular vitamins, minerals, amino acids, herbals, enzymes, and other supplements are covered in this updated and indexed guide.

Botanical Safety Handbook: Guidelines for the Safe Use and Labeling for Herbs in Commerce
McGuffin M, Hobbs C, Upton R, Goldberg A (editors).
American Herbal Products Association. New York, NY, CRC Press, 1997. 256 pp.
ISBN: 0849316758
Web site: http://www.ahpa.org/
Description: Provides safety data for more than 600 commonly sold herbs and includes information on international regulatory status, standard dosage, and toxicity issues.

The 5-Minute Herb and Dietary Supplement Clinical Consult
Adriane Fugh-Berman
Lippincott, Williams and Wilkins, 2003. 475 pp.
ISBN: 0683302736
Description: Includes herbs, minerals, vitamins, amino acids, and enzymes and their uses to treat common problems and improve health.

The ABC Clinical Guide to Herbs
Mark Blumenthal, Josef Brinckmann, Bernd Wollschlaeger
Austin, TX: American Botanical Council, 2003. 480 pp.
ISBN: 1588901572

Description: Provides health professionals with information on 29 of the most popular herbs, and other herbal products. Information includes usage, dosage, contraindication, adverse effects, drug interactions, and pharmacological effects.

The Handbook of Clinically Tested Herbal Remedies
Marilyn Barrett
Haworth Herbal Press, 2004, 2-volume set
ISBN: 0789027232
Description: A thorough, informative, in-depth text for clinicians searching for accurate information on herbal clinical trials.

Encyclopedia of Dietary Supplements
Paul M. Coates, Marc R. Blackman, Gordon M. Cragg, Mark Levine, Joel Moss, Jeffrey D. White (editors)
New York, NY: Marcel Dekker, 2005. 819 pp.
ISBN: 0824755049
Description: Provides detailed scientific information on over 75 dietary supplements including description and chemical composition, mechanisms of action, pharmacology, usage and dosage, safety and adverse effects, and regulatory issues.

Tyler's Honest Herbal: A Sensible Guide to the Use of Herbs and Related Remedies, 4th Edition
Steven Foster, Varro E. Tyler.
New York: Pharmaceutical Products Press, 1999. 442 pp.
ISBN: 0789008750
Description: Reviews uses of herbal medicinals, efficacy, and safety.

Nutrition in Clinical Practice. A Comprehensive, Evidence-Based Manual for the Practioner, 2nd Edition
Philadelphia, PA: Lippincott Williams & Wilkins, 2007. 480 pp.
ISBN: 1582558213
Description: Nutrition information provided in concert with information on supplements (nutraceuticals). Nutrient/supplement reference tables included.

Rational Phytotherapy: A Physician's Guide to Herbal Medicine, 5th Edition
Volker Schulz, Varro E. Tyler, V. E. Tyler, Rudolf Hansel, Rudolf Hdnsel, Mark Blumenthal
New York, NY: Springer Verlag, 2004. 400 pp.
ISBN: 3540408320
Description: This book is a practice-oriented introduction into phythotherapy and reviews the pharmaceutical aspects of phytotherapy.

EVIDENCED-BASED REVIEWS

Effect of Supplemental Antioxidants Vitamin C, Vitamin E, and Coenzyme Q10 for the Prevention and Treatment of Cardiovascular Disease
Agency for Healthcare Research and Quality
Evidence report/technology assessment: number 83, June 2003
Summary (publication no. 03-E042)
Evidence report (publication no. 03-E043)
Web site: http://www.ahrq.gov/clinic/epcsums/antioxsum.htm
Description: A paper which reviews what research has been done on the use of vitamin C, vitamin E, and coenzyme Q10 for the prevention and treatment of cardiovascular disease.

Garlic: Effects on Cardiovascular Risks and Disease, Protective Effects Against Cancer, and Clinical Adverse Effects
Agency for Healthcare Research and Quality
Evidence report/technology assessment: number 20, October, 2000
Summary (publication no. 01-E022)
Evidence report (publication no. 01-E023)
Web site: http://www.ahrq.gov/clinic/epcsums/garlicsum.htm
Description: A paper which reviews what research has been done on the use of garlic and its effect on cardiovascular disease and cancer.

Omega-3 Fatty Acids
Office of Dietary Supplements, National Institutes of Health
Web site: http://dietary-supplements.info.nih.gov/Health_Information/omega_3_fatty_acids.aspx
Description: Provides information on omega-3 fatty acids including links to reports from the Agency for Healthcare Research and Quality.

Effects of Soy on Health Outcomes
Agency for Healthcare Research and Quality
Evidence report/technology assessment: number 126, August 2005
Summary (publication no. 05-E024-1)
Evidence report (publication no. 05-E024-2)
Web site http://www.ahrq.gov/clinic/epcsums/soysum.htm
Description: Systematic review to describe the range of soy products and their effects on a wide variety of medical conditions in healthy adults.

DATABASES

AltMedDex System
Thomson Micromedex
Web site: http://www.micromedex.com/products/altmeddex/ (by subscription)
Description: Referenced information on herbals, vitamins, minerals, other dietary supplements, Chinese medicine, acupuncture, and more. Includes data on dosing, pharmacokinetics, and clinical applications.

International Bibliographic Information on Dietary Supplements (IBIDS) Database
National Institutes of Health, Office of Dietary Supplements and the
  National Agricultural Library, Food and Nutrition Information Center
Web site: ods.od.nih.gov/Health_Information/IBIDS.aspx.
Description: IBIDS is a comprehensive bibliographic database that helps
  health-care providers, researchers, and consumers find credible, scientific
  literature on dietary supplements. Currently, the database contains dietary
  supplements citations/abstracts from MEDLINE, AGRICOLA, and
  AGRIS, and selected nutrition journals from CAB abstracts and CAB's
  Global Health databases dating from 1986 to the present.

Natural Medicines Comprehensive Database
The Pharmacist's Letter/The Prescriber's Letter; 1999, updated yearly.
Web site: www.NaturalDatabase.com (by subscription)
Description: Referenced, peer reviewed, continuously updated online
  database. Search by keyword or by brand name products. Includes
  drug-herb interactions and conditions.

MEDLINEPlus for Herbal Information
MEDLINEPlus Health Information, National Library of Medicine,
  National Institutes of Health
Web site: http://www.nlm.nih.gov/medlineplus/herbalmedicine.html
Description: Contains up-to-date, quality health care information on herbs
  and herbal medicine from the National Library of Medicine at the
  National Institutes of Health.

MEDLINEPlus for Dietary Supplements
MEDLINEPlus Health Information, National Library of Medicine, National
  Institutes of Health
Web site: http://www.nlm.nih.gov/medlineplus/dietarysupplements.html
Description: Links, including the latest research, on dietary supplements
  from the National Library of Medicine at the National Institutes of
  Health.

PDA-COMPATIBLE PROGRAMS

Epocrates Rx Pro
Epocrates, Inc.
Web site: http://www2.epocrates.com/products/rxpro/ (by subscription)
Description: Drug and formulary reference including more than 400
  alternative medicine (herbal) monographs. Includes information on uses,
  doses, cautions, interactions, adverse reactions, and more.

mobileMicromedex
Thomson Micromedex
Web site: http://www.micromedex.com/products/mobilemicromedex/
(by subscription)
Description: Clinical information, including over 300 of the most popular
herbals and dietary supplements, to help support and confirm treatment
decisions. Includes information on indications, dosage, contraindications,
drug interactions, adverse effects, and more.

INDEX